NEUROSCIENTIFIC FOUNDATIONS OF ANESTHESIOLOGY

NEUROSCIENTIFIC FOUNDATIONS OF ANESTHESIOLOGY

EDITED BY

George A. Mashour, MD, PhD

DIRECTOR, DIVISION OF NEUROANESTHESIOLOGY
ASSISTANT PROFESSOR OF
ANESTHESIOLOGY & NEUROSURGERY
UNIVERSITY OF MICHIGAN MEDICAL SCHOOL
ANN ARBOR, MICHIGAN

EDITED BY

Ralph Lydic, PhD

BERT LA DU PROFESSOR OF ANESTHESIOLOGY
PROFESSOR OF PHYSIOLOGY
ASSOCIATE CHAIR FOR ANESTHESIA RESEARCH
UNIVERSITY OF MICHIGAN MEDICAL SCHOOL
ANN ARBOR, MICHIGAN

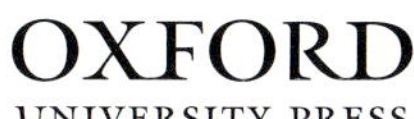

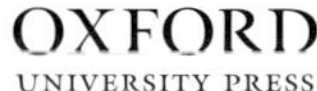

Oxford University Press, Inc., publishes works that further Oxford University's objective of excellence in research, scholarship, and education.

Oxford New York
Auckland Cape Town Dar es Salaam Hong Kong Karachi
Kuala Lumpur Madrid Melbourne Mexico City Nairobi
New Delhi Shanghai Taipei Toronto

With offices in
Argentina Austria Brazil Chile Czech Republic France Greece
Guatemala Hungary Italy Japan Poland Portugal Singapore
South Korea Switzerland Thailand Turkey Ukraine Vietnam

Published by Oxford University Press, Inc.
198 Madison Avenue, New York, New York 10016
www.oup.com

Library of Congress Cataloging-in-Publication Data

Mashour, George A. (George Alexander)
Neuroscientific foundations of anesthesiology / George A. Mashour, Ralph Lydic.
p. ; cm.
Includes bibliographical references and index.
ISBN 978-0-19-539824-3
1. Anesthesia. 2. Anesthetics. I. Lydic, Ralph. II. Title.
[DNLM: 1. Anesthesia. 2. Anesthetics—pharmacology. 3. Nervous System Physiological Phenomena. WO 200]
RD81.M35 2011
617.9'6—dc22 2011012544

---

9 8 7 6 5 4 3 2 1
Printed in China
on acid-free paper

FOREWORD

I am flattered to be invited to provide a foreword for this well-crafted textbook, coedited by an eminent basic scientist and a clinician-scientist in the neurosciences. This symbiotic relationship has provided a bidirectional flow that reflects the type of partnership required to produce the paradigm-shifting breakthroughs that have enabled the neurosciences to progress so rapidly in the last decade.

While the clinical management of patients that fall within the realm of anesthesiology, perioperative care, and pain management is based on principles that are physiologic and pharmacologic in nature, its *foundation* is steeped in the neurosciences. The targets for our therapeutic interventions reside largely within the central and peripheral nervous systems; the invariable side effects that arise in other organ systems are the result of "collateral damage" (e.g., myocardial depressant effect of volatile agents) because similar processes are present outside of the nervous system. Hence, investigation has focused on identifying what is the exclusive domain of the nervous system in order to yield evermore specific targets.

By necessity, those engaged in clinical practice are required to have more than a passing knowledge of the intricate workings of the nervous system. Formerly, for this to be clinically meaningful, the data had to be derived from investigation of in vitro and *ex vivo* models of material of human origin. Fortunately, techniques have evolved to the point that precise functional measurements of neurobiological processes in vivo in humans are now attainable. The current array of imaging technologies has provided unique insights into the workings of the nervous system in ways that we had not previously contemplated. Not only are we able to delineate regions of interest, but we can also discern the connectivity involved in transducing the processes enabling the complex responses that differentiate *Homo sapiens* from other nonhuman primates. Coupled with the long-awaited dividends from the human genome project and the new promise of nanotechnology, we are encountering disruptive technologies that require us to rethink previously considered sacrosanct tenets. For example, with optogenetics, neuroscientists can now activate discrete nuclei with a precisely directed light source and record the consequences using imaging techniques. Using this approach, functional magnetic resonance imaging has been validated and the conclusions based on this technology can now be accepted beyond plausibility.

This is not the end—rather this is the end of the beginning! We are on the cusp of bringing to our specialty previously undreamed of advances in the neurosciences that will enable clinicians to provide a quality of care that can become the paragon for other clinical specialties. This textbook is an exemplar that leads not only by being a pathfinder, but by assembling the best to contribute to this burgeoning field.

Mervyn Maze, MB, ChB
Chair, Department of Anesthesia and Perioperative Care
University of California, San Francisco

CONTENTS

CONTRIBUTORS

Michael T. Alkire, MD
Staff Physician
VA Long Beach Health Care System
Long Beach, CA
and
Associate Professor in Residence,
Department of Anesthesiology & Perioperative Care
Fellow, Center for the Neurobiology of Learning and Memory
University of California, Irvine
Irvine, CA

Timothy Angelotti, MD, PhD
Associate Professor
Department of Anesthesia/CCM
Stanford University School of Medicine
Stanford, CA

Joseph F. Antognini, MD, MBA
Professor of Anesthesiology and Pain Medicine
Professor of Neurobiology, Physiology, and Behavior
University of California, Davis School of Medicine
Davis, CA

Helen A. Baghdoyan, PhD
Director of Laboratory Research
Professor of Anesthesiology
Professor of Pharmacology
University of Michigan
Ann Arbor, MI

Robert Bonin, PhD
Department of Physiology
University of Toronto
Toronto, Ontario, Canada

Timothy J. Brennan, PhD, MD
Samir Gergis Professor and Vice Chair for Research
Departments of Anesthesia and Pharmacology
University of Iowa Hospitals and Clinics
Iowa City, IA

Sorin J. Brull, MD
Professor of Anesthesiology
Mayo Clinic College of Medicine
Jacksonville, FL

Chad M. Brummett, MD
Assistant Professor
Department of Anesthesiology
Director, Adult Pain Research
University of Michigan Medical School
Ann Arbor, MI

Adam J. Carinci, MD
Instructor
Division of Pain Medicine
Department of Anesthesia, Critical Care and Pain Medicine
Harvard Medical School
Massachusetts General Hospital
Boston, MA

Daniel J. Clauw, MD
Professor
Division of Rheumatology
Director, Chronic Pain and Fatigue Research Center
University of Michigan Medical School
Ann Arbor, MI

François Donati, PhD, MD, FRCPC
Professor
Department of Anesthesiology
Université de Montréal
Staff anesthesiologist
Hôpital Maisonneuve-Rosemont
Montréal, Québec, Canada

Michael Erdek, MD
Assistant Professor
Department of Anesthesiology and Critical Care Medicine and Oncology
Director of Quality Improvement
Department of Anesthesiology
Division of Pain Medicine
Johns Hopkins University School of Medicine
Baltimore, MD

David B. Glick, MD, MBA
Associate Professor
Anesthesia and Critical Care
University of Chicago, Pritzker School of Medicine
Chicago, IL

Gerald Glick, MD
Professor Emeritus of Medicine
Rush Medical College
Chicago, IL

Haroon Hameed, MD
Fellow
Division of Pain Medicine
Department of Anesthesia and Critical Care Medicine
Johns Hopkins University, School of Medicine
Baltimore, MD

Mariam Hameed, MD
Resident
Department of Physical Medicine and Rehabilitation
Johns Hopkins University, School of Medicine
Baltimore, MD

Richard E. Harris, PhD
Assistant Professor of Anesthesiology
Chronic Pain and Fatigue Research Center
University of Michigan
Ann Arbor, MI

Anthony G. Hudetz, DBM, PhD
Professor of Anesthesiology, Physiology, and Biophysics
Department of Anesthesiology
Medical College of Wisconsin
Milwaukee, WI

Vesna Jevtovic-Todorovic, MD, PhD, MBA
Harold Carron Professor of Anesthesiology and Neuroscience
Department of Anesthesiology and Neuroscience
University of Virginia Health System
Charlottesville, VA

Steven L. Jinks, PhD
Associate Professor of Anesthesiology and Pain Medicine
University of California, Davis School of Medicine
Davis, CA

Mihir M. Kamdar, MD
Co-Director
Massachusetts General Hospital Cancer Pain Clinic
and
Instructor
Division of Pain Medicine
Department of Anesthesia, Critical Care and Pain Medicine
Harvard Medical School
Massachusetts General Hospital
Boston, MA

Sinyoung Kang, MD, PhD
Clinical Fellow in Regional Anesthesia
Department of Anesthesia
University of Iowa Hospitals and Clinics
Iowa City, IA

Max Kelz, MD, PhD
Assistant Professor of Anesthesiology and Critical Care
Member, Mahoney Institute of Neurological Sciences
University of Pennsylvania School of Medicine
Philadelphia, PA

Smith C. Manion, MD
Instructor
Division of Pain Medicine
Department of Anesthesia, Critical Care and Pain Medicine
Harvard Medical School
Massachusetts General Hospital
Boston, MA

Jianren Mao, MD, PhD
Director, MGH Center for Translational Pain Research
Associate Professor, Harvard Medical School
Division of Pain Medicine
Department of Anesthesia, Critical Care and Pain Medicine,
Harvard Medical School
Massachusetts General Hospital
Boston, MA

Terri G. Monk, MD, MS
Professor
Department of Anesthesiology
Duke University Medical Center
Durham VA Medical Center
Durham, NC

Jason Moore, B.S.
M.D., Ph.D. Candidate
University of Pennsylvania School of Medicine
Philadelphia, PA

Mohamed Naguib, MB, BCh, MSc, FFARCSI, MD
Professor of Anesthesiology, Cleveland Clinic
Lerner College of Medicine of Case
Western Reserve University
Department of General Anesthesiology,
Cleveland Clinic
Cleveland, OH

Dhananjay Namjoshi, MPharm, MSc
Graduate Student (Neuroscience Program)
Faculty of Medicine
The University of British Columbia
Vancouver, Canada

Beverley A. Orser, MD, PhD
Canada Research Chair in Anesthesia
Professor, Departments of Anesthesia and Physiology
University of Toronto
and
Department of Anesthesia
Sunnybrook Health Sciences Centre
Toronto, Ontario, Canada

Catherine C. Price, PhD
Assistant Professor
Clinical and Health Psychology and
Department of Anesthesiology
University of Florida
Gainesville, FL

Kane O. Pryor, MD
Assistant Professor of Anesthesiology
Assistant Professor of Anesthesiology in Psychiatry
Weill Cornell Medical College
New York, NY

Srinivasa Raja, MD
Professor
Department of Anesthesiology and Critical
Care Medicine and Oncology
Division Chief, Pain Medicine
Department of Anesthesiology
Johns Hopkins University School of Medicine
Baltimore, MD

Raul Sanoja, MD, PhD
Research Associate
Faculty of Pharmaceutical Sciences
University of British Columbia
Vancouver, Canada

Tobias Schmidt-Wilcke, MD
Department of Neurology
University of Regensburg
Regensburg, Germany

Peter J. Soja, PhD
Professor, Pharmacology and Neuroscience
Faculty of Pharmaceutical Sciences
The University of British Columbia
Vancouver, Canada

Jared J. Tanner, MS
Graduate Student
Clinical and Health Psychology
University of Florida
Gainesville, FL

Pablo Torterolo, MD, PhD
Assistant Professor
Department of Physiology
School of Medicine
Universidad de la República
Montevideo, Uruguay

Giancarlo Vanini, MD
Research Investigator
Department of Anesthesiology
University of Michigan
Ann Arbor, MI

Robert A. Veselis, MD
Professor of Clinical Anesthesiology
Memorial Sloan-Kettering Cancer Center
New York, NY

Sanja Vukicevic, BScPharm, RPh
Medical Student
Faculty of Medicine
The University of British Columbia
Vancouver, Canada

Marnie B.Welch, MD
Staff Anesthesiologist
Department of Anesthesiology
Gundersen Lutheran Hospital
Lacrosse, WI

Zhongcong Xie, MD, PhD
Associate Professor in Anesthesia
Harvard Medical School
Boston, MA

Jun Xu, MD, PhD
Senior Scientist
Neuroscience Research
Global Pharmaceutical Research and Development
Abbott Laboratories
Abbott Park, IL

Yiying (Laura) Zhang, MD, MS
Research Fellow in Anesthesia
Harvard Medical School
Boston, MA

PART I

INTRODUCTION

INTRODUCTION

George A. Mashour and Ralph Lydic

The first public demonstration of a surgery under general anesthesia on October 16, 1846, was a seminal event in the history of medicine. Indeed, it has been argued that the discovery of general anesthesia was one of the most important advances in medicine in the past thousand years.[1] Clinically, anesthesiology has advanced and diversified significantly since the nineteenth century, with an elaboration of drugs, interventional techniques, and clinical domains. Anesthesiology now plays a key role across the spectrum of patient care, and the scope of perioperative medicine has widened.

But what is the *scientific* identity of anesthesiology? This question may give pause to those who understand the diversity of clinical practice but who overlook the fact that anesthesiology does have a single organ system of interest. *Neuroscientific Foundations of Anesthesiology* is offered as an answer: anesthesiology is a clinical branch of neuroscience. Perhaps even more routinely than neurologists or neurosurgeons, anesthesia providers are modulating the brain, spinal cord, peripheral nerves, autonomic nervous system, and neuromuscular junction—often all in the course of a single surgical intervention. Although anesthesiologists are also adept at the modulation of other physiological systems, it should be recognized that many of these critically important skills have been developed to address the *secondary* effects of general anesthesia that, from the scientific perspective, are merely derivative.

Neuroscientific Foundations of Anesthesiology was organized to reflect the fact that the clinical practice of anesthesiology targets virtually every component of the nervous system. The structure of the book is primarily systems based. Each major division focuses on a different part of the nervous system and begins with an introductory chapter that prepares the reader for the subsequent discussion. For example, in Chapter 1 Moore and Kelz give an overview of the brain that provides a context for more detailed discussions of topics such as the thalamocortical system (Chapter 4, Hudetz and Alkire) or the mediotemporal lobe (Chapter 5, Pryor and Veselis). The content is intended to be scientific in nature, while maintaining relevance to clinical practice. Indeed, we as editors of this volume bring perspectives from both bench (Lydic) and bedside (Mashour). The last section of the book departs from the systems-based approach to explore a topic of current controversy and importance—anesthetic neurotoxicity. The degree to which anesthetics impair the subsequent function of the nervous system—especially at the extremes of age—will be a critically important one to answer.

We thank all of the contributing authors for the time and scholarship devoted to writing for this volume. The authors were selected based on their leadership role in research or clinical practice. Readers will recognize a number of highly respected scientists as well as a number of editorial board members of high impact journals. In keeping with the goal of maintaining relevance to the general practice of anesthesiology, there are also important contributions by authors who are more clinically focused. Although the roster of contributors surely contains many of the best and brightest, it is not a comprehensive list. Publication mandates for an edited volume invariably result in a list of potential authors and topics that are not included. We apologize for egregious omissions and welcome input from readers regarding topics of emerging importance. There are many remarkable scholars who bridge the fields of neuroscience and anesthesiology that are not represented here, but whose work nonetheless informs the content.

Finally, the goal of this book is to provide a broad overview of the neuroscientific basis of anesthesiology that is readable, scientifically grounded, and clinically relevant. It is our hope that *The Neuroscientific Foundations* itself will be a foundation for future and more extensive books on the subject. What should be clear from the present volume is that anesthesiology *is* a clinical branch of neuroscience and that the investigation of anesthesia and analgesia *is* a form of neuroscience. The discipline of neuroscience has experienced explosive growth, making it one of the most vibrant areas of biomedical research. A content analysis of this book demonstrates the positive valence between exciting developments in neuroscience and clinically relevant problems in anesthesiology.

REFERENCES

1. Looking back on the millennium in medicine. *N Engl J Med*. 2000; 342(1):42–49.

PART II

BRAIN

1

BRAIN ANATOMY OF RELEVANCE TO THE ANESTHESIOLOGIST

Jason Moore and Max Kelz

INTRODUCTION

General anesthetics are administered to millions of patients annually in the United States alone, yet they remain one of the most toxic and least understood classes of drugs that are in widespread clinical use. To this day—more than sixteen decades after the first public demonstration of ether anesthesia—the central questions of where and how anesthetics act to produce their disparate effects remain unanswered. For much of the history of modern anesthesia it was assumed that all anesthetics had the same mechanism of action, since there is a remarkable amount of apparent overlap in the behavioral state that results from the administration of any general anesthetic compound, whether it be a gaseous, volatile, or intravenous anesthetic agent. Most general anesthetics produce behavioral effects in a dose-dependent manner: relatively low dosages produce amnesia, whereas increasingly higher dosages produce sedation/hypnosis, analgesia, and finally immobilization (Figure 1.1). This overall dose-effect order is consistent across all anesthetics even though some anesthetics do not produce each behavioral endpoint or have slight differences in MAC-adjusted potency. For example, the minimum alveolar concentration needed to cause immobility (MAC) in 40-year-olds is 0.76% for halothane, 1.19% for isoflurane, 1.88% for sevoflurane, and 6.45% for desflurane. Suppression of response to commands (MAC-Awake), a widely used clinical marker of unconsciousness, requires a dose of roughly one-third of a MAC for the halogenated ethers. However, for halothane the concentration needed to produce unconsciousness is closer to two-thirds of a MAC.[1] While the similar ratios of MAC-Awake/MAC for isoflurane, sevoflurane, and desflurane may argue for a common physiological mechanism of action, it is clear that agent-specific differences exist.

Agent-specific differences aside, recent research indicates that the common effects of anesthetic agents may not reside at the molecular or cellular level. Ion channels located in the cellular membranes of neurons have become promising molecular targets of general anesthetics, with several molecules (most notably, the γ-aminobutyric acid $[GABA]_A$ and K_{2P} receptors) emerging as likely targets for many anesthetics (see Chapter 2). However, each drug binds and modulates a large number of different proteins, and no currently known ion channel is bound by clinically relevant doses of all anesthetics. One alternate possibility suggests that although anesthetics may have different molecular targets, they may all work by specifically targeting the same anatomic loci throughout the neuroaxis. This is unlikely, however, as anesthetics freely distribute and bind to targets almost uniformly throughout the cerebrum.[2] Some hypothesize that global actions of anesthetic drugs ubiquitously suppress the activity of neurons leading to widespread and nonspecific central nervous system failure (the wet blanket theory).[3] In fact, recent research into the cause of anesthetic-induced hypnosis has revealed that some anesthetics target entirely different subsets of nuclei than others. One must therefore consider a third possibility that might explain how anesthetics produce a relatively similar behavioral state: different anesthetics may be acting on different molecular targets located in different anatomic loci, but these loci may be part of a common neural network that underlies the behavioral endpoints observed in general anesthesia.[4] Thus, a neuroanatomical understanding of the neural systems that are affected by anesthetics is critical to understanding the state of general anesthesia.

For the remainder of this chapter, we will be discussing the cerebral neural networks involved in three of the primary endpoints of general anesthesia—amnesia, hypnosis, and immobility—as well as surveying the current neuroscientific evidence as to how general anesthetics may be interacting with these networks to produce the behavioral state of anesthesia. This chapter is meant to serve as an introduction and overview for the material that is presented in the rest of this section.

AMNESIA

All anesthetics, given at a sufficiently high dose, will cause amnesia due to the inextricable link between unconsciousness and amnesia—a patient who is not fully conscious will necessarily have some deficit in forming or retrieving

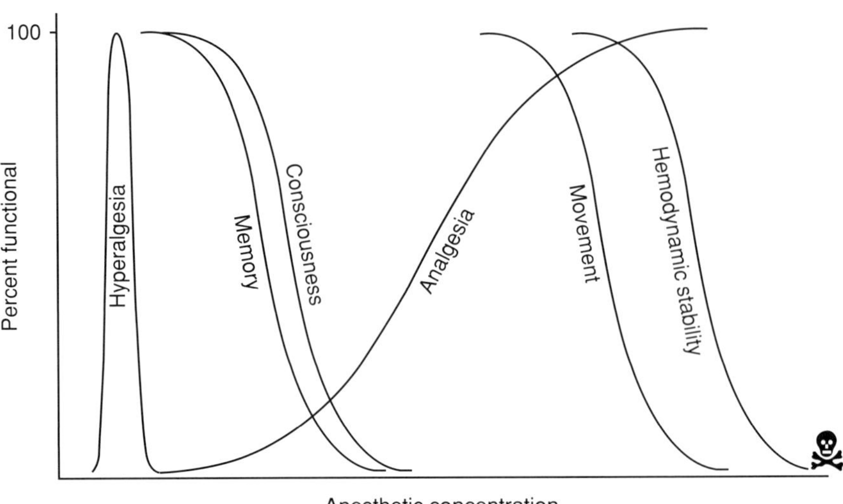

Figure 1.1 Schematic depicting the dose-response curves for each of the anesthetic endpoints for an idealized complete general anesthetic. Note that not every anesthetic agent is capable of producing every endpoint. Increasing anesthetic doses are shown toward the right. MAC is the concentration at which 50% of a population ceases movement in response to a surgical incision and is illustrated by the movement curve. MAC-awake is the concentration at which 50% of a population loses the ability to follow a command and may be found by tracing the consciousness curve. At very low doses, on the order of 0.1 MAC, inhaled anesthetics possess hyperalgesic properties. The amnesic doses for most anesthetics occur around 0.1–0.3 MAC. Reprinted from Alkire MT, Miller J. General anesthesia and the neural correlates of consciousness. *Prog Br Res*. 2005;150:229–244, with permission from Elsevier.

memories. However, many (but not all) anesthetics have amnesic effects at subhypnotic concentrations, suggesting that these drugs directly interfere with the brain's memory systems.[5]

In order to understand the amnesic effects of anesthetics, one must first understand the hierarchy of memories and how that corresponds to the anatomic representation of memory systems. Short-term memories only persist for seconds to hours unless they are consolidated into long-term memories. There is no centralized short-term memory store, but, in general, short-term memory relies on the parietal and frontal cortices. Studies in patients with localized cortical lesions show that it is possible to have a deficit in short-term memory specific to a sensory modality (e.g., normal ability to remember a phone number when it is heard, but not when it is seen).[6,7] Likewise, there is no centralized store for long-term memories, but a number of structures have been identified that play critical roles in certain types of long-term memories. The medial temporal lobe (including the hippocampus) and portions of the diencephalon are involved in explicit memories (memories that can be consciously recalled, such as facts and events),[8] while implicit memories depend on structures such as the striatum (habits and procedures) and the amygdala (emotional responses). Furthermore, the storage and retrieval of very long-term memories is also dependent on the anterior cingulate cortex.[9,10] Because of the distributed nature of circuits involved in memory, amnesia in the conscious subject is never complete and the type of amnesia that is observed is dependent on the brain areas that are affected.

While anesthetics can affect explicit and implicit memory,[11] explicit memories appear to be the most susceptible to anesthetic-induced amnesia, so the effects of anesthetics on the medial temporal lobe have been relatively well-characterized. The effects of anesthetics impairing hippocampus-dependent memory have been well studied in both rodents and humans for a wide array of anesthetics.[11–19] Most notably, long-term potentiation (LTP) and long-term depression—two cellular processes that are thought to be critical components of the cellular model of memory[20,21]—are impaired in the hippocampus by a wide range of anesthetics,[22–24] as are the hippocampal electrical rhythms that are believed to be a key component of the network model of memory.[25] The amygdala has also been implicated in anesthetic-induced amnesia, especially as a component of impairments in hippocampus-independent implicit memories.[14,26] In particular, the basolateral nucleus of the amygdala is necessary for the production of amnesia by propofol, sevoflurane, and benzodiazepines,[27–29] although this may have as much to do with the anatomic vicinity of the amygdala to the hippocampus and the high degree of interconnectedness between these two structures as with the sole importance of the basolateral nucleus to anesthetic-induced amnesia.

In summary, anesthetics can produce amnesia either indirectly, by inducing a hypnotic state, or directly, by interfering with one of the many brain regions that are critical for normal formation and recall of memories. Through mechanisms that are detailed in Chapter 5, many anesthetics that have subhypnotic amnesic effects interfere with the normal cellular and network physiology in the medial temporal lobe. Clinically, it is fortuitous that memory is the most sensitive and easily disrupted of the anesthetic endpoints.

HYPNOSIS

Although sedation, which is believed to be a part of the same behavioral and physiological continuum as hypnosis (or unconsciousness), often co-occurs with amnesia for many anesthetics, amnesia, sedation, and hypnosis are dissociable and have clearly separate mechanisms.[5,30] Because of the importance of maintaining an unconscious state during surgery, hypnosis is perhaps the second best studied behavioral endpoint after anesthetic-induced immobility. However, the nature of anesthetic-induced hypnosis remains mysterious, largely due to our rudimentary knowledge of the neural basis of consciousness. Since it is logical to assume that anesthetics likely interact with the same neural circuits that maintain consciousness, anesthetic drugs could be useful in understanding the neurological basis of consciousness.[31] This fact was recognized by Henry Beecher in the first half of the twentieth century when he astutely pointed to anesthesia's second power—probing the neurophysiology of consciousness itself.[32]

ENDOGENOUS AROUSAL CIRCUITRY AS A POSSIBLE SUBSTRATE FOR ANESTHETIC-INDUCED HYPNOSIS

One possible mechanism by which general anesthetics induce hypnosis is by acting on the endogenous arousal neural circuitry[33,34] (Figure 1.2). Anesthetic-induced unconsciousness is a nonarousable behavioral state that shares many commonalities with non–rapid eye movement (NREM) sleep. Both behavioral states produce a functional loss in cortical connectivity,[35–40] which produces similar cortical EEG patterns,[34] and makes both states amenable to processed EEG monitoring to approximate the level of consciousness.[41] Moreover, both anesthesia and sleep show an inhibition of thalamic nuclei.[42–45] and of the wake-active nuclei historically known as the reticular activating system.[42] Furthermore, in some paradigms anesthesia can substitute for sleep. Prolonged periods of propofol-induced unconsciousness do not incur a sleep debt,[46] and may actually relieve previously incurred sleep debts.[47,48] Furthermore, both sleep deprivation and administration of endogenous somnogens reduce the dose of anesthetic required to reach hypnosis.[48,49] Conversely, induction and maintenance of anesthesia itself has the capacity to alter the levels of endogenous somnogens.[50] Because of these and other similar findings, an increasingly popular theory for anesthetic action is that anesthetic-induced hypnosis may arise at least in part from the specific actions of anesthetics on the arousal neural circuitry that underlies endogenous sleep-wake control.[51]

Preservation of the finely tuned regulation of arousal state is an essential feature for an individual's and species' survival. Were the critical neuroanatomic substrates confined to a single area, damage to that region of the brain would have catastrophic consequences. Hence, it should not be surprising that the responsibility for regulation of sleep and wakefulness is widely distributed with substantial redundancy engineered as a defining feature.[52] As discussed below, the neural circuits involved in arousal control are quite complex, so the knowledge of how the activity of each nucleus is affected by anesthetics will undoubtedly be critical to understanding the basis of anesthetic-induced hypnosis.[53]

Homeostasis between sleep and wakefulness is maintained through interactions among dozens of disparate nuclei spread along the entire neuroaxis. One hypothesis is that the neural circuits regulating arousal state form a flip-flop switch, in which at any given time only sleep- or wake-active neurons fire predominantly. Arousal-promoting nuclei (located predominantly in the pons, midbrain, and basal forebrain) and sleep-promoting nuclei (located predominantly in the preoptic hypothalamus) mutually antagonize each other via reciprocal inhibitory connections. Thus, in the absence of pathology, an organism is either stably in a state of wakefulness or sleep, with rapid and complete transitions occurring between states.[54]

AROUSAL PROMOTING NUCLEI IN THE RETICULAR ACTIVATING SYSTEM

While the definitive studies that will undoubtedly prove a causative association between behavioral state and neural activity in the wake-promoting regions of brain are finally within reach,[55] decades of accumulating evidence have established strong correlations between firing rates of discrete populations of neurons dispersed across the neuroaxis and an organism's state of arousal. Wake-active neurons display increased rates of discharge during wakefulness and slow or become virtually quiescent during NREM and REM sleep, respectively. Such neurons are classified both by the neurotransmitters that they contain as well as by their location within the brain and are discussed in turn below.

Locus Coeruleus (LC)

The LC is the site of the brain's largest collection of noradrenergic neurons. As with many of the other monoaminergic systems, the LC diffusely innervates the brain by projecting directly to the cortex, thalamus, hypothalamus, basal forebrain, amygdala, hippocampus, and other subcortical systems. State-dependent modulation of activity within the LC has long been proposed as an essential means of regulating arousal; changes in the activity of LC neurons occur before and are predictive of changes in an organism's behavioral state.[56] Through its actions on alpha$_1$ and beta receptors, firing of LC neurons is thought to promote wakefulness in part through actions on the medial septum, the medial preoptic area, and the substantia innominata within the basal forebrain. Moreover, LC activity modulates activity within thalamocortical circuits, switching the tone of

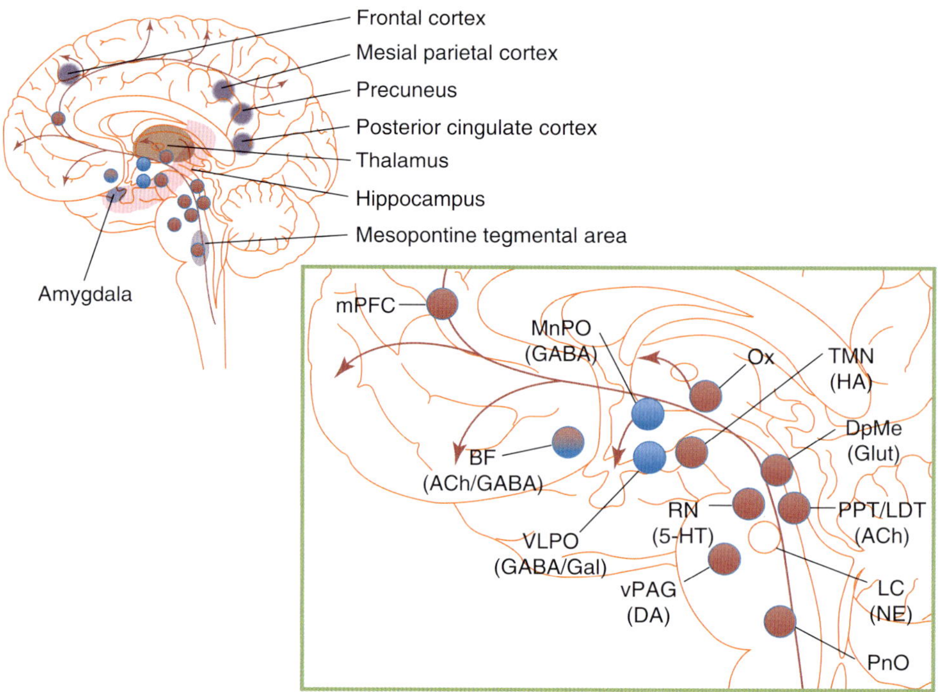

Figure 1.2 Schematic sagittal view of a human brain demonstrating the approximate locations of important cortical and subcortical regions involved in the generation of anesthetic-induced amnesia, hypnosis, and immobility. The inset highlights key arousal systems along with their neurotransmitters involved in the generation and maintenance of sleep or wakefulness. Ascending projections traverse either a dorsal pathway through the thalamus, or a ventral pathway through the hypothalamus and basal forebrain. Sleep-active loci are shown in light blue. When wake-active systems (shown in red) are firing they antagonize the sleep-active groups. Conversely, when sleep-active neurons are active, they mutually antagonize the wake-active regions to further reinforce sleep. Anesthetic drugs are known to interact with this circuitry to produce hypnosis. 5-HT: serotonin; ACh: acetylcholine; DA: dopamine; GABA: γ-aminobutyric acid; Gal: galanin; HA: histamine; Glut: glutamate; NE: norepinephrine; BF: basal forebrain; DpME: deep mesencephalic reticular formation; LC: locus coeruleus; LDT laterodorsal tegmentum; MnPO: Median preoptic nucleus; mPFC: medial prefrontal cortex; Ox: orexin/hypocretin neurons in lateral, perifornical, and posterior hypothalamus; PnO: pontine reticular nucleus oral part; PPT pedunculopontine tegmentum; RN: raphe nuclei; SCN: suprachiasmatic nucleus; TMN: tuberomammillary nucleus; VLPO ventrolateral preoptic nucleus; vPAG: ventral periaqueductal gray.

thalamocortical neurons from the burst pattern that defines slow wave sleep to a spiking pattern that characterizes wakefulness.[56] However it must also be mentioned that additional noradrenergic populations outside of the LC, such as the A1 and A2 brainstem groups, may also contribute to the regulation of sleep, wakefulness, and anesthesia.[57–59]

Raphe Nuclei (RN)

As with the noradrenergic system, serotonergic neurons in the raphe nuclei diffusely innervate the neuroaxis and display state-dependent activity similar to that of the noradrenergic LC system. The RN form the brain's major source of serotonin. A number of studies have demonstrated that serotonergic neurons in the RN fire maximally during wakefulness, decrease their firing during NREM sleep, and cease firing during REM sleep. However the role of the RN in arousal state regulation is not as clear as with the LC, since single unit studies demonstrate that firing rates of serotonergic neurons do not anticipate spontaneous changes in arousal state. Hence activity of serotonergic neurons may not be causally linked to changes in behavioral state. Nonetheless, pharmacologic, genetic, and lesion studies do confirm a complex contribution of serotonergic signaling to wakefulness. Through its seven major receptor subtypes, and distinct efferent projection systems, serotonin may exert biphasic influences on arousal, promoting either sleep or wakefulness. This is typified by serotonin's effects on the sleep-active ventrolateral preoptic nucleus (VLPO), where serotonin inhibits roughly half and excites the other half of VLPO neurons in contrast to norepinephrine and acetylcholine, which uniformly inhibit all VLPO neurons.[60]

Ventral Periaqueductal Gray (vPAG)

Accumulating evidence over the years suggested a dopaminergic contribution to wakefulness. However, the best-studied populations of dopaminergic neurons in the ventral tegmental area and substantia nigra do not display state-dependent activity. Hence the discovery of a wake-active subset of dopaminergic neurons in the vPAG helps to reconcile the observations that drugs that block dopamine (but not norepinephrine) reuptake promote wakefulness and that global loss of dopaminergic neurons is associated with sleepiness in Parkinson's disease. In fact, specific lesions of the vPAG dopaminergic neurons were also shown to cause increased sleepiness in rodents.[61] The vPAG efferent targets include multiple areas associated with arousal state regulation including the basal forebrain, orexinergic neurons in the perifornical hypothalamus, midline thalamic and intralaminar thalamus, laterodorsal tegmentum (LDT), as well as the sleep-active VLPO. Such circuitry places the vPAG in a prime position to modulate levels of arousal.

Laterodorsal Tegmentum (LDT) and Pedunculopontine Tegmentum (PPT)

These nuclei comprise two major cholinergic populations in the brainstem with the ability to regulate arousal state and promote wakefulness or REM sleep. These cholinergic neurons densely innervate the midline and intralaminar thalamic nuclei and thalamic reticular nucleus and alter thalamic activity from bursting to spiking. Additionally, the LDT and PPT are classically described as REM-ON populations that fire most rapidly during REM sleep, sending cholinergic projections into the pontine reticular formation.[62–64] However, the LDT and PPT also contain important subsets of GABAergic neurons. Microinjection of muscimol (a $GABA_A$ agonist) into the PPT increases REM sleep and decreases wakefulness. Conversely, microinjection of bicuculline, a $GABA_A$ antagonist, induces the opposite behavioral changes: increasing wakefulness and decreasing both REM and NREM sleep.[65]

Pontine Reticular Nucleus, Oral Part (PnO)

Neurons in this large region (which includes the sublaterodorsal nucleus) receive cholinergic, orexinergic, and GABAergic inputs. Within this area, REM-ON generating neurons are found. However, the region also has the capacity to promote wakefulness in addition to REM sleep. Moreover, anesthetics are known to exert important actions on neurons here.[66,67] The PnO illustrates a critical point about the importance of neuroanatomic and neurochemical compartments: unlike most other regions of brain, increased GABA levels in the PnO promote wakefulness. Moreover, wakefulness can be impaired by local delivery of adenosine or acetylcholine into PnO or alternatively promoted by local delivery of orexin or GABA.[68–70] Cholinergic input to the PnO originates from the LDT and PPT, while the orexinergic input arises from the hypothalamus. However, the opposing responses to adenosine and GABA suggest that simple disinhibition of a single population of PnO neurons will not be sufficient to understand the actions of these neuromodulators. Clearly, a more complex local microcircuitry is awaiting discovery.

Deep Mesencephalic Reticular Formation (DpMe)

Over the decades, many studies have demonstrated that electrical stimulation in the DpMe reliably induces cortical activation in anesthetized animals. These presumptively glutamatergic neurons project to the thalamus, hypothalamus, and basal forebrain, where they increase their firing rates prior to the onset of wakefulness and fire more slowly during NREM sleep.[71]

Tuberomammillary Nucleus (TMN)

The brain's sole source of histaminergic signaling originates from the TMN. Although spatially confined to a discrete region of the hypothalamus, the histaminergic innervation stemming from the TMN is widespread. TMN neurons display state-dependent firing patterns with maximal rates of discharge occurring during wakefulness, slower firing in NREM sleep, and minimal activity during REM sleep.[72] Fluctuating levels of GABA modulate activity of TMN neurons, which are known to receive inhibitory projections from sleep-active VLPO neurons. Local microinjection of the $GABA_A$ agonist muscimol into the TMN has been shown to be sufficient to cause hypnosis, although microinjection of propofol or pentobarbital only caused sedation, arguing that localized inhibition of the TMN by anesthetics isn't sufficient for loss of consciousness.[73] Nonetheless, modulation of histaminergic neurotransmission is capable of facilitating arousal and modifying the anesthetized state as well.[74,75]

Hypocretin/Orexin Neurons (Ox)

Initially discovered in the late 1990s, the hypocretin/orexin signaling system exerts potent wake-promoting and stabilizing effects. As with the aforementioned monoaminergic wake-active systems, the hypocretin/orexin system displays state-dependent firing patterns with maximal activity during active wakefulness.[76,77] The neurons are silent during NREM sleep but occasionally burst during REM sleep. Anatomically, these neurons project to all of the monoaminergic groups along with arborizing to the basal forebrain, midline thalamic nuclei, and other regions known to participate in the regulation of arousal.[78] When signaling in these neurons is impaired, narcolepsy with cataplexy ensues. However, in addition to their critical role in maintaining arousal, these neurons integrate other physiological inputs. They can directly sense levels of glucose, carbon dioxide, and acidity, giving them the ability to rouse a sleeping individual to feed should energy levels plummet or breathe more deeply to maintain a normal blood pH level.[79] Of direct relevance to clinical anesthesiology, orexin/hypocretin neurons play an important role in modulating emergence from several anesthetics.[80,81] Local application of orexin excites target neurons expressing either of the two orexin G_q-coupled neurotransmitter receptors, including the LDT, LC, RN, basal forebrain (BF), and thalamocortical neurons.[79]

Cholinergic Neurons of the Basal Forebrain (BF)

The basal forebrain sits atop the ventral extrathalamic relay and receives integrated arousal inputs from caudal structures. The BF can be further subdivided into the nucleus basalis, the vertical and diagonal bands, and the septal area. Within the BF, there are wake-active cholinergic neurons, sleep-active GABAergic neurons (discussed below), and state-indifferent neurons. The cholinergic neurons receive afferents from the LC, DpME, TMN, and orexinergic neurons and send widespread efferent projections to the cortex and hippocampus as well as back to the hypothalamus. Increased activity of the basal forebrain cholinergic neurons during wakefulness is responsible for the fluctuations in cortical acetylcholine levels. The cholinergic neurons stimulate cortical activation and their increased discharge underlies the desynchronized EEG that typifies wakefulness as well as REM sleep.[82] Modulation of BF activity is known to affect the anesthetized state[83] as discussed in Chapter 3.

SLEEP-ACTIVE NUCLEI IN THE ANTERIOR HYPOTHALAMUS

One means to establish state bistability is through interconnected positive and negative feedback loops. Within the flip-flop switch that underlies regulation of sleep and arousal in mammals, hypnogenic sleep-promoting centers mutually antagonize wake-promoting ones, creating the negative feedback component of mutual inhibition. The majority of sleep-active neurons utilize the inhibitory neurotransmitter GABA. However, a recently discovered cortical population of sleep-active interneurons is also distinguished by the presence of neuronal nitric oxide synthase.[84] Details surrounding the sleep-active nuclei follow below.

Ventrolateral Preoptic (VLPO) Nucleus

The VLPO lies within the anterior hypothalamus positioned on the ventral floor at the level of the optic chiasm. Its discovery caused a paradigm shift in the field of sleep neurobiology, as VLPO neurons were shown to become more active specifically during both REM and NREM sleep.[85–87] Moreover, changes in VLPO activity precede the changes in an organism's behavioral state. Destruction of VLPO was also shown to cause long-lasting insomnia.[88] Retrograde and anterograde labeling studies demonstrated that the VLPO is reciprocally interconnected with many of the wake-promoting nuclei, including the histaminergic TMN, serotonergic RN, noradrenergic LC, cholinergic LDT and PPT, as well as the orexinergic neurons of the hypothalamus.[54] VLPO neurons contain the inhibitory neurotransmitters GABA and galanin and are thus ideally positioned to coordinate and reciprocally inhibit wake-active ascending reticular activating nuclei. Evidence discussed in Chapter 3 will highlight the known effects of anesthetics and their capacity to recruit the VLPO, either directly or indirectly through disinhibition.

Median Preoptic (MnPO) Nucleus

In the earliest attempts to identify specific populations of sleep-promoting neurons, a definitive role was assigned to the preoptic anterior hypothalamus—a broad region that encompasses the VLPO. However, additional neurons with state-dependent activity patterns similar to VLPO and inverse to the monoaminergic populations were recognized in the MnPO, which straddles the decussation of the anterior commissure. Similar to the VLPO, MnPO sleep-active neurons are GABAergic and fire more rapidly several seconds prior to sleep onset.[89] Due to the activity pattern of MnPO, it has been assigned an important role in the initiation of sleep. Endogenous somnogens such as adenosine, prostaglandin D2 (PGD2), interleukin 1 beta (IL1B), and growth hormone releasing hormone (GHRH) all activate MnPO as well as VLPO. Moreover, like VLPO, MnPO is known to send inhibitory projections to multiple arousal systems, including the orexinergic neurons in the hypothalamus.[90] Unlike the VLPO, MnPO neurons also appear to play a critical role in regulation of temperature as well as in serum osmolarity; however it remains unknown the degree to which these functions are dissociable from the sleep-promoting functions of the MnPO.

GABAergic Neurons of the Basal Forebrain (BF)

A subset of GABAergic neurons within the heterogeneous BF exhibit specific increases in local unit activity during slow wave sleep (the deepest stage of NREM sleep) and have been hypothesized to be another sleep-active group.[91] Such neurons are found in the magnocellular preoptic area and substantia innominata regions of the basal forebrain. While this collection of neurons is intermingled with adjacent neurons that do not display sleep-active firing patterns, a majority of the sleep-active subset is GABAergic and expresses the noradrenergic α_{2A} receptor subtype.

THALAMOCORTICAL SYSTEM

Nearly two decades of research points toward the thalamus as a critical site for toggling between the conscious and unconscious states. Thalamic nuclei receive input from the dorsal pathway and from wake-active regions in the hypothalamus (Figure 1.2). The architecture within the thalamus can be schematized by three neuronal types with interlocking positive and negative feedback systems. Thalamocortical neurons (TC) send excitatory glutamatergic input to the other two populations: the reticular thalamic neurons and the corticothalamic neurons. The corticothalamic neurons send depolarizing glutamatergic feedback to the TC (forming the positive feedback loop) and excitatory input to the reticular neurons (forming the negative feedback loop, since the reticular neurons are GABAergic and innervate the TC neurons). Both reticular and thalamocortical neurons receive monoaminergic and cholinergic input from the brainstem but with opposing results. TC neurons are depolarized, while reticular neurons are hyperpolarized. These interlocking loops translate into behavioral state regulation as follows. During wakefulness, ongoing depolarization of the TC neurons is marked by their tonic firing and ensuing faithful gating of afferent input to the cortex. However, with the onset of NREM sleep, TC neurons undergo prolonged periods of hyperpolarization followed by increased membrane conductance leading to a bursting pattern of activity during NREM sleep. This bursting activity transiently interrupts sensory stimuli from being passed to the cortex and forms the neuronal correlate for "closing of the thalamic gates."[45] A wide spectrum of general anesthetics disrupt the tonic firing pattern of corticothalamic neurons.[42,92–96] Within the midline thalamic nuclei that receive ascending reticular activating inputs, presumptive depolarization of corticothalamic neurons with restoration of their tonic activity has been shown to be sufficient to antagonize sevoflurane hypnosis.[97] Together with neuroimaging work, these results have led to speculation that thalamocortical circuits form an essential switch for modulating consciousness.[42]

CEREBRAL CORTEX

Although most anesthetics reduce the global cerebral metabolic rate (with ketamine and nitrous oxide being two of the most notable exceptions), the effects of anesthetics on the cerebral cortex are very heterogeneous. Primary sensory cortices—the regions of cortex that first receive information from sensory afferents—maintain nearly identical evoked potentials across the awake, asleep, and anesthetized states. While these cortices remain receptive to incoming sensory information, their ability to communicate with other functionally related regions of cortex (such as the same modality's contralateral primary sensory cortex) is impaired during anesthetic-induced hypnosis (Figure 1.3).[38] Indeed, the cortical regions that are most uniformly affected by anesthetics are largely midline structures that play key roles in information transfer across the cortex. These medial structures (which include the mesial parietal cortex, posterior cingulate cortex, and precuneus) are largely deactivated during both sleep[98] and anesthesia.[99,100] During anesthesia, the deactivation of these

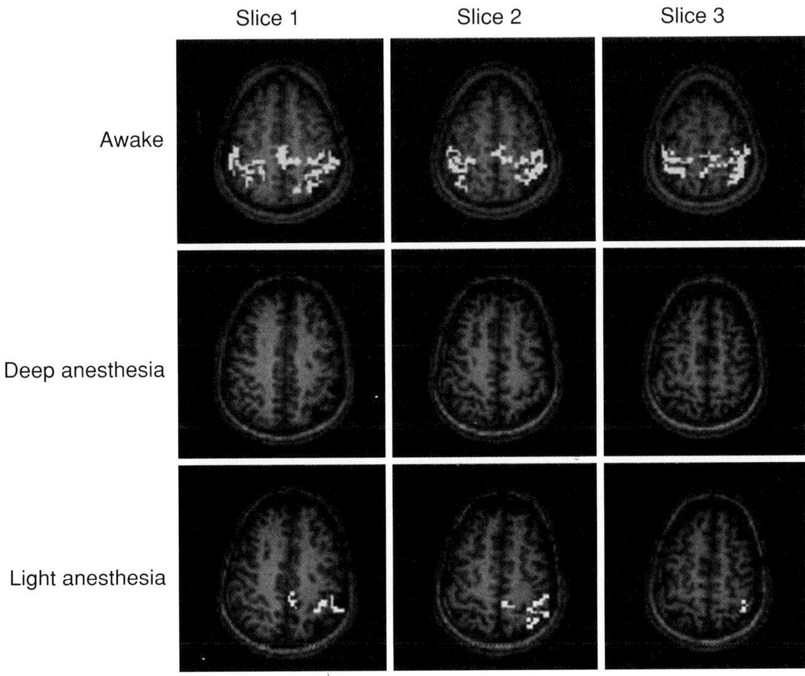

Figure 1.3 Sample functional MRI connectivity maps from a human volunteer showing a loss of functional connectivity between cortical areas during administration of sevoflurane. Functional connectivity is approximated here as the amount of correlation between cortical regions in low-frequency oscillations (< 0.08 Hz). Functionally related areas, such as the left and right primary motor cortices, have low-frequency oscillations that are highly temporally correlated (top row). As increasing dosages of the anesthetic are applied to the volunteer (bottom row: 1.0% sevoflurane; middle row: 2.0% sevoflurane), the amount of functional connectivity greatly diminishes. All significant voxels have a $p < 2.5 \times 10^{-5}$. Reprinted with permission from Peltier S, Kerssens C, Hamann S, et al. Functional connectivity changes with concentration of sevoflurane anesthesia. *Neuroreport.* 2005;16(3):285–288.

structures is thought to lead to an attenuated state of information transfer across the cortex with relative preservation of frontoparietal feed-forward mechanisms,[101,102] but degradation of frontoparietal feedback, leading to the idea that the unconscious state is one in which information is received, but not perceived.[103] However, not all higher-order cortical areas are affected by anesthetics. For example, activity in the frontal cortex, which is critical for many higher mental functions, is preserved during thiopental-induced hypnosis,[104] and lesions of the frontal cortex are insufficient to induce unconsciousness.[105] Therefore, the regions of cortex that are most affected by anesthetics are those that are involved in providing cortical connectivity. Such data is supported by modeling studies of network activity,[106,107] by in vitro work with isolated cortical networks[108] as well as in vivo and is in concordance with many recent theories of consciousness that hypothesize that unconsciousness results from a breakdown in the ability to integrate information across the cerebrum.[35,36,109]

IMMOBILITY

Unlike amnesia and hypnosis, immobility is primarily a consequence of anesthetics acting on sites located in the spinal cord, not in the cerebrum (see Chapter 8). For volatile anesthetics, the MAC is unchanged in decerebrated animals[110] and in animals where the anesthetic is selectively delivered extracerebrally (by taking advantage of the specialized cardiovascular system of the goat, where the brain and spinal column are served by independent circulations).[111,112] However, volatile anesthetics can also cause immobility when only administered to the cerebrum at a dose 2.5–4 times MAC in a normal animal,[112] and some anesthetics such as barbiturates produce immobility by acting supraspinally.[113] Thus, although immobility is largely thought to be a result of anesthetic actions on the spinal cord, there is evidence for modulation of motor tone by descending signals arising from cerebral sites of action. Microinjection of barbiturates into the mesopontine tegmental area rapidly elicits surgical levels of immobility together with hypnosis.[114] Detailed knowledge of this intriguing supraspinal site of anesthetic-induced immobility and hypnosis is beginning to emerge.[115,116]

CONCLUSION

Amnesia, hypnosis, and immobility form the core components of the anesthetic state. While individual anesthetic drugs may selectively interact with specific molecular targets (as in the case of etomidate and the $GABA_A$ receptor) or may be widely promiscuous (as in the case of the volatile anesthetics) convergence of diverse agents has been demonstrated within the central nervous system at the circuit level. The chapters that follow will explore the molecular, cellular, and circuit level effects of anesthetics in greater depth.

REFERENCES

1. Eger EI. Age, minimum alveolar anesthetic concentration, and minimum alveolar anesthetic concentration-awake. *Anesth Analg.* 2001;93(4):947–953.
2. Eckenhoff MF, Eckenhoff RG. Quantitative autoradiography of halothane binding in rat brain. *J Pharmacol Exp Ther.* 1998; 285(1):371–376.
3. Sukhotinsky I, et al. Neural pathways associated with loss of consciousness caused by intracerebral microinjection of GABA(A)-active anesthetics. *Eur J Neurosci.* 2007;25(5):1417–1436.
4. Rudolph U, Antkowiak B. Molecular and neuronal substrates for general anaesthetics. *Nat Rev Neurosci.* 2004;5(9):709–720.
5. Veselis RA, Reinsel RA, Feshchenko VA. Drug-induced amnesia is a separate phenomenon from sedation: electrophysiologic evidence. *Anesthesiology.* 2001;95(4):896–907.
6. Fastenau PS, Conant LL, Lauer RE. Working memory in young children: evidence for modality-specificity and implications for cerebral reorganization in early childhood. *Neuropsychologia.* 1998; 36(7):643–652.
7. Kim JJ, Fanselow MS. Modality-specific retrograde amnesia of fear. *Science.* 1992;256(5057):675–677.
8. Squire LR, Zola SM. Structure and function of declarative and nondeclarative memory systems. *Proc Natl Acad Sci USA.* 1996;93(24):13515–13522.
9. Frankland PW, Bontempi B. The organization of recent and remote memories. *Nat Rev Neurosci.* 2005;6(2):119–130.
10. Frankland PW, et al. The involvement of the anterior cingulate cortex in remote contextual fear memory. *Science.* 2004;304(5672): 881–883.
11. Reinsel RA, et al. Midazolam decreases cerebral blood flow in the left prefrontal cortex in a dose-dependent fashion. *Int J Neuropsychopharmacol.* 2000;3(2):117–127.
12. Andrade J. Learning during anaesthesia: a review. *Br J Psychol.* 1995; 86 (Pt 4):479–506.
13. Andrade J, Baddeley A. Depth of anesthesia: human memory and anesthesia. *Int Anesthesiol Clin.* 1993;31(4):39–51.
14. Dutton RC, et al. The concentration of isoflurane required to suppress learning depends on the type of learning. *Anesthesiology.* 2001;94(3):514–519.
15. Ghoneim MM, Block RI. Learning and consciousness during general anesthesia. *Anesthesiology.* 1992;76(2):279–305.
16. Ghoneim MM, Block RI. Depth of anesthesia: learning during anesthesia. *Int Anesthesiol Clin.* 1993;31(4):53–65.
17. Ghoneim MM, Block RI. Learning and memory during general anesthesia: an update. *Anesthesiology.* 1997;87(2):387–410.
18. Lubke GH, et al. Dependence of explicit and implicit memory on hypnotic state in trauma patients. *Anesthesiology.* 1999;90(3):670–680.
19. Veselis RA. Memory: a guide for anaesthetists. *Best Pract Res Clin Anaesthesiol.* 2007;21(3):297–312.
20. Bliss TV, Collingridge GL. A synaptic model of memory: long-term potentiation in the hippocampus. *Nature.* 1993;361(6407):31–39.
21. Martin SJ, Grimwood PD, Morris RG. Synaptic plasticity and memory: an evaluation of the hypothesis. *Annu Rev Neurosci.* 2000;23:649–711.
22. Akhondzadeh S, Stone TW. Potentiation of muscimol-induced long-term depression by benzodiazepines and prevention or reversal by pregnenolone sulfate. *Pharmacol Res.* 1998;38(6):441–448.
23. Nagashima K, Zorumski CF, Izumi Y. Propofol inhibits long-term potentiation but not long-term depression in rat hippocampal slices. *Anesthesiology.* 2005;103(2):318–326.
24. Simon W, et al. Isoflurane blocks synaptic plasticity in the mouse hippocampus. *Anesthesiology.* 2001;94(6):1058–1065.

25. Perouansky M, et al. Amnesic concentrations of the nonimmobilizer 1,2-dichlorohexafluorocyclobutane (F6, 2N) and isoflurane alter hippocampal theta oscillations in vivo. *Anesthesiology*. 2007; 106(6):1168–1176.
26. Dutton RC, et al. Isoflurane causes anterograde but not retrograde amnesia for Pavlovian fear conditioning. *Anesthesiology*. 2002; 96(5):1223–1229.
27. Alkire MT, Nathan SV. Does the amygdala mediate anesthetic-induced amnesia? Basolateral amygdala lesions block sevoflurane-induced amnesia. *Anesthesiology*. 2005;102(4):754–760.
28. Alkire MT, Nathan SV, McReynolds JR. Memory enhancing effect of low-dose sevoflurane does not occur in basolateral amygdala-lesioned rats. *Anesthesiology*. 2005;103(6):1167–1173.
29. Alkire MT, et al. Lesions of the basolateral amygdala complex block propofol-induced amnesia for inhibitory avoidance learning in rats. *Anesthesiology*. 2001;95(3):708–715.
30. Zeller A, et al. Distinct molecular targets for the central respiratory and cardiac actions of the general anesthetics etomidate and propofol. *FASEB J*. 2005;19(12):1677–1679.
31. Crick F, Koch C. A framework for consciousness. *Nat Neurosci*. 2003;6(2):119–126.
32. Beecher HK. Anesthesia's second power: probing the mind. *Science*. 1947;105(2720):164–166.
33. Franks NP. General anaesthesia: from molecular targets to neuronal pathways of sleep and arousal. *Nat Rev Neurosci*. 2008;9(5): 370–386.
34. Lydic R, Baghdoyan HA. Sleep, anesthesiology, and the neurobiology of arousal state control. *Anesthesiology*. 2005;103(6): 1268–1295.
35. John ER, et al. Invariant reversible QEEG effects of anesthetics. *Conscious Cogn*. 2001;10(2):165–183.
36. Mashour G. Consciousness unbound: toward a paradigm of general anesthesia. *Anesthesiology*. 2004;100(2):428–433.
37. Pack CC, Berezovskii VK, Born RT. Dynamic properties of neurons in cortical area MT in alert and anaesthetized macaque monkeys. *Nature*. 2001;414(6866):905–908.
38. Peltier SJ, et al. Functional connectivity changes with concentration of sevoflurane anesthesia. *Neuroreport*. 2005;16(3):285–288.
39. Mashour G. Integrating the science of consciousness and anesthesia. *Anesth Analg*. 2006;103(4):975–982.
40. Massimini M, et al. Breakdown of cortical effective connectivity during sleep. *Science*. 2005;309(5744):2228–2232.
41. Sleigh JW, et al. The bispectral index: a measure of depth of sleep? *Anesth Analg*. 1999;88(3):659–661.
42. Alkire MT, Haier RJ, Fallon JH. Toward a unified theory of narcosis: brain imaging evidence for a thalamocortical switch as the neurophysiologic basis of anesthetic-induced unconsciousness. *Conscious Cogn*. 2000;9(3):370–386.
43. Detsch O, et al. Increased responsiveness of cortical neurons in contrast to thalamic neurons during isoflurane-induced EEG bursts in rats. *Neurosci Lett*. 2002;317(1):9–12.
44. Vahle-Hinz C, et al. Local GABA(A) receptor blockade reverses isoflurane's suppressive effects on thalamic neurons in vivo. *Anesth Analg*. 2001;92(6):1578–1584.
45. Steriade M. The corticothalamic system in sleep. *Front Biosci*. 2003;8:d878–899.
46. Tung A, Lynch JP, Mendelson WB. Prolonged sedation with propofol in the rat does not result in sleep deprivation. *Anesth Analg*. 2001;92(5):1232–1236.
47. Tung A, Mendelson WB. Anesthesia and sleep. *Sleep Med Rev*. 2004;8(3):213–225.
48. Tung A, et al. Sleep deprivation potentiates the onset and duration of loss of righting reflex induced by propofol and isoflurane. *Anesthesiology*. 2002;97(4):906–911.
49. Kaputlu I, Sadan G, Ozdem S. Exogenous adenosine potentiates hypnosis induced by intravenous anaesthetics. *Anaesthesia*. 1998; 53(5):496–500.
50. Sato T, et al. Decreased hypothalamic prostaglandin D2 and prostaglandin E2 contents during isoflurane anaesthesia in rats. *Can J Anaesth*. 1995;42(11):1031–1034.
51. Lydic R, Biebuyck JF. Sleep neurobiology: relevance for mechanistic studies of anaesthesia. *Br J Anaesth*. 1994;72(5):506–508.
52. Jones BE, Arousal systems. *Front Biosci*. 2003;8:s438–451.
53. Dong HL, et al. Excitatory and inhibitory actions of isoflurane on the cholinergic ascending arousal system of the rat. *Anesthesiology*. 2006;104(1):122–133.
54. Saper CB, Chou TC, Scammell TE. The sleep switch: hypothalamic control of sleep and wakefulness. *Trends Neurosci*. 2001;24(12):726–731.
55. Adamantidis AR, et al. Neural substrates of awakening probed with optogenetic control of hypocretin neurons. *Nature*. 2007;450(7168): 420–424.
56. Berridge, CW. Noradrenergic modulation of arousal. *Brain Res Rev*. 2008;58(1):1–17.
57. Hirota K, Kushikata T. Central noradrenergic neurones and the mechanism of general anaesthesia. *Br J Anaesth*. 2001;87(6):811–813.
58. Kubota T, et al. Effects of ketamine and pentobarbital on noradrenaline release from the medial prefrontal cortex in rats. *Can J Anaesth*. 1999;46(4):388–392.
59. Yoshida H, et al. Xenon inhalation increases norepinephrine release from the anterior and posterior hypothalamus in rats. *Can J Anaesth*. 2001;48(7):651–655.
60. Gallopin T, et al. The endogenous somnogen adenosine excites a subset of sleep-promoting neurons via A2A receptors in the ventrolateral preoptic nucleus. *Neuroscience*. 2005;134(4):1377–1390.
61. Lu J, Jhou TC, Saper CB. Identification of wake-active dopaminergic neurons in the ventral periaqueductal gray matter. *J Neurosci*. 2006;26(1):193–202.
62. Steriade M, et al. Neuronal activities in brain-stem cholinergic nuclei related to tonic activation processes in thalamocortical systems. *J Neurosci*. 1990;10(8):2541–2559.
63. Steriade M, et al. Different cellular types in mesopontine cholinergic nuclei related to ponto-geniculo-occipital waves. *J Neurosci*. 1990;10(8):2560–2579.
64. Greene RW, Gerber U, McCarley RW. Cholinergic activation of medial pontine reticular formation neurons in vitro. *Brain Res*. 1989;476(1):154–159.
65. Fuller PM, Saper CB, Lu J. The pontine REM switch: past and present. *J Physiol (Lond)*. 2007;584(Pt 3):735–741.
66. Vanini G, et al. Gamma-aminobutyric acid-mediated neurotransmission in the pontine reticular formation modulates hypnosis, immobility, and breathing during isoflurane anesthesia. *Anesthesiology*. 2008;109(6):978–988.
67. Nelson AM, et al. Opioid-induced decreases in rat brain adenosine levels are reversed by inhibiting adenosine deaminase. *Anesthesiology*. 2009;111(6):1327–1333.
68. Coleman CG, Baghdoyan HA, Lydic R. Dialysis delivery of an adenosine A2A agonist into the pontine reticular formation of C57BL/6J mouse increases pontine acetylcholine release and sleep. *J Neurochem*. 2006;96(6):1750–1759.
69. Tanase D, Baghdoyan HA, Lydic R. Dialysis delivery of an adenosine A1 receptor agonist to the pontine reticular formation decreases acetylcholine release and increases anesthesia recovery time. *Anesthesiology*. 2003;98(4):912–920.
70. Watson CJ, et al. Pontine reticular formation (PnO) administration of hypocretin-1 increases PnO GABA levels and wakefulness. *Sleep*. 2008;31(4).453–464.
71. Datta S, Maclean RR. Neurobiological mechanisms for the regulation of mammalian sleep-wake behavior: reinterpretation of historical evidence and inclusion of contemporary cellular and molecular evidence. *Neurosci Biobehav Rev*. 2007;31(5):775–824.
72. John J, et al. Cataplexy-active neurons in the hypothalamus: implications for the role of histamine in sleep and waking behavior. *Neuron*. 2004;42(4):619–634.

73. Nelson LE, et al. The sedative component of anesthesia is mediated by GABA(A) receptors in an endogenous sleep pathway. *Nat Neurosci*. 2002;5(10):979–984.
74. Luo T, Leung LS. Basal forebrain histaminergic transmission modulates electroencephalographic activity and emergence from isoflurane anesthesia. *Anesthesiology*. 2009;111(4):725–733.
75. Zecharia AY, et al. The involvement of hypothalamic sleep pathways in general anesthesia: testing the hypothesis using the GABAA receptor {beta}3N265M knock-in mouse. *J Neurosci*. 2009;29(7): 2177–2187.
76. Mileykovskiy BY, Kiyashchenko LI, Siegel JM. Behavioral correlates of activity in identified hypocretin/orexin neurons. *Neuron*. 2005;46(5):787–798.
77. Lee MG, Hassani OK, Jones BE. Discharge of identified orexin/ hypocretin neurons across the sleep-waking cycle. *J Neurosci*. 2005;25(28):6716–6720.
78. Peyron C, et al. Neurons containing hypocretin (orexin) project to multiple neuronal systems. *J Neurosci*. 1998;18(23):9996–10015.
79. Ohno K, Sakurai T. Orexin neuronal circuitry: role in the regulation of sleep and wakefulness. *Front Neuroendocrinol*. 2008;29(1): 70–87.
80. Kelz MB, et al. An essential role for orexins in emergence from general anesthesia. *Proc Natl Acad Sci USA*. 2008;105(4): 1309–1314.
81. Yasuda Y, et al. Orexin a elicits arousal electroencephalography without sympathetic cardiovascular activation in isoflurane-anesthetized rats. *Anesth Analg*. 2003;97(6):1663–1666.
82. Jones BE. Activity, modulation and role of basal forebrain cholinergic neurons innervating the cerebral cortex. *Prog Brain Res*. 2004; 145:157–169.
83. Ma J, et al. The septohippocampal system participates in general anesthesia. *J Neurosci*. 2002;22(2):RC200.
84. Gerashchenko D, et al. Identification of a population of sleep-active cerebral cortex neurons. *Proc Natl Acad Sci USA*. 2008; 105(29):10227–10232.
85. Szymusiak R, et al. Sleep-waking discharge patterns of ventrolateral preoptic/anterior hypothalamic neurons in rats. *Brain Res*. 1998; 803(1–2):178–188.
86. Sherin JE, et al. Innervation of histaminergic tuberomammillary neurons by GABAergic and galaninergic neurons in the ventrolateral preoptic nucleus of the rat. *J Neurosci*. 1998;18(12): 4705–4721.
87. Sherin JE, et al. Activation of ventrolateral preoptic neurons during sleep. *Science*. 1996;271(5246):216–219.
88. Lu J, et al. Effect of lesions of the ventrolateral preoptic nucleus on NREM and REM sleep. *J Neurosci*. 2000;20(10):3830–3842.
89. Suntsova N, et al. Sleep-waking discharge patterns of median preoptic nucleus neurons in rats. *J Physiol (Lond)*. 2002; 543(Pt 2):665–677.
90. Szymusiak R, Gvilia I, McGinty D. Hypothalamic control of sleep. *Sleep Med*. 2007;8(4):291–301.
91. Manns ID, Alonso A, Jones BE. Discharge properties of juxtacellularly labeled and immunohistochemically identified cholinergic basal forebrain neurons recorded in association with the electroencephalogram in anesthetized rats. *J Neurosci*. 2000;20(4):1505–1518.
92. White NS, Alkire MT. Impaired thalamocortical connectivity in humans during general-anesthetic-induced unconsciousness. *Neuroimage*. 2003;19(2 Pt 1):402–411.
93. Velly L, et al. Differential dynamic of action on cortical and subcortical structures of anesthetic agents during induction of anesthesia. *Anesthesiology*. 200;107(2):202–212.
94. Massopust LC, Wolin LR, Albin MS. Electrophysiologic and behavioral responses to ketamine hydrochloride in the Rhesus monkey. *Anesth Analg*. 1972;51(3):329–341.
95. Sparks DL, et al. Further studies of the neural mechanisms of ketamine-induced anesthesia in the rhesus monkey. *Anesth Analg*. 1975;54(2):189–195.
96. Gottschalk A, Miotke SA. Volatile anesthetic action in a computational model of the thalamic reticular nucleus. *Anesthesiology*. 2009;110(5):996–1010.
97. Alkire MT, et al. Thalamic microinjection of nicotine reverses sevoflurane-induced loss of righting reflex in the rat. *Anesthesiology*. 2007;107(2):264–272.
98. Maquet P. Functional neuroimaging of normal human sleep by positron emission tomography. *J Sleep Res*. 2000;9(3):207–231.
99. Kaisti KK, et al. Effects of sevoflurane, propofol, and adjunct nitrous oxide on regional cerebral blood flow, oxygen consumption, and blood volume in humans. *Anesthesiology*. 2003;99(3): 603–613.
100. Kaisti KK, et al. Effects of surgical levels of propofol and sevoflurane anesthesia on cerebral blood flow in healthy subjects studied with positron emission tomography. *Anesthesiology*. 2002;96(6): 1358–1370.
101. Imas OA, et al. Volatile anesthetics disrupt frontal-posterior recurrent information transfer at gamma frequencies in rat. *Neurosci Lett*. 2005;387(3):145–150.
102. Lee U, et al. The directionality and functional organization of frontoparietal connectivity during consciousness and anesthesia in humans. *Conscious Cogn*. 2009;18(4):1069–1078.
103. Hudetz AG. Feedback suppression in anesthesia: is it reversible? *Conscious Cogn*. 2009;18(4):1079–1081.
104. Veselis RA, et al. Thiopental and propofol affect different regions of the brain at similar pharmacologic effects. *Anesth Analg*. 2004;99(2):399–408.
105. Markowitsch HJ, Kessler J. Massive impairment in executive functions with partial preservation of other cognitive functions: the case of a young patient with severe degeneration of the prefrontal cortex. *Exp Brain Res*. 2000;133(1):94–102.
106. Judge O, Hill S, Antognini JF. Modeling the effects of midazolam on cortical and thalamic neurons. *Neurosci Lett*. 2009;464(2): 135–139.
107. Talavera JA, et al. Modeling the GABAergic action of etomidate on the thalamocortical system. *Anesth Analg*. 2009;108(1): 160–167.
108. Antkowiak B. Different actions of general anesthetics on the firing patterns of neocortical neurons mediated by the GABA(A) receptor. *Anesthesiology*. 1999;91(2):500–511.
109. Ferrarelli F, et al. Breakdown in cortical effective connectivity during midazolam-induced loss of consciousness. *Proc Natl Acad Sci USA*. 2010;107(6):2681–2686.
110. Rampil IJ, Mason P, Singh H. Anesthetic potency (MAC) is independent of forebrain structures in the rat. *Anesthesiology*. 1993;78(4):707–712.
111. Antognini JF, Schwartz K. Exaggerated anesthetic requirements in the preferentially anesthetized brain. *Anesthesiology*. 1993;79(6): 1244–1249.
112. Antognini JF, Carstens E, Atherley R. Does the immobilizing effect of thiopental in brain exceed that of halothane? *Anesthesiology*. 2002;96(4):980–986.
113. Stabernack C, et al. Thiopental produces immobility primarily by supraspinal actions in rats. *Anesth Analg*. 2005;100(1):128–136.
114. Devor M, Zalkind V. Reversible analgesia, atonia, and loss of consciousness on bilateral intracerebral microinjection of pentobarbital. *Pain*. 2001;94(1):101–112.
115. Reiner K, Sukhotinsky I, Devor M. Mesopontine tegmental anesthesia area projects independently to the rostromedial medulla and to the spinal cord. *Neuroscience*. 2007;146(3):1355–1370.
116. Reiner K, Sukhotinsky I, Devor M. Bulbospinal neurons implicated in mesopontine-induced anesthesia are substantially collateralized. *J Comp Neurol*. 2008;508(3):418–436.

2

CELLULAR AND MOLECULAR EFFECTS OF GENERAL ANESTHETICS IN THE BRAIN

Robert P. Bonin and Beverley A. Orser

INTRODUCTION

Each year, more than 234 million surgical operations are performed worldwide.[1] The introduction of safe general anesthesia has dramatically relieved human suffering and laid the foundation for the modern surgical era. Most major advances in anesthetic care have evolved from an understanding of *what* anesthetics do, rather than *how* they work. The challenge remains to identify the receptors and neuronal networks that are necessary and sufficient to produce general anesthesia. Such mechanistic insights are important because the expectation remains that identification of specific targets will promote the development of new anesthetics and will allow optimization in the use of currently available drugs.

Why, after centuries of use, do the mechanisms of anesthesia continue to perplex scientists? Major obstacles to understanding the neuronal substrates of anesthetic actions include the structural diversity of anesthetic compounds, the low potency of some classes of drugs, and a lack of specific antagonists. Anesthetic molecules range in structural complexity from single elements, such as xenon, to complex organic compounds, such as halogenated hydrocarbons and neurosteroids. The anesthetic state itself is highly complex, with multiple components that include memory blockade, loss of consciousness, analgesia, and immobility.[2] Finally, the biology of the cognitive processes that are modulated by anesthetics remains poorly defined. In this regard, anesthetics have proven to be powerful tools for dissecting the molecular substrates of learning, memory, and consciousness.

Despite the complexity of the anesthetic state, increasing evidence suggests that the desirable therapeutic actions of anesthetics are due to a limited number of molecular targets. Moreover, anesthetics appear to target receptors that are expressed in the endogenous pathways that usually regulate memory and consciousness. For example, memory blockade results from interactions of the anesthetic with drug receptors in the memory circuits of the hippocampus and cortex,[3–5] and loss of consciousness results from anesthetic actions in the neuronal networks that regulate sleep and wakefulness.[6–7] In this chapter, we will first review the major discoveries that led to the contemporary protein-based theory of anesthesia. Then, we will describe the receptors in the mammalian central nervous system that likely contribute to the major therapeutic properties of anesthetics.

EVOLUTION OF ANESTHETIC THEORY

Meyer and Overton proposed the first widely accepted theory of anesthesia in 1899. These two investigators independently and simultaneously described the striking correlation between the potency of an anesthetic and its solubility in olive oil.[8–9] The observation that most anesthetics are lipophilic and highly hydrophobic led to the hypothesis that these agents act via a common mechanism to perturb the lipid cell membrane of neurons.

Over the past 60 years, however, a surge of experimental evidence has strongly implicated membrane proteins, rather than the lipid bilayer, as primary sites of anesthetic action. According to the protein model, there are no single, universal targets for anesthetics, but rather drug interactions that are limited to a number of specific receptors. In 1984, Franks and Lieb showed that a variety of anesthetics inhibit the function of a soluble protein. Specifically, the luminescence of a firefly enzyme, luciferase, was reduced by the application of a variety of anesthetics and the potency of inhibition was correlated with the lipid solubility of the anesthetic.[10] Other studies showed that stereoisomers of isoflurane differ in their anesthetic potency, an observation that had not been predicted from lipid-based models of anesthesia.[11–12] Furthermore, it was observed that some compounds that were predicted on the basis of their chemical structure and lipid solubility to cause immobility did not inhibit motor reflexes ("nonimmobilizers").[13–14] Finally, long-chain alcohols lose their anesthetic potency above a certain critical chain length, which suggests that anesthetics interact with specific binding sites within proteins.[15–16] These findings, along with a growing understanding of the role of synapse and neurotransmitter receptors, fueled the search for specific molecular targets.

Certain criteria have been proposed to identify sites that are relevant to the clinical effects of anesthetics.[17]

For example, at clinically relevant concentrations, the function of the proposed target must be reversibly altered by anesthetics. In addition, the proposed target must be expressed in appropriate anatomic locations to mediate a relevant behavioral effect of the anesthetic. Any stereoselective behavioral actions of the anesthetic must be mirrored by the in vitro stereoselective effects of the drugs at the proposed target. Also, the proposed target must be insensitive to the effects of "nonimmobilizers." According to these criteria, there is strong evidence for the involvement of only a few targets in mediating the actions of anesthetics.[17–18]

Key receptors reviewed in this chapter include the γ-aminobutyric acid subtype A ($GABA_A$ receptor), the glycine receptors, the glutamate receptors (particularly the N-methyl-D-asparate [NMDA] subtype receptor), several families of potassium channels including hyperpolarization-activated, cyclic nucleotide-gated (HCN) "pacemaker" channels and two-pore "leak" channels, and voltage-gated sodium channels. These molecular targets and other less well characterized molecular targets are summarized in Table 2.1.

$GABA_A$ RECEPTORS

$GABA_A$ receptors are the major inhibitory receptors in the mammalian brain. These ubiquitous receptors are expressed in nearly one-third of all synapses, where they generate fast synaptic inhibition.[19] Each $GABA_A$ receptor is a pentameric complex containing an integral anion channel that is permeable to chloride and, to a lesser extent, bicarbonate ions.[20–21] Binding of GABA to the receptor causes a conformational change, which leads to channel opening and a flux of anions across the cell membrane. In most mature neurons, an increase in permeability to anions generally causes membrane hyperpolarization and a reduction in the effectiveness of an excitatory input in evoking an action potential. Anesthetics that target $GABA_A$ receptors include barbiturates, etomidate, propofol, inhaled anesthetics, and neurosteroids, as well as the sedative and hypnotic benzodiazepines.[4,22–24] These drugs typically bind at different sites to allosterically facilitate channel opening.

STRUCTURE

The $GABA_A$ receptor itself is a heteromeric structure composed of multiple subunits. At least 19 mammalian genes encode for the various subunits (α_{1-6}, β_{1-3}, γ_{1-3}, δ, ε, θ, π, and ρ_{1-3}).[25–26] The subunit composition of a $GABA_A$ receptor determines its cellular expression pattern and its biophysical and pharmacological properties. Typically, the $GABA_A$ receptor is a combination of α, β, and γ subunits in a ratio of 2:2:1; however, in some brain regions, the γ subunit may be absent or may be replaced by a δ, θ, π, or ε subunit.[27–29] Some $GABA_A$ receptor subtypes are widely expressed, including those containing the γ subunit and δ subunit. The γ subunit–containing receptors are typically clustered in the postsynaptic membrane of the inhibitory synapses.[30] In contrast, $GABA_A$ receptors containing the δ subunit are expressed predominantly outside of the synapse.[31] One major exception to this pattern is the $\alpha_5\beta_3\gamma_2$ receptor, which is located predominantly outside the synapse in the hippocampus and olfactory bulb.[32–34]

It has become apparent that the subunit composition of the $GABA_A$ receptors strongly determines their sensitivity to inhaled and intravenous anesthetics.[4,35–36] Many recent studies have been aimed at determining which $GABA_A$ receptor subtypes underlie the different behavioral endpoints of the anesthetic state.

SYNAPTIC AND TONIC INHIBITION

$GABA_A$ receptors generate two distinct forms of inhibition: synaptic and tonic (Figure 2.1). As summarized below, recent studies have shown that tonic inhibition is particularly vulnerable to clinically relevant concentrations of anesthetics. Furthermore, $GABA_A$ receptors that generate a tonic conductance are frequently expressed in the information-processing regions of the brain.

The release of GABA into the synapse generates fast, transient inhibitory postsynaptic currents. $GABA_A$ receptors clustered at postsynaptic terminals are briefly activated by very high, near-saturating concentrations of GABA.[37] At the level of the neuronal networks, this form of synaptic or "phasic" inhibition is thought to be critical for high-fidelity neuronal communication, the precise timing of action potentials, and the synchronization of neuronal rhythms.[38–39] For many years, enhancement of synaptic inhibition was thought to be the primary mechanism underlying the activity of most anesthetics. Indeed, many anesthetics, including etomidate, pentobarbital, propofol, and isoflurane, slow the rate of decay of synaptic currents, thereby increasing GABAergic inhibition.[23,36]

More recently, a persistent form of tonic inhibition has been identified, which is putatively generated by high-affinity, slowly desensitizing $GABA_A$ receptors located mainly outside the synapse.[29] This low concentration of GABA may arise from nonvesicular sources, such as the reverse operation of GABA transporters,[40–41] or from the spillover of GABA from GABAergic synapses.[42–44] Tonic GABAergic inhibition is present in a cell-type and regionally specific manner, and is found throughout the mammalian brain,[45] particularly in cerebellar granule cells,[46–47] the hippocampus,[48–50] thalamocortical relay neurons of the ventral basal complex,[51–54] and neocortex.[55–56]

A tonic inhibition has been described in several major cell types of the hippocampus, including the principal excitatory neurons (pyramidal neurons)[57–60] and the inhibitory interneurons[50,61] in the CA1 region, and the granule cells in the dentate gyrus.[49] Anesthetics such as isoflurane, etomidate, neurosteroids, and propofol have been shown to

Table 2.1 THE NEURONAL, PHYSIOLOGICAL AND PHARMACOLOGICAL ROLES OF PUTATIVE ANESTHETIC TARGETS IN THE CENTRAL NERVOUS SYSTEM

MOLECULAR TARGET	CELLULAR FUNCTION	BEHAVIOR AND PHARMACOLOGY
	Ligand–Gated Ion Channels	
$GABA_A$ receptors	Increase Cl^- permeability	Enhanced activity associated with anxiolysis, sedation, and amnesia
	Hyperpolarize membrane	
	Inhibit neuronal excitability	Important role in epilepsy
Glycine receptors	Increase Cl^- permeability	Inhibitory receptor in the spinal cord
	Hyperpolarize membrane	Modulates spinal reflexes and startle response
	Inhibit neuronal excitability	
Glutamate receptors (NMDA subtype)	Fast excitatory neurotransmission	Important receptor in perception, learning and memory.
	Increase permeability to Na^+, K^+, and Ca^{2+}	
	Synaptic plasticity	
Neuronal nicotinic acetylcholine receptors	Increase permeability to sodium, potassium, and calcium	Regulates arousal, memory, nociception, and autonomic function
	Modulates neurotransmitter release	
Serotonin receptors	Increase cation conductance (5-HTR_3)	Regulates neuronal excitation and emesis
	Increase K^+ conductance (5-HTR_2)	
	Other Ion Channels	
Two-pore-domain K^+ channels	Increase K^+ permeability	Regulates neuronal excitability
	Can be activated by pH, chemical, or mechanical stimulation	Chemosensation
ATP-activated K^+ channels	Activated by metabolic activity	Neuroprotection, insulin secretion
Hyperpolarization-activated cyclic-nucleotide gated channels	Activates nonspecific cation current during membrane hyperpolarization	Regulates resting membrane potential
		Modulates dendritic function, neuronal oscillation, and action potential bursting
Voltage activated K^+ channels	Regulation of resting membrane potential and recovery from action potential	Essential for nerve transmission

(Continued)

Table 2.1 (CONTINUED)

MOLECULAR TARGET	CELLULAR FUNCTION	BEHAVIOR AND PHARMACOLOGY
Voltage activated Na^+ channels	**Initiate action potentials**	**Essential for nerve transmission and neurotransmitter release**
Voltage-gated Ca^{2+} channels	**Increase permeability to Ca^{2+} during depolarization** **Neurotransmitter release**	**Essential for neurotransmitter release Regulates nociception**

Reprinted from Mashour GA, Forman SA, Campagna JA. Mechanisms of general anesthesia: from molecules to mind. *Best Pract Res Clin Anaesthesiol.* 2005;19(3):349–364, with permission from Elsevier.

enhance the tonic conductance. Furthermore, the effects of propofol, midazolam,[48] etomidate,[62] and gaboxadol[52] on tonic current compared to synaptic current consistently showed several-fold greater enhancement of the tonic conductance.

Preferential enhancement of the tonic current relative to the synaptic current probably results from two important factors. Anesthetics typically increase the affinity of the $GABA_A$ receptor for GABA, which results in an increase in the GABA current evoked by low concentrations of GABA.[63] Extrasynaptic receptors are exposed to low concentrations of GABA that are typically present in the extrasynaptic space.[44,64–65] Because the extrasynaptic concentration of GABA does not fully saturate the extrasynaptic population of $GABA_A$ receptors, an increase in agonist affinity by anesthetics can greatly increase GABAergic current. This situation contrasts with that of postsynaptic $GABA_A$ receptors, which are activated by near-saturating concentrations of GABA.[37,66] In this case, increasing the receptor affinity for GABA does not appreciably increase GABA current as the receptors are saturated or near saturation. Second, extrasynaptic receptors desensitize to a lesser extent than their synaptic counterparts.[48,67–69] This means that the extrasynaptic $GABA_A$ receptors, which are continuously activated by ambient GABA, would remain open longer than synaptic receptors. When considered over time,

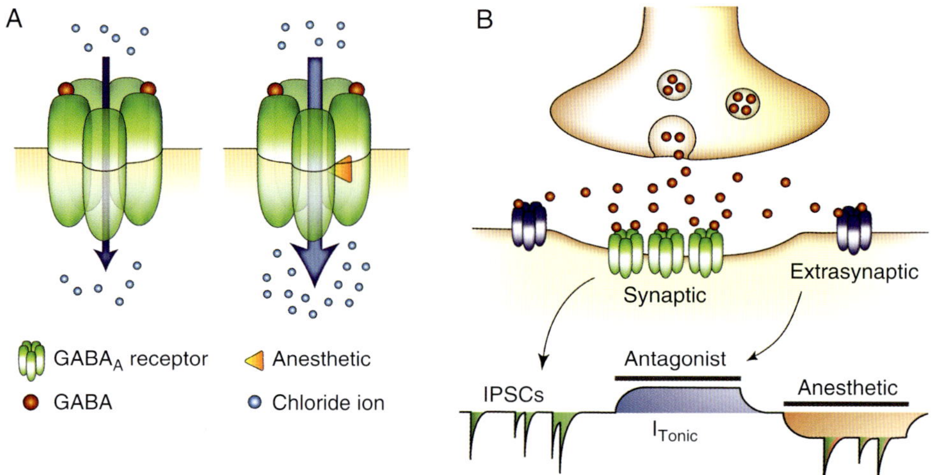

Figure 2.1 Effect of anesthetics on inhibitory neurotransmission in the brain. A) When γ-aminobutryic acid (GABA) binds to the $GABA_A$ receptor it causes a conformational change that opens the channel pore and allows the flux of Cl- ions across the cell membrane. Many general anesthetics, neuroactive steroids, and benzodiazepines increase the potency of GABA at the $GABA_A$ receptor level and thereby increase Cl- flux. B) Action potential–dependent release of GABA into the synaptic cleft transiently activates $GABA_A$ receptors in the postsynaptic membrane. This generates inhibitory postsynaptic currents, which are typically of a brief duration due to GABA diffusion and uptake, and the desensitization of synaptic receptors. Extrasynaptic $GABA_A$ receptors are activated by low concentrations of GABA in the extracellular space arising from synaptic spillover or other nonsynaptic release mechanisms. These receptors have low desensitization rates and can produce a continuous or "tonic" current. The tonic current is revealed by application of a $GABA_A$ antagonist, which inhibits the current. Many anesthetics potently enhance the tonic current at clinically relevant concentrations. © Orser BA, Mazer CD, Baker AJ. Awareness during anesthesia. *CMAJ.* 2008;178(2):185–188. This work is protected by copyright and the making of this copy was with the permission of Access Copyright. Any alteration of its content or further copying in any form whatsoever is strictly prohibited unless otherwise permitted by law.

the net increase in tonic current caused by anesthetics is often larger than the synaptic current, which leaves the extrasynaptic $GABA_A$ receptors with far greater influence over neuronal excitability than the synaptic receptors.[52,57,62,70]

ANESTHETIC BINDING POCKET

The $GABA_A$ receptor contains binding sites for neuroactive steroids, benzodiazepines, and intravenous and volatile anesthetics[4,22,35–36] (Figure 2.2). The binding site for etomidate and volatile anesthetics was first isolated to a domain 45 amino acids in length within the $GABA_A$ receptor subunit in transmembrane domains 2 and 3 in the α and β subunits. The identity of key residues was later refined to Ser-270 in the α_1 subunit for the binding of volatile anesthetics,[71] and Asn-289 in the β_3 subunit for etomidate binding.[72] Recently, a photoreactive, radiolabeled analog of etomidate, [(3)H]azietomidate has been used to directly label amino acids of the $GABA_A$ receptor that are in proximity to the etomidate binding site.[73–74] In these studies, two amino acids, the Met-236 in α_1 and Met-286 in the β subunit were labeled by azietomidate. This suggests that an anesthetic binding pocket is located at the transmembrane interface between α and β subunits in the $GABA_A$ receptor.

MEMORY BLOCKADE

Memory blockade or amnesia is arguably the most important effect of any anesthetic. The molecular basis of memory blockade is of clinical interest because some patients experience explicit recall of events that occurred during general anesthesia,[75] whereas others, particularly

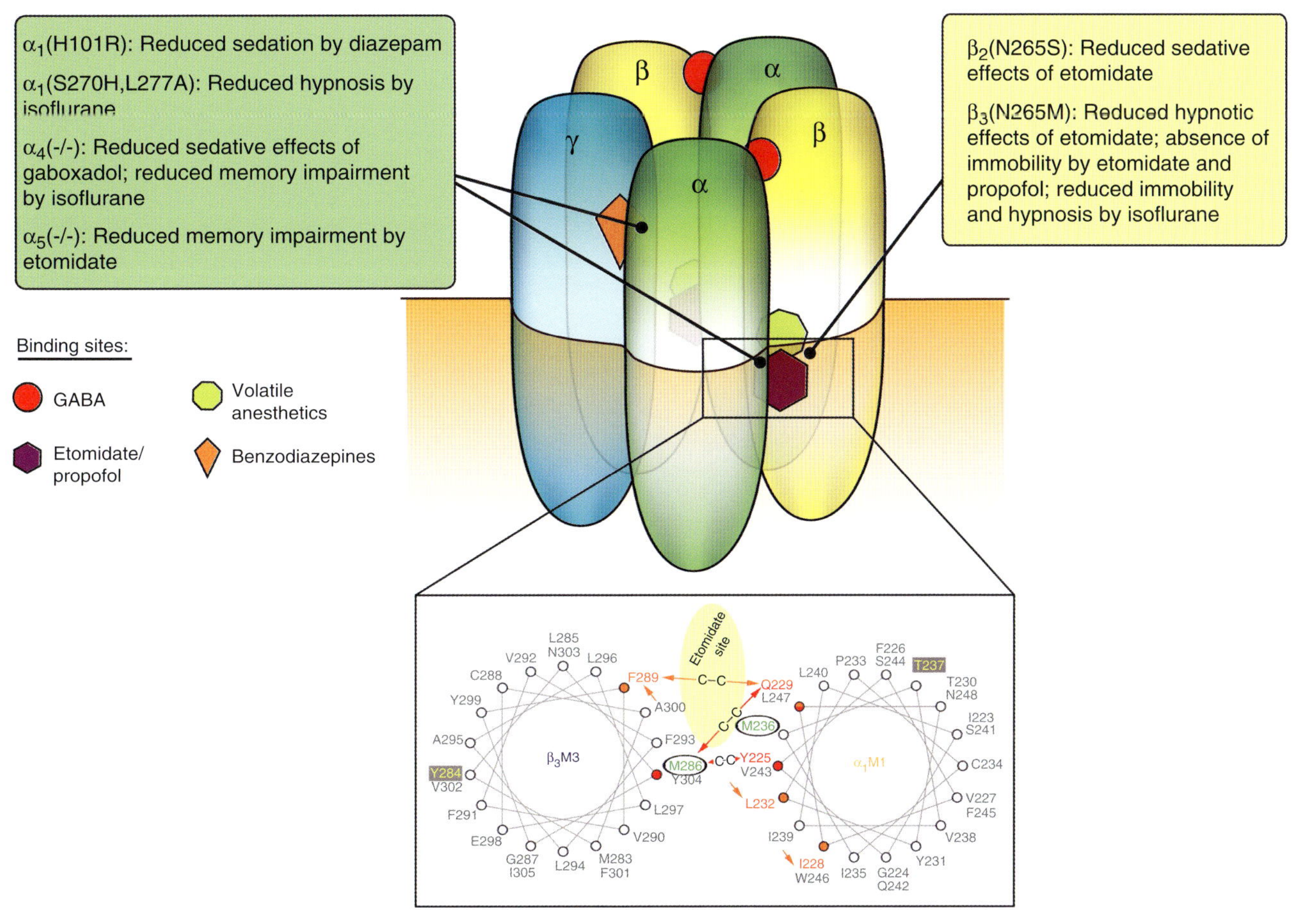

Figure 2.2 Anesthetic binding sites on the $GABA_A$ receptor. The $GABA_A$ receptor is a site of action for many general anesthetics and neurodepressive drugs. The approximate binding sites for several anesthetics on the $GABA_A$ receptor are indicated in the cartoon. The subunit composition of the $GABA_A$ receptor isoforms produces receptors with unique biophysical and pharmacological properties. Anesthetic action at select receptor isoforms may selectively produce several of the behavioral endpoints associated with the anesthetic state, such as amnesia or hypnosis. The evidence for this is largely provided through the study of mutant $GABA_A$ receptors that are insensitive to anesthetics or through the genetic deletion of specific $GABA_A$ receptor subunits. The mutations can reduce or eliminate some behavioral effects of anesthetics and the effects of these genetic manipulations on anesthetic action are indicated in the boxes. See text for further details. Inset: Etomidate is proposed to interact with a common anesthetic binding pocket at the interface of the $GABA_A$ receptor α and β subunits. Reprinted with permission from Li GD, Chiara DC, Cohen JB, Olsen RW. Neurosteroids allosterically modulate binding of the anesthetic etomidate to gamma-aminobutyric acid type A receptors. *J Biol Chem.* 2009;284(18):11771–11775. © 2009 The American Society for Biochemistry and Molecular Biology.

the elderly, experience persistent postoperative memory deficits.[76–77] In addition, memory blockade is one of the most potent effects of an anesthetic and occurs at low doses.[2] Studies have identified a $GABA_A$ receptor subtype in the hippocampus that is particularly sensitive to low concentrations of most intravenous anesthetics.

In hippocampal pyramidal neurons, the tonic inhibitory conductance is generated primarily by $GABA_A$ receptors containing the α_5 subunit (α_5GABA_A) receptors. The α_5 receptor subunit is of particular interest for the study of anesthetic-induced memory impairment as this subunit is expressed predominantly in the hippocampus, where it is incorporated into about 20% of all $GABA_A$ receptors.[34]

Several lines of evidence have implicated the α_5GABA_A receptor in learning and memory processes. Inverse agonists that selectively inhibit the activity of α_5GABA_A receptors improve performance in animal tests of memory function[78–79] and improve word recall in humans with ethanol-induced memory impairment.[80] Thus, the activity of these receptors appears to constrain memory performance. In support of this, genetic deletion of the α_5GABA_A receptor subunit in mice improves hippocampal-dependent learning relative to normal littermates.[81] The expression of the α_5 subunit was also reduced in mice expressing a point mutation of the α_5 subunit (His105Arg).[82] These α_5His105Arg mice also had enhanced memory performance for trace fear conditioning, which supports a role for these receptors in memory function.

In vitro studies have shown that α_5GABA_A receptors are highly sensitive to anesthetics. The tonic conductance generated by α_5GABA_A receptors in hippocampal pyramidal neurons is enhanced by low concentrations of several anesthetics, including propofol,[83] isoflurane,[84] and etomidate.[62] The increase in tonic inhibitory conductance can strongly influence a form of neuronal memory called long-term potentiation. Long-term potentiation is an increase in the amplitude of excitatory neurotransmission, which in the hippocampus is widely considered to be a molecular substrate for memory. In particular, long-term plasticity was reduced by etomidate in hippocampal slices from wild-type but not null mutant mice lacking the $\alpha5$ subunit (α_5−/−).[62,85] The above findings correlate with behavioral studies showing that a low, clinically relevant dose of etomidate impaired the performance of wild-type but not α_5−/−mice for hippocampal-dependent learning and memory tasks.[62,85] However, a low dose of etomidate produced similar impairment of motor coordination, loss of righting reflex, and anxiolysis in the two genotypes. Together, these results strongly support the suggestion that α_5GABA_A receptors are involved in the memory-impairing effects of general anesthetics but may not be involved in their sedative or hypnotic effects. These results also demonstrate that the amnestic effects of anesthetics can be dissociated from behavioral components of the anesthetic state, which supports the current hypothesis that general anesthesia results from the activity of anesthetics at several specific molecular targets.

The α_4 subunit is implicated in the amnestic effects of volatile anesthetics. The potency of isoflurane to inhibit fear memory was reduced in both male and female mice lacking the α_4 subunit.[86] However, the hypnotic and immobilizing effects of isoflurane were not changed in the $\alpha4$ knockout mice.[86]

SEDATION

Sedation is a decreased level of arousal in humans, as indicated by longer response times, decreased motor activity, and slurred speech. These behaviors are harder to characterize in animals, and surrogate measures of sedation include a reduction in motor activity and decreased arousal.[2] The identity of the $GABA_AR$ subtypes that contribute to the sedative actions of several intravenous drugs was revealed through a series of elegant studies using genetically modified knockin mouse models. In those models, the substitution of a single amino acid in a particular $GABA_A$ receptor subunit rendered the $GABA_A$ receptor subtype insensitive to certain anesthetics, as typically evidenced by in vitro electrophysiological studies. Behavioral assays were then used to determine whether anesthetic actions at $GABA_A$ receptors containing the modified subunit contributed to the various behavioral effects. For example, replacement of the asparagine residue at position 265 in the β_2 or β_3 $GABA_A$ receptor subunit with serine or methionine, respectively, rendered $GABA_A$ receptors containing these subunits relatively insensitive to etomidate or propofol.[87–88] A low dose of etomidate that impairs the motor performance of wild-type mice on the rotating rod apparatus along with their spontaneous locomotor activity did not impair the function mutant β_2(Asn265Ser) mice.[87]

Similarly, the α_1 subunit has been implicated in mediating the sedative properties of benzodiazepines, including diazepam. $GABA_A$ receptors that contain a mutation of histidine to arginine at position 101 of the α_1 subunit were less sensitive to positive allosteric enhancement by diazepam in vitro.[89] Behavioral studies showed that the sedative properties of diazepam were eliminated in knockin mice that expressed the α_1(His101Arg) mutation.[89]

The thalamus is critically involved in sleep and waking processes.[90] A subpopulation of $GABA_A$ receptors in this brain region is implicated in the sedative actions of gaboxadol. Although gaboxadol is not commonly used as an anesthetic,[91] it promotes slow wave sleep and produces the analgesic, sedative, and hypnotic ataxic effects that are similarly induced by other anesthetics.[91–92] $GABA_A$ receptors that generate a tonic current in neurons of the thalamic ventrobasal complex may contribute to the sedative action of gaboxadol. The tonic current is generated by $GABA_A$ receptors containing both α_4 and δ subunits in the ventrobasal neurons.[93] At low concentrations, gaboxadol strongly activated these $GABA_A$ receptors.[94] Accordingly, gaboxadol enhanced the tonic but not the phasic current in ventrobasal neurons.[87] Behavioral studies showed that motor performance in the rotarod task and spontaneous locomotor activity were impaired by gaboxadol in wild-type but not α_4 subunit knockout mice,[93] which suggests that $\alpha_4\delta$ subunit-containing $GABA_A$ receptors are necessary for the sedative and ataxic effects of gaboxadol.

HYPNOSIS

Hypnosis refers to a loss of consciousness. In animal studies, loss of the righting reflex is used as an indicator of the hypnotic state.[95] The induction of hypnosis typically requires higher doses of anesthetic than those that produce sedation.[95] Both β_2 and β_3 subunit-containing $GABA_A$ receptors contribute to hypnosis, as the loss of righting reflex caused by etomidate was of reduced duration but was not absent in β_2(Asn265Ser) mice.[87] Also, the duration of impairment of the righting reflex by etomidate or propofol was reduced in β_3(Asn265Met) mice relative to wild-type mice.[88] Interestingly, the electroencephalographic patterns observed during etomidate anesthesia were similar for β_2(Asn265Ser) and wild-type mice, which suggests that $GABA_A$ receptors containing the β_2 subunit do not entirely contribute to the loss of consciousness associated with loss of the righting reflex.[87]

The $\delta GABA_A$ receptor subunit has also been implicated in hypnosis. Neuroactive steroids including allopregnanalone, pregnanalone, and tetrahydrodeoxycorticosterone preferentially enhance the activity of $GABA_A$ receptors containing the δ subunit.[94,96] The synthetic neuroactive steroid alphaxalone and the endogenous steroid pregnanalone prevented the loss-of-righting reflex for shorter durations in mice lacking the δ subunit.[97] However, midazolam, etomidate, propofol, ketamine, and halothane all produced comparable loss-of-righting reflex in mice lacking the δ subunit compared to controls,[97] demonstrating that several $GABA_AR$ isoforms contribute to anesthetic-induced hypnosis.

IMMOBILITY

A lack of response to noxious stimuli is a defining characteristic of anesthesia. Indeed, the potency of volatile anesthetics is quantified through the concept of minimal alveolar concentration (MAC),[98] which is related to the partial pressure of a volatile anesthetic that is required to prevent movement during a painful surgical stimulus in 50% of patients. In animal studies, immobilization by anesthetics is indicated by the suppression of the withdrawal reflex to a noxious stimulus. The immobilizing properties of anesthetics predominantly arise from anesthetic effects at spinal sites of action.[18,95] The relative importance of spinal and brain sites of action in the immobilizing effects of anesthetics have been explored through the use of a goat model that allows volatile anesthetics to be selectively delivered to the brain or torso.[99–101] In this goat model, the delivery of isoflurane to the torso was much more effective at inhibiting movement to noxious stimuli than brain delivery,[101–102] suggesting that volatile anesthetics act at molecular targets in the spinal cord to produce immobility. Additional studies in rats have provided further evidence for the contribution of spinal targets to anesthetic immobility.[103–105] Although this chapter focuses on anesthetic targets in the brain, we will provide an overview of the contribution of $GABA_A$ receptors to this anesthetic endpoint.

The immobilizing effect of anesthetics parallels their hypnotic effect, yet these two phenomena are likely mediated by distinct molecular targets. For example, the immobilizing effect of etomidate was similar between β_2(Asn265Ser) and wild-type mice,[87] whereas the immobilizing effects on wild-type mice of both propofol and etomidate were absent in β_3(Asn265Met) mice.[88,106] These results contrast with the combined contribution of β_2 and β_3 subunit-containing $GABA_A$ receptors to hypnosis and suggest that $GABA_A$ receptors containing the β_3 subunit are predominantly responsible for immobilization by etomidate and propofol.

VOLATILE ANESTHETICS

It is worth noting that determining the molecular sites of action of volatile anesthetics is generally more challenging than studying intravenous anesthetics. First, volatile anesthetics have lower potency and influence a variety of receptors at clinically relevant concentrations,[2] and second, behavioral testing for a variety of endpoints with volatile anesthetics is technically more difficult. Nonetheless, several carefully designed studies have shown that volatile anesthetics modify $GABA_A$ receptor subtypes to produce some behavioral anesthetic endpoints.

A discrete anesthetic-binding cavity for volatile anesthetics involving the α_1 subunit of the $GABA_A$ receptor has been identified in studies using site-directed mutagenesis.[107–109] Two amino acids in the α_1 subunit are critical for potentiating the actions of volatile anesthetics: serine 270 and alanine 291.[109] The substitution of large amino acid residues at Ser270 reduced the sensitivity of $GABA_A$ receptors to volatile anesthetics,[71,108] whereas substitution with smaller-volume amino acids had the opposite effect.[108] Moreover, replacing the α_1 Ser270 residue with histidine eliminated the sensitivity of $GABA_A$ receptors to isoflurane.[108] The α_1(Ser270His) mutation also increased the potency of GABA at the $GABA_A$ receptor, which complicates interpretation of the results.[110] However, this change in potency was reversed by replacing the leucine residue at position 277 in the α_1 subunit with alanine.[111] The combination of these two mutations in a double knockin mouse, α_1(Ser270His, Leu277Ala) laid the foundation for studying the contribution of $\alpha_1 GABA_A$ receptors to isoflurane anesthesia.

Isoflurane caused less impairment of the righting reflex of double-mutant α_1(Ser270His, Leu277Ala) mice compared with wild-type mice.[112] This observation suggests that the hypnotic actions of isoflurane are dependent on the α_1 subunit. In contrast, the immobilizing and memory-blocking effects of isoflurane were similar in the double knockin and wild-type mice, which suggested that α_1 subunit-containing $GABA_A$ receptors do not contribute to these endpoints in isoflurane anesthesia. Interestingly, the memory-blocking effects of isoflurane were impaired in mice in which the α_1 subunit had been knocked out either globally or in the forebrain.[113]

The β subunit of the $GABA_A$ receptors also contributes to the binding site for volatile anesthetics and the behavioral effects of these agents.[109,114] The potentiation of GABA current by enflurane was reduced by substituting the asparagine residue at position 265 on the β_3 subunit with methionine.[114] Additionally, isoflurane is slightly less potent at inhibiting the righting reflex in mice that express the β_3(Asn265Met) knockin mutation,[115] which suggests that the β_3 subunit plays a small role in isoflurane hypnosis. However, the immobilizing effects of isoflurane are greatly reduced in the knockin mice.[115–116] Of interest, cardiovascular depression by isoflurane was also blunted in β_3(Asn265Met) mice.[106]

Together, these results suggest that distinct subpopulations of $GABA_A$ receptors contribute to the anesthetic actions of volatile anesthetics. However, it is clear that $GABA_A$ receptors are not the sole molecular target of volatile anesthetics. The actions of these drugs involve a wider array of molecular targets, including voltage-gated ion channels and excitatory neurotransmitter receptors.

GLUTAMATE RECEPTORS

There is strong evidence that the inhibition of excitatory neurotransmitter receptors contributes to the neurodepressive effects of anesthetics.[23–24,36] Glutamate is the major excitatory neurotransmitter in the mammalian brain. It activates two broad subclasses of ion-permeable receptors: the *N*-methyl-D-aspartate (NMDA) receptors and the non-NMDA receptors, which are further subdivided into α-amino-3-hydroxy-5-methyl-4-isoxazole propionic acid (AMPA) and kainate receptors.[117–118]

The AMPA and kainate receptors are permeable to Na^+ and K^+, have rapid kinetics, and mediate the fast component of excitatory postsynaptic potentials.[118] These two types of receptor are largely insensitive to anesthetics[119–121] and are not considered further here. In contrast, the NMDA receptors are permeable to Na^+, K^+, and Ca^{2+} and mediate the slow component of excitatory postsynaptic potentials.[118] The kinetic regulation of the NMDA receptors is complex. Their activation requires binding of both glutamate and either glycine or D-serine.[122–123] NMDA receptors do not conduct ionic current at hyperpolarized or resting membrane potentials because, under these conditions, the ion pore of these channels is blocked by a Mg^{2+} ion.[124] Depolarization of the membrane, which can be achieved through activation of non-NMDA receptors, relieves the Mg^{2+} block and allows ion flux through the NMDA receptor. Thus, NMDA receptors conduct Ca^{2+} in response to simultaneous pre- and postsynaptic glutamatergic activity, which allows them to function as "coincidence detectors."[117] NMDA receptors are heteromeric complexes comprised of three subtypes of subunits: GluN1, GluN2, and GluN3. There are eight different GluN1 subunits generated by alternative gene splicing, four different GluN2 subunits (A, B, C and D), and two GluN3 subunits (A and B)[118,125] (Figure 2.2). Functional NMDA receptors are formed from a combination of obligatory GluN1 subunits with GluN2 and/or GluN3 subunits.[118] As is the case for the $GABA_A$ receptors, the subunit composition of NMDA receptors determines their subcellular distribution, as well as their pharmacological and kinetic properties, and varies with cell type.[117]

KETAMINE

The NMDA receptors are targets of several general anesthetics, including ketamine, xenon, and nitrous oxide. Ketamine is a widely used NMDA receptor antagonist and dissociative anesthetic. In addition to loss of consciousness, ketamine produces a number of effects in humans, including profound amnesia, analgesia, and hallucinations.[126–127] Ketamine is a noncompetitive inhibitor of NMDA receptors and acts by either blocking the channel pore or by stabilizing a closed nonconducting state of the receptor.[128–129] The anesthetic potency of ketamine stereoisomers in behavioral studies parallels the stereoselective inhibition of the NMDA receptor by ketamine,[130] which implies that this receptor is likely a key mediator of ketamine anesthesia. However, the hypnotic effects of ketamine may also involve the inhibition of voltage-gated ion channels,[131] or $GABA_A$ receptors containing the α_6 and δ subunits.[132]

INHALED ANESTHETICS

The NMDA receptors are also sensitive to the inhaled anesthetics xenon and nitrous oxide. Both of these compounds potently inhibit the activity of NMDA receptors.[119,133–138] Since these gases have little or no effect on the $GABA_A$ receptors, it is likely that their anesthetic effects are mediated through actions on the NMDA receptor. Both xenon and isoflurane can compete with the co-agonist glycine at the NMDA receptor, which reduces receptor activation.[133] The ability of xenon to inhibit the function of the NMDA receptors appears to be nonselective to the subunit composition of the receptor, and this drug produces similar inhibition of GluN2A and GluN2B subunit-containing NMDA receptors.[139–140] It has been predicted

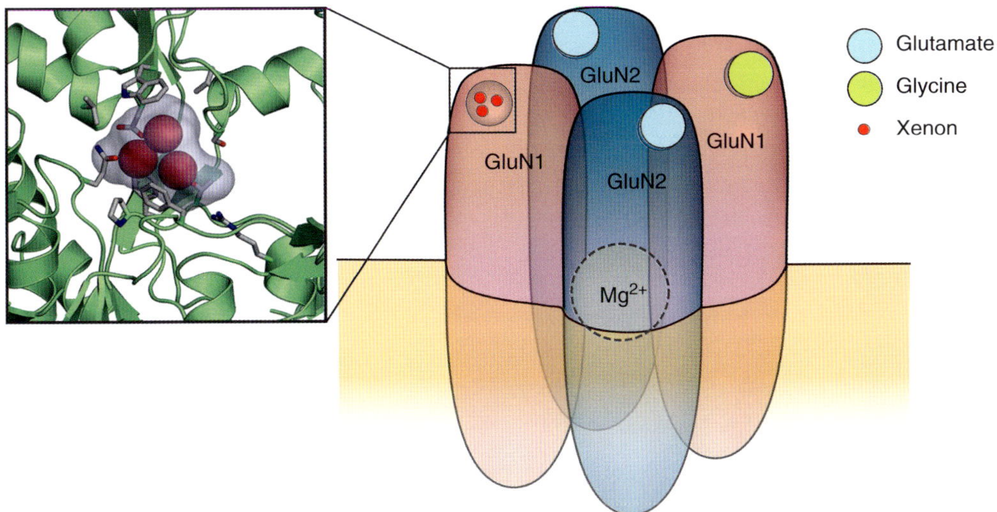

Figure 2.3 Xenon inhibition of M-methyl-D-aspartate (NMDA) receptors. The NMDA receptor is a ligand-gated ion channel that is permeable to Na^+, K^+, and Ca^{2+}. Activation of the NMDA receptor requires the binding of the neurotransmitter glutamate and the co-agonist glycine (or D-serine). At resting membrane potentials, the pore of the channel is blocked by Mg^{2+}, preventing ion flux. The Mg^{2+} block is relieved by membrane depolarization, which repels the Mg^{2+} ion and allows ion flux when the channel is activated. The NMDA receptor is a molecular site of action for the anesthetic effects of xenon. Xenon can bind to the glycine binding site on the GluN1 subunit to prevent glycine binding and prevent NMDA receptor activation. Inset: ribbon diagram showing the interaction of xenon with the glycine binding site. Reprinted with permission from Dickinson R, Peterson B, Banks P, et al. Competitive inhibition at the glycine site of the N-Methyl-d-aspartate receptor by the anesthetics xenon and isoflurane. *Anesthesiology*. 2007;107(5):756–767.

that xenon binds to the glycine binding site of the GluN1 subunit of NMDA receptors.[133] A mutation in the GluN1 subunit that increases the receptor's affinity for glycine (F639A) prevents the inhibition of the NMDA receptor by xenon and isoflurane[133] (Figure 2.3).

These data demonstrate a role for NMDA-type glutamate receptors in mediating the anesthetic effects of some volatile anesthetics. It is notable that the anesthetic effects of NMDA antagonists are qualitatively different from those of other general anesthetics such as propofol and etomidate, which largely act at the $GABA_A$ receptors. For example, ketamine induces psychological abnormalities at subanesthetic concentrations, and the electroencephalograph patterns of brain activity that accompany ketamine anesthesia are markedly different from those induced by other general anesthetics.[141]

CATION CHANNELS AS ANESTHETIC TARGETS

Several types of K^+ channels are implicated in the actions of anesthetics. The outward current generated by the flux of K^+ ions through K^+ channels inhibits neuronal activity. The activation of a persistent K^+ conductance by isoflurane was first identified in the snail *Lymnaea stagnalis*.[142] This persistent or "leak" current is generated by potassium channels that belong to the two-pore-domain K^+ channels. The two-pore-domain family of potassium channels encompasses 15 members that are expressed across many species, including a variety of mammals.[143–144] Volatile anesthetics can directly activate or enhance the activity of several members of the two-pore-domain family of K^+ channels.[145–148] Mice that do not express the leak K^+ channel TREK-1 are resistant to the anesthetic effects of halothane, sevoflurane, desflurane, and chloroform, as indicated by increased MAC in the knockout mice.[149] Mice lacking the type 3 but not the type 1 acid-sensitive leak K^+ channel (TASK-3 and TASK-1, respectively) were profoundly less sensitive to the hypnotic effects of halothane.[150]

HYPERPOLARIZATION-ACTIVATED, CYCLIC NUCLEOTIDE-GATED CHANNELS

The hyperpolarization-activated, cyclic nucleotide-gated (HCN) channels represent another anesthetic target. The HCN channels are activated by membrane hyperpolarization to conduct a mixed current of Na^+ and K^+ that reverses near 0 mV and depolarizes the neuron.[151] Because this inward current is uniquely activated at hyperpolarized potentials, it has been variously termed I_f, I_q, or I_h, for funny, queer, and hyperpolarization activated current. The kinetics of HCN activation are regulated by intracellular cyclic adenosine monophosphate (cAMP).[151–152] The I_h current regulates many important components of neuronal activity, including stabilization of resting membrane potential, modulation of the firing of action potential, modification of the properties of dendritic cables and the synchrony of neuronal networks, and generation of spontaneous rhythmic activity in "pacemaker" neurons.[151–153]

The HCN channels are modulated by both volatile and injectable anesthetics. The volatile anesthetic halothane changes the activation kinetics of I_h such that this current is activated at more hyperpolarized membrane potentials, which results in less depolarizing I_h current at rest and reduces action potential firing.[154] Similarly, isoflurane produces a hyperpolarized shift in the activation kinetics of the I_h current and inhibits the maximal I_h current generated by HCN subtype 1 channels[155] (Figure 2.4). The inhibition of HCN1 channels by isoflurane was associated with enhanced synaptic summation and an increase in neuronal excitability.[155] The inhibitory effects of propofol on I_h have also been well described. Propofol causes both a reduction in the amplitude of I_h and a hyperpolarized shift in the I_h activation kinetics.[131,156–160] Low concentrations of ketamine can also inhibit I_h to produce membrane hyperpolarization and enhance synaptic summation.[131] Notably, ketamine- and propofol-induced loss of the righting reflex was reduced in mice lacking the HCN1 channel,[131] suggesting that HCN channels may contribute to anesthetic hypnosis.

VOLTAGE-GATED Na^+ CHANNELS

Voltage-gated Na^+ channels are critical for the generation of action potentials in neurons, but, these channels are typically not considered as major anesthetic targets. Early research indicated that the generation and conductance of action potentials in axons is not affected by clinically relevant concentrations of volatile anesthetics.[161] Additionally, voltage-dependent Na^+ currents in large invertebrate axons are not inhibited by volatile anesthetics.[162–163] Recently, it was observed that volatile anesthetics could reduce axonal conductance velocity in the small, unmyelinated axons of mammalian hippocampal neurons.[164–165] Thus, there may be a selective role for voltage-gated Na^+ channels in mediating the neurodepressive effects of general anesthetics.

The family of voltage-gated Na^+ channels contains 10 subtypes, each with unique neuronal and subcellular distributions.[166–167] Volatile anesthetics inhibit the peak current of the $Na_v1.2$ isoform expressed in neurons and shifts the inactivation kinetics of these channels to more negative potentials, causing a further reduction in Na^+ current during neuronal depolarization.[168] Several other isoforms, including the $Na_v1.4$, $Na_v1.5$, and $Na_v1.6$ isoforms, are also inhibited by volatile anesthetics.[168–170] In contrast, the persistently active $Na_v1.8$ isoform is not inhibited by anesthetics.[169–170] The inhibition of voltage-gated Na^+ channels by volatile anesthetics may regulate the presynaptic release of neurotransmitter.[171–172] In the calyx of Held, a large synapse that is widely used to study the mechanisms of

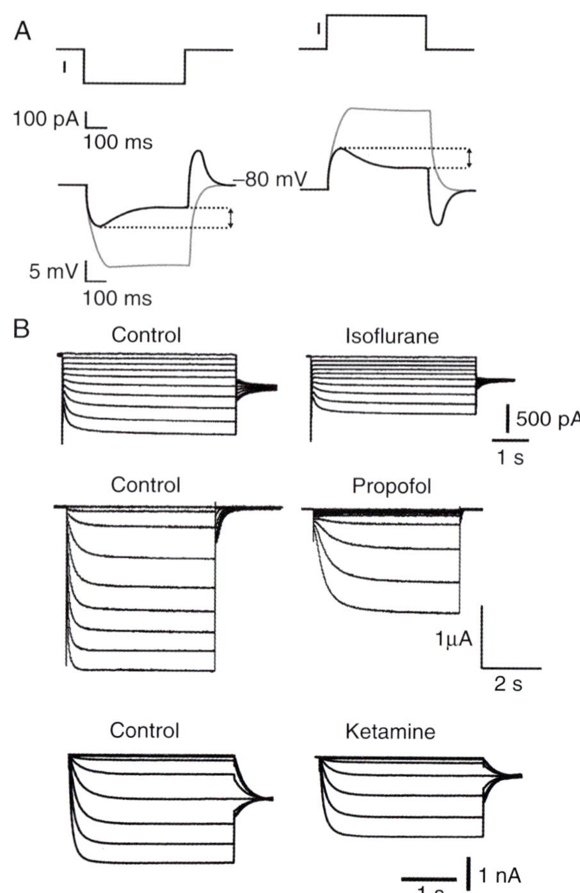

Figure 2.4 Anesthetic inhibition of hyperpolarization-activated cyclic nucleotide-gated (HCN) channels. HCN channels are voltage activated, nonselective cation channels that are directly regulated by intracellular cyclic adenosine monophosphate. A) The depolarizing current generated by HCN channels (Ih) activates during membrane hyperpolarization and inactivates during membrane depolarization. Thus, hyperpolarizing a neuron with a negative current injection (left) produces a depolarizing current sag as Ih activates, while depolarizing a neuron with a positive current injection (right) produces a hyperpolarizing voltage sag as Ih inactivates. B) The amplitude and activation kinetics of Ih is modulated by several general anesthetics, including isoflurane, propofol, and ketamine. **Sources: (1)** With kind permission from Springer Science+Business Media: Wahl-Schott C, Biel M. HCN channels: structure, cellular regulation and physiological function. *Cell Mol Life Sci*. 2009;66(3):470–494. **(2)** Reprinted with permission from Chen X, Shu S, Kennedy DP, Willcox SC, Bayliss DA. Subunit-specific effects of isoflurane on neuronal Ih in HCN1 knockout mice. *J Neurophysiol*. Jan 2009;101(1):129–140. **(3)** Reprinted with permission from Cacheaux LP, Topf N, Tibbs GR, et al. Impairment of hyperpolarization-activated, cyclic nucleotide-gated channel function by the intravenous general anesthetic propofol. *J Pharmacol Exp Ther*. 2005;315(2):517–525. **(4)** Reprinted with permission from Chen X, Shu S, Bayliss DA. HCN1 channel subunits are a molecular substrate for hypnotic actions of ketamine. *Journal of Neuroscience*. Jan 21 2009;29(3):600–609.

vesicular release, isoflurane reduces the number of vesicles released during presynaptic depolarization.[173] This effect is independent of the Ca^{2+} current and was associated with a small reduction in the amplitude of the action potential. Taken together, these findings indicate that the inhibition of voltage-gated Na^+ channels may mediate some of the neurodepressive effects of general anesthetics, although this contribution appears to be modest.

ANESTHETIC MODULATION OF NEURONAL ACTIVITY

NEURONAL EXCITABILITY

Neurons communicate information in neuronal networks primarily through the generation of action potentials. Whether a neuron generates an action potential depends on the balance of the excitatory and inhibitory drives that are present. Enhancing the magnitude of GABAergic inhibition with anesthetics can reduce the excitability of neurons and prevent the transfer of information between connected neurons. This is particularly true for the enhancement of tonic GABAergic inhibition, which can strongly regulate neuronal excitability[59,61,70,174–175] and control the flow of information through neuronal networks.[176] Reducing the excitability of neurons is likely a major mechanism by which anesthetics depress neural function.

SYNAPTIC PLASTICITY

Neurons are typically stimulated to generate action potentials through excitatory synaptic activity. One critical mechanism by which information is stored in neuronal networks is through plastic changes in the strength of excitatory synapses between neurons, called long-term synaptic potentiation (LTP). The coincident firing of pre- and postsynaptic neurons can strengthen the excitatory synapse through the recruitment of glutamate receptors to the postsynaptic membrane and their subsequent stabilization and the growth of new synapses.[177–178] The overall effect of these changes is to increase the probability that a postsynaptic neuron will fire by increasing the excitatory drive generated by a presynaptic neuron and hence to increase the strength of the connection between the two neurons in a form of neuronal "memory."[179] Anesthetics can disrupt the formation or maintenance of LTP by reducing excitatory neurotransmission[180–183] or increasing GABAergic inhbition.[62,85,184–185] Injectable anesthetics such as propofol[184–185] and etomidate[62,85] primarily inhibit LTP by enhancing GABAergic activity. The inhibition of LTP by volatile anesthetics such as halothane,[180] isoflurane,[183,186] and sevoflurane[181–182] can be attributed to both a depression of excitatory synaptic activity and an enhancement of inhibitory synaptic activity. For example, isoflurane depresses excitatory postsynaptic potentials, but the inhibition of LTP by isoflurane is dependent on $GABA_A$ receptor activity.[183] The dual nature by which volatile anesthetics inhibit LTP is not surprising given the broad array of molecular targets these drugs modulate.

Notably, the inhibition of LTP may be one mechanism through which anesthetics disrupt memory. The enhancement of tonic GABAergic inhibition and the inhibition of LTP by low concentrations of etomidate in hippocampal pyramidal neurons was shown to depend on the expression of the $\alpha_5 GABA_A$ receptor subunit.[62,85] Low concentrations of etomidate prevented the development and maintenance of LTP, but the etomidate-induced inhibition could be blocked by genetically or pharmacologically preventing the activity of the $\alpha_5 GABA_A$ receptors. This effect paralleled the amnestic effects of low doses of etomidate. Etomidate inhibited fear conditioning performance in normal mice but not in mice that did not express the $\alpha_5 GABA_A$ receptor subunit.[62]

NEURONAL NETWORK ACTIVITY

Neurons function within highly interconnected networks that can generate coordinated brain rhythms through the synchronization of neuronal activity. Coherent oscillations may have important functions within the brain related to the representation of information, the regulation of information transfer between brain regions, and to the storage and retrieval of information.[187–188] Synchronized oscillatory activity is maintained through a balance of excitation and inhibition within neuronal networks. Pyramidal neurons in neuronal networks receive excitatory input from recurrent synaptic connects within the neuronal network or from networks in other brain regions.[189] The activity of pyramidal neurons is constrained and regulated by synaptic GABAergic inhibition from interneurons, and the reciprocal connections between pyramidal neurons and interneurons can give rise to coherent oscillatory activity.[187–188]

The balance of excitatory and inhibitory activity in neuronal networks can be disrupted by anesthetics, leading to changes in network oscillatory activity.[190–191] Propofol[192–193] and isoflurane[194] prolong the duration of inhibitory GABAergic events, leading to changes in the stability and pattern of oscillations in small neuronal networks. Anesthetics can also act on non-GABAergic targets to alter network oscillations as well. For example, halothane can induce strong oscillations in the theta frequency by enhancing the activity of TASK-3 K^+ channels,[150] and propofol inhibition of I_h decreases rhythmic bursting in thalamic tissue slices.[156] Finally, anesthetic use is commonly associated with the development of epileptiform activity, as indicated by the development of network "hypersynchrony" within small cortical areas during anesthesia.[189]

SUMMARY

Knowledge of the mechanisms by which general anesthetics produce anesthesia has advanced considerably over the past decade. The identification of specific protein targets for anesthetic action has distinguished the contributions of these individual proteins to the anesthetic state. Genetic manipulation and subunit-selective drugs have been used to identify discrete $GABA_A$ receptor populations and other protein targets that mediate anesthesia endpoints such as sedation, hypnosis, and amnesia. Understanding how anesthetics modify the activity of these proteins enables us to predict how they will affect the activity of neurons at the cellular and network levels and furthers our understanding of what changes in brain activity contribute to anesthesia.

REFERENCES

1. Weiser TG, Regenbogen SE, Thompson KD, et al. An estimation of the global volume of surgery: a modelling strategy based on available data. *Lancet.* Jul 12 2008;372(9633):139–144.
2. Campagna JA, Miller KW, Forman SA. Mechanisms of actions of inhaled anesthetics. *N Engl J Med.* 2003;348(21):2110–2124.
3. Orser BA, Mazer CD, Baker AJ. Awareness during anesthesia. *CMAJ.* Jan 15 2008;178(2):185–188.
4. Bonin RP, Orser BA. GABA(A) receptor subtypes underlying general anesthesia. *Pharmacol Biochem Behav.* Jul 2008;90(1):105–112.
5. Orser BA. Extrasynaptic GABAA receptors are critical targets for sedative-hypnotic drugs. *J Clin Sleep Med.* Apr 15 2006;2(2):S12–18.
6. Alkire MT, Hudetz AG, Tononi G. Consciousness and anesthesia. *Science.* Nov 7 2008;322(5903):876–880.
7. Mashour GA. Integrating the science of consciousness and anesthesia. *Anesth Analg.* Oct 2006;103(4):975–982.
8. Overton E. *Studien über die Narkose, zugleich ein Beitrag zur allgemeinen Pharmakologie.* Jena, Germany: Fischer Verlag; 1901.
9. Meyer HH. Zur Theorie der Alkoholnarkose, I: Welche Eigenschaft der Anästhetica bedingt ihre narkotische Wirkung? *Arch Exp Pathol Pharmakol.* 1899;42:109–118.
10. Franks NP, Lieb WR. Do general anaesthetics act by competitive binding to specific receptors? *Nature.* 1984;310(5978):599–601.
11. Lysko GS, Robinson JL, Casto R, Ferrone RA. The stereospecific effects of isoflurane isomers in vivo. *Eur J Pharmacol.* Sep 22 1994;263(1–2):25–29.
12. Dickinson R, White I, Lieb WR, Franks NP. Stereoselective loss of righting reflex in rats by isoflurane. *Anesthesiology.* Sep 2000; 93(3):837–843.
13. Fang Z, Sonner J, Laster MJ, et al. Anesthetic and convulsant properties of aromatic compounds and cycloalkanes: implications for mechanisms of narcosis. *Anesth Analg.* Nov 1996;83(5): 1097–1104.
14. Koblin DD, Chortkoff BS, Laster MJ, Eger EI 2nd, Halsey MJ, Ionescu P. Polyhalogenated and perfluorinated compounds that disobey the Meyer-Overton hypothesis. *Anesth Analg.* Dec 1994; 79(6):1043–1048.
15. Raines DE, Korten SE, Hill AG, Miller KW. Anesthetic cutoff in cycloalkanemethanols: a test of current theories. *Anesthesiology.* May 1993;78(5):918–927.
16. Raines DE, Miller KW. On the importance of volatile agents devoid of anesthetic action. *Anesth Analg.* Dec 1994;79(6):1031–1033.
17. Hemmings HC Jr, Akabas MH, Goldstein PA, Trudell JR, Orser BA, Harrison NL. Emerging molecular mechanisms of general anesthetic action. *Trends Pharmacol Sci.* 2005;26(10):503–510.
18. Sonner JM, Antognini JF, Dutton RC, et al. Inhaled anesthetics and immobility: mechanisms, mysteries, and minimum alveolar anesthetic concentration. *Anesth Analg.* 2003;97(3):718–740.
19. Bloom FE, Iversen LL. Localizing 3H-GABA in nerve terminals of rat cerebral cortex by electron microscopic autoradiography. *Nature.* Feb 26 1971;229(5287):628–630.
20. Moss SJ, Smart TG. Constructing inhibitory synapses. *Nat Rev Neurosci.* 2001;2(4):240–250.
21. Macdonald RL, Olsen RW. GABAA receptor channels. *Ann Rev Neurosci.* 1994;17:569–602.
22. Belelli D, Lambert JJ. Neurosteroids: endogenous regulators of the GABA(A) receptor. *Nat Rev Neurosci.* 2005;6(7):565–576.
23. Franks NP. General anaesthesia: from molecular targets to neuronal pathways of sleep and arousal. *Nat Rev Neurosci.* May 2008;9(5): 370–386.
24. Kopp Lugli A, Yost CS, Kindler CH. Anaesthetic mechanisms: update on the challenge of unravelling the mystery of anaesthesia. *Eur J Anaesthesiol.* Oct 2009;26(10):807–820.
25. Olsen RW, Sieghart W. GABA A receptors: subtypes provide diversity of function and pharmacology. *Neuropharmacology.* Jan 2009;56(1):141–148.
26. Olsen RW, Sieghart W. International Union of Pharmacology, LXX: Subtypes of gamma-aminobutyric acid(A) receptors: classification on the basis of subunit composition, pharmacology, and function. Update. *Pharmacol Rev.* Sep 2008;60(3):243–260.
27. Sieghart W. Structure and pharmacology of gamma-aminobutyric acidA receptor subtypes. *Pharmacol Rev.* Jun 1995;47(2):181–234.
28. Hevers W, Luddens H. The diversity of GABAA receptors: pharmacological and electrophysiological properties of GABAA channel subtypes. *Mol Neurobiol.* Aug 1998;18(1):35–86.
29. Farrant M, Nusser Z. Variations on an inhibitory theme: phasic and tonic activation of GABA(A) receptors. *Nat Rev Neurosci.* 2005;6(3):215–229.
30. Nusser Z, Sieghart W, Benke D, Fritschy JM, Somogyi P. Differential synaptic localization of two major gamma-aminobutyric acid type A receptor alpha subunits on hippocampal pyramidal cells. *Proc Natl Acad Sci U S A.* 1996;93(21):11939–11944.
31. Nusser Z, Sieghart W, Somogyi P. Segregation of different GABAA receptors to synaptic and extrasynaptic membranes of cerebellar granule cells. *J Neurosci.* 1998;18(5):1693–1703.
32. Brunig I, Scotti E, Sidler C, Fritschy JM. Intact sorting, targeting, and clustering of gamma-aminobutyric acid A receptor subtypes in hippocampal neurons in vitro. *J Comp Neurol.* 2002;443(1): 43–55.
33. Pirker S, Schwarzer C, Wieselthaler A, Sieghart W, Sperk G. GABA(A) receptors: immunocytochemical distribution of 13 subunits in the adult rat brain. *Neuroscience.* 2000;101(4): 815–850.
34. Sur C, Fresu L, Howell O, McKernan RM, Atack JR. Autoradiographic localization of alpha5 subunit-containing GABAA receptors in rat brain. *Brain Res.* 1999;822(1–2):265–270.
35. Korpi ER, Grunder G, Luddens H. Drug interactions at GABA(A) receptors. *Prog Neurobiol.* 2002;67(2):113–159.
36. Franks NP. Molecular targets underlying general anaesthesia. *Br J Pharmacol.* Jan 2006;147 Suppl 1:S72–81.
37. Maconochie DJ, Zempel JM, Steinbach JH. How quickly can GABAA receptors open? *Neuron.* 1994;12(1):61–71.
38. Cobb SR, Buhl EH, Halasy K, Paulsen O, Somogyi P. Synchronization of neuronal activity in hippocampus by individual GABAergic interneurons. *Nature.* 1995;378(6552):75–78.
39. Pouille F, Scanziani M. Enforcement of temporal fidelity in pyramidal cells by somatic feed-forward inhibition. *Science.* Aug 10 2001;293(5532):1159–1163.
40. Wu Y, Wang W, Richerson GB. Vigabatrin induces tonic inhibition via GABA transporter reversal without increasing vesicular GABA release. *J Neurophysiol.* 2003;89(4):2021–2034.
41. Rossi DJ, Hamann M, Attwell D. Multiple modes of GABAergic inhibition of rat cerebellar granule cells. *J Physiol.* 2003;548(Pt 1): 97–110.
42. Hamann M, Rossi DJ, Attwell D. Tonic and spillover inhibition of granule cells control information flow through cerebellar cortex. *Neuron.* 2002;33(4):625–633.
43. Rossi DJ, Hamann M. Spillover-mediated transmission at inhibitory synapses promoted by high affinity alpha6 subunit GABA(A) receptors and glomerular geometry. *Neuron.* 1998;20(4):783–795.
44. Glykys J, Mody I. The main source of ambient GABA responsible for tonic inhibition in the mouse hippocampus. *J Physiol (Online).* 2007;582(3):1163–1178.

45. Kullmann DM, Ruiz A, Rusakov DM, Scott R, Semyanov A, Walker MC. Presynaptic, extrasynaptic and axonal GABAA receptors in the CNS: where and why? *Prog Biophys Mol Biol.* 2005;87(1):33–46.
46. Brickley SG, Cull-Candy SG, Farrant M. Development of a tonic form of synaptic inhibition in rat cerebellar granule cells resulting from persistent activation of GABA(A) receptors. *J Physiol.* 1996;497(Pt 3):753–759.
47. Wall MJ, Usowicz MM. Development of action potential-dependent and independent spontaneous GABAA receptor-mediated currents in granule cells of postnatal rat cerebellum. *Eur J Neurosci.* 1997;9(3):533–548.
48. Bai D, Zhu G, Pennefather P, Jackson MF, MacDonald JF, Orser BA. Distinct functional and pharmacological properties of tonic and quantal inhibitory postsynaptic currents mediated by g-aminobutyric acid(A) receptors in hippocampal neurons. *Mol Pharmacol.* 2001;59(4):814–824.
49. Nusser Z, Mody I. Selective modulation of tonic and phasic inhibitions in dentate gyrus granule cells. *J Neurophysiol.* 2002; 87(5):2624–2628.
50. Stell BM, Mody I. Receptors with different affinities mediate phasic and tonic GABA(A) conductances in hippocampal neurons. *J Neurosci.* 2002;22 RC223:1–5.
51. Belelli D, Peden DR, Rosahl TW, Wafford KA, Lambert JJ. Extrasynaptic GABAA receptors of thalamocortical neurons: a molecular target for hypnotics. *J Neurosci.* 2005;25(50):11513–11520.
52. Cope DW, Hughes SW, Crunelli V. GABAA receptor-mediated tonic inhibition in thalamic neurons. *J Neurosci.* 2005;25(50): 11553–11563.
53. Jia F, Pignataro L, Schofield CM, Yue M, Harrison NL, Goldstein PA. An extrasynaptic GABAA receptor mediates tonic inhibition in thalamic VB neurons. *J Neurophysiol.* 2005;94(6): 4491–4501.
54. Porcello DM, Huntsman MM, Mihalek RM, Homanics GE, Huguenard JR. Intact synaptic GABAergic inhibition and altered neurosteroid modulation of thalamic relay neurons in mice lacking delta subunit. *J Neurophysiol.* 2003;89(3):1378–1386.
55. Drasbek KR, Hoestgaard-Jensen K, Jensen K. Modulation of extrasynaptic THIP conductances by GABAA-receptor modulators in mouse neocortex. *J Neurophysiol.* 2007;97(3):2293–2300.
56. Salin PA, Prince DA. Spontaneous GABAA receptor-mediated inhibitory currents in adult rat somatosensory cortex. *J Neurophysiol.* 1996;75(4):1573–1588.
57. Bai D, Zhu G, Pennefather P, Jackson MF, MacDonald JF, Orser BA. Distinct functional and pharmacological properties of tonic and quantal inhibitory postsynaptic currents mediated by gamma-aminobutyric acid(A) receptors in hippocampal neurons. *Mol Pharmacol.* 2001;59(4):814–824.
58. Caraiscos VB, Elliott EM, You T, et al. Tonic inhibition in mouse hippocampal CA1 pyramidal neurons is mediated by a5 subunit-containing gamma-aminobutyric acid type A receptors. *Proc Natl Acad Sci.* 2004;101 (10):3662–3667.
59. Marchionni I, Omrani A, Cherubini E. In the developing rat hippocampus a tonic GABAA-mediated conductance selectively enhances the glutamatergic drive of principal cells. *J Physiol.* 2007;581(Pt 2):515–528.
60. Petrini EM, Marchionni I, Zacchi P, Sieghart W, Cherubini E. Clustering of extrasynaptic GABA(A) receptors modulates tonic inhibition in cultured hippocampal neurons. *J Biol Chem.* 2004;279(44):45833–45843.
61. Semyanov A, Walker MC, Kullmann DM. GABA uptake regulates cortical excitability via cell type-specific tonic inhibition. *Nat Neurosci.* 2003;6(5):484–490.
62. Cheng VY, Martin LJ, Elliott EM, et al. Alpha5GABAA receptors mediate the amnestic but not sedative-hypnotic effects of the general anesthetic etomidate. *J Neurosci.* Apr 5 2006;26(14):3713–3720.
63. Orser BA, McAdam LC, Roder S, MacDonald JF. General anaesthetics and their effects on GABA(A) receptor desensitization. *Toxicol Lett.* 1998;100–101:217–224.
64. Lerma J, Herranz AS, Herreras O, Abraira V, Martin dR. In vivo determination of extracellular concentration of amino acids in the rat hippocampus: a method based on brain dialysis and computerized analysis. *Brain Res.* 1986;384(1):145–155.
65. Cavelier P, Hamann M, Rossi D, Mobbs P, Attwell D. Tonic excitation and inhibition of neurons: ambient transmitter sources and computational consequences. *Prog Biophys Mol Biol.* 2005;87(1):3–16.
66. Mody I, De Koninck Y, Otis TS, Soltesz I. Bridging the cleft at GABA synapses in the brain. *Trends Neurosci.* 1994;17(12):517–525.
67. Bianchi MT, Haas KF, Macdonald RL. Alpha1 and alpha6 subunits specify distinct desensitization, deactivation and neurosteroid modulation of GABA(A) receptors containing the delta subunit. *Neuropharmacology.* 2002;43(4):492–502.
68. Haas KF, Macdonald RL. GABAA receptor subunit gamma2 and delta subtypes confer unique kinetic properties on recombinant GABAA receptor currents in mouse fibroblasts. *J Physiol (Lond).* 1999;514(Pt 1):27–45.
69. Yeung JY, Canning KJ, Zhu G, Pennefather P, MacDonald JF, Orser BA. Tonically activated GABAA receptors in hippocampal neurons are high-affinity, low-conductance sensors for extracellular GABA. *Mol Pharmacol.* 2003;63(1):2–8.
70. Bonin RP, Martin LJ, MacDonald JF, Orser BA. Alpha5GABAA receptors regulate the intrinsic excitability of mouse hippocampal pyramidal neurons. *J Neurophysiol.* Oct 2007;98(4):2244–2254.
71. Nishikawa K, Jenkins A, Paraskevakis I, Harrison NL. Volatile anesthetic actions on the GABAA receptors: contrasting effects of alpha 1(S270) and beta 2(N265) point mutations. *Neuropharmacology.* 2002;42(3):337–345.
72. Belelli D, Lambert JJ, Peters JA, Wafford K, Whiting PJ. The interaction of the general anesthetic etomidate with the gamma-aminobutyric acid type A receptor is influenced by a single amino acid. *Proc Natl Acad Sci U S A.* 1997;94(20):11031–11036.
73. Li GD, Chiara DC, Cohen JB, Olsen RW. Neurosteroids allosterically modulate binding of the anesthetic etomidate to gamma-aminobutyric acid type A receptors. *J Biol Chem.* May 1 2009; 284(18):11771–11775.
74. Li GD, Chiara DC, Sawyer GW, Husain SS, Olsen RW, Cohen JB. Identification of a GABAA receptor anesthetic binding site at subunit interfaces by photolabeling with an etomidate analog. *J Neurosci.* Nov 8 2006;26(45):11599–11605.
75. Sebel PS, Bowdle TA, Ghoneim MM, et al. The incidence of awareness during anesthesia: a multicenter United States study. *Anesth Analg.* 2004;99(3):833–839, table.
76. Hudetz JA, Iqbal Z, Gandhi SD, et al. Postoperative cognitive dysfunction in older patients with a history of alcohol abuse. *Anesthesiology.* 2007;106(3):423–430.
77. Moller JT, Cluitmans P, Rasmussen LS, et al. Long-term postoperative cognitive dysfunction in the elderly ISPOCD1 study. ISPOCD investigators. International Study of Post-Operative Cognitive Dysfunction. *Lancet.* 1998;351(9106):857–861.
78. Chambers MS, Atack JR, Carling RW, et al. An orally bioavailable, functionally selective inverse agonist at the benzodiazepine site of GABAA alpha5 receptors with cognition enhancing properties. *J Med Chem.* 2004;47(24):5829–5832.
79. Chambers MS, Atack JR, Broughton HB, et al. Identification of a novel, selective GABAA à5 receptor inverse agonist which enhances cognition. *J Med Chem.* 2003;46(11):2227–2240.
80. Nutt DJ, Besson M, Wilson SJ, Dawson GR, Lingford-Hughes AR. Blockade of alcohol's amnestic activity in humans by an alpha5 subtype benzodiazepine receptor inverse agonist. *Neuropharmacology.* 2007;53(7):810–820.
81. Collinson N, Kuenzi FM, Jarolimek W, et al. Enhanced learning and memory and altered GABAergic synaptic transmission in mice lacking the alpha 5 subunit of the GABAA receptor. *J Neurosci.* 2002;22(13):5572–5580.
82. Crestani F, Keist R, Fritschy JM, et al. Trace fear conditioning involves hippocampal alpha5 GABA(A) receptors. *Proc Natl Acad Sci U S A.* 2002;99(13):8980–8985.

83. Bieda MC, MacIver MB. Major role for tonic GABAA conductances in anesthetic suppression of intrinsic neuronal excitability. *J Neurophysiol.* Sep 2004;92(3):1658–1667.
84. Caraiscos VB, Newell JG, You T, et al. Selective enhancement of tonic GABAergic inhibition in murine hippocampal neurons by low concentrations of the volatile anesthetic isoflurane. *J Neurosci.* 2004;24 (39):8454–8458.
85. Martin LJ, Oh GHT, Orser BA. Etomidate targets alpha5 gamma-aminobutyric acid subtype A receptors to regulate synaptic plasticity and memory blockade. *Anesthesiology.* Nov 2009;111(5): 1025–1035.
86. Rao Y, Wang YL, Chen YQ, Zhang WS, Liu J. Protective effects of emulsified isoflurane after myocardial ischemia-reperfusion injury and its mechanism in rabbits. *Chin J Traumatol.* Feb 2009;12(1):18–21.
87. Reynolds DS, Rosahl TW, Cirone J, et al. Sedation and anesthesia mediated by distinct GABA(A) receptor isoforms. *J Neurosci.* 2003;23(24):8608–8617.
88. Jurd R, Arras M, Lambert S, et al. General anesthetic actions in vivo strongly attenuated by a point mutation in the GABA(A) receptor beta3 subunit. *FASEB J.* 2003;17(2):250–252.
89. Rudolph U, Crestani F, Benke D, et al. Benzodiazepine actions mediated by specific gamma-aminobutyric acid(A) receptor subtypes. *Nature.* 1999;401(6755):796–800.
90. Steriade M. Sleep, epilepsy and thalamic reticular inhibitory neurons. *Trends Neurosci.* 2005;28(6):317–324.
91. Wafford KA, Ebert B. Gaboxadol—a new awakening in sleep. *Curr Opin Pharmacol.* Feb 2006;6(1):30–36.
92. Krogsgaard-Larsen P, Frolund B, Liljefors T, Ebert B. GABA(A) agonists and partial agonists: THIP (Gaboxadol) as a non-opioid analgesic and a novel type of hypnotic. *Biochem Pharmacol.* Oct 15 2004;68(8):1573–1580.
93. Chandra D, Jia F, Liang J, et al. GABAA receptor α4 subunits mediate extrasynaptic inhibition in thalamus and dentate gyrus and the action of gaboxadol. *Proc Natl Acad Sci.* 2006;103(41): 15230–15235.
94. Brown N, Kerby J, Bonnert TP, Whiting PJ, Wafford KA. Pharmacological characterization of a novel cell line expressing human alpha(4)beta(3)delta GABA(A) receptors. *Br J Pharmacol.* 2002;136(7):965–974.
95. Rudolph U, Antkowiak B. Molecular and neuronal substrates for general anaesthetics. *Nat Rev Neurosci.* 2004;5(9):709–720.
96. Wohlfarth KM, Bianchi MT, Macdonald RL. Enhanced neurosteroid potentiation of ternary GABA(A) receptors containing the delta subunit. *J Neurosci.* 2002;22(5):1541–1549.
97. Mihalek RM, Banerjee PK, Korpi ER, et al. Attenuated sensitivity to neuroactive steroids in gamma -aminobutyrate type A receptor delta subunit knockout mice. *Proc Natl Acad Sci.* 1999;96(22): 12905–12910.
98. Eger EI, Saidman LJ, Brandstater B. Minimum alveolar anesthetic concentration: a standard of anesthetic potency. *Anesthesiology.* 1965;26(6):756–763.
99. Antognini JF, Jinks S, Buzin V, Carstens E. A method for differential delivery of intravenous drugs to the head and torso of the goat. *Anesth Analg.* Dec 1998;87(6):1450–1452.
100. Antognini JF, Carstens E, Tabo E, Buzin V. Effect of differential delivery of isoflurane to head and torso on lumbar dorsal horn activity. *Anesthesiology.* Apr 1998;88(4):1055–1061.
101. Antognini JF, Schwartz K. Exaggerated anesthetic requirements in the preferentially anesthetized brain. *Anesthesiology.* 1993;79(6): 1244–1249.
102. Borges M, Antognini JF. Does the brain influence somatic responses to noxious stimuli during isoflurane anesthesia? *Anesthesiology.* Dec 1994;81(6):1511–1515.
103. King BS, Rampil IJ. Anesthetic depression of spinal motor neurons may contribute to lack of movement in response to noxious stimuli. *Anesthesiology.* 1994;81(6):1484–1492.
104. Rampil IJ. Anesthetic potency is not altered after hypothermic spinal cord transection in rats. *Anesthesiology.* 1994;80(3): 606–610.
105. Rampil IJ, Mason P, Singh H. Anesthetic potency (MAC) is independent of forebrain structures in the rat. *Anesthesiology.* 1993;78(4):707–712.
106. Zeller A, Arras M, Jurd R, Rudolph U. Mapping the contribution of beta3-containing GABAA receptors to volatile and intravenous general anesthetic actions. *BMC Pharmacol.* 2007;7:2.
107. Jenkins A, Greenblatt EP, Faulkner HJ, et al. Evidence for a common binding cavity for three general anesthetics within the GABA(A) receptor. *J Neurosci.* 2001;21(6):U7–U10.
108. Koltchine VV, Finn SE, Jenkins A, Nikolaeva N, Lin A, Harrison NL. Agonist gating and isoflurane potentiation in the human gamma-aminobutyric acid type A receptor determined by the volume of a second transmembrane domain residue. *Mol Pharmacol.* 1999;56(5):1087–1093.
109. Mihic SJ, Ye Q, Wick MJ, et al. Sites of alcohol and volatile anaesthetic action on GABA(A) and glycine receptors [see comments]. *Nature.* 1997;389(6649):385–389.
110. Hall AC, Rowan KC, Stevens RJ, Kelley JC, Harrison NL. The effects of isoflurane on desensitized wild-type and alpha 1(S270H) gamma-aminobutyric acid type A receptors. *Anesth Analg.* May 2004;98(5):1297–1304, table of contents.
111. Borghese CM, Werner DF, Topf N, et al. An isoflurane- and alcohol-insensitive mutant GABA(A) receptor alpha(1) subunit with near-normal apparent affinity for GABA: characterization in heterologous systems and production of knockin mice. *J Pharmacol Exp Ther.* Oct 2006;319(1):208–218.
112. Sonner JM, Werner DF, Elsen FP, et al. Effect of isoflurane and other potent inhaled anesthetics on minimum alveolar concentration, learning, and the righting reflex in mice engineered to express alpha1 gamma-aminobutyric acid type A receptors unresponsive to isoflurane. *Anesthesiology.* Jan 2007;106(1):107–113.
113. Sonner JM, Xing Y, Zhang Y, et al. Administration of epinephrine does not increase learning of fear to tone in rats anesthetized with isoflurane or desflurane. *Anesth Analg.* May 2005;100(5): 1333–1337, table of contents.
114. Siegwart R, Jurd R, Rudolph U. Molecular determinants for the action of general anesthetics at recombinant alpha(2)beta(3) gamma(2) gamma-aminobutyric acid(A) receptors. *J Neurochem.* 2002;80(1):140–148.
115. Lambert S, Arras M, Vogt KE, Rudolph U. Isoflurane-induced surgical tolerance mediated only in part by beta3-containing GABA(A) receptors. *Eur J Pharmacol.* May 23 2005;516(1): 23–27.
116. Liao M, Sonner JM, Jurd R, et al. Beta3-containing gamma-aminobutyric acidA receptors are not major targets for the amnesic and immobilizing actions of isoflurane. *Anesth Analg.* Aug 2005; 101(2):412–418, table of contents.
117. Cull-Candy S, Brickley S, Farrant M. NMDA receptor subunits: diversity, development and disease. *Curr Opin Neurobiol.* Jun 2001; 11(3):327–335.
118. Dingledine R, Borges K, Bowie D, Traynelis SF. The glutamate receptor ion channels. *Pharmacol Rev.* 1999;51(1):7–61.
119. de Sousa SL, Dickinson R, Lieb WR, Franks NP. Contrasting synaptic actions of the inhalational general anesthetics isoflurane and xenon. *Anesthesiology.* Apr 2000;92(4):1055–1066.
120. Perouansky M, Baranov D, Salman M, Yaari Y. Effects of halothane on glutamate receptor-mediated excitatory postsynaptic currents: a patch-clamp study in adult mouse hippocampal slices. *Anesthesiology.* 1995;83(1):109–119.
121. Plested AJ, Wildman SS, Lieb WR, Franks NP. Determinants of the sensitivity of AMPA receptors to xenon. *Anesthesiology.* Feb 2004;100(2):347–358.
122. Wolosker H. D-serine regulation of NMDA receptor activity. *Sci STKE.* Oct 10 2006;2006(356):pe41.

123. McBain CJ, Mayer ML. N-methyl-D-aspartic acid receptor structure and function. *Physiol Rev.* 1994;74(3):723–760.
124. Nowak L, Bregestovski P, Ascher P, Herbet A, Prochiantz A. Magnesium gates glutamate-activated channels in mouse central neurones. *Nature.* 1984;307(5950):462–465.
125. Collingridge GL, Olsen RW, Peters J, Spedding M. A nomenclature for ligand-gated ion channels. *Neuropharmacology.* Jan 2009; 56(1):2–5.
126. Lahti AC, Koffel B, LaPorte D, Tamminga CA. Subanesthetic doses of ketamine stimulate psychosis in schizophrenia. *Neuropsychopharmacology.* Aug 1995;13(1):9–19.
127. Krystal JH, Karper LP, Seibyl JP, et al. Subanesthetic effects of the noncompetitive NMDA antagonist, ketamine, in humans. Psychotomimetic, perceptual, cognitive, and neuroendocrine responses. *Arch Gen Psychiatry.* Mar 1994;51(3):199–214.
128. MacDonald JF, Miljkovic Z, Pennefather P. Use-dependent block of excitatory amino acid currents in cultured neurons by ketamine. *J Neurophysiol.* 1987;58(2):251–266.
129. Orser BA, Pennefather PS, MacDonald JF. Multiple mechanisms of ketamine blockade of N-methyl-D-aspartate receptors. *Anesthesiology.* 1997;86(4):903–917.
130. Franks NP, Lieb WR. Molecular and cellular mechanisms of general anaesthesia. *Nature.* 1994;367(6464):607–614.
131. Chen X, Shu S, Bayliss DA. HCN1 channel subunits are a molecular substrate for hypnotic actions of ketamine. *J Neurosci.* Jan 21 2009;29(3):600–609.
132. Hevers W, Hadley SH, Luddens H, Amin J. Ketamine, but not phencyclidine, selectively modulates cerebellar GABA(A) receptors containing alpha6 and delta subunits. *J Neurosci.* May 14 2008;28(20):5383–5393.
133. Dickinson R, Peterson BK, Banks P, et al. Competitive inhibition at the glycine site of the N-methyl-D-aspartate receptor by the anesthetics xenon and isoflurane: evidence from molecular modeling and electrophysiology. *Anesthesiology.* Nov 2007;107(5): 756–767.
134. Franks NP, Dickinson R, de Sousa SL, Hall AC, Lieb WR. How does xenon produce anaesthesia? *Nature.* Nov 26 1998; 396(6709):324.
135. Yamakura T, Harris RA. Effects of gaseous anesthetics nitrous oxide and xenon on ligand-gated ion channels: comparison with isoflurane and ethanol. *Anesthesiology.* Oct 2000;93(4): 1095–1101.
136. Ogata J, Shiraishi M, Namba T, Smothers CT, Woodward JJ, Harris RA. Effects of anesthetics on mutant N-methyl-D-aspartate receptors expressed in Xenopus oocytes. *J Pharmacol Exp Ther.* Jul 2006;318(1):434–443.
137. Jevtovic-Todorovic V, Todorovic SM, Mennerick S, et al. Nitrous oxide (laughing gas) is an NMDA antagonist, neuroprotectant and neurotoxin. *Nat Med.* Apr 1998;4(4):460–463.
138. Ranft A, Kurz J, Becker K, et al. Nitrous oxide (N2O) pre- and postsynaptically attenuates NMDA receptor-mediated neurotransmission in the amygdala. *Neuropharmacology.* Mar 2007;52(3): 716–723.
139. Haseneder R, Kratzer S, Kochs E, et al. The xenon-mediated antagonism against the NMDA receptor is non-selective for receptors containing either NR2A or NR2B subunits in the mouse amygdala. *Eur J Pharmacol.* Oct 1 2009;619(1–3):33–37.
140. Haseneder R, Kratzer S, Kochs E, Eckle VS, Zieglgansberger W, Rammes G. Xenon reduces N-methyl-D-aspartate and alpha-amino-3-hydroxy 5 methyl-4-isoxazolepropionic acid receptor-mediated synaptic transmission in the amygdala. *Anesthesiology.* Dec 2008;109(6):998–1006.
141. Langsjo JW, Maksimow A, Salmi E, et al. S-ketamine anesthesia increases cerebral blood flow in excess of the metabolic needs in humans. *Anesthesiology.* Aug 2005;103(2):258–268.
142. Franks NP, Lieb WR. Stereospecific effects of inhalational general anesthetic optical isomers on nerve ion channels. *Science.* Oct 18 1991;254(5030):427–430.
143. Patel AJ, Honore E. Anesthetic-sensitive 2P domain K^+ channels. *Anesthesiology.* Oct 2001;95(4):1013–1021.
144. Patel AJ, Honore E. Properties and modulation of mammalian 2P domain K^+ channels. *Trends Neurosci.* Jun 2001;24(6):339–346.
145. Gray AT, Winegar BD, Leonoudakis DJ, Forsayeth JR, Yost CS. TOK1 is a volatile anesthetic stimulated K^+ channel. *Anesthesiology.* Apr 1998;88(4):1076–1084.
146. Gray AT, Zhao BB, Kindler CH, et al. Volatile anesthetics activate the human tandem pore domain baseline K^+ channel KCNK5. *Anesthesiology.* Jun 2000;92(6):1722–1730.
147. Patel AJ, Honore E, Lesage F, Fink M, Romey G, Lazdunski M. Inhalational anesthetics activate two-pore-domain background K^+ channels. *Nat Neurosci.* May 1999;2(5):422–426.
148. Winegar BD, Owen DF, Yost CS, Forsayeth JR, Mayeri E. Volatile general anesthetics produce hyperpolarization of Aplysia neurons by activation of a discrete population of baseline potassium channels. *Anesthesiology.* Oct 1996;85(4):889–900.
149. Heurteaux C, Guy N, Laigle C, et al. TREK-1, a K^+ channel involved in neuroprotection and general anesthesia. *EMBO J.* Jul 7 2004;23(13):2684–2695.
150. Pang DS, Robledo CJ, Carr DR, et al. An unexpected role for TASK-3 potassium channels in network oscillations with implications for sleep mechanisms and anesthetic action. *Proc Natl Acad Sci U S A.* Oct 13 2009;106(41):17546–17551.
151. Wahl-Schott C, Biel M. HCN channels: structure, cellular regulation and physiological function. *Cell Mol Life Sci.* Feb 2009; 66(3):470–494.
152. Biel M, Wahl-Schott C, Michalakis S, Zong X. Hyperpolarization-activated cation channels: from genes to function. *Physiol Rev.* Jul 2009;89(3):847–885.
153. Santoro B, Baram TZ. The multiple personalities of h-channels. *Trends Neurosci.* Oct 2003;26(10):550–554.
154. Chen X, Sirois JE, Lei Q, Talley EM, Lynch C 3rd, Bayliss DA. HCN subunit-specific and cAMP-modulated effects of anesthetics on neuronal pacemaker currents. *J Neurosci.* Jun 15 2005;25(24):5803–5814.
155. Chen X, Shu S, Kennedy DP, Willcox SC, Bayliss DA. Subunit-specific effects of isoflurane on neuronal Ih in HCN1 knockout mice. *J Neurophysiol.* Jan 2009;101(1):129–140.
156. Ying S-W, Abbas SY, Harrison NL, Goldstein PA. Propofol block of I(h) contributes to the suppression of neuronal excitability and rhythmic burst firing in thalamocortical neurons. *Eur J Neurosci.* Jan 2006;23(2):465–480. [Erratum appears in Eur J Neurosci. Mar 2006;23(5):1403].
157. Chen X, Shu S, Bayliss DA. Suppression of Ih contributes to propofol-induced inhibition of mouse cortical pyramidal neurons. *J Neurophysiol.* Dec 2005;94(6):3872–3883.
158. Cacheaux LP, Topf N, Tibbs GR, et al. Impairment of hyperpolarization-activated, cyclic nucleotide-gated channel function by the intravenous general anesthetic propofol. *J Pharmacol Exp Ther.* Nov 2005;315(2):517–525.
159. Funahashi M, Higuchi H, Miyawaki T, Shimada M, Matsuo R. Propofol suppresses a hyperpolarization-activated inward current in rat hippocampal CA1 neurons. *Neurosci Lett.* 2001;311(3):177–180.
160. Funahashi M, Mitoh Y, Matsuo R. The sensitivity of hyperpolarization-activated cation current (Ih) to propofol in rat area postrema neurons. *Brain Res.* Jul 23 2004;1015(1–2):198–201.
161. Larrabee MG, Posternak JM. Selective action of anesthetics on synapses and axons in mammalian sympathetic ganglia. *J Neurophysiol.* Mar 1952;15(2):91–114.
162. Haydon DA, Kimura JE. Some effects of n-pentane on the sodium and potassium currents of the squid giant axon. *J Physiol (Lond).* 1981;312:57–70:57–70.
163. Bean BP, Shrager P, Goldstein DA. Modification of sodium and potassium channel gating kinetics by ether and halothane. *J Gen Physiol.* Mar 1981;77(3):233–253.
164. Berg-Johnsen J, Langmoen IA. The effect of isoflurane on unmyelinated and myelinated fibres in the rat brain. *Acta Physiol Scand.* May 1986;127(1):87–93.

165. Mikulec AA, Pittson S, Amagasu SM, Monroe FA, MacIver MB. Halothane depresses action potential conduction in hippocampal axons. *Brain Res.* Jun 15 1998;796(1–2):231–238.
166. Yu FH, Catterall WA. The VGL-chanome: a protein superfamily specialized for electrical signaling and ionic homeostasis. *Sci STKE.* Oct 5 2004;2004(253):re15.
167. Catterall WA. Structure and function of voltage-gated ion channels. *Annu Rev Biochem.* 1995;64:493–531:493–531.
168. Rehberg B, Xiao YH, Duch DS. Central nervous system sodium channels are significantly suppressed at clinical concentrations of volatile anesthetics. *Anesthesiology.* May 1996;84(5):1223–1233; discussion 1227A.
169. Stadnicka A, Kwok WM, Hartmann HA, Bosnjak ZJ. Effects of halothane and isoflurane on fast and slow inactivation of human heart hH1a sodium channels. *Anesthesiology.* Jun 1999; 90(6):1671–1683.
170. Shiraishi M, Harris RA. Effects of alcohols and anesthetics on recombinant voltage-gated Na+ channels. *J Pharmacol Exp Ther.* Jun 2004;309(3):987–994.
171. Schlame M, Hemmings HC Jr. Inhibition by volatile anesthetics of endogenous glutamate release from synaptosomes by a presynaptic mechanism. *Anesthesiology.* Jun 1995;82(6):1406–1416.
172. Westphalen RI, Hemmings HC Jr. Selective depression by general anesthetics of glutamate versus GABA release from isolated cortical nerve terminals. *J Pharmacol Exp Ther.* 2003;304(3): 1188–1196.
173. Wu XS, Sun JY, Evers AS, Crowder M, Wu LG. Isoflurane inhibits transmitter release and the presynaptic action potential. *Anesthesiology.* Mar 2004;100(3):663–670.
174. Brickley SG, Revilla V, Cull-Candy SG, Wisden W, Farrant M. Adaptive regulation of neuronal excitability by a voltage-independent potassium conductance. *Nature.* 2001;409(6816): 88–92.
175. Mitchell SJ, Silver RA. Shunting inhibition modulates neuronal gain during synaptic excitation. *Neuron.* 2003;38(3):433–445.
176. Chadderton P, Margrie TW, Hausser M. Integration of quanta in cerebellar granule cells during sensory processing. *Nature.* 2004; 428(6985):856–860.
177. Malenka RC. Synaptic plasticity and AMPA receptor trafficking. *Ann N Y Acad Sci.* 2003;1003:1–11.
178. Malenka RC, Bear MF. LTP and LTD: an embarrassment of riches. *Neuron.* 2004;44(1):5–21.
179. Bliss TV, Collingridge GL. A synaptic model of memory: long-term potentiation in the hippocampus. *Nature.* 1993;361(6407): 31–39.
180. MacIver MB, Tauck DL, Kendig JJ. General anaesthetic modification of synaptic facilitation and long-term potentiation in hippocampus. *Br J Anaesth.* Mar 1989;62(3):301–310.
181. Ishizeki J, Nishikawa K, Kubo K, Saito S, Goto F. Amnestic concentrations of sevoflurane inhibit synaptic plasticity of hippocampal CA1 neurons through gamma-aminobutyric acid-mediated mechanisms. *Anesthesiology.* Mar 2008;108(3): 447–456.
182. Otsubo T, Maekawa M, Nagai T, Sakio H, Hori Y. Facilitatory effects of subanesthetic sevoflurane on excitatory synaptic transmission and synaptic plasticity in the mouse hippocampal CA1 area. *Brain Res.* Mar 4 2008;1197:32–39.
183. Simon W, Hapfelmeier G, Kochs E, Zieglgansberger W, Rammes G. Isoflurane blocks synaptic plasticity in the mouse hippocampus. *Anesthesiology.* Jun 2001;94(6):1058–1065.
184. Wang W, Wang H, Gong N, Xu T-L. Changes of K^{+} -Cl- cotransporter 2 (KCC2) and circuit activity in propofol-induced impairment of long-term potentiation in rat hippocampal slices. *Brain Res Bull.* Oct 16 2006;70(4–6):444–449.
185. Takamatsu I, Sekiguchi M, Wada K, Sato T, Ozaki M. Propofol-mediated impairment of CA1 long-term potentiation in mouse hippocampal slices. *Neurosci Lett.* Dec 9 2005;389(3):129–132.
186. Rammes G, Starker LK, Haseneder R, et al. Isoflurane anaesthesia reversibly improves cognitive function and long-term potentiation (LTP) via an up-regulation in NMDA receptor 2B subunit expression. *Neuropharmacology.* Mar 2009;56(3):626–636.
187. Sejnowski TJ, Paulsen O. Network oscillations: emerging computational principles. *J Neurosci.* Feb 8 2006;26(6):1673–1676.
188. Buzsaki G, Draguhn A. Neuronal oscillations in cortical networks. *Science.* Jun 25 2004;304(5679):1926–1929.
189. Voss LJ, Sleigh JW, Barnard JP, Kirsch HE. The howling cortex: seizures and general anesthetic drugs. *Anesth Analg.* Nov 2008; 107(5):1689–1703.
190. Dickinson R, Awaiz S, Whittington MA, Lieb WR, Franks NP. The effects of general anaesthetics on carbachol-evoked gamma oscillations in the rat hippocampus in vitro. *Neuropharmacology.* 2003;44(7):864–872.
191. Faulkner HJ, Traub RD, Whittington MA. Disruption of synchronous gamma oscillations in the rat hippocampal slice: a common mechanism of anaesthetic drug action. *Br J Pharmacol.* 1998;125(3):483–492.
192. Baker PM, Pennefather PS, Orser BA, Skinner FK. Disruption of coherent oscillations in inhibitory networks with anesthetics: role of GABA(A) receptor desensitization. *J Neurophysiol.* 2002; 88(5):2821–2833.
193. Hutt A, Longtin A. Effects of the anesthetic agent propofol on neural populations. *Cogn Neurodyn.* Mar 2010;4(1):37–59.
194. Antkowiak B, Hentschke H. Cellular mechanisms of gamma rhythms in rat neocortical brain slices probed by the volatile anaesthetic isoflurane. *Neurosci Lett.* 1997;231(2):87–90.
195. Mashour GA, Forman SA, Campagna JA. Mechanisms of general anesthesia: from molecules to mind. *Best Pract Res Clin Anaesthesiol.* Sep 2005;19(3):349–364.

3

THE SHARED CIRCUITS OF SLEEP AND ANESTHESIA

Giancarlo Vanini, Pablo Torterolo,

Helen A. Baghdoyan, and Ralph Lydic

INTRODUCTION

Anesthetic drugs are safely administered to thousands of patients on a daily basis, yet the mechanisms by which these drugs generate loss of consciousness remain enigmatic. Two hypotheses that are not mutually exclusive subsume research efforts aiming to elucidate the mechanisms of action of general anesthetics. One hypothesis proposes that neural networks that evolved to generate sleep are preferentially modulated by general anesthetics. This shared circuits hypothesis[1] is now supported by evidence from numerous laboratories.[2–14] The cognitive binding hypothesis[15] proposes that anesthetic drugs cause cognitive unbinding and loss of consciousness by disrupting effective connectivity between high-order cortical areas (Figure 3.1). Features of cognitive binding directly relevant to anesthesia include information integration among anatomically distributed neuronal networks and temporal integration expressed as synchronization of neuronal excitability.[16] The utility of the cognitive unbinding hypothesis has been supported by recent studies of propofol[17,18] and midazolam[19] in humans. Disrupted transmission of cortical information in humans during non–rapid eye movement sleep[20] provides additional support for the hypothesis that shared neural circuits generate loss of consciousness during sleep and anesthesia. This chapter focuses on the shared circuits hypothesis by reviewing studies demonstrating that some anesthetics can cause loss of consciousness by actions on neuronal networks known to generate states of sleep and wakefulness.

SLEEP HOMEOSTASIS AND GENERAL ANESTHESIA

The temporal organization of sleep stages has been mathematically modeled as the interaction between homeostatic and circadian factors.[21] The homeostatic process, named Process S, describes the build-up in sleep propensity during wakefulness and its subsequent dissipation during sleep. The circadian process, Process C, is independent of the duration of prior sleep and wakefulness and describes the oscillation between periods of high and low sleep propensity. A third factor, referred to as an ultradian process, represents the cycling between the behavioral states of non–rapid eye movement (NREM) sleep and rapid eye movement (REM) sleep. The cellular discharge profiles from selected groups of aminergic and cholinergic neurons was used to construct the first neuronally based, mathematical model able to predict the temporal organization of the NREM and REM phases of sleep.[22,23]

Data now support the interpretation that the purine nucleoside adenosine is one molecular substrate of the homeostatic Process S. The role of adenosine in mediating the homeostatic sleep drive is supported by evidence that brain extracellular levels of adenosine increase during wakefulness, when there is a high level of neuronal activity, and decrease during sleep.[24] Specifically, adenosine levels in the basal forebrain and cortex increase during prolonged wakefulness and decrease during recovery sleep.[25,26] Indeed, high levels of adenosine in the basal forebrain during recovery sleep after sleep restriction are associated with biomarkers of sleep propensity such as high electroencephalographic (EEG) delta power (0.5 to 4 Hz) and greater duration of NREM sleep episodes.[27] Adenosine signaling has been shown to promote sleep, in part, by actions within the preoptic,[28,29] posterior,[30] and perifornical[31] hypothalamic regions, pontine reticular formation,[32–34] and prefrontal cortex.[5]

Of relevance to the shared circuits hypothesis are data showing that sleep deprivation decreases the time to loss of righting response and increases the time to recovery of righting response caused by propofol or isoflurane.[35] Similarly, administration of adenosine receptor antagonists into the basal forebrain partially reverses the enhancement

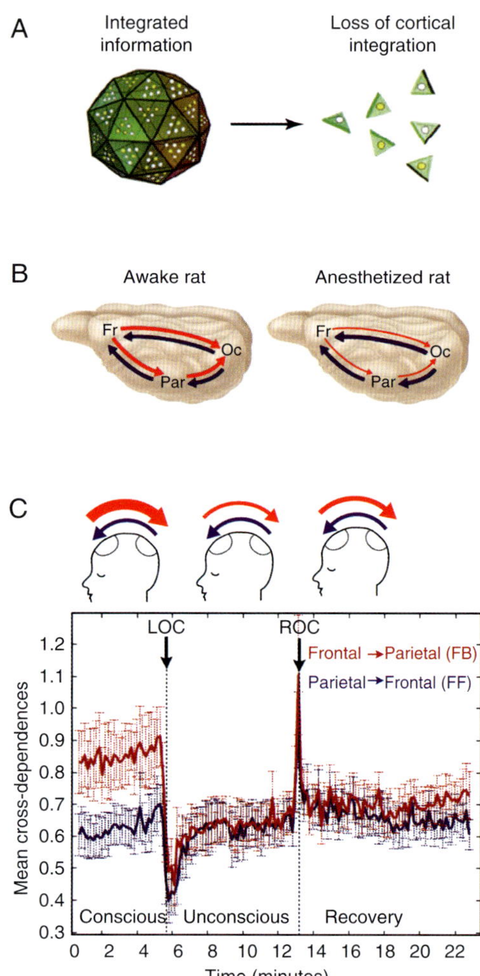

Figure 3.1 Loss of consciousness induced by anesthesia as described by the cortical integration and cognitive unbinding hypotheses. A. During wakefulness, information is integrated by effective connectivity between the thalamocortical system and high-order association areas. During general anesthesia and sleep, the process of integrating information is disrupted, causing unconsciousness. B. During wakefulness, the transfer of information between frontal (Fr), occipital (Oc), and parietal (Par) cortices is balanced between the feedforward (blue arrows) and feedback (red arrows) directions. The thickness of the arrows represents the amount of information transferred between each cortical region. During isoflurane anesthesia the feedback process is reduced, implying a substantial disruption in front-to-back cortical connectivity and thus disruption of integration. Modified from Alkire et al., Consciousness and anesthesia. *Science*. 2008;322:876–880. C. Frontoparietal interactions as a function of state of consciousness in humans. The feedback (FB, red) interaction is reduced during propofol-induced loss of consciousness, whereas the feedforward (FF, blue) interaction remains relatively constant across states of consciousness, except during the transitions to loss (LOC) and recovery (ROC) of consciousness. Thus, diminished cortical functional connectivity (unbinding) is one mechanism underlying the loss of consciousness induced by anesthetic drugs in humans. Reprinted from Lee U, Kim S, Noh G, et al. The directionality and functional organization of frontoparietal connectivity during consciousness and anesthesia in humans. *Conscious Cogn*. 2009;18:1069–1078, with permission from Elsevier.

of anesthetic-induced loss of righting response caused by prior sleep deprivation.[36] At present, there is no clinical evidence supporting the idea that the induction of, depth of, or recovery from general anesthesia can be significantly impacted by administering anesthetics to patients who have been deprived of sleep (Process S), or who are at different phases of their circadian cycles (Process C). Possibly, the combination of drugs and the doses used clinically overcome any potential effects of an increased sleep drive due to prior deprivation or circadian phase.

Opioids are major analgesic drugs commonly used to treat perioperative pain and are known to disrupt sleep homeostasis.[37,38] Microdialysis delivery of opioids to the substantia innominata region of the basal forebrain and to the pontine reticular formation causes a significant decrease in adenosine levels in both of these brain regions.[39] These data are consistent with the interpretation that causing a decrease in adenosine levels in these sleep-modulating brain areas is one mechanism by which opioids disrupt the temporal organization of sleep and wakefulness.[37] Opioid induced sleep disruption is directly relevant to anesthesiology because sleep disruption, even in pain free humans, causes hyperalgesia[40] that leads to an increase in opioid requirement for adequate pain management.

NEUROCHEMISTRY OF SLEEP, WAKEFULNESS, AND GENERAL ANESTHESIA

Restrictions on chapter length preclude reviewing data from all brain regions known to be relevant for the regulation of sleep and anesthesia. Readers are referred elsewhere[22,41–43] for information on additional brain regions that regulate sleep. Although the spinal cord is not necessary for generating sleep, spinal mechanisms participate in generating characteristic traits of anesthetic states such as immobility and analgesia.[44]

THE FOREBRAIN

Prefrontal Cortex

The prefrontal cortex (PFC) mediates motor and cognitive functions, is highly active during wakefulness, (Figure 3.2a), and is deactivated during sleep.[45–47] Activity in the PFC and cognitive performance are critically impaired by prolonged wakefulness. Preclinical pharmacological data are consistent with the view that the PFC also contributes to the regulation of arousal. Direct administration of an adenosine A_1 receptor agonist to the PFC decreases acetylcholine release in the PFC and increases recovery time from anesthesia.[5] Similarly, blocking adenosine receptors in the PFC increases acetylcholine release in the PFC, decreases recovery time from anesthesia, and increases time spent in wakefulness at

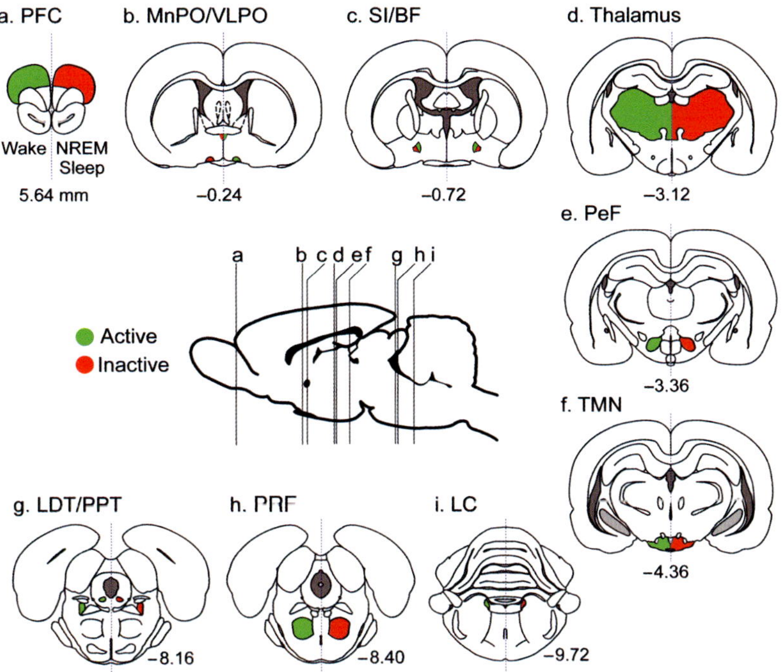

Figure 3.2 Major brain regions that regulate sleep and wakefulness. Vertical lines on the schematic sagittal view of the rat brain (center) indicate the rostral-to-caudal span of the coronal drawings of brain sections (a to i). The distance from bregma (mm) is indicated below each schematic. Brain areas described in this chapter are identified by colors. Active brain areas are shown in green, and inactive brain areas are shown in red. Activity during wakefulness is indicated on the left half of the brain, and activity during sleep is indicated on the right side of the coronal brain drawings. Abbreviations: LC, locus coeruleus; LDT/PPT, laterodorsal and pedunculopontine tegmental nuclei; PeF, perifornical region of the hypothalamus; PFC, prefrontal cortex (frontal association area, rat homologue of prefrontal cortex); PRF, pontine reticular formation; SI/BF, substantia innominata region of the basal forebrain; TMN, tuberomammillary nucleus of the hypothalamus; MnPO/VLPO, median preoptic nucleus and ventrolateral preoptic area of the hypothalamus.

the expense of time spent asleep.[5] These findings are consistent with the interpretation that adenosine in the PFC functions to inhibit arousal. Moreover, acetylcholine release within the pontine reticular formation is increased or decreased, respectively, by dialysis delivery of adenosine receptor agonists or antagonists to the PFC.[5] Collectively, these data support the idea that a descending system that inhibits wakefulness originates, in part, in the PFC and is modulated by adenosine A_1 receptors. These data encourage future studies to further characterize the mechanisms by which adenosine in the PFC modulates sleep and wakefulness, as well as anesthesia-induced loss and resumption of consciousness.

Basal Forebrain

The basal forebrain (Figure 3.2c) comprises a bilateral group of brain structures including the medial septal nuclei, the diagonal band of Broca, the basal nucleus of Meynert, and the substantia innominata. Two major populations of projection neurons that are located within the basal forebrain include acetylcholine-containing neurons and GABA-containing neurons. Acetylcholine-containing neurons of the basal forebrain play a role in the generation of cortical activation, behavioral arousal, and attention.[48,49] These cholinergic neurons receive excitatory projections from brainstem and hypothalamic arousal-promoting nuclei, and project to the entire cerebral cortex.[50–52]

Recording the discharge patterns of single neurons across the sleep-wake cycle revealed that identified cholinergic neurons are active during wakefulness and REM sleep.[53] Expression of the immediate early gene Fos is a marker of cell activity, and Fos expression in basal forebrain cholinergic neurons is lowest during NREM sleep.[54] Consistent with these data are findings showing that acetylcholine release in the basal forebrain[55] and cortex[56] is greater during wakefulness and REM sleep than during NREM sleep. Measures of attention and cognitive function combined with functional neuroanatomy using MRI show that acetylcholine regulates attention, and that administration of the muscarinic receptor antagonist scopolamine decreases brain activation in the anterior cingulate cortex and disrupts information processing.[57]

In humans, the acetylcholinesterase inhibitor physostigmine reverses the hypnotic effect of sevoflurane anesthesia.[58] Morphine decreases acetylcholine release in the prefrontal cortex, and this effect is mediated, in part, at the level of the basal forebrain.[59] Thus, anesthetic drugs and opioids may blunt or disrupt consciousness by decreasing cortical acetylcholine release.

GABAergic neurons are codistributed with cholinergic neurons within the basal forebrain and project in parallel with cholinergic neurons to cortical areas.[60] These basal forebrain GABAergic neurons innervate cortical GABAergic interneurons[61] that modulate the activity of large populations of pyramidal cells. GABAergic cells in the basal forebrain express Fos in association with NREM sleep and contain alpha-2 receptors, suggesting that these sleep active neurons are inhibited during wakefulness by noradrenergic projections that originate in the locus coeruleus.[54] Electrophysiological recordings of identified basal forebrain GABAergic neurons across the sleep-wake cycle revealed that these cells are functionally heterogeneous. For example, similar to cholinergic neurons, some GABAergic cells exhibited greatest discharge rates during wakefulness and REM sleep, others discharged maximally during NREM sleep, and a third group fired fastest during REM sleep.[62] These data suggest that GABAergic neurons in the basal forebrain modulate arousal state.

Preoptic Area of the Hypothalamus

Since the early 20th century the hypothalamus has been proposed to contain mutually antagonistic centers that drive either sleep or wakefulness, with the anterior hypothalamus being sleep promoting.[63,64] The suprachiasmatic nucleus (SCN) and the preoptic area (POA) are two critical regions within the anterior hypothalamus that regulate states of sleep and wakefulness. The SCN generates circadian rhythms, and there are studies suggesting a direct role of the SCN in sleep regulation.[65,66,67] There is, however, no evidence indicating that the SCN mediates anesthesia-induced loss of consciousness.

Electrolytic and neurotoxin-induced lesions, as well as electrical and neurochemical stimulation studies have demonstrated that the POA (Figure 3.2b) participates in the generation of NREM sleep.[68] Based on Fos expression studies, a cluster of neurons in the ventrolateral division of rat preoptic area (VLPO) has been shown to be sleep-active.[69] Recordings from VLPO (Figure 3.2b) neurons that revealed an increase in firing rates during NREM sleep compared to wakefulness reinforced this concept.[68] Most of the NREM sleep-active neurons in the VLPO are GABAergic and galaninergic.[68] However, Fos studies failed to identify this NREM sleep-active cluster of neurons in cat VLPO, perhaps because neurons with sleep- and wakefulness-related discharge patterns are intermingled in different regions of cat POA.[67,70] In addition, a cluster of cells located dorsally and medially to the VLPO in the rat (named extended-VLPO; eVLPO), showed increased Fos expression during REM sleep, but not during NREM sleep.[71] Lesions of the eVLPO area produced a significant decrease in the amount of REM sleep but caused only minor reductions in NREM sleep.[71] This REM sleep–related area has not been identified in cat.[67] A separate aggregate of neurons that express Fos immunoreactivity during NREM sleep has been identified in the median preoptic nucleus (MnPO) of rat and cat.[67,72] MnPO (Figure 3.2b) neurons increase their firing rates during sleep, and chemical stimulation or inhibition of this nucleus in rat generates or inhibits NREM sleep, respectively.[73,74] Several lines of evidence suggest that the POA contributes to sleep regulation by inhibitory projections to wakefulness-promoting neurons of the hypothalamus and brainstem.[68]

The POA has been carefully investigated as a possible site of action for general anesthetic and hypnotic drugs. Intra-POA administration of propofol, pentobarbital, and triazolam increases sleep in the rat.[75–77] Moreover, administering drugs that enhance GABAergic transmission, such as pentobarbital or the selective alpha-2 adrenoceptor agonist dexmedetomidine, increases the activity of VLPO neurons.[9,78] These results suggest that the VLPO may inhibit arousal-promoting neuronal networks during anesthesia. Contrasting with this interpretation is the fact that systemic administration of the benzodiazepine triazolam to POA-lesioned rats causes hypnosis.[79] This finding is consistent with the interpretation that there is more than one anatomical site by which general anesthetic and hypnotic drugs act to cause loss of consciousness.

Perifornical Region and Posterior Hypothalamus

The posterolateral region of the hypothalamus (including the perifornical region; Figure 3.2e) comprises a large area containing small to middle sized neurons that utilize several types of neurotransmitters. The tuberomammillary nucleus (Figure 3.2f) is also located within the hypothalamus.[80] Specific neuronal groups within these regions that contribute to the control of sleep and wakefulness are discussed below.

Hypocretin/Orexin Neurons

Neurons that synthesize and release the neuropeptides hypocretin-1 and 2 (also called orexin-A and B) are localized within the perifornical, dorsal, and posterior subregions of the lateral hypothalamus.[81] Hypocretins/orexins are excitatory neuropeptides that exert their biological effects through two metabotropic receptors. Numerous publications have posited that the hypocretin/orexin system is involved in the regulation of sleep and wakefulness. Disruption of this system results in the sleep disorder narcolepsy in which hypersomnia is the most common symptom.[82,83] Fos staining and extracellular recordings of identified neurons have demonstrated that hypocretin/orexin neurons are active during wakefulness characterized by motor activity.[84–87] The wakefulness-promoting effects of hypocretin/orexin-containing neurons are mediated by direct projections to the thalamocortical system, as well as by interactions with other wakefulness-promoting systems.[88,89]

Many studies suggest that general anesthetics modulate the hypocretin/orexin system to induce loss of consciousness. Several anesthetic drugs inhibit c-Fos expression in hypocretin/orexin neurons.[8,9] Hypocretin/orexin receptor agonists decrease the duration and depth of anesthesia, whereas administration of a hypocretin/orexin receptor-1 antagonist increases the duration of anesthesia.[90,91] Consistent with the shared circuits hypothesis,[1] hypocretin/orexin acts on multiple neural networks that are important for generating states of sleep and anesthesia. Hypocretin/orexin interacts with the basal forebrain cholinergic system to modulate the link between attention and arousal.[92] Sleep is strongly modulated by adenosine, and hypocretin/orexin neurons in the hypothalamus express adenosine A1 receptors.[93] Genetic ablation of hypocretin/orexin neurons, which causes murine narcolepsy, delays emergence from isoflurane and sevoflurane anesthesia without changing anesthetic induction time.[8] Administering a hypocretin-1 receptor antagonist delayed emergence as well, lending additional support to the interpretation that hypocretin/orexin promotes wakefulness.[8] These data also indicate that anesthetic induction and emergence are different, rather than mirror image, processes.[8] Mice lacking hypocretin/orexin neurons, however, did not show delayed emergence from halothane anesthesia.[94] The findings demonstrate that anesthetic drugs exert their effects by modulating distinct neurotransmitter systems and diverse brain areas. Microinjecting hypocretin-1/orexin-A into the pontine reticular formation, a sleep regulating brain region, also causes antinociception.[95] This finding raises the possibility that some anesthetic drugs may cause analgesia by modulating the effects of hypocretins/orexins within brain areas that participate in pain processing.

Melanin Concentrating Hormone-Containing Neurons

Melanin-concentrating hormone (MCH) is a 19-amino acid cyclic neuropeptide contained in neurons localized in the lateral hypothalamus and incertohypothalamic area, where the zona incerta merges with the medial hypothalamus.[96,97] These neurons send projections throughout the central nervous system. There are particularly dense MCHergic projections and MCH receptors in hypothalamic and brainstem areas that are involved in the regulation of sleep and wakefulness.[96,98] A number of physiological studies support the concept that MCHergic neurons promote sleep. Two independent groups have shown that MCHergic neurons express c-Fos during sleep.[99,100] Intraventricular and intracerebral microinjection of MCH promotes REM sleep,[100–102] and systemically applied MCH receptor-1 antagonists decrease both NREM sleep and REM sleep.[103] Future studies are needed to determine whether MCHergic neurons are causally involved in generating states of general anesthesia.

Histaminergic Neurons

Neurons that utilize histamine as a neurotransmitter are exclusively localized in the tuberomammillary nucleus (TMN; Figure 3.2f) of the posterior hypothalamus.[104] Several studies have shown that histaminergic neurons are involved in the maintenance of wakefulness. Accordingly, sleepiness is a side effect of clinically used antihistaminergic drugs.[105] Systemic administration of the alpha-2 adrenoceptor agonist dexmedetomidine decreases Fos immunoreactivity within the TMN. Drugs that cause sedation or anesthesia by activation of $GABA_A$ receptors also increase Fos expression in the TMN. These data suggested that the sedative/anesthetic effects are mediated, in part, by inhibiting wakefulness-promoting histaminergic neurons of the TMN. This inhibition is thought to be mediated by GABAergic/galaninergic projections to the TMN that originate in the VLPO.[9,78] In support of this hypothesized mechanism of action, microinjection of a $GABA_A$ receptor antagonist into the TMN attenuates the sedative responses to GABAergic drugs and dexmedetomidine.[78,106]

Delivery of histamine into the basal forebrain (Figure 3.2c) causes a significant increase in wakefulness and decrease in NREM sleep.[107] Pharmacological activation of histamine type 1 (H1) receptors in the basal forebrain increases EEG activation, increases respiratory rates, and decreases time to emergence from anesthesia with isoflurane. These data suggest that the wakefulness promoting effect of histamine is mediated by H1 receptors in the basal forebrain.[108]

Thalamus

The thalamus (Figure 3.2d) is the major gateway for the flow of sensory information from the periphery into the cortex, and the thalamus receives inputs from the cerebellum, basal ganglia, cortex, and reticular formation.[109] The thalamus and its strong reciprocal connections with the neocortex are the main substrates for the EEG rhythms that occur in wakefulness and sleep.[22] During wakefulness, networks promoting EEG and behavioral arousal depolarize thalamic neurons that project to the cortex (thalamocortical neurons) allowing sensory information to be faithfully transmitted to the cortex. In this depolarized condition thalamic neurons are in the "transmission mode."[22] During the transition to sleep, spindles are generated by a reverberation between thalamocortical and thalamic reticular neurons.[110] As deep NREM sleep develops, thalamocortical neurons hyperpolarize due to the loss of excitatory inputs and enter into a low-frequency (1–4 Hz) bursting mode set by intrinsic conductances (I_T and I_h).[22] This hyperpolarization and fixed pattern of discharge impair sensory transmission toward the cortex. In addition, because of extensive lateral connectivity, this pattern of activity spreads to large groups of thalamic and cortical neurons and causes the large amplitude synchronous slow oscillations of the EEG that characterize NREM sleep.[22]

The thalamus and its network interactions with the cerebral cortex play a critical role in the generation of conscious awareness. One of the more consistent regional effects produced by anesthetics at the onset of loss of consciousness is a reduction of thalamic metabolism and blood flow.[111] Some investigators conceptualize this as a "thalamic switch" during which a hyperpolarization block of thalamocortical neurons mediates sleep and anesthetic-induced loss of wakefulness.[112] This thalamic suppressive action has also been proposed as a part of the hypothesized cascade of events produced by general anesthetics.[113] Available data caution that thalamic gating varies as a function of sensory modality, anesthetic agent, dose, and species. During deep anesthesia produced by isoflurane, desflurane, or propofol, visual stimuli can still cause cortical activation in rat.[114] Human imaging studies show that during loss of consciousness caused by propofol the auditory cortex remained responsive to auditory stimuli while higher-level processing of the auditory signal was eliminated.[115] Commentaries on the elegant study by Plourde and colleagues point to evidence for the existence of unconscious processing of auditory input during anesthesia.[116] This commentary demonstrates the importance of differentiating loss of consciousness caused by propofol from loss of consciousness characteristic of physiological sleep.

GABA agonists microinjected into the centromedial thalamic nucleus produce sleep.[117] The medial, centromedial, and intralaminar thalamic nuclei have widespread projections to the cortex and are especially important for maintaining wakefulness. In fact, rats anesthetized with sevoflurane can be awakened by microinjecting nicotine into the centromedial thalamic nucleus.[118] These results suggest that suppression of cholinergic inputs to the midline thalamus may be one of the mechanisms by which anesthetics produce loss of consciousness. Nevertheless, quantitative analyses from simultaneous cortical and subcortical electrophysiological recordings during induction of anesthesia revealed that, at loss of consciousness, the cerebral cortex is significantly deactivated whereas there is little effect on subcortical (i.e., "mainly thalamic") parameters.[119] These data can be contrasted with the finding that deactivation or inhibition of the thalamus caused by anesthetic drugs is sufficient to cause loss of consciousness.[6,118] These studies point to an important future research opportunity to determine the extent to which anesthetics cause loss of consciousness by actions on the cortex and/or the thalamus.

THE BRAINSTEM

Cholinergic Nuclei in the Mesopontine Tegmentum

The laterodorsal and pedunculopontine tegmental nuclei (LDT/PPT; Figure 3.2g) are localized at the level of the pontomesencephalic junction and contain large cholinergic and noncholinergic neurons.[120,121] Cholinergic LDT/PPT neurons cause cortical activation during wakefulness and REM sleep by ascending projections via a ventral extrathalamic pathway to the hypothalamus and basal forebrain, and via a dorsal pathway to the thalamus.[122,123] Descending projections from the LDT/PPT to a cholinoceptive area of the pontine reticular formation are key for REM sleep generation.[124,125] Electrophysiological recordings from single neurons show that presumably cholinergic neurons in the LDT/PPT discharge in a state-dependent manner and are classified into two distinctive groups, a REM-on subpopulation, and a Wake-on/REM-on subpopulation.[126,127] Cholinergic neurons in the LDT/PPT express Fos during the sleep rebound after selective REM sleep deprivation,[128] and neurotoxic lesion of cholinergic neurons in the LDT/PPT cause a reduction in REM sleep.[129] Acetylcholine release in the pontine reticular formation is greater during REM sleep than during wakefulness and NREM sleep,[130,131] and microinjection of cholinomimetics generates a REM sleep–like state.[132] Taken together, this evidence supports the conclusion that acetylcholine released from LDT-PPT neurons that project to the pontine reticular formation contributes to the generation of REM sleep.

Acetylcholine release in the pontine reticular formation is decreased by halothane anesthesia[133] and by systemic administration of ketamine.[134] In addition, generation of cortical EEG spindles occurs in association with decreased acetylcholine release in the pontine reticular formation during halothane anesthesia.[133] Opioids obtund wakefulness and disrupt normal sleep[37] in part by decreasing acetylcholine release in the pontine reticular formation.[134] Thus, general anesthetics and opioids eliminate wakefulness and disrupt natural sleep by decreasing cholinergic transmission within the pontine reticular formation.

Locus Coeruleus

The locus coeruleus (LC; Figure 3.2i) is localized in the dorsolateral mesopontine region of the brainstem and is defined by norepinephrine-containing neurons. LC neurons project diffusely to the forebrain, neocortex, brainstem, and spinal cord to promote wakefulness and facilitate muscle tone.[135] LC neurons discharge tonically during wakefulness[136] when norepinephrine release in the cortex is maximal,[137] decrease their discharge rates during NREM sleep, and stop firing during REM sleep.

The selective alpha-2 adrenoceptor agonist dexmedetomidine is thought to cause hypnosis, in part, by inhibiting the firing of LC neurons.[78,138] The sedative effects of dexmedetomidine are suggested to result from the inhibition of LC and histaminergic neurons, with the subsequent disinhibition of sleep-promoting VLPO neurons.[78] Sevoflurane and isoflurane increase norepinephrine release in the preoptic area.[139] A possible mechanism for the high incidence of emergence agitation after sevoflurane anesthesia may be related to a direct excitatory effect of sevoflurane on LC neurons.[140] In addition, it is becoming clear that alpha-2 adrenoceptors on nonadrenergic neurons also mediate the sedating effect of alpha-2 agonists.[141]

Pontine Reticular Formation

The pontine reticular formation (PRF; Figure 3.2h) comprises a part of the ascending reticular activating system.[142] The midbrain and rostral portions of the pontine reticular formation send ascending projections, presumably glutamatergic, that activate thalamocortical and basalocortical systems. The caudal pons and medulla contain reticulospinal neurons that facilitate maintenance of skeletal muscle tone during wakefulness.[143]

The PRF contributes to the generation of sleep and wakefulness,[22] and general anesthesia.[10] Although the synaptic mechanisms remain to be specified for specific anesthetic agents, several lines of research support the conclusion that GABA acts in the PRF to generate wakefulness. Microinjection of $GABA_A$ receptor agonists into the PRF increases wakefulness and suppresses sleep.[144,145] Conversely, microinjection of $GABA_A$ antagonists into the same pontine area decreases wakefulness and increases REM sleep.[145] Accordingly, increasing pontine GABA levels by blocking GABA uptake mechanisms or decreasing GABA levels by interfering with the synthesis of GABA increases or decreases wakefulness, respectively.[146] The data suggest that an endogenous sleep promoting network is tonically modulated by GABAergic mechanisms within the PRF. Local and systemic administration of the mu opioid receptor agonist morphine disrupts normal sleep, decreases wakefulness, and decreases GABA levels in the PRF.[147] In agreement with a wakefulness-promoting role for GABA in the PRF, isoflurane anesthesia significantly decreases GABA levels in the PRF.[12] The isoflurane-induced decrease in GABA levels occurs in association with cortical deactivation and reduced dorsal neck muscle tone.

Studies using rodents to investigate mechanisms of anesthetic action commonly use time to loss of righting reflex as an index of unconsciousness and time to resumption of righting reflex as a measure of time needed to recover from anesthesia.[8,12,118] Figure 3.3 illustrates that microinjection of receptor agonists and antagonists into specific brain regions can be used to alter loss and resumption of righting in response to anesthetic administration. Such studies permit inferences about the roles of the receptor subtypes and brain regions that regulate anesthetic states. For example, in the PRF pharmacologically increasing or decreasing GABA levels increases or decreases, respectively, the time required to induce anesthesia with isoflurane.[12] These results support the interpretation that isoflurane causes loss of consciousness, in part, by decreasing GABA levels in the PRF.[12]

OPPORTUNITIES FOR ANESTHESIA RESEARCH

Calls for the convergence of research on mechanisms of anesthetic action with studies of sleep neurobiology are as recent as 1994.[148] The 16-year interval from 1994 to the present chapter represents only about 10% of the total time since the 1846 discovery of anesthesia. Although the convergence of anesthesia research and sleep research is recent, it is conceptually based, and research convergence is clinically relevant.

The conceptual value of linking investigations into the mechanisms of general anesthesia to cognitive neuroscience has been described elsewhere.[16,17] The 2009 celebration of the 150th anniversary of Charles Darwin's publication of *On the Origin of Species* also provides a reminder that during the course of evolution, exposure to halogenated ether did not impact brain development. Convergent, divergent,

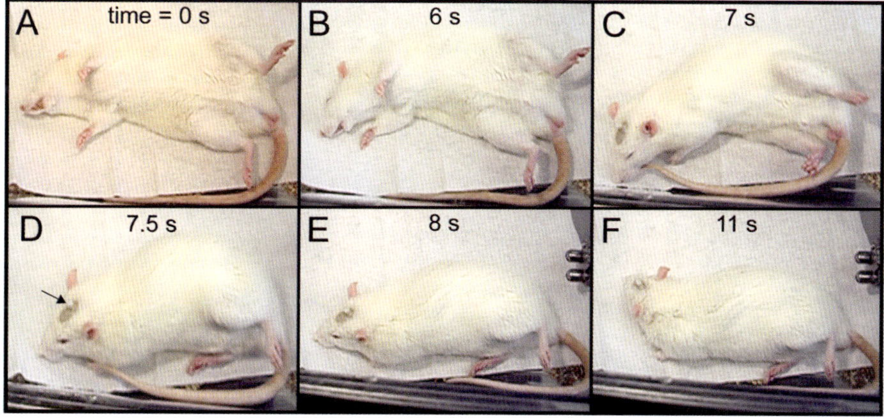

Figure 3.3 Time to resumption of righting response in rodents is an accepted surrogate measure for the time needed to regain consciousness after general anesthesia. The sequence of photographs (from A to F) shows a typical resumption of righting response in rat. Animals are placed in dorsal recumbency (A; time = 0 seconds) and resumption of righting is complete when animals regain consciousness and turn over (F). This rat was implanted with a microinjection guide cannula (arrow in frame D) used to deliver drugs into the pontine reticular formation.

or parallel evolutionary schemes offer no justification for evolutionary development of an "anesthesia center" in the brain. The hypothesis of a single brain region causing sleep or anesthesia is a throwback to an 1850s postulate by Flourens that a single "vital node" generates the oscillations between inspiratory and expiratory phases of the respiratory cycle.[149] Environmental[150] and metabolic[151] pressures did push the mammalian nervous system to evolve neural networks that generate periodic states of behavioral activity (wakefulness) and inactivity (sleep). The data selectively reviewed here and elsewhere[95,152] support the interpretation that neural circuits generating sleep are the cellular substrates that are preferentially altered by anesthetics.

Efforts to understand states of anesthesia and sleep are also conceptually linked by the insight that these states can be identified and classified based on a constellation of physiological and behavioral traits. A systematic trait analysis was the basis of Guedel's classic system for evaluating anesthetic depth.[153] Trait analysis was also the thesis of Hobson's 1978 paper operationally defining the behavioral state concept for integrative neuroscience.[154] As Hobson defined it, "the state of a system at a given instant is the set of numerical values which its variables have at that instant." Guedel succeeded in choosing the variables (traits) providing a reliable index for depth of anesthesia. The foregoing concepts are the basis for ongoing research opportunities to develop systems that can objectively assess anesthetic states using a simple trait such as a numerically transformed single EEG recording.[155]

The clinical relevance for convergence of anesthesiology research and sleep research is encouraged by the fact that loss of wakefulness causes disruptions in autonomic physiology.[156] Pain prevention and management is the raison d'être for anesthesiology. Anatomically distributed neuronal networks cause pain.[157,158] Thus, anesthetics are effective at blocking pain in part because of their anatomically distributed actions. Human imaging data show that isoflurane,[159] opioids,[160] and propofol[161] alter activity in multiple neuronal circuits. The unwanted side effect of autonomic disruption occurs because many of these neuronal circuits also regulate autonomic function. Research on the brain mechanisms underlying sleep-related autonomic disruption will aid in the rational, as opposed to empiric, development of anesthetic drugs that cause minimal autonomic disruption. The convergence of sleep research and anesthesia research is also an opportunity to enhance care for patients with sleep-disordered breathing who are known to be at risk for adverse anesthetic outcome.[162,163]

ACKNOWLEDGMENTS

Support: National Institutes of Health Grant numbers: HL40881, MH45361, HL57120, HL65272 and the Department of Anesthesiology.

REFERENCES

1. Lydic R, Reticular modulation of breathing during sleep and anesthesia. *Curr Opin Pulm Med.* 1996;2:474–481.
2. Mashour GA, Lipinski WJ, Matlen LB, et al. Isoflurane anesthesia does not satisfy the homeostatic need for rapid eye movement sleep. *Anesth Analg.* 2010;110:1283–1289.
3. Abulafia R, Zalkind V, Devor M. Cerebral activity during the anesthesia-like state induced by mesopontine microinjection of pentobarbital. *J Neurosci.* 2009;29:7053–7064.
4. Zecharia AY, Nelson LE, Gent TC, et al. Involvement of hypothalamic sleep pathways in general anesthesia: testing the hypothesis using the GABA-A receptor β3N265N knock-in mouse. *J Neurosci.* 2009;29:2177–2187.
5. Van Dort CJ, Baghdoyan HA, Lydic R. Adenosine A(1) and A(2A) receptors in mouse prefrontal cortex modulate acetylcholine release and behavioral arousal. *J Neurosci.* 2009;29:871–881.
6. Alkire MT, Hudetz AG, Tononi G. Consciousness and anesthesia. *Science.* 2008;322:876–880.
7. Franks NP. General anaesthesia: from molecular targets to neuronal pathways of sleep and arousal. *Nat Rev Neurosci.* 2008;9:370–386.
8. Kelz MB, Sun Y, Chen J, et al. An essential role for orexins in emergence from general anesthesia. *Proc Natl Acad Sci U S A.* 2008;105:1309–1314.
9. Lu J, Nelson LE, Franks N, et al. Role of endogenous sleep-wake and analgesic systems in anesthesia. *J Comp Neurol.* 2008;508:648–662.
10. Lydic R, Baghdoyan HA. Sleep, anesthesiology, and the neurobiology of arousal state control. *Anesthesiology.* 2005;103:1268–1295.
11. Tung A, Mendelson WB. Anesthesia and sleep. *Sleep Med Rev.* 2004;8:213–225.
12. Vanini G, Watson CJ, Lydic R, et al. Gamma-aminobutyric acid-mediated neurotransmission in the pontine reticular formation modulates hypnosis, immobility, and breathing during isoflurane anesthesia. *Anesthesiology.* 2008;109:978–988.
13. Ma J, Shen B, Stewart LS, et al. The septohippocampal system participates in general anesthesia. *J Neurosci.* 2002;22:1–6.
14. Lee RS, Steffensen SC, Henriksen SJ. Discharge profiles of ventral tegmental area GABA neurons during movement, anesthesia, and the sleep-wake cycle. *J Neurosci.* 2001;21:1757–1766.
15. Mashour GA. Consciousness unbound: toward a paradigm of general anesthesia. *Anesthesiology.* 2004;100:428–433.
16. Mashour GA. Integrating the science of consciousness and anesthesia. *Anesth Analg.* 2006;103:975–982.
17. Lee U, Mashour GA, Kim S, et al. Propofol induction reduces the capacity for neural information integration: implications for the mechanisms of consciousness and general anesthesia. *Conscious Cogn.* 2009;18:56–64.
18. Lee U, Kim S, Noh GJ, et al. The directionality and functional organization of frontoparietal connectivity during consciousness and anesthesia in humans. *Conscious Cogn.* 2009;18:1069–1078.
19. Ferrarelli F, Massimini M, Sarasso S, et al. Breakdown in cortical effective connectivity during midazolam-induced loss of consciousness. *Proc Natl Acad Sci U S A.* 2010;107(6):2681–2686.
20. Massimini M, Ferrarelli F, Huber R, et al. Breakdown of cortical effective connectivity during sleep. *Science.* 2005;309:2228–2232.
21. Achermann P, Borbely AA. Mathematical models of sleep regulation. *Front Biosci.* 2003;8:683–693.
22. Steriade M, McCarley RW. *Brain Control of Wakefulness and Sleep.* New York: Kluwer Academic/Plenum Press; 2005.
23. McCarley R. Neurobiology of REM and NREM sleep. *Sleep Med Rev.* 2007;8:302–330.
24. Radulovacki M. Adenosine sleep theory: how I postulated it. *Neurol Res.* 2005;27:137–138.
25. Porkka-Heiskanen T, Strecker RE, McCarley RW. Brain site-specificity of extracellular adenosine concentration changes during sleep deprivation and spontaneous sleep: an in vivo microdialysis study. *Neuroscience.* 2000;99:507–517.

26. Porkka-Heiskanen T, Strecker RE, Thakkar M, et al. Adenosine: a mediator of the sleep-inducing effects of prolonged wakefulness. *Science.* 1997;276:1265–1268.
27. McKenna JT, Tartar JL, Ward CP, et al. Sleep fragmentation elevates behavioral, electrographic and neurochemical measures of sleepiness. *Neuroscience.* 2007;146:1462–1473.
28. Methippara MM, Kumar S, Alam MN, et al. Effects on sleep of microdialysis of adenosine A1 and A2a receptor analogs into the lateral preoptic area of rats. *Am J Physiol Regul Integr Comp Physiol.* 2005;289:1715–1723.
29. Morairty S, Rainnie D, McCarley R, et al. Disinhibition of ventrolateral preoptic area sleep-active neurons by adenosine: a new mechanism for sleep promotion. *Neuroscience.* 2004;123:451–457.
30. Hong ZY, Huang ZL, Qu WM, et al. An adenosine A receptor agonist induces sleep by increasing GABA release in the tuberomammillary nucleus to inhibit histaminergic systems in rats. *J Neurochem.* 2005;92:1542–1549.
31. Thakkar MM, Engemann SC, Walsh KM, et al. Adenosine and the homeostatic control of sleep: effects of A1 receptor blockade in the perifornical lateral hypothalamus on sleep-wakefulness. *Neuroscience.* 2008;153:875–880.
32. Tanase D, Baghdoyan HA, Lydic R. Dialysis delivery of an adenosine A1 receptor agonist to the pontine reticular formation decreases acetylcholine release and increases anesthesia recovery time. *Anesthesiology.* 2003;98:912–920.
33. Marks GA, Shaffery JP, Speciale SG, et al. Enhancement of rapid eye movement sleep in the rat by actions at A1 and A2a adenosine receptor subtypes with a differential sensitivity to atropine. *Neuroscience.* 2003;116:913–920.
34. Coleman CG, Baghdoyan HA, Lydic R. Dialysis delivery of an adenosine A2A agonist into the pontine reticular formation of C57BL/6J mouse increases pontine acetylcholine release and sleep. *J Neurochem.* 2006;96:1750–1759.
35. Tung A, Szafran MJ, Bluhm B, et al. Sleep deprivation potentiates the onset and duration of loss of righting reflex induced by propofol and isoflurane. *Anesthesiology.* 2002;97:906–911.
36. Tung A, Herrera S, Szafran MJ, et al. Effect of sleep deprivation on righting reflex in the rat is partially reversed by administration of adenosine A1 and A2 receptor antagonists. *Anesthesiology.* 2005;102: 1158–1164.
37. Lydic R, Baghdoyan HA. Neurochemical mechanisms mediating opioid-induced REM sleep disruption. In: Lavigne G, Sessle BJ, Choiniere M, Soja PJ, eds. *Sleep and Pain*. Seattle: IASP Press; 2007.
38. Bonafide CP, Aucutt-Walter N, Divittore N, et al. Remifentanil inhibits rapid eye movement sleep but not the nocturnal melatonin surge in humans. *Anesthesiology.* 2008;108:627–633.
39. Nelson AM, Battersby AS, Baghdoyan HA, et al. Opioid-induced decreases in rat brain adenosine levels are reversed by inhibiting adenosine deaminase. *Anesthesiology.* 2009;111:1327–1333.
40. Chhangani BS, Roehrs TA, Harris EJ, et al. Pain sensitivity in sleepy pain-free normals. *Sleep.* 2009;32:1011–1017.
41. Monti JM, Pandi-Perumal SR, Sinton CM, eds. *The Neurochemistry of Sleep and Wakefulness*. Cambridge, UK: Cambridge University Press; 2008.
42. Hudetz AG, Pearce RA, eds. *Suppressing the Mind: Anesthetic Modulation of Memory and Consciousness*. Totowa, NJ: Humana/ Springer; 2009.
43. Mashour GA, ed. *Consciousness, Awareness, and Anesthesia*. New York, NY: Cambridge University Press; 2010.
44. Antognini JF, Carstens E. In vivo characterization of clinical anaesthesia and its components. *Br J Anaesth.* 2002;89:156–166.
45. Muzur A, Pace-Schott EF, Hobson JA. The prefrontal cortex in sleep. *Trends Cogn Sci.* 2002;6:475–481.
46. Nofzinger EA, Mintun MA, Wiseman M, et al. Forebrain activation in REM sleep: an FDG PET study. *Brain Res.* 1997;770:192–201.
47. Nofzinger EA, Buysse DJ, Miewald JM, et al. Human regional cerebral glucose metabolism during non-rapid eye movement sleep in relation to waking. *Brain.* 2002;125:1105–1115.
48. Semba K. The cholinergic basal forebrain: a critical role in cortical arousal. *Adv Exp Med Biol.* 1991;295:197–218.
49. Sarter M, Hasselmo ME, Bruno JP, et al. Unraveling the attentional functions of cortical cholinergic inputs: interactions between signal-driven and cognitive modulation of signal detection. *Brain Res Rev.* 2005;48:98–111.
50. Jones BE, Cuello AC. Afferents to the basal forebrain cholinergic cell area from pontomesencephalic—catecholamine, serotonin, and acetylcholine—neurons. *Neuroscience.* 1989;31:37–61.
51. Semba K, Reiner PB, McGeer EG, et al. Brainstem afferents to the magnocellular basal forebrain studied by axonal transport, immunohistochemistry, and electrophysiology in the rat. *J Comp Neurol.* 1988;267:433–453.
52. Semba K. Multiple output pathways of the basal forebrain: organization, chemical heterogeneity, and roles in vigilance. *Behav Brain Res.* 2000;115:117–141.
53. Lee MG, Manns ID, Alonso A, et al. Sleep-wake related discharge properties of basal forebrain neurons recorded with micropipettes in head-fixed rats. *J Neurophysiol.* 2004;92:1182–1198.
54. Modirrousta M, Mainville L, Jones BE. Gabaergic neurons with alpha2-adrenergic receptors in basal forebrain and preoptic area express c-Fos during sleep. *Neuroscience.* 2004;129:803–810.
55. Vazquez J, Baghdoyan HA. Basal forebrain acetylcholine release during REM sleep is significantly greater than during waking. *Am J Physiol Regul Integr Comp Physiol.* 2001;280:598–601.
56. Jasper HH, Tessier J. Acetylcholine liberation from cerebral cortex during paradoxical (REM) sleep. *Science.* 1971;172:601–602.
57. Thienel R, Kellermann T, Schall U, et al. Muscarinic antagonist effects on executive control of attention. *Int J Neuropsychopharm.* 2009;12:1307–1317.
58. Plourde G, Chartrand D, Fiset P, et al. Antagonism of sevoflurane anaesthesia by physostigmine: effects on the auditory steady-state response and bispectral index. *Br J Anaesth.* 2003;91:583–586.
59. Osman NI, Baghdoyan HA, Lydic R. Morphine inhibits acetylcholine release in rat prefrontal cortex when delivered systemically or by microdialysis to basal forebrain. *Anesthesiology.* 2005;103: 779–787.
60. Gritti I, Mainville L, Mancia M, et al. GABAergic and other noncholinergic basal forebrain neurons, together with cholinergic neurons, project to the mesocortex and isocortex in the rat. *J Comp Neurol.* 1997;383:163–177.
61. Freund TF, Meskenaite V. Gamma-Aminobutyric acid-containing basal forebrain neurons innervate inhibitory interneurons in the neocortex. *Proc Natl Acad Sci U S A.* 1992;89:738–742.
62. Hassani OK, Lee MG, Henny P, et al. Discharge profiles of identified GABAergic in comparison to cholinergic and putative glutamatergic basal forebrain neurons across the sleep-wake cycle. *J Neurosci.* 2009;29:11828–11840.
63. Nauta W. Hypothalamic regulation of sleep in rats. *J Neurophysiol.*1946;283–316.
64. von Economo C. Sleep as a problem of localization. *Journal of Nervous and Mental Disease.* 1930;71:249–259.
65. Deboer T, Vansteensel MJ, Detari L, et al. Sleep states alter activity of suprachiasmatic nucleus neurons. *Nat Neurosci.* 2003;6: 1086–1090.
66. Mistlberger RE. Circadian regulation of sleep in mammals: role of the suprachiasmatic nucleus. *Brain Res Rev.* 2005;49:429–454.
67. Torterolo P, Benedetto L, Lagos P, et al. State-dependent pattern of Fos protein expression in regionally-specific sites within the preoptic area of the cat. *Brain Res.* 2009;1267:44–56.
68. Szymusiak R, McGinty D. Hypothalamic regulation of sleep and arousal. *Ann N Y Acad Sci.* 2008;1129:275–286.
69. Sherin JE, Shiromani PJ, McCarley RW, et al. Activation of ventrolateral preoptic neurons during sleep. *Science.* 1996;271:216–219.
70. Wagner D, Salin-Pascual R, Greco MA, et al. Distribution of hypocretin-containing neurons in the lateral hypothalamus and C-fos-immunoreactive neurons in the VLPO. *Sleep Res Online.* 2000;3:35–42.

71. Lu J, Bjorkum AA, Xu M, et al. Selective activation of the extended ventrolateral preoptic nucleus during rapid eye movement sleep. *J Neurosci.* 2002;22:4568–4576.
72. Gong H, Szymusiak R, King J, et al. Sleep-related c-Fos protein expression in the preoptic hypothalamus: effects of ambient warming. *Am J Physiol Regul Integr Comp Physiol.* 2000;279:2079–2088.
73. Suntsova N, Szymusiak R, Alam MN, et al. Sleep-waking discharge patterns of median preoptic nucleus neurons in rats. *J Physiol.* 2002;543:665–677.
74. Suntsova N, Guzman-Marin R, Kumar S, et al. The median preoptic nucleus reciprocally modulates activity of arousal-related and sleep-related neurons in the perifornical lateral hypothalamus. *J Neurosci.* 2007;27:1616–1630.
75. Tung A, Bluhm B, Mendelson WB. The hypnotic effect of propofol in the medial preoptic area of the rat. *Life Sci.* 2001;69:855–862.
76. Mendelson WB. Sleep induction by microinjection of pentobarbital into the medial preoptic area in rats. *Life Sci.* 1996;59:1821–1828.
77. Mendelson WB, Martin JV, Perlis M, et al. Enhancement of sleep by microinjection of triazolam into the medial preoptic area. *Neuropsychopharmacology.* 1989;2:61–66.
78. Nelson LE, Lu J, Guo T, et al. The alpha2-adrenoceptor agonist dexmedetomidine converges on an endogenous sleep-promoting pathway to exert its sedative effects. *Anesthesiology.* 2003;98:428–436.
79. Mendelson WB. Effects of parenterally administered triazolam on sleep in rats with lesions of the preoptic area. *Pharmacol Biochem Behav.* 1998;61:81–86.
80. Simerly RB. Anatomical substrates of hypothalamic integration. In: Paxinos G, ed. *The Rat Nervous System.* San Diego, CA: Academic Press; 1995.
81. Peyron C, Tighe DK, van den Pol AN, et al. Neurons containing hypocretin (orexin) project to multiple neuronal systems. *J Neurosci.* 1998;18:9996–10015.
82. Fronczek R, Baumann CR, Lammers GJ, et al. Hypocretin/orexin disturbances in neurological disorders. *Sleep Med Rev.* 2009; 13:9–22.
83. Nunez A, Rodrigo-Angulo ML, Andres ID, et al. Hypocretin/orexin neuropeptides: participation in the control of sleep-wakefulness cycle and energy homeostasis. *Curr Neuropharmacol.* 2009;7:50–59.
84. Torterolo P, Yamuy J, Sampogna S, et al. Hypothalamic neurons that contain hypocretin (orexin) express c-fos during active wakefulness and carbachol-induced active sleep. *Sleep Res Online.* 2001;4(1): 25–32.
85. Torterolo P, Yamuy J, Sampogna S, et al. Hypocretinergic neurons are primarily involved in activation of the somatomotor system. *Sleep.* 2003;26:25–28.
86. Lee MG, Hassani OK, Jones BE. Discharge of identified orexin/hypocretin neurons across the sleep-waking cycle. *J Neurosci.* 2005;25:6716–6720.
87. Mileykovskiy BY, Kiyashchenko LI, Siegel JM. Behavioral correlates of activity in identified hypocretin/orexin neurons. *Neuron.* 2005;46:787–798.
88. Bernard R, Lydic R, Baghdoyan HA. Hypocretin-1 activates G proteins in arousal-related brainstem nuclei of rat. *Neuroreport.* 2002;13:447–450.
89. Govindaiah G, Cox CL. Modulation of thalamic neuron excitability by orexins. *Neuropharmacology.* 2006;51:414–425.
90. Kushikata T, Hirota K, Yoshida H, et al. Orexinergic neurons and barbiturate anesthesia. *Neuroscience.* 2003;121:855–863.
91. Yasuda Y, Takeda A, Fukuda S, et al. Orexin a elicits arousal electroencephalography without sympathetic cardiovascular activation in isoflurane-anesthetized rats. *Anesth Analg.* 2003;97:1663–1666.
92. Fadel J, Burk JA. Orexin/hypocretin modulation of the basal forebrain cholinergic system: Role in attention. *Brain Res.* 2009;1341: 112–123.
93. Thakkar MM, Winston S, McCarley RW. Orexin neurons of the hypothalamus express adenosine A1 receptors. *Brain Res.* 2002; 944:190–194.
94. Gompf H, Chen J, Sun Y, et al. Halothane-induced hypnosis is not accompanied by inactivation of orexinergic output in rodents. *Anesthesiology.* 2009;111:1001–1009.
95. Watson SL, Watson CJ, Baghdoyan HA, et al. Thermal nociception is decreased by hypocretin-1 and an adenosine-A1 receptor agonist microinjected into the pontine reticular formation of Sprague Dawley rat. *J Pain* 2010;11(6):535–544.
96. Bittencourt JC, Presse F, Arias C, et al. The melanin-concentrating hormone system of the rat brain: an immuno- and hybridization histochemical characterization. *J Comp Neurol.* 1992;319: 218–245.
97. Torterolo P, Sampogna S, Morales FR, et al. MCH-containing neurons in the hypothalamus of the cat: searching for a role in the control of sleep and wakefulness. *Brain Res.* 2006;1119:101–114.
98. Kilduff TS, de Lecea L. Mapping of the mRNAs for the hypocretin/orexin and melanin-concentrating hormone receptors: networks of overlapping peptide systems. *J Comp Neurol.* 2001; 435:1–5.
99. Verret L, Goutagny R, Fort P, et al. A role of melanin-concentrating hormone producing neurons in the central regulation of paradoxical sleep. *BMC Neurosci.* 2003;4:19.
100. Modirrousta M, Mainville L, Jones BE. Orexin and MCH neurons express c-Fos differently after sleep deprivation vs recovery and bear different adrenergic receptors. *Eur J Neurosci.* 2005;21: 2807–2816.
101. Lagos P, Torterolo P, Jantos H, et al. Effects on sleep of melanin-concentrating hormone (MCH) microinjections into the dorsal raphe nucleus. *Brain Res.* 2009;1265:103–110.
102. Torterolo P, Sampogna S, Chase MH. MCHergic projections to the nucleus pontis oralis participate in the control of active (REM) sleep. *Brain Res.* 2009;1268:76–87.
103. Ahnaou A, Drinkenburg WH, Bouwknecht JA, et al. Blocking melanin-concentrating hormone MCH1 receptor affects rat sleep-wake architecture. *Eur J Pharmacol.* 2008;579:177–188.
104. Haas HL, Sergeeva OA, Selbach O. Histamine in the nervous system. *Physiol Rev.* 2008;88:1183–1241.
105. Lin JS. Brain structures and mechanisms involved in the control of cortical activation and wakefulness, with emphasis on the posterior hypothalamus and histaminergic neurons. *Sleep Med Rev.* 2000; 4:471–503.
106. Nelson LE, Guo TZ, Lu J, et al. The sedative component of anesthesia is mediated by $GABA_A$ receptors in an endogenous sleep pathway. *Nat Neurosci.* 2002;5:979–984.
107. Ramesh V, Thakkar MM, Strecker RE, et al. Wakefulness-inducing effects of histamine in the basal forebrain of freely moving rats. *Behav Brain Res.* 2004;152:271–278.
108. Luo T, Leung LS. Basal forebrain histaminergic transmission modulates electroencephalographic activity and emergence from isoflurane anesthesia. *Anesthesiology.* 2009;111:725–733.
109. Price JL. Thalamus. In: Paxinos G, ed. *The Rat Nervous System.* San Diego, CA: Academic Press; 1995.
110. De Gennaro L, Ferrara M. Sleep spindles: an overview. *Sleep Med Rev.* 2003;7:423–440.
111. Alkire MT, Miller J. General anesthesia and the neural correlates of consciousness. *Prog Brain Res.* 2005;150:229–244.
112. Alkire MT, Haier RJ, Fallon JH. Toward a unified theory of narcosis: brain imaging evidence for a thalamocortical switch as the neurophysiologic basis of anesthetic-induced unconsciousness. *Conscious Cogn.* 2000;9:370–386.
113. John ER, Prichep LS. The anesthetic cascade: a theory of how anesthesia suppresses consciousness. *Anesthesiology.* 2005;102: 447–471.
114. Hudetz AG, Imas OA. Burst activation of the cerebral cortex by flash stimuli during isoflurane anesthesia in rats. *Anesthesiology.* 2007;107:983–991.
115. Plourde G, Belin P, Chartrand D, et al. Cortical processing of complex auditory stimuli during alterations of consciousness with the general anesthetic propofol. *Anesthesiology.* 2006;104:448–457.

116. Veselis RA. To sleep, perchance to decode? *Anesthesiology.* 2006;105:1278–1279.
117. Miller JW, Ferrendelli JA. Characterization of GABAergic seizure regulation in the midline thalamus. *Neuropharmacology.* 1990; 29:649–655.
118. Alkire MT, McReynolds JR, Hahn EL, et al. Thalamic microinjection of nicotine reverses sevoflurane-induced loss of righting reflex in the rat. *Anesthesiology.* 2007;107:264–272.
119. Velly LJ, Rey MF, Bruder NJ, et al. Differential dynamic of action on cortical and subcortical structures of anesthetic agents during induction of anesthesia. *Anesthesiology.* 2007;107:202–212.
120. Kimura H, McGeer PL, Peng JH, et al. The central cholinergic system studied by choline acetyltransferase immunohistochemistry in the cat. *J Comp Neurol.* 1981;200:151–201.
121. Wang HL, Morales M. Pedunculopontine and laterodorsal tegmental nuclei contain distinct populations of cholinergic, glutamatergic and GABAergic neurons in the rat. *Eur J Neurosci.* 2009;29:340–358.
122. Datta S, Maclean RR. Neurobiological mechanisms for the regulation of mammalian sleep-wake behavior: reinterpretation of historical evidence and inclusion of contemporary cellular and molecular evidence. *Neurosci Biobehav Rev.* 2007;31:775–824.
123. Hallanger AE, Wainer BH. Ascending projections from the pedunculopontine tegmental nucleus and the adjacent mesopontine tegmentum in the rat. *J Comp Neurol.* 1988;274:483–515.
124. Mitani A, Ito K, Hallanger AE, et al. Cholinergic projections from the laterodorsal and pedunculopontine tegmental nuclei to the pontine gigantocellular tegmental field in the cat. *Brain Res.* 1988;451:397–402.
125. Semba K, Fibiger HC. Afferent connections of the laterodorsal and the pedunculopontine tegmental nuclei in the rat: a retro- and antero-grade transport and immunohistochemical study. *J Comp Neurol.* 1992;323:387–410.
126. el Mansari M, Sakai K, Jouvet M. Unitary characteristics of presumptive cholinergic tegmental neurons during the sleep-waking cycle in freely moving cats. *Exp Brain Res.* 1989;76:519–529.
127. Thakkar MM, Strecker RE, McCarley RW. Behavioral state control through differential serotonergic inhibition in the mesopontine cholinergic nuclei: a simultaneous unit recording and microdialysis study. *J Neurosci.* 1998;18:5490–5497.
128. Maloney KJ, Mainville L, Jones BE. Differential c-Fos expression in cholinergic, monoaminergic, and GABAergic cell groups of the pontomesencephalic tegmentum after paradoxical sleep deprivation and recovery. *J Neurosci.* 1999;19:3057–3072.
129. Webster HH, Jones BE. Neurotoxic lesions of the dorsolateral pontomesencephalic tegmentum-cholinergic cell area in the cat, II: effects upon sleep-waking states. *Brain Res.* 1988;458: 285–302.
130. Kodama T, Takahashi Y, Honda Y. Enhancement of acetylcholine release during paradoxical sleep in the dorsal tegmental field of the cat brain stem. *Neurosci Lett.* 1990;114:277–282.
131. Leonard TO, Lydic R. Nitric oxide synthase inhibition decreases pontine acetylcholine release. *Neuroreport.* 1995;6:1525–1529.
132. Lydic R, Baghdoyan HA. Acetylcholine modulates sleep and wakefulness: a synaptic perspective. In: Monti JM, Pandi-Perumal SR, Sinton CM, eds. *Neurochemistry of Sleep and Wakefulness.* Cambridge, UK: Cambridge University Press; 2008.
133. Keifer JC, Baghdoyan HA, Becker L, et al. Halothane decreases pontine acetylcholine release and increases EEG spindles. *Neuroreport.* 1994;5:577–580.
134. Lydic R, Baghdoyan HA. Ketamine and MK-801 decrease acetylcholine release in the pontine reticular formation, slow breathing, and disrupt sleep. *Sleep.* 2002;25:617–622.
134. Lydic R, Keifer JC, Baghdoyan HA, et al. Microdialysis of the pontine reticular formation reveals inhibition of acetylcholine release by morphine. *Anesthesiology.* 1993;79:1003–1012.
135. Berridge CW. Noradrenergic modulation of arousal. *Brain Res Rev.* 2008;58:1–17.
136. Aston-Jones G, Bloom FE. Activity of norepinephrine-containing locus coeruleus neurons in behaving rats anticipates fluctuations in the sleep-waking cycle. *J Neurosci.* 1981;1:876–886.
137. Berridge CW, Abercrombie ED. Relationship between locus coeruleus discharge rates and rates of norepinephrine release within neocortex as assessed by in vivo microdialysis. *Neuroscience.* 1999;93:1263–1270.
138. Correa-Sales C, Rabin BC, Maze M. A hypnotic response to dexmedetomidine, an alpha 2 agonist, is mediated in the locus coeruleus in rats. *Anesthesiology.* 1992;76:948–952.
139. Anzawa N, Kushikata T, Ohkawa H, et al. Increased noradrenaline release from rat preoptic area during and after sevoflurane and isoflurane anesthesia. *Can J Anaesth.* 2001;48:462–465.
140. Yasui Y, Masaki E, Kato F. Sevoflurane directly excites locus coeruleus neurons of rats. *Anesthesiology.* 2007;107:992–1002.
141. Gilsbach R, Roser C, Beetz N, et al. Genetic dissection of alpha-2 adrenoceptor functions in adrenergic versus nonadrenergic cells. *Mol Pharmacol.* 2009;75:1160–1170.
142. Moruzzi G, Magoun HW. Brain stem reticular formation and activation of the EEG. *Electroencephalog Clin Neurophysiol.* 1949;1: 455–473.
143. Jones BE. Basic mechanisms of sleep-wake states. In: Kryger MH, Roth T, Dement WC, eds. *Principles and Practice of Sleep Medicine.* 4th ed. Philadelphia, PA: Elsevier Saunders; 2005.
144. Camacho-Arroyo I, Alvarado R, Manjarrez J, et al. Microinjections of muscimol and bicuculline into the pontine reticular formation modify the sleep-waking cycle in the rat. *Neurosci Lett.* 1991;129:95–97.
145. Xi MC, Morales FR, Chase MH. Evidence that wakefulness and REM sleep are controlled by a GABAergic pontine mechanism. *J Neurophysiol.* 1999;82:2015–2019.
146. Watson CJ, Soto-Calderon H, Lydic R, et al. Pontine reticular formation (PnO) administration of hypocretin-1 increases PnO GABA levels and wakefulness. *Sleep.* 2008;31:453–464.
147. Watson CJ, Lydic R, Baghdoyan HA. Sleep and GABA levels in the oral part of rat pontine reticular formation are decreased by local and systemic administration of morphine. *Neuroscience.* 2007;144:375–386.
148. Lydic R, Biebuyck JF. Sleep neurobiology: relevance for mechanistic studies of anaesthesia. *Br J Anaesth.* 1994;72:506–508.
149. Pitts RF. Organization of the respiratory center. *Physiol Rev.* 1946;26:609–630.
150. Allison T, Cicchetti DV. Sleep in mammals: ecological and constitutional correlates. *Science.* 1976;194:732–734.
151. Gettys GC, Lydic R. Bioenergetics of sleep. In: Koob G, Thompson RF, LeMoal M, eds. *Encyclopedia of Behavioral Neuroscience.* New York, NY: Elsevier; 2010.
152. Vanini G, Baghdoyan HA, Lydic R. Relevance of sleep neurobiology for cognitive neuroscience and anesthesia. In: Mashour GA, ed. *Consciousness, Awareness, and Anesthesia.* Cambridge, UK: Cambridge University Press; 2010.
153. Guedel AE. Third stage ether anesthesia: A subclassification regarding the significance of the position and movements of the eyeball. *Am J Surg.* 1920;34:53–57.
154. Hobson JA. What is a behavioral state? In: Ferrendelli JA, ed. *Aspects of Behavioral Neurobiology.* Bethesda, MD: Society for Neuroscience; 1978. *Behavioral Neurobiology*; vol. 3.
155. Avidan MS, Zhang L, Burnside BA, et al. Anesthesia awareness and the bispectral index. *N Engl J Med.* 2008;358:1097–1108.
156. Lydic R. State-dependent aspects of regulatory physiology. *FASEB J.* 1987;1:6–15.
157. Bingel U, Tracey I. Imaging CNS modulation of pain in humans. *Physiology.* 2008;23:317–380.
158. Jensen MP. A neuropsychological model of pain: research and clinical implications. *J Pain.* 2010;11:2–12.
159. Heinke W, Schwarzbauer C. In vivo imaging of anesthetic action in humans: approaches with positron emission tomography (PET) and functional magnetic resonance imaging (fMRI). *Br J Anaesth.* 2002;89:112–122.

160. Firestone LL, Gyulai F, Mintun M, et al. Human brain activity response to fentanyl imaged by positron emission tomography. *Anesth Analg.* 1996;82:1247–1251.
161. Fiset P, Plourde G, Backman SB. Brain imaging in research on anesthetic mechanisms: studies with propofol. *Prog Brain Res.* 2005;150:245–250.
162. Chung F, Yegneswaran B, Liao P, et al. STOP questionnaire: a tool to screen patients for obstructive sleep apnea. *Anesthesiology.* 2008;108:812–821.
163. Ramachandran S, Josephs L. A meta-analysis of clinical screening tests for obstructive sleep apnea. *Anesthesiology.* 2009;110:928–939.

4

THALAMOCORTICAL SYSTEM AND ANESTHETIC-INDUCED UNCONSCIOUSNESS

Anthony G. Hudetz and Michael T. Alkire

MODERN PHRENOLOGY: NEUROIMAGING OF ANESTHESIA

From a neuroscience perspective, the German physician Franz Joseph Gall (1758–1828) nearly had it all completely right, about two centuries ahead of his time. In fact, his major contribution to modern neuroscience is readily visible today in nearly every neuroimaging study published in the scientific literature. It was Dr. Gall who hypothesized that brain structure and brain function are intimately linked together and as such could form the basis for explaining the intellectual faculties present within any particular individual. Indeed, it was Dr. Gall who believed that the brain is the organ of all the propensities, sentiments, and faculties of any individual; as eloquently detailed in his seminal work published in 1819, *The Anatomy and Physiology of the Nervous System in General, and of the Brain in Particular, with Observations upon the Possibility of Ascertaining the Several Intellectual and Moral Dispositions of Man and Animal, by the Configuration of Their Heads.* The idea that we are the sum total of our brain's abilities and functions predates the modern neuroscientific study of consciousness by some 175 years, as reflected by the publication of Sir Francis H. C. Crick's book *The Astonishing Hypothesis: The Scientific Search for the Soul*, in 1994. Of course, Dr. Gall made one small mistaken assumption in his neuroscientific study of the mind (or, from the Greek word for mind, "phrēn"). He thought the structure of the brain would be reflected in the shape of a person's skull. Thus, he became known as the father of phrenology; the study of how bumps on a person's skull might be related to their underlying personality. Had he not made that one correlational misstep, perhaps he would more rightfully be recognized as the father of modern cognitive neuroscience.

To get to a more modern basis for cognitive neuroscience and the study of consciousness we have to move forward in history to the seminal work of Korbinian Brodmann (1868–1918). He was a German neurologist who became famous for his meticulous and detailed work clarifying the cytoarchitectonic organization of the human cerebral cortex. The work allowed him to classify and segregate the areas of the human cortex into 52 regions, which are now commonly known as Brodmann's areas. Wisely, unlike Gall, he made no extra assumptions about what his structural brain findings might mean and he was content with simply making a map of cortical structure.

The functional aspects of the human cerebral cortex and its correspondence with Brodmann's structural nomenclature became well established in concert with the growth of modern neurosurgical techniques. Neurosurgeon Wilder Penfield (1891–1976) and neurobiologist Herbert Jasper (1909–1999) mapped out many of the localized functional responses that occurred in awake patients having epilepsy surgery when pinpoint electrical stimulations were applied to various portions of their cerebral cortex. Penfield's work, among others, led to our modern understanding and mapping of the sensory and motor cortices of the human brain and how they are functionally connected with the various limbs and organs of the body. This work was published in part in the 1954 landmark book, *Epilepsy and the Functional Anatomy of the Human Brain*.

Yet the noninvasive study of human brain structure-function relationships and the real arrival of cognitive neuroscience as a prelude to the study of consciousness had to await the development of modern neuroimaging techniques that would allow researchers to watch the human brain at work. Among the first of such techniques was positron emission tomography. By 1980, when experiments were properly controlled for using the cognitive subtraction technique,[1] the measurement of incremental regional cerebral blood flow changes (a reflection of increased neuronal work being conducted by various brain regions) could be visualized as they occurred in response to specific cognitive tasks. This allowed researchers to link the functioning of the living human brain to its underlying structural components on a time scale of minutes. In 1990, it was discovered that functional images of brain activity could also be obtained using magnetic resonance imaging (MRI) machines if they were tuned to looking at changes in regional blood-oxygen-level-dependent (BOLD) signals.[2] Regional changes in BOLD signals could now form a link that would represent regional neuronal responses to cognitive tasks on a time scale of seconds. At last, it seemed that

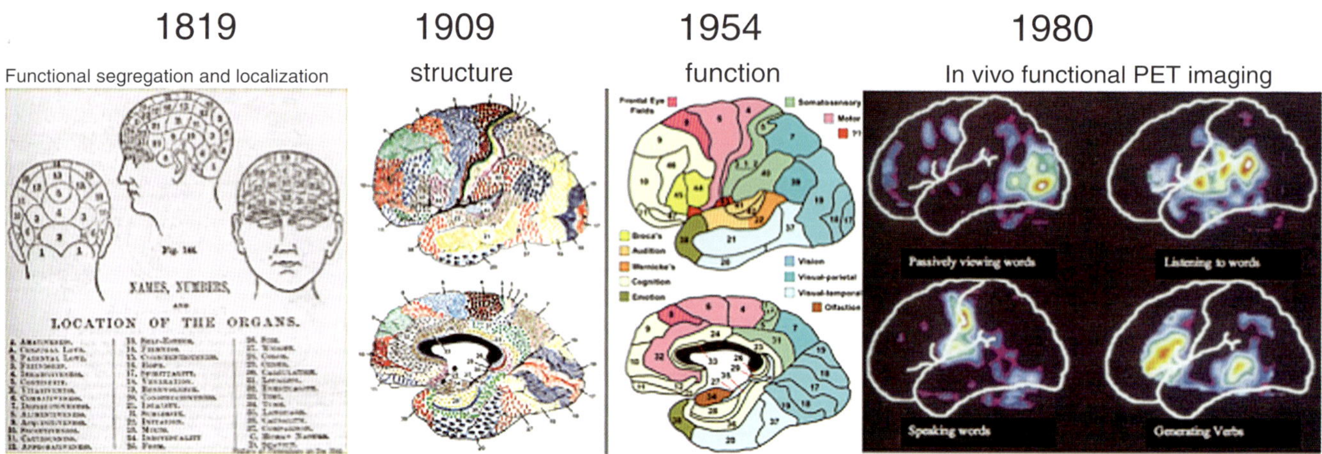

Figure 4.1 Milestones of phrenology: localization by structural, functional, and neuroimaging techniques. Brain PET scan taken from the book *Images of Mind* by Michael I. Posner and Marcus E. Raichle. Copyright © 1994, 1997 by Scientific American Library. Reprinted by permission of Henry Holt and Company, LLC.

the era of cognitive neuroimaging was born and the neuroimaging search for the neural correlates of consciousness could begin in earnest. The mentioned milestones in brain phrenology are illustrated in Figure 4.1.

EARLY ANESTHESIA STUDIES

As cognitive neuroscience was advancing and evolving, so too was the study of anesthetic mechanisms. It was well known by the 1970s and early 1980s that most anesthetics greatly suppressed global brain metabolism in a dose-dependent manner and often at the same time increased cerebral blood flow (especially for those agents that were inhaled).[3] Indeed, with the introduction of the Sokoloff method for measuring local cerebral glucose utilization and metabolism in 1974,[4–6] a plethora of animal studies were shortly performed, by numerous investigators, that characterized the nature of the anesthetic state and the resultant changes in regional brain functioning caused by nearly all of the various anesthetic drugs.[7–18] Due to many small variations in technical methods and slight differences in the drug doses studied, the overall pattern of results from all of these studies were hard to interpret, and a single focus of anesthetic action could not be clearly identified. One of the few reliable effects of anesthetics on regional brain activity was noted by Ori in 1986, when he stated that most, if not all agents greatly reduced the amount of regional metabolic activity occurring in the somatosensory cortex of anesthetized animals.[17,19]

The first study to use positron emission tomography (PET) in humans to try to link regional brain effects of anesthesia to the loss of consciousness was conducted by Alkire and his colleagues at the University of California, Irvine, in 1995.[20] Their study looked at the regional cerebral metabolic effects of propofol anesthesia in volunteers that were studied on two different occasions, once while they were awake to provide a baseline for comparison and once while they were unresponsive during a near-steady state infusion of propofol anesthesia. The results of the study basically confirmed in humans what was previously found to be the effects of propofol on regional cerebral metabolism in animals,[9] but it also served to add a few new technical considerations to the study of consciousness with anesthesia and neuroimaging.

First, it showed that individual subjects had vastly different baseline brain metabolic rates of glucose utilization. In fact, within the six subjects studied the metabolic baseline of some subjects was nearly twice that of other subjects. This means that if the data had been pooled within condition and across the subjects, as was always done in animal studies of that time by necessity (because the deoxyglucose technique requires sectioning an animal's brain), it might have appeared that some brain regions could have shown an increase in their absolute metabolic rate above the awake condition, if by chance a skewed sample of subjects (with high baseline metabolism) had just happened to be studied in the anesthesia condition. However, because each subject was studied twice, each could be compared to himself, and this clearly revealed that propofol always decreases brain metabolism in every region of the brain, by as much as 30–70% at the loss of consciousness endpoint. As it would turn out, once other anesthetic agents had been tested in humans with PET,[20–24] this global metabolic suppression effect of anesthesia was found to be dose-dependent and a common property of all other anesthetics yet tested, with the one exception being ketamine anesthesia.[25] This global metabolic suppression effect of anesthesia is illustrated in Figure 4.2.

Second, the study revealed that the pattern of regional metabolic suppression caused by propofol was remarkably consistent from person to person. This means that no matter where a person starts on the scale of global metabolic rate, the drug essentially "turns off" the brain in the same way

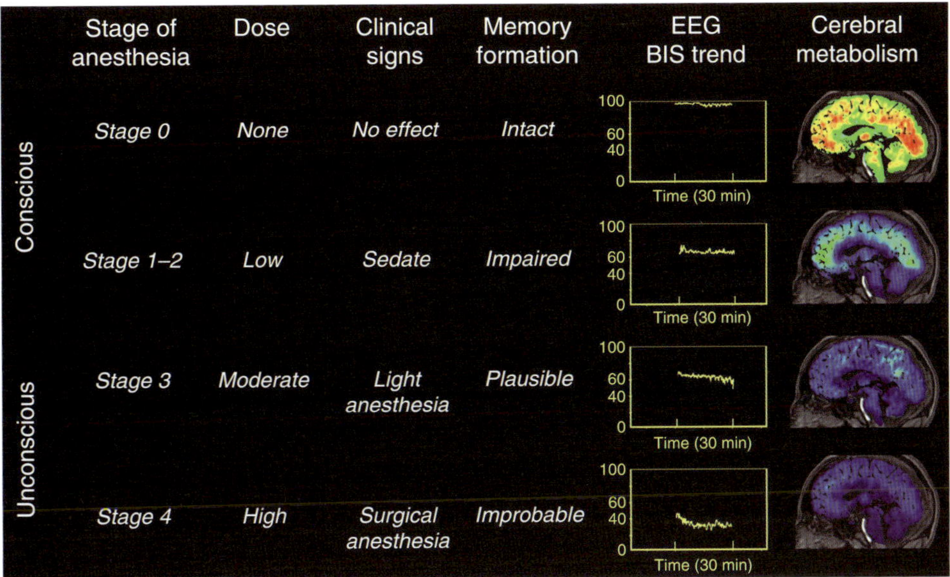

Figure 4.2 Dose-dependent effect of general anesthetics on clinical signs, EEG bispectral index (BIS), memory formation, and global brain metabolism. Reproduced after Figure 10.3 from Steven Laureys and Giulio Tononi, 2009, *The Neurology of Consciousness: Cognitive Neuroscience and Neuropathology*, p. 122, Academic Press, London.

for everyone. Indeed, the largest and most consistent change was found to occur in the cortical parietal lobes, which seemed to be "turned-off" almost twice as much as the other cortical areas. Subsequent PET studies of propofol anesthesia would later confirm this finding and, using more evolved image analysis methods, reveal that this parietal cortical effect was usually accompanied by a similar cortical suppression in parts of the frontal lobes.[26,27]

Third and finally, the study used a region of interest analysis technique because neuroimaging analysis methods were still in their infancy and most animal data reported findings as metabolic rate per specific structure. Thus, to make the data more comparable to previous animal work the findings were reported as regions of interest. Yet, this method limited the real power of neuroimaging to find new and unanticipated regional effects that might span the border between two different functional areas. Indeed, when propofol was studied again by the Montreal group with PET using the cerebral blood flow technique and analyzed with a three-dimensional analysis method it became clear that a relatively localized effect of propofol occurs in the thalamus, posterior parietal areas, and some frontal lobe areas when consciousness is lost.[22,28]

REGIONAL THALAMIC SUPPRESSION WITH ANESTHESIA

Shortly after the report on propofol appeared, another study reported that the effects of halothane and isoflurane anesthesia in humans had a common site of regional suppression when both agents were examined using three-dimensional analysis methods that investigated common regional metabolic suppression activity.[29,30] That common site of apparent action between these two agents was primarily localized to the thalamus. This effect, coupled with other findings of the day, suggested that a localized effect of anesthesia could contribute to a loss of consciousness by interfering with the proper functioning of the thalamocortical system. This idea was often overinterpreted to imply that the authors were suggesting the site of action of anesthesia for causing a loss of consciousness was the thalamus. However, the real intent of the work was to focus attention on the thalamocortical system (i.e., thalamocortical-corticothalamic-reticulothalamic) in the process of anesthesia and to try to understand how its interactions with various cortical and subcortical networks might change when consciousness is lost. This change in functioning was thought to occur through an anesthetic effect that contributed to cellular hyperpolarization (taking neurons farther away from the firing threshold) of the relevant network neurons. This was thought to possibly occur either through direct drug effects on the neurons of importance, or through indirect effects at the network level that would then impact the functioning of the whole thalamocortical system. Of course, the possibility that both effects, direct and indirect, might also play a role in changing the functioning of the system was also entertained.

As further neuroimaging studies of anesthesia were performed, they did little to refute the idea that a common effect of anesthesia was the suppression of thalamic activity. However, two possible exceptions to this idea did emerge. Ketamine, as previously mentioned, does not cause a global metabolic suppression and, in fact, it actually causes a relative increase in thalamic metabolic activity. Additionally, thiopental in one study did not seem to have a regional suppressive effect on the thalamus.[27] Indeed, it seemed to have a pattern of change that was different from that of propofol's, when both were titrated to similar clinical endpoints. Yet and still, the regional suppression of thalamic activity appears to be a relatively robust finding in multiple neuroimaging studies. This effect is shown in Figure 4.3.

Despite this regional similarity between agents, this still does not mean that the anesthetics were not also suppressing global activity throughout the brain. In connection with each drug's global metabolic suppression effect it appeared that another common regional suppression effect could be seen in the anesthesia data. It appears that suppression of a parietal-frontal cortical network also accompanies the changes in regional thalamic activity. Thus, a number of cortical areas also seem to be depressed in common between different states of unconsciousness, such as sleep, coma, anesthesia, and even with seizures (Figure 4.4).[31]

Taken together, the thalamus and cortex emerge from the anesthesia neuroimaging data as the brain sites most consistently affected by anesthesia when consciousness is lost. In fact, a small but specific lesion of the medial thalamus

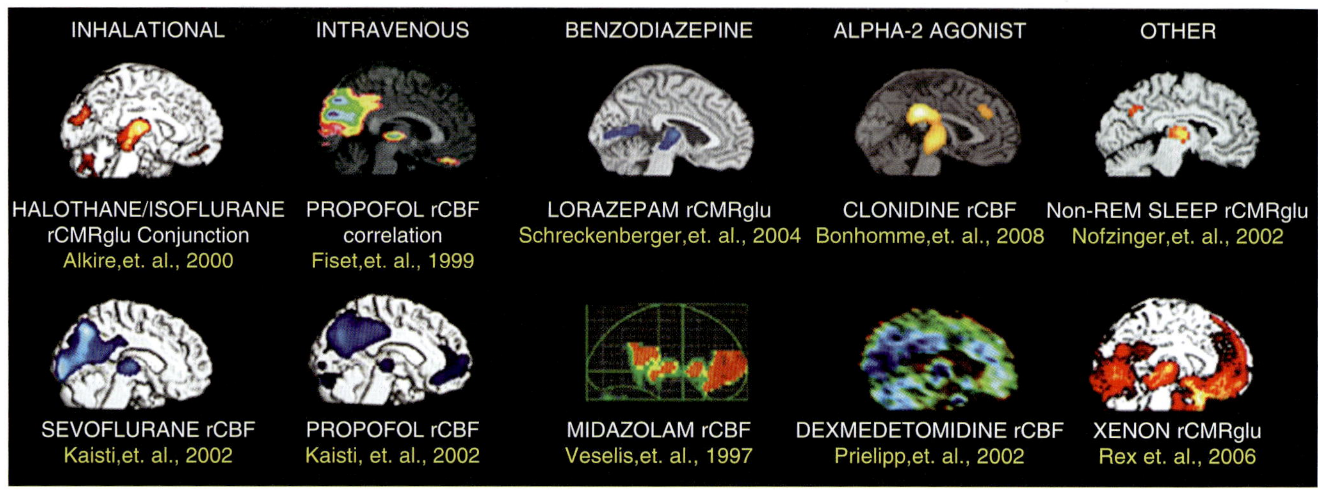

Figure 4.3 Suppression of thalamic activity as a common effect of various anesthetic agents.[22,23,26,29,201–205]

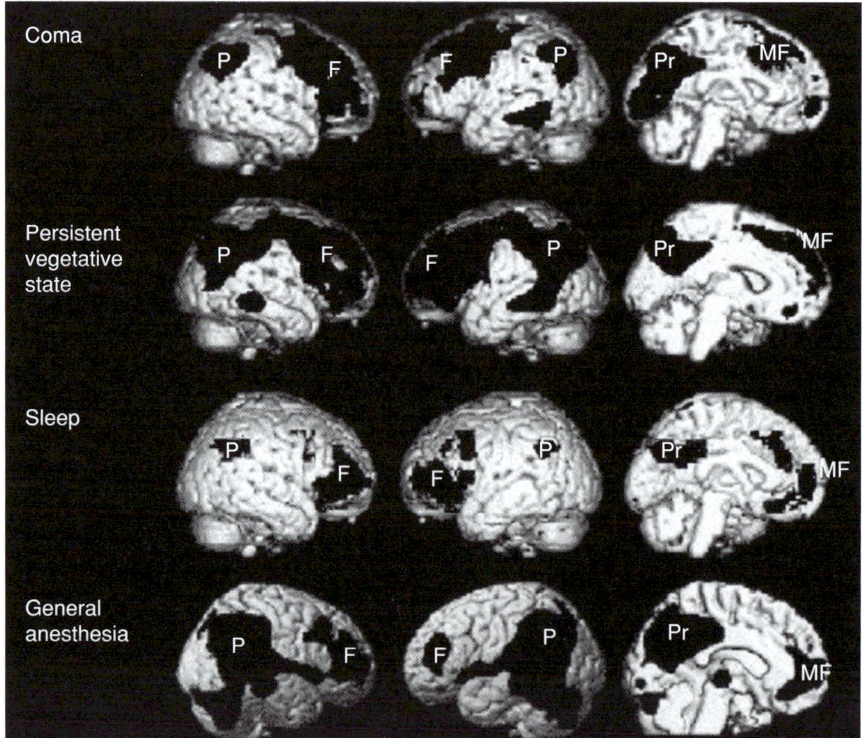

Figure 4.4 Suppression of frontoparietal brain regions in various forms of unconsciousness. Reprinted from Baars BJ, Ramsøy TZ, Laureys S. Brain, conscious experience and the observing self. *Trends Neurosci*. 2003;26(12): 671–675, with permission from Elsevier.

or a global failure of cortical integrity will render patients unconscious.[32] On the other hand, several principal structures including the basal ganglia, tectum, basal forebrain, hippocampus, and cerebellum, that play important roles in cognitive functions, have been ruled unnecessary for mediating consciousness due to their fundamentally parallel architecture and due to the fact that selective lesions of these regions do not produce unconsciousness.[33]

The thalamus and cortex form a system that functions as an integrated unit. In fact, the thalamus is viewed by some as the seventh layer of the cortex.[34] The thalamus not only relays ascending and descending information en route to and from the cortex but it also relays information among various regions of the cerebral cortex.[35] Moreover, the thalamus also engages in the modulation and selection of distributed information processing across the cortex.[36] The thalamus and cortex are both capable of activity in isolation. However, their normal functions are carried out in unison.[37] This functional interdependence makes it difficult to tease apart the relative roles of each, and to understand the mechanism of functional derangements caused by exogenous factors such as anesthesia due to the multiplicity of cellular and molecular targets of anesthetic agents. Thus, a fundamental question is if anesthetics exert a critical effect in the thalamus, cortex, or elsewhere, leading to a disruption of the thalamocortical function through an indirect route.

EFFECT OF ANESTHETICS ON THALAMIC AND CORTICAL NEURONS

Neuroimaging provides a window on the activity of a large population of neurons. To understand the neurophysiological events underlying the metabolic and hemodynamic changes as seen by neuroimaging, one has to directly examine the effect of anesthetics on the neurons themselves. Anesthetics are thought to produce a general decrease in neuronal excitability.[38,39] This effect follows the reduced nonspecific drive from the brainstem. Ogawa et al[40,41] found that the volatile anesthetics halothane, isoflurane, enflurane, and sevoflurane suppressed multiunit activity in the reticular formation.

Several investigators suggested that anesthetics suppress the reactivity of thalamocortical neurons.[42–44] Decades ago, Angel[42,45] proposed that the anesthetic state was due to a corticothalamic block of information transfer. Angel tested several older anesthetic agents, and his study was limited to somatosensory stimulation. Later, other types of anesthetics, particularly isoflurane, were found to attenuate the thalamic transfer of somatosensory signals in vitro.[43] This effect is tied to a hyperpolarization of thalamocortical cells and shunting in part through voltage-gated Na^+ and Ca^{2+} currents.[44,46]

Detsch and colleagues also found that the effect of anesthetics on neuronal excitability depended on the stimulus presentation frequency.[43] They showed that isoflurane at > 0.8% concentration suppressed the responsiveness of thalamocortical cells especially when driven by high-frequency (30–100 Hz) somatosensory stimuli but not when stimulated at long interstimulus intervals. With high-frequency driving, the initial response to the onset of the stimulus train was present, but the responses to subsequent stimuli were quickly attenuated.

General anesthetics are also known to reduce spontaneous neuron firing in the cerebral cortex.[39,47–50] Their effect on the reactivity of cortical neurons is more controversial. Ikeda and Wright[51] found that halothane at 2.2% reduced the sensitivity of cat striate cortex neurons to stimulus orientation, spatial frequency, and contrast. Armstrong-James and colleagues found that cortical neuronal receptive fields were expanded in light anesthesia and suppressed at deeper levels.[49] Tigwell and Sauter[52] found reliable neuron responses in monkey striate cortex at isoflurane concentrations up to 0.9%. Villeneuve and Casanova[50] compared the concentration-dependent effects of halothane/nitrous oxide and isoflurane/nitrous oxide on cat striate cortex neuron responses and found that isoflurane produced a greater suppression (50% at 0.8 MAC) than did halothane. Neither anesthetic influenced the orientation sensitivity, direction sensitivity, or receptive field organization of the neurons.

Few studies have examined the effect of volatile anesthetics on cortical unit reactivity at latencies longer than 100 ms. Robson[53] noted that the late components (200–500 ms) of unit response to flash in cat visual cortex were more sensitive to anesthesia than was the primary response within the 100 ms. Ikeda and Wright[54] studied the reactivity of neurons in cat visual cortex and found that in stage III anesthesia, characterized by slow-wave electroencephalogram, the sustained response component (up to 5 seconds) of certain neurons was suppressed during halothane/nitrous oxide while the primary response was preserved. Likewise, Chapin et al[55] found that 0.75% halothane depressed the long-latency (300 ms) excitatory firing of rat somatosensory cortical neurons following cutaneous stimulation of the forepaw while short-latency responses within 50 ms were little affected. Tigwell and Sauter[52] reported that the sustained response up to 300 ms of monkey striate cortex neurons was preserved under anesthesia with 0.5–0.9% isoflurane and 73% nitrous oxide. While the exact reason for this discrepancy is unclear, it may have been due to the difference in chosen stimulus parameters (prolonged vs. brief stimuli).

Recently, Hudetz et al[56] found that under desflurane anesthesia at 2%–8%, visual cortex neurons remained responsive to flash stimulation, demonstrating a strong, transient increase in firing within the first 100 ms poststimulus. However, the subsequent long-latency (> 150 ms) components of their response was attenuated in a concentration-dependent manner. In some cases, the early unit

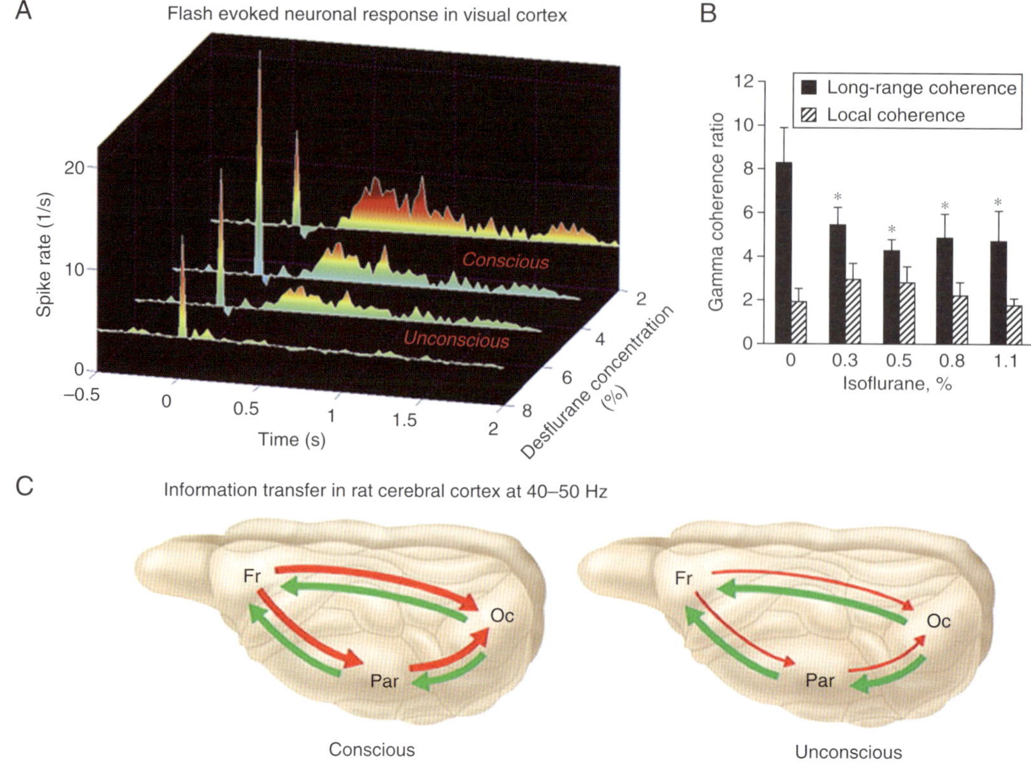

Figure 4.5 Effect of volatile anesthetic agents on cortical reactivity, gamma oscillations and information exchange. A: Neuronal response to visual flash stimulation in conscious and unconscious rats. B: Frontal-occipital coherence and frontal local coherence of field potential gamma oscillations. C: Feedforward and feedback information transfer estimated from the transfer entropy of cortical gamma field potentials. Reproduced from Alkire MT, Hudetz AG, Tononi G. Consciousness and anesthesia. *Science.* 2008; 322: 876–880.

response was even augmented at the highest examined anesthetic concentrations (desflurane, 8%–10%) suggesting a form of neuronal hypersensitivity (Figure 4.5A).

The reason for the preservation of the early cortical neuronal reactivity during anesthesia is unclear. Erchova et al[57] suggested that sensory specificity may increase with increasing anesthetic depth due to a reduction of associative inputs. Another possibility is that feedforward inhibition through GABA-mediated effects are suppressed.[58] The neuronal response may be also augmented by increased spike synchronization.

The attenuation of the long-latency response is more understandable. Chapin et al[55] suggested that the cortical long-latency response was brought about by nonspecific spinoreticulothalamic pathways. In awake animals this response was exhibited by cells with large receptive fields, it attenuated rapidly to high stimulus frequencies (> 2 Hz), and could be elicited by nonspecific, arousing stimuli. Long-latency responses could be selectively abolished by cryogenic blockade of the centromedian thalamic nuclei.[59] Therefore, the attenuation of the long-latency response of cortical neurons may have been due to a reduced nonspecific input, while the specific inputs may have been augmented due to reduced lateral or feedforward inhibition.

These observations also appear to be valid in humans and for other types of anesthetic agents. A recent study demonstrated that during loss of consciousness achieved by midazolam in human subjects, transcranial magnetic stimulation failed to evoke the long-latency, traveling waves in EEG that are normally seen during waking.[60] The failure of wave propagation during loss of consciousness resembled previous observations made during non–rapid eye movement sleep.[61]

FEEDBACK MAY BE A KEY TO PERCEPTION

Corticocortical associational projections are bidirectional throughout the hierarchy of modality-specific, multimodal, and supramodal regions.[62] The feedback projections greatly outnumber the feedforward projections, suggesting their functional importance.[63] This reciprocal connectivity has been proposed as an essential substrate for conscious perception and conscious behavior.[64–66] As suggested, the forward connections represent and analyze incoming sensory data, whereas the feedback projections play a modulating role in the selection and contextual interpretation of information.[67–69]

Studies of conscious perception confirm that neural activities in primary visual cortex within the first 100 ms after stimulus presentation indicate stimulus registration, whereas those that follow the stimulus by more than 100 ms reflect feedback signaling from higher visual processing regions.[70–72] Only the latter components correlate with conscious perception,[72] and differentiate between explicit and implicit retrieval.[73] Backward masking studies of Bachmann[74,75] suggest a similar time scale (100–150 ms) for the development of conscious experience.

To the extent that conscious information processing depends on long-latency feedback effects, these findings suggest that an important component of anesthetic-induced unconsciousness may be mediated by anesthetic effects on feedback networks.[76,77] Based on experiments with halothane, Chapin et al[55] suggested earlier that the selective reduction of long-latency responses may play a role in the loss of consciousness associated with anesthesia. Our recent data extend these findings to other inhalational anesthetics, and advance the theory of anesthetic-induced unconsciousness to the network level. Consciousness may be removed by a "top-down" process rather than a "bottom-up" process.

Certain anesthetics, such as urethane, produce a pattern of spontaneous activity of cortical neurons similar to that seen in natural slow-wave sleep. This state is characterized by a slow, 1 Hz oscillation in neuronal membrane potential, such that in the depolarized "up" state, neurons fire rapidly and in the hyperpolarized "down" state they are silent.[78] The mechanism of slow oscillation during urethane anesthesia has not been determined with certainty, but possibilities include spontaneous cortical phase transition,[79] bistability of thalamic relay[80] or reticular neurons,[81] or an interaction of these. Cortical–cortical interactions may also be playing a role in the generation and maintenance of this oscillation.[82] The importance of this phenomenon is that it carries with it the possibility that under anesthesia, information processing capacity of the cortex is not permanently blocked, but transiently recovers about once a minute. Each up state could allow a window of the brain to briefly open to the world, for a fraction of a second that, in principle, is long enough to generate a fragment of conscious experience. Of course, urethane is a unique anesthetic that produces very little depression of spontaneous neuronal activity as compared to other, commonly used anesthetic agents. The generality of these findings for anesthesia with other agents remains to be established.

Interestingly, at deep levels of anesthesia, characterized by partially or fully suppressed spontaneous EEG, the cortical neurons become hyperexcitable. In this state, sensory stimuli elicit brief bursts of cortical activity from an isoelectric baseline. This is surprising because in states with burst-suppressed EEG, patients are always nonresponsive and are considered totally unconscious. Nevertheless, such EEG bursts have been elicited by visual, auditory, and micromechanical stimuli.[83–88] Since the bursts exhibit long latencies (100–300 ms), they are unlikely to be mediated by thalamocortical relays. It is more likely that the bursts are produced by transiently increased neuronal excitability through polysynaptic or nonsynaptic reticular, basal forebrain, or nonspecific thalamic pathways.[86,87]

THALAMIC CONTROL OF CONSCIOUSNESS

The involvement of the thalamus in controlling consciousness is at least twofold. On the one hand, the thalamus is involved in the exchange of specific information with the cortex and thus participates in the formation of conscious representations. On the other hand, its role is likely more modulatory in nature, regulating the level of cortical arousal under the influence of the brainstem. The latter function is most likely tied to the medial or intralaminar thalamic nuclei.

The traditional view has been that anesthesia removes consciousness by suppressing the activity of the ascending arousal system.[89] The ascending arousal system modulates the activity of the cerebral cortex via pathways that originate in the brainstem and follow dorsal and ventral ascending pathways.[90] The dorsal pathway extends through the intralaminar nuclei (ILN) of the thalamus, on its way to the cortex, and the ventral pathway targets the basal forebrain through the subthalamus and hypothalamus.[91]

It was recognized about half a century ago, that the intralaminar thalamic nuclei were essential to maintain cortical arousal, implicating their role in enabling consciousness.[92,93] The intralaminar nuclei project heavily on both the striatum and the cerebral cortex.[94,95] The frontal medial and dorsolateral aspects of the cortex are especially favored, although at least a few intralaminar cells project to every cortical area. The cortical projections are not entirely diffuse or "nonspecific," but clusters of intralaminar cells project to regional zones of the cortex. The main projection of the central medial nucleus is to the medial and basal areas of the cortex—areas previously implicated in having high resting state activity and metabolism.

The brainstem afferents of the intralaminar nuclei arise from the Raphe nuclei, peribrachial nucleus, and locus coeruleus. All subcortical efferents terminate on thalamostriatal cells; thus brainstem modulation likely drives striatal behavior patterns. Also prevalent are inputs from the cholinergic basal forebrain and amygdala. Finally, all intralaminar nuclei receive organized input from cerebral cortex; specifically, the central medial nucleus receives fibers from the prefrontal and medial limbic cortices. This is consistent with its role in cognitive-emotional arousal.

In addition to its cortical projections, the thalamostriatal projections of the intralaminar nuclei are topographically organized and target the calbindin-rich matrix compartment of the striatum. Striatal targets of the anterior intralaminar nuclei, including the central medial nucleus, are closely associated with corticostriatal input. The central medial nucleus itself projects mainly to the limbic striatum. According to Van Der Werf[96] the anterior section of the central medial nucleus in rats is involved in cognitive functions, whereas the posterior part is involved in multimodal sensory processing. Many cells in the midline of the anterior intralaminar group also project to the amygdala. Thus, these projections of the central medial nucleus are consistent with limbic, cognitive, and multisensory arousal—together plausibly taken as a hallmark for conscious awakening.

Selective lesions of the medial thalamus can produce coma or vegetative state,[32] and behavioral responsiveness was restored in a minimally conscious patient following electrical stimulation of the central thalamus.[97] Recently, Alkire and colleagues showed that stimulation of the central medial nucleus of the thalamus (CMT) by the microinjection of nicotine could awaken rats kept under light anesthesia with sevoflurane.[98] A similar effect during either sevoflurane or desflurane anesthesia was achieved by microinjection of a blocking antibody to voltage-gated potassium channels.[99] These findings suggest that the CMT may be an activator or "on-switch" of consciousness that is able to overcome the more global suppressive effects of anesthesia.

Miller and colleagues found that microinfusion of various GABA agonists into the midline thalamus could induce sedation and, in some cases, loss of the righting reflex in rats.[100–102] More recently Alkire and colleagues found similar evidence with relevance to general anesthesia.[103] Injection of the GABA agonist muscimol into the CMT of rats anesthetized with sevoflurane produced a dose-dependent, site-specific decrease of the sevoflurane dose needed to suppress the righting reflex. Interestingly, the nonspecific inhibition of the CMT with the local anesthetic marcaine produced no change in the anesthetic concentration required for loss of righting. These findings support the possibility for an active, specific, GABAergic thalamic consciousness "off-switch" in the CMT.

The intralaminar nuclei are of course part of an elaborate network of the arousal control system involved in complex regulation of sleep-wake states, attention, orienting, etc. The CMT most likely works in parallel with other arousal centers of the forebrain that control corticothalamic interaction and cortical function. A loss of righting in rats can also be induced by GABAergic inactivation of the septohippocampal area, supramammillary area, nucleus accumbens, ventral pallidum, the mesopontine ventral tegmentum,[104,105] or the tuberomammillary nucleus of the hypothalamus.[106] The Hudetz group recently obtained evidence that pharmacological stimulation of the nucleus basalis can also produce transient behavioral activation in rats under inhalational anesthesia (Anesthesiology, submitted).

Finally, several investigations suggest that the effect of anesthesia on the thalamus may be indirect and driven by actions on the cortex or other brain areas that project to the thalamus.[29,76,107] Spontaneous thalamic firing during anesthesia is largely driven by feedback from cortical neurons,[107] especially anesthetic-sensitive layer V cells.[45] Many of these cells project through the thalamus onto brainstem arousal centers, providing a pathway through which anesthetic-induced cortical suppression can also act to reduce overall arousal.[108] The metabolic and electrophysiological effects of anesthetics on the thalamus are no longer present if the overlying feedback portions of the cerebral cortex are removed.[16] In patients with implanted brain electrodes that were undergoing a second surgery for the placement of a deep brain stimulator unit, the cortical EEG changed dramatically when the patients lost consciousness.[109] However, thalamic EEG activity did not appear to change much until almost 10 minutes later. Finally, recent results from mathematical modeling of the effect of midazolam on cortical and thalamic neurons suggested that the predicted change in thalamic firing was insufficient to account for the drug's sedative/hypnotic effect and that the principal neuronal target of midazolam for loss of consciousness was in fact cortical.[110]

These observations suggest that the anesthetic effect on the thalamus may reflect the overall global suppression of cortical functioning. Given that under general anesthesia sensory stimuli continue to excite the cerebral cortex, anesthetic-induced unconsciousness cannot be explained by cortical deafferentation or a lack of cortical responsiveness. This does not negate the proposal that the thalamus and the cortex should be intimately coupled to mediate consciousness. Rather, the role of the thalamus in general anesthesia may be in the modulation of the cortical state and its capacity to process information. In fact, thalamocortical functional disconnection during general anesthesia has been supported by human neuroimaging data[30] and similar results were obtained in a vegetative state patient.[111]

GAMMA OSCILLATIONS AND THALAMOCORTICAL SYNCHRONY

It is also possible that neither the thalamus nor the cortex can be singled out as an exclusive anesthetic target; instead, the key effect may be a disruption of the functional coordination of these intimately coupled structures. The thalamus and cortex are coupled by multiple bidirectional pathways, involving the specific relay nuclei, the nonspecific nuclei, and the nucleus reticularis. Parvalbumin-immunoreactive core cells, which dominate in the thalamic relay nuclei, project to cortical layers III and IV, and receive feedback from layer VI. The calbindin-immunoreactive matrix cells, which dominate the intralaminar nuclei, mainly project to cortical layer I, and receive feedback from layer V. These parallel loops generate coupled oscillatory activity at 40 Hz gamma frequency that has been postulated to be critical for consciousness.[37,112,113] The oscillations are controlled by the reticular nucleus, which is under the control of ascending and descending nerve traffic via collaterals and under the control of brainstem arousal centers. The nonspecific feedforward projections and the corticothalamic feedback connections are relatively divergent and play a role in the synchronization of oscillations across larger thalamic and cortical territories that may serve an integrative role.[94,95] The secondary and higher order thalamic relays[35] also play a role in corticocortical communications and are now considered driving as opposed to modulatory. These synchronization mechanisms may help couple the distributed units of a specific neuronal ensemble that exists for a brief amount of time to serve a specific step in information processing in a perceptual, motor, or cognitive function.

Oscillations in the EEG or cortical local field potentials at gamma frequency (30–80 Hz) have enjoyed considerable interest because they have been thought to play an important role in conscious information processing in the brain. Event-related gamma oscillations in the EEG, local field potentials, and neuronal firing rates are involved in various cognitive functions, including attention,[114–118] short-term memory,[119] feature binding,[120] conscious perception,[121–123] and voluntary action.[124–127] Moreover, gamma oscillations in local field potentials or unit discharges tend to synchronize each other in a network of brain regions participating in a given perceptual or motor task.[128–136] When comparing consciously perceived and unperceived stimuli, only the consciously perceived stimuli were associated with long-distance gamma synchronization.[137]

Nearly twenty years ago, it was proposed that a suppression of 40 Hz gamma oscillations may underlie anesthetic-induced loss of consciousness,[138] and a number of observations in humans have supported this contention.[139–144] However, experimental studies in animals have not revealed a consistent effect of anesthetics on gamma oscillations. Several investigators noted that spontaneous gamma or beta band power can be either decreased or increased in the anesthetized state.[145–151] In particular, Imas and coworkers[150,151] found that the visual evoked gamma frequency response was not attenuated by volatile anesthetics. These results contrast with the observation that in human patients, general anesthetics decrease the amplitude and prolong the latency of sensory evoked potentials.[152] The difference is most likely due to the fact that evoked potentials are usually tested with stimuli delivered at relatively high frequency (10–40 Hz). As mentioned before, anesthesia prolongs the recovery of neuronal excitability after each stimulus, which leads to frequency-dependent attenuation of the averaged evoked response.[43] The same effect is seen with steady state evoked responses with numerous anesthetics.[143,153–155] With long stimulus intervals (5s) used by Imas et al, there is ample time for neuronal excitability to recover, and thus the direct cortical response is preserved. These findings suggest that under general anesthesia, cortical processing circuits are reactive but cannot be driven at as high a frequency as during wakefulness. Indeed, Osa et al[156] found that halothane did not attenuate human visual evoked potentials when tested at low-frequency (0.5 or 1 Hz) stimuli.

Hudetz and coworkers recently reexamined the effects of isoflurane on spontaneous cortical gamma activity in the rat model.[157] They found no significant change in the power of low-frequency (30–50 Hz) gamma oscillations; however, the power of high-frequency (70–140 Hz) gamma oscillations was attenuated in a concentration-dependent manner. This observation suggests that a distinction between various gamma frequency bands is important when evaluating the effect of anesthesia. In fact, different cognitive functions are carried out at various gamma frequency bands.[158]

In contrast to gamma power, the coherence of 40–50 Hz gamma oscillations among distant regions has been shown to be reduced by anesthesia. John and coworkers[159] found that the critical change in the EEG that correlated with the loss and return of consciousness was a decrease in gamma coherence between the frontal hemispheres as well as between the frontal and occipital regions of the same hemisphere. Based on these findings, Mashour[160,161] proposed that the mechanism of anesthetic-induced loss of consciousness is "cognitive unbinding" of conscious sensory representations that result from the suppression of gamma coherence at 40 Hz. Hameroff[162] also emphasized the importance of gamma synchrony for consciousness. Hudetz and coworkers found that anterior-posterior EEG coherence was decreased by isoflurane in rats while local gamma coherence within the frontal region was unchanged (Figure 4.5B).[163] Thus, the answer to unconsciousness probably lies in the disruption of corticocortical and thalamocortical oscillatory ensembles.

INFORMATION INTEGRATION IN THE CORTEX

Conscious cognition depends on information integration across wide regions of the cerebral cortex. We know that consciousness survives injuries to fairly large portions of the cerebral cortex, although specific functional deficits occur. We also know that lesions to specific subcortical structures, particularly those along the midline pontothalamic axis, can produce an immediate and full loss of consciousness.[32] The efficacy of these lesions may lie in their unimpeded and complete disruption of cortical integrative function, either due to a diminution of cortical arousal that normally enables consciousness or to a disconnection of cooperating cortical regions. Thus, we entertain the hypothesis that unconsciousness during anesthesia is due to the inability of the brain to integrate or interpret the sensory information it receives.[77]

Cortical integration assumes the cooperation of multiple specific brain regions although different spatial configurations may establish conscious processes. These configurations are dynamic as shown by the spatiotemporal EEG patterns in the resting brain that repeatedly shift from one network to another at every 80 ms, on average.[164] Corticocortical connectivity is key to integration, although part of the connectivity may be corticothalamocortical. The latter provides fast integration, probably most important for sensory motor responses and coordination. The slower, polysynaptic corticocortical networks may allow elaboration of the cortical representations, giving rise to conscious contents.

An integrative model of consciousness was developed by Tononi in the Information Integration Theory. Tononi[165] suggested that consciousness derives from "the brain's capacity to integrate information." At any moment, the brain can be in one of a great many configurational states; the realization of a specific state represents a reduction of prior uncertainty and, therefore, equates to a large amount of information. At the same time, components of the brain as a system at any level (functional regions, neurons, synapses, molecules, etc) are not independent but closely linked (integrated). Tononi states that consciousness requires both a "large repertoire of brain states" (information) and their "availability to the system as a whole" (integration). From this postulate it follows that consciousness may be suppressed in two principle ways: by reducing the repertoire of available brain states (reducing the amount of information) or by disrupting the communication among the system components (reducing integration). Subsequently, Alkire and colleagues have shown that either or both of these can occur during general anesthesia.[76] There has been experimental evidence to support this hypothesis as discussed in the next section. Another question to be addressed is whether there are cortical regions whose participation is more important for unconsciousness than that of others.

THE FRONTOPARIETAL NETWORK AND CONSCIOUSNESS

It has been suggested that specific regions of the lateral frontal and parietal association cortices play a critical role in conscious perception, attention, working memory, episodic retrieval, and intelligence.[72,166–168] Frontoparietal regions are preferentially deactivated in patients in a vegetative state[111] and during propofol anesthesia.[22] Alkire[76] recently described a hypothesized "consciousness circuit" consisting of the implicated frontoparietal regions and the posterior cingulate cortex. This system shows a certain degree of homology with the so-called default network of the brain,[169] which is highly active in the unstimulated brain but exhibits a decrease in activity during goal-directed behavior. Spontaneous activity in the default-mode network is reduced but not eliminated in states of unconsciousness produced by general anesthesia,[170–172] during sedation,[173] or in vegetative state,[174] consistent with the suggestion that the default network is anatomically determined.[175,176] However, the latter observations are based on fluctuations in blood-oxygen-dependent signals of MRI and therefore may not reflect all aspects of neuronal activity. Thus, further electrophysiological studies are necessary to determine the significance of these cortical regions in supporting the conscious state.

In an experimental study, Hudetz and coworkers estimated the information exchange between anterior and posterior cortical sites using *transfer entropy* that allows for a nonlinear, model-free estimation of directional information flow.[177] Multiple recording electrodes were chronically implanted in various regions of the visual system, in the adjoining parietal and temporal association areas, and in the frontal region at various locations to record local field potentials from which transfer entropy was then calculated. They found that the effect of volatile anesthetics on transfer entropy was asymmetrical. At critical anesthetic concentrations that produced unconsciousness, feedback transfer entropies in the frontoparietal, fronto-occipital, and parieto-occipital directions were significantly reduced (Figure 4.5C). Moreover, these reductions were significantly larger than the change in transfer entropies in the corresponding feedforward directions, suggesting that the critical anesthetic effect associated with unconsciousness (loss of the righting reflex) was the preferential reduction in feedback information transfer as carried by gamma oscillations.

Additional experimental support for the frontoparietal feedback hypothesis of anesthesia was recently obtained from human subjects undergoing general anesthesia. Lee et al[178] showed that directed feedback connectivity derived from multichannel EEG measurements was diminished upon the loss of consciousness in patients anesthetized with propofol. The effect was reversed when patients began to respond to verbal commands. In a parallel paper, Lee et al[179] calculated the capacity of the cortex for neural information integration based on Tononi's information theory. They found that propofol significantly reduced information integration capacity, especially in the EEG gamma band. In a different study, Heinke and coworkers[180] found that propofol suppressed frontal lobe activity before it suppressed temporal lobe activity during a language task when subjects became unresponsive, suggesting that fronto-temporal communication was impaired by anesthesia.

The cause of the preferential disruption of cortical feedback by anesthetics is not clear. The dependence of feedback connections on polysynaptic pathways could contribute to their enhanced sensitivity to anesthetics.[152] Anesthetic depression of synaptic transmission may result in a cumulative loss of signaling such that the more synapses involved, the greater overall suppression is produced. In turn, complex information processing that relies on high synaptic connectivity would be affected the most. Another mechanism may be that general anesthetics impede axonal conduction along unmyelinated fibers.[181,182] As these effects may not occur uniformly in the brain, there is the potential to disrupt the timing and synchronization of neuronal messages, thus impeding communication within functional neuronal assemblies that integrate sensory information.

In spite of their membership in the core functional networks of the brain, the role of frontal cortical sites in consciousness remains questionable.[183] Stuss et al[184] suggested that the frontal lobe is critical for self-awareness. However, frontal injury from stroke may produce an akinetic syndrome rather than loss of consciousness.[185] It is possible that the critical change in cortical information transfer for loss of consciousness occurs within the local feedback loops of the posterior parietal cortex, including sensory and association regions, leading to a generalized failure of information integration. Observations from epilepsy, stroke, vegetative state, and anesthesia converge, suggesting that a common cortical area, the region of posterior cingulate, retrosplenial and precuneus, has a critical role in consciousness.[186] With some anesthetics, such as ketamine, motor suppression may be the primary effect, dissociated from the smaller influence on sensory functions.[29,187] Thus, an agent-invariant "final common pathway" to unconsciousness may reside with the disruption of information integration in a network of the posterior cortex.

CAN WE FIND THE NEURAL CORRELATES OF UNCONSCIOUSNESS?

It is certainly the most miraculous fact that we have conscious experience. Its elusive nature, to even defy adequate definition, has led many thinkers into deep philosophical problems. To make progress, we and many others have followed the suggestion of Crick and Koch[188] to limit our investigation to the *neural correlates of consciousness*. For our purposes, the neural correlate of consciousness is defined as the "minimal neuronal function necessary and sufficient for consciousness" as a state. Being in a state of consciousness then is a necessary condition for being able to carry out conscious functions such as perception, mentation, reflection, thinking, etc.

When we can call a person conscious depends on one's definition of consciousness. In anesthesia practice, consciousness is often equated to wakefulness because a healthy wakeful person shows behavioral evidence for being conscious. However it is easy to see that this definition fails for certain brain-injured patients who are locked-in (motor incapacity), akinetic (volitional incapacity), or vegetative (integrative incapacity).[111,189–191] In these contexts, consciousness is often described as consisting of two components: wakefulness and awareness. Here wakefulness is related to behavioral arousal, and awareness is related to the contents of consciousness. However, if dreaming is considered a conscious experience, which often occurs during anesthesia,[192–195] then it is difficult to accept wakefulness as a necessary condition for consciousness, although the level of wakefulness clearly modulates the contents of conscious experience.

We contend that a two-dimensional partition of consciousness into awareness and wakefulness is still too simplistic. Sleepwalking does not fit the schema—because these patients have high level, cortex-dependent sensory and motor functions but no awareness of self and have, perhaps, a distorted sense of time. They lack agency and self-control. They are probably not aware of their actions. Are they conscious? In the operating room, we would say yes. Their neurologists or psychiatrists would say no.

These considerations lead to the conclusion that consciousness is best viewed to exist in multiple psychophysical dimensions: perceptual, interoceptual, volitional, conceptual, emotional, etc. How each of these dimensions may be influenced by anesthetic agents remains a challenge for future research.

The differentiation between wakefulness and consciousness is even more difficult to determine in animals for whom voluntary communication is essentially impossible. In animal experiments we can only observe behavior, so we have to go on the assumption that waking behavior entails conscious experience. This may be misleading. Decerebrate rats recover and are able to right themselves, groom, and move around, although they are unable to forage food for themselves.[196] Mesencephalic transected cats also display elaborate waking behaviors including sitting, standing, walking, and climbing. They show orientation and avoidance, and can learn through conditioning. There is little doubt that the isolated neocortex has no knowledge of these behaviors. It is possible that such animals are in a "zombie"-like state, similar to sleepwalking and not accompanied by conscious reflection. However, in decerebrate animals, the isolated forebrain normally displays alternating states of synchronized and desynchronized electrocortical activity, suggesting that it may be able to sustain information processing and perhaps even consciousness. This may be an endogenous form of consciousness, similar to dreaming,[197,198] but nevertheless, a subjective state. Whether a form of isolated consciousness may be present in the cortex cannot be determined with certainty at this time.

CONCLUDING THOUGHTS

One of the currently influential theories of anesthesia is that anesthetic agents activate sleep-promoting and deactivate wake-promoting centers in the brainstem and diencephalon.[199] This effect may be likened to turning off the power switch to the forebrain as it is accompanied by electroencephalographic changes suggesting sleep. However, in spite of a profound suppression of spontaneous activity, the cortex remains reactive and arousable by sensory stimuli. Cortical arousal during anesthesia is not expressed behaviorally due to the simultaneous suppression of descending and spinal motor pathways. Thus, we cannot be certain whether or not the transient and covert arousal events may occasionally be accompanied by momentary conscious experiences and, possibly, subsequent memories.

For decades, the regulation of natural sleep has been viewed as an essentially bottom-up mechanism. It is now believed that the regulation of sleep-wake states is hierarchical; it is organized in a rostrocaudal manner such that telencephalic control overrides diencephalic control, which in turn overrides brainstem control.[200] A person's state can thus be controlled relatively independently, by forebrain and by brainstem structures. Parts of the brain may be asleep or awake, questioning the validity of sleep and waking as unitary descriptors of state. In the hierarchical relationship of state control centers, the descending control from the telencephalon is essentially inhibitory, involved in voluntary maintenance of alertness and overriding the lower centers that are more autonomous and simple. The actual state switching occurs at the intermediate, thalamic–basal forebrain level, via both ascending and descending influences, but this too is under cortical control. Since general anesthetics simultaneously target multiple levels of integrated control, a delineation of their action into primary and secondary effects is more difficult. Nevertheless, the behavioral expression of patients during anesthesia induction and emergence, most often seen as drowsy disinhibition, suggest that the cortical voluntary component that controls attention, working memory and purposeful action is suppressed first. Cortical suppression then releases the midbrain switching circuits and the automaticity of brainstem control that favors sleep, atonia, and other corresponding physiological traits.

So how important is the thalamus itself for consciousness? If both thalami are surgically removed, olfactory, auditory, and visual stimuli can still activate the cortex through extrathalamic routes,[200] but it is unlikely that these activations can form a conscious percept. Athalamic animals cannot locate the source of stimuli and their EEG is dominated by high-voltage slow waves. Thus, the thalamus is a key component of the consciousness circuit not only relaying but also controlling information flow and integration within the cortex. It is the latter capacity of the thalamus that is compromised in anesthesia when consciousness is lost. Thus, in many respects, the thalamic suppression seen in neuroimaging studies of anesthesia might turn out to be the modern equivalent of neuroimaging phrenology. It is simply a reflection of an underlying process that is much more complex and actually likely to be occurring elsewhere in the structure of the brain.

ACKNOWLEDGMENTS

Part of this work was supported by the grant R01 GM-56398 from the Institute of General Medical Sciences, National Institutes of Health, Bethesda, Maryland, USA. The help from Jeannette Vizuete, B.S. preparing Panel A of Figure 5 is appreciated.

REFERENCES

1. Raichle ME. Visualizing the mind. *Sci Am.* Apr 1994;270(4): 58–64.
2. Ogawa S, Lee TM, Nayak AS, Glynn P. Oxygenation-sensitive contrast in magnetic resonance image of rodent brain at high magnetic fields. *Magn Reson Med.* Apr 1990;14(1):68–78.
3. Stullken EH Jr., Milde JH, Michenfelder JD, Tinker JH. The nonlinear responses of cerebral metabolism to low concentrations of halothane, enflurane, isoflurane, and thiopental. *Anesthesiology.* Jan 1977; 46(1):28–34.
4. Kennedy C, des Rosiers M, Reivich M, Sokoloff L. Mapping of functional pathways in brain by autoradiographic survey of local cerebral metabolism. *Trans Am Neurol Assoc.* 1974;99:143–147.
5. Reivich M, Sokoloff L, Shapiro H, des Rosiers M, Kennedy C. Validation of an autoradiographic method for the determination of the rates of local cerebral glucose utilization. *Trans Am Neurol Assoc.* 1974;99:238–240.
6. Sokoloff L. [1-14C]-2-deoxy-d-glucose method for measuring local cerebral glucose utilization: mathematical analysis and determination of the "lumped" constants. *Neurosci Res Program Bull.* Sep 1976;14(4):466–468.
7. Crosby G, Crane AM, Jehle J, Sokoloff L. The local metabolic effects of somatosensory stimulation in the central nervous system of rats given pentobarbital or nitrous oxide. *Anesthesiology.* Jan 1983; 58(1):38–43.
8. Crosby G, Crane AM, Sokoloff L. Local changes in cerebral glucose utilization during ketamine anesthesia. *Anesthesiology.* Jun 1982; 56(6):437–443.
9. Dam M, Ori C, Pizzolato G, et al. The effects of propofol anesthesia on local cerebral glucose utilization in the rat. *Anesthesiology.* Sep 1990;73(3):499–505.
10. Davis DW, Hawkins RA, Mans AM, Hibbard LS, Biebuyck JF. Regional cerebral glucose utilization during Althesin anesthesia. *Anesthesiology.* Oct 1984;61(4):362–368.
11. Davis DW, Mans AM, Biebuyck JF, Hawkins RA. Regional brain glucose utilization in rats during etomidate anesthesia. *Anesthesiology.* Jun 1986;64(6):751–757.
12. Dudley RE, Nelson SR, Samson F. Influence of chloralose on brain regional glucose utilization. *Brain Res.* Feb 4 1982;233(1): 173–180.
13. Ito M, Miyaoka M, Ishii S. Alterations in local cerebral glucose utilization during various anesthesia—the effect of urethane and a review [in Japanese]. *No To Shinkei.* Dec 1984;36(12): 1191–1199.
14. Lenz C, Rebel A, van Ackern K, Kuschinsky W, Waschke KF. Local cerebral blood flow, local cerebral glucose utilization, and flow-metabolism coupling during sevoflurane versus isoflurane anesthesia in rats. *Anesthesiology.* Dec 1998;89(6):1480–1488.
15. Maekawa T, Tommasino C, Shapiro HM, Keifer-Goodman J, Kohlenberger RW. Local cerebral blood flow and glucose utilization during isoflurane anesthesia in the rat. *Anesthesiology.* 1986;65(2): 144–151.
16. Nakakimura K, Sakabe T, Funatsu N, Maekawa T, Takeshita H. Metabolic activation of intercortical and corticothalamic pathways during enflurane anesthesia in rats. *Anesthesiology.* May 1988; 68(5):777–782.

17. Ori C, Dam M, Pizzolato G, Battistin L, Giron G. Effects of isoflurane anesthesia on local cerebral glucose utilization in the rat. *Anesthesiology.* Aug 1986;65(2):152–156.
18. Savaki HE, Desban M, Glowinski J, Besson MJ. Local cerebral glucose consumption in the rat, I: effects of halothane anesthesia. *J Comp Neurol.* Jan 1 1983;213(1):36–45.
19. Freo U, Dam M, Ori C. The time-dependent effects of midazolam on regional cerebral glucose metabolism in rats. *Anesth Analg.* May 2008;106(5):1516–1523.
20. Alkire MT, Haier RJ, Barker SJ, Shah NK, Wu JC, Kao YJ. Cerebral metabolism during propofol anesthesia in humans studied with positron emission tomography. *Anesthesiology.* 1995;82(2): 393–403; 327A.
21. Bonhomme V, Fiset P, Meuret P, et al. Propofol anesthesia and cerebral blood flow changes elicited by vibrotactile stimulation: a positron emission tomography study. *J Neurophysiol.* 2001;85(3): 1299–1308.
22. Fiset P, Paus T, Daloze T, et al. Brain mechanisms of propofol-induced loss of consciousness in humans: a positron emission tomographic study. *J Neurosci.* 1999;19(13):5506–5513.
23. Veselis RA, Reinsel RA, Beattie BJ, et al. Midazolam changes cerebral blood flow in discrete brain regions: an H2(15)O positron emission tomography study. *Anesthesiology.* 1997;87(5):1106–1117.
24. Alkire MT, Haier RJ, Shah NK, Anderson CT. Positron emission tomography study of regional cerebral metabolism in humans during isoflurane anesthesia. *Anesthesiology.* 1997;86(3):549–557.
25. Langsjo JW, Maksimow A, Salmi E, et al. S-ketamine anesthesia increases cerebral blood flow in excess of the metabolic needs in humans. *Anesthesiology.* Aug 2005;103(2):258–268.
26. Kaisti KK, Metsahonkala L, Teras M, et al. Effects of surgical levels of propofol and sevoflurane anesthesia on cerebral blood flow in healthy subjects studied with positron emission tomography. *Anesthesiology.* Jun 2002;96(6):1358–1370.
27. Veselis RA, Feshchenko VA, Reinsel RA, Dnistrian AM, Beattie B, Akhurst TJ. Thiopental and propofol affect different regions of the brain at similar pharmacologic effects. *Anesth Analg.* Aug 2004; 99(2):399–408.
28. Fiset P, Plourde G, Backman SB. Brain imaging in research on anesthetic mechanisms: studies with propofol. *Prog Brain Res.* 2005; 150:245–250.
29. Alkire MT, Haier RJ, Fallon JH. Toward a unified theory of narcosis: brain imaging evidence for a thalamocortical switch as the neurophysiologic basis of anesthetic- induced unconsciousness. *Conscious Cogn.* 2000;9(3):370–386.
30. White NS, Alkire MT. Impaired thalamocortical connectivity in humans during general-anesthetic-induced unconsciousness. *Neuroimage.* Jun 2003;19(2 Pt 1):402–411.
31. Baars BJ, Ramsoy TZ, Laureys S. Brain, conscious experience and the observing self. *Trends Neurosci.* Dec 2003;26(12):671–675.
32. Schiff ND. Central thalamic contributions to arousal regulation and neurological disorders of consciousness. *Ann N Y Acad Sci.* 2008; 1129:105–118.
33. Tononi G, Koch C. The neural correlates of consciousness: an update. *Ann N Y Acad Sci.* Mar 2008;1124:239–261.
34. LaBerge D. Attention, awareness, and the triangular circuit. *Conscious Cogn.* Jun 1997;6(2/3):149–181.
35. Guillery RW, Sherman SM. Thalamic relay functions and their role in corticocortical communication: generalizations from the visual system. *Neuron.* Jan 17 2002;33(2):163–175.
36. Sillito AM, Jones HE. Corticothalamic interactions in the transfer of visual information. *Philos Trans R Soc Lond B Biol Sci.* Dec 29 2002;357(1428):1739–1752.
37. Llinas RR, Steriade M. Bursting of thalamic neurons and states of vigilance. *J Neurophysiol.* Jun 2006;95(6):3297–3308.
38. Berg-Johnsen J, Langmoen IA. Mechanisms concerned in the direct effect of isoflurane on rat hippocampal and human neocortical neurons. *Brain Res.* Jan 15 1990;507(1):28–34.
39. Hentschke H, Schwarz C, Antkowiak B. Neocortex is the major target of sedative concentrations of volatile anaesthetics: strong depression of firing rates and increase of GABAA receptor-mediated inhibition. *Eur J Neurosci.* Jan 2005;21(1):93–102.
40. Ogawa T, Shingu K, Shibata M, Osawa M, Mori K. The divergent actions of volatile anaesthetics on background neuronal activity and reactive capability in the central nervous system in cats. *Can J Anaesth.* Oct 1992;39(8):862–872.
41. Osawa M, Shingu K, Murakawa M, et al. Effects of sevoflurane on central nervous system electrical activity in cats. *Anesth Analg.* Jul 1994;79(1):52–57.
42. Angel A. The G. L. Brown lecture. Adventures in anaesthesia. *Exp Physiol.* 1991;76(1):1–38.
43. Detsch O, Vahle-Hinz C, Kochs E, Siemers M, Bromm B. Isoflurane induces dose-dependent changes of thalamic somatosensory information transfer. *Brain Res.* 1999;829(1–2):77–89.
44. Ries CR, Puil E. Mechanism of anesthesia revealed by shunting actions of isoflurane on thalamocortical neurons. *J Neurophysiol.* 1999;81(4):1795–1801.
45. Angel A. Central neuronal pathways and the process of anaesthesia. *Br J Anaesth.* Jul 1993;71(1):148–163.
46. Ries CR, Puil E. Ionic mechanism of isoflurane's actions on thalamocortical neurons. *J Neurophysiol.* 1999;81(4):1802–1809.
47. Adams AD, Forrester JM. The projection of the rat's visual field on the cerebral cortex. *Q J Exp Physiol Cogn Med Sci.* Jul 1968; 53(3):327–336.
48. Mountcastle VB, Davies PW, Berman AL. Response properties of neurons of cat's somatic sensory cortex to peripheral stimuli. *J Neurophysiol.* Jul 1957;20(4):374–407.
49. Armstrong-James M, George MJ. Influence of anesthesia on spontaneous activity and receptive field size of single units in rat Sm1 neocortex. *Exp Neurol.* Feb 1988;99(2):369–387.
50. Villeneuve MY, Casanova C. On the use of isoflurane versus halothane in the study of visual response properties of single cells in the primary visual cortex. *J Neurosci Methods.* Oct 15 2003;129(1):19–31.
51. Ikeda H, Wright MJ. Sensitivity of neurones in visual cortex (area 17) under different levels of anaesthesia. *Exp Brain Res.* 1974; 20(5):471–484.
52. Tigwell DA, Sauter J. On the use of isofluorane as an anaesthetic for visual neurophysiology. *Exp Brain Res.* 1992;88(1):224–228.
53. Robson JG. The effects of anesthetic drugs on cortical units. *Anesthesiology.* Jan-Feb 1967;28(1):144–154.
54. Ikeda H, Wright MJ. Effect of halothane-nitrous oxide anaesthesia on the behaviour of "sustained" and "transient" visual cortical neurones. *J Physiol.* Mar 1974;237(2):20P–21P.
55. Chapin JK, Waterhouse BD, Woodward DJ. Differences in cutaneous sensory response properties of single somatosensory cortical neurons in awake and halothane anesthetized rats. *Brain Res Bull.* Jan 1981;6(1):63–70.
56. Hudetz AG, Vizuete JA, Imas OA. Desflurane selectively suppresses long-latency cortical neuronal response to flash in the rat. *Anesthesiology.* Aug 2009;111(2):231–239.
57. Erchova IA, Lebedev MA, Diamond ME. Somatosensory cortical neuronal population activity across states of anaesthesia. *Eur J Neurosci.* Feb 2002;15(4):744–752.
58. Nishikawa K, MacIver MB. Excitatory synaptic transmission mediated by NMDA receptors is more sensitive to isoflurane than are non-NMDA receptor-mediated responses. *Anesthesiology.* Jan 2000; 92(1):228–236.
59. O'Brien JH, Rosenblum SM. Contribution of nonspecific thalamus to sensory evoked activity in cat postcruciate cortex. *J Neurophysiol.* May 1974;37(3):430–442.
60. Ferrarelli F, Massimini M, Sarasso S, et al. Breakdown in cortical effective connectivity during midazolam-induced loss of consciousness. *Proc Natl Acad Sci U S A.* Feb 9 2010;107(6):2681–2686.
61. Massimini M, Ferrarelli F, Huber R, Esser SK, Singh H, Tononi G. Breakdown of cortical effective connectivity during sleep. *Science.* Sep 30 2005;309(5744):2228–2232.
62. Coogan TA, Burkhalter A. Conserved patterns of cortico-cortical connections define areal hierarchy in rat visual cortex. *Exp Brain Res.* 1990;80(1):49–53.

63. Bullier J. Integrated model of visual processing. *Brain Res Rev.* Oct 2001;36(2–3):96–107.
64. Cauller LJ, Kulics AT. The neural basis of the behaviorally relevant N1 component of the somatosensory-evoked potential in SI cortex of awake monkeys: evidence that backward cortical projections signal conscious touch sensation. *Exp Brain Res.* 1991;84(3): 607–619.
65. Jackson ME, Cauller LJ. Neural activity in SII modifies sensory evoked potentials in SI in awake rats. *Neuroreport.* 1998;9(15): 3379–3382.
66. Cauller L. Layer I of primary sensory neocortex: where top-down converges upon bottom-up. *Behav Brain Res.* 1995;71(1–2): 163–170.
67. Shao Z, Burkhalter A. Different balance of excitation and inhibition in forward and feedback circuits of rat visual cortex. *J Neurosci.* 1996;16(22):7353–7365.
68. Lamme VA, Roelfsema PR. The distinct modes of vision offered by feedforward and recurrent processing. *Trends Neurosci.* Nov 2000; 23(11):571–579.
69. Pascual-Leone A, Walsh V. Fast backprojections from the motion to the primary visual area necessary for visual awareness. *Science.* Apr 20 2001;292(5516):510–512.
70. Heinke W, Schwarzbauer C. Subanesthetic isoflurane affects task-induced brain activation in a highly specific manner: a functional magnetic resonance imaging study. *Anesthesiology.* 2001;94(6): 973–981.
71. Garrido MI, Kilner JM, Kiebel SJ, Friston KJ. Evoked brain responses are generated by feedback loops. *Proc Natl Acad Sci U S A.* Dec 26 2007;104(52):20961–20966.
72. Del Cul A, Baillet S, Dehaene S. Brain dynamics underlying the non-linear threshold for access to consciousness. *PLoS Biol.* Oct 2007; 5(10):e260.
73. Badgaiyan RD. Conscious awareness of retrieval: an exploration of the cortical connectivity. *Int J Psychophysiol.* Feb 2005;55(2): 257–262.
74. Aru J, Bachmann T. Occipital EEG correlates of conscious awareness when subjective target shine-through and effective visual masking are compared: bifocal early increase in gamma power and speed-up of P1. *Brain Res.* May 19 2009;1271:60–73.
75. Aru J, Bachmann T. Boosting up gamma-band oscillations leaves target-stimulus in masking out of awareness: explaining an apparent paradox. *Neurosci Lett.* Feb 6 2009;450(3):351–355.
76. Alkire MT, Hudetz AG, Tononi G. Consciousness and anesthesia. *Science.* Nov 7 2008;322(5903):876–880.
77. Hudetz AG. Suppressing consciousness: mechanisms of general anesthesia. *Seminars in Anesthesia, Perioperative Medicine and Pain.* 2006;25(4):196–204.
78. Clement EA, Richard A, Thwaites M, Ailon J, Peters S, Dickson CT. Cyclic and sleep-like spontaneous alternations of brain state under urethane anaesthesia. *PLoS One.* 2008;3(4):e2004.
79. Wilson MT, Barry M, Reynolds JN, Hutchison EJ, Steyn-Ross DA. Characteristics of temporal fluctuations in the hyperpolarized state of the cortical slow oscillation. *Phys Rev E Stat Nonlin Soft Matter Phys.* Jun 2008;77(6 Pt 1):061908.
80. Timofeev I, Grenier F, Bazhenov M, Sejnowski TJ, Steriade M. Origin of slow cortical oscillations in deafferented cortical slabs. *Cereb Cortex.* Dec 2000;10(12):1185–1199.
81. Fuentealba P, Timofeev I, Bazhenov M, Sejnowski TJ, Steriade M. Membrane bistability in thalamic reticular neurons during spindle oscillations. *J Neurophysiol.* Jan 2005;93(1): 294–304.
82. Hill S, Tononi G. Modeling sleep and wakefulness in the thalamo-cortical system. *J Neurophysiol.* Mar 2005;93(3):1671–1698.
83. Hartikainen K, Rorarius M, Makela K, Perakyla J, Varila E, Jantti V. Visually evoked bursts during isoflurane anaesthesia. *Br J Anaesth.* 1995;74(6):681–685.
84. Hartikainen KM, Rorarius M, Perakyla JJ, Laippala PJ, Jantti V. Cortical reactivity during isoflurane burst-suppression anesthesia. *Anesth Analg.* 1995;81(6):1223–1228.
85. Hartikainen K, Rorarius MG. Cortical responses to auditory stimuli during isoflurane burst suppression anaesthesia. *Anaesthesia.* 1999;54(3):210–214.
86. Hudetz AG, Imas OA. Burst activation of the cerebral cortex by flash stimuli during isoflurane anesthesia in rats. *Anesthesiology.* Dec 2007;107(6):983–991.
87. Kroeger D, Amzica F. Hypersensitivity of the anesthesia-induced comatose brain. *J Neurosci.* Sep 26 2007;27(39):10597–10607.
88. Rojas MJ, Navas JA, Greene SA, Rector DM. Discrimination of auditory stimuli during isoflurane anesthesia. *Comp Med.* Oct 2008;58(5):454–457.
89. French JD, Livingston RB, Hernandez-Peon R. Cortical influences upon the arousal mechanism. *Trans Am Neurol Assoc.* 1953;3(78th Meeting):57–58; 58–59.
90. Moruzzi G, Magoun HW. Brain stem reticular formation and activation of the EEG. *Electroencephalogr Clin Neurophysiol.* Nov 1949;1(4):455–473.
91. Dringenberg HC, Olmstead MC. Integrated contributions of basal forebrain and thalamus to neocortical activation elicited by pedunculopontine tegmental stimulation in urethane-anesthetized rats. *Neuroscience.* 2003;119(3):839–853.
92. Jasper HH. Sensory information and conscious experience. *Adv Neurol.* 1998;77:33–48.
93. Jasper HH. Historical perspective. *Adv Neurol.* 1998;77:1–6.
94. Jones EG. A new view of specific and nonspecific thalamocortical connections. *Adv Neurol.* 1998;77:49–71.
95. Jones EG. Viewpoint: the core and matrix of thalamic organization. *Neuroscience.* 1998;85(2):331–345.
96. Van der Werf YD, Witter MP, Groenewegen HJ. The intralaminar and midline nuclei of the thalamus. Anatomical and functional evidence for participation in processes of arousal and awareness. *Brain Res Rev.* Sep 2002;39(2–3):107–140.
97. Schiff ND. Central thalamic deep-brain stimulation in the severely injured brain: rationale and proposed mechanisms of action. *Ann N Y Acad Sci.* Mar 2009;1157:101–116.
98. Alkire MT, McReynolds JR, Hahn EL, Trivedi AN. Thalamic microinjection of nicotine reverses sevoflurane-induced loss of righting reflex in the rat. *Anesthesiology.* Aug 2007;107(2): 264–272.
99. Alkire MT, Asher CD, Franciscus AM, Hahn EL. Thalamic microinfusion of antibody to a voltage-gated potassium channel restores consciousness during anesthesia. *Anesthesiology.* Apr 2009; 110(4):766–773.
100. Miller JW. The role of mesencephalic and thalamic arousal systems in experimental seizures. *Prog Neurobiol.* Aug 1992;39(2): 155–178.
101. Miller JW, Ferrendelli JA. The central medial nucleus: thalamic site of seizure regulation. *Brain Res.* Feb 5 1990;508(2): 297–300.
102. Miller JW, Ferrendelli JA. Characterization of GABAergic seizure regulation in the midline thalamus. *Neuropharmacology.* Jul 1990; 29(7):649–655.
103. Van Lierop D, Alkire M. Evidence for a localized consciousness "off-switch": Microinfusion of the GABA agonist muscimol into the central medial thalamus reduces the dose of sevoflurane required to produce unconsciousness. *FAER Medical Student Anesthesia Research Fellowship Symposium*, Orlando, FL 2008, p 34.
104. Ma J, Shen B, Stewart LS, Herrick IA, Leung LS. The septohippocampal system participates in general anesthesia. *J Neurosci.* 2002 Jan 15;22(2):RC200.
105. Ma J, Leung LS. Limbic system participates in mediating the effects of general anesthetics. *Neuropsychopharmacology.* 2006 Jun;31(6):1177–1192.
106. Nelson LE, Guo TZ, Lu J, Saper CB, Franks NP, Maze M. The sedative component of anesthesia is mediated by GABA(A) receptors in an endogenous sleep pathway. *Nat Neurosci.* 2002 Oct;5(10):979–984.
107. Vahle-Hinz C, Detsch O, Siemers M, Kochs E. Contributions of GABAergic and glutamatergic mechanisms to isoflurane-induced

suppression of thalamic somatosensory information transfer. *Exp Brain Res.* Jan 2007;176(1):159–172.
108. French JD, Hernandez-Peon R, Livingston RB. Projections from cortex to cephalic brain stem (reticular formation) in monkey. *J Neurophysiol.* Jan 1955;18(1):74–95.
109. Velly LJ, Rey MF, Bruder NJ, et al. Differential dynamic of action on cortical and subcortical structures of anesthetic agents during induction of anesthesia. *Anesthesiology.* Aug 2007;107(2): 202–212.
110. Judge O, Hill S, Antognini JF. Modeling the effects of midazolam on cortical and thalamic neurons. *Neurosci Lett.* Oct 23 2009; 464(2):135–139.
111. Laureys S. The neural correlate of (un)awareness: lessons from the vegetative state. *Trends Cogn Sci.* Dec 2005;9(12):556–559.
112. Llinas R, Ribary U, Contreras D, Pedroarena C. The neuronal basis for consciousness. *Philos Trans R Soc Lond B Biol Sci.* Nov 29 1998;353(1377):1841–1849.
113. Llinas R, Ribary U. Consciousness and the brain: the thalamocortical dialogue in health and disease. *Ann N Y Acad Sci.* Apr 2001; 929:166–175.
114. Fries P, Reynolds JH, Rorie AE, Desimone R. Modulation of oscillatory neuronal synchronization by selective visual attention. *Science.* 2001;291(5508):1560–1563.
115. Bouyer JJ, Montaron MF, Rougeul A, Buser P. Parietal electrocortical rhythms in the cat: their relation to a behavior of focused attention and possible mesencephalic control through a dopaminergic pathway [in French]. *C R Seances Acad Sci D.* 1980;291(9): 779–783.
116. Steinmetz PN, Roy A, Fitzgerald PJ, Hsiao SS, Johnson KO, Niebur E. Attention modulates synchronized neuronal firing in primate somatosensory cortex. *Nature.* 2000;404(6774):187–190.
117. Tiitinen H, Sinkkonen J, Reinikainen K, Alho K, Lavikainen J, Naatanen R. Selective attention enhances the auditory 40-Hz transient response in humans. *Nature.* 1993;364(6432):59–60.
118. Muller MM, Gruber T, Keil A. Modulation of induced gamma band activity in the human EEG by attention and visual information processing. *Int J Psychophysiol.* 2000;38(3):283–299.
119. Tallon-Baudry C, Kreiter A, Bertrand O. Sustained and transient oscillatory responses in the gamma and beta bands in a visual short-term memory task in humans. *Vis Neurosci.* 1999;16(3): 449–459.
120. Treisman A. The binding problem. *Curr Opin Neurobiol.* Apr 1996;6(2):171–178.
121. Srinivasan R, Russell DP, Edelman GM, Tononi G. Increased synchronization of neuromagnetic responses during conscious perception. *J Neurosci.* 1999;19(13):5435–5448.
122. Keil A, Muller MM, Ray WJ, Gruber T, Elbert T. Human gamma band activity and perception of a gestalt. *J Neurosci.* 1999; 19(16):7152–7161.
123. Tallon-Baudry C, Bertrand O. Oscillatory gamma activity in humans and its role in object representation. *Trends Cogn Sci.* 1999;3(4):151–162.
124. Donoghue JP, Sanes JN, Hatsopoulos NG, Gaal G. Neural discharge and local field potential oscillations in primate motor cortex during voluntary movements. *J Neurophysiol.* 1998;79(1):159–173.
125. Riehle A, Grammont F, Diesmann M, Grun S. Dynamical changes and temporal precision of synchronized spiking activity in monkey motor cortex during movement preparation. *J Physiol Paris.* 2000;94(5–6):569–582.
126. Pfurtscheller G, Flotzinger D, Neuper C. Differentiation between finger, toe and tongue movement in man based on 40 Hz EEG. *Electroencephalogr Clin Neurophysiol.* 1994;90(6):456–460.
127. Bressler SL, Coppola R, Nakamura R. Episodic multiregional cortical coherence at multiple frequencies during visual task performance. *Nature.* 1993;366(6451):153–156.
128. Rodriguez E, George N, Lachaux JP, Martinerie J, Renault B, Varela FJ. Perception's shadow: long-distance synchronization of human brain activity. *Nature.* 1999;397(6718):430–433.
129. Roelfsema PR, Engel AK, Konig P, Singer W. Visuomotor integration is associated with zero time-lag synchronization among cortical areas. *Nature.* 1997;385(6612):157–161.
130. Maloney KJ, Cape EG, Gotman J, Jones BE. High-frequency gamma electroencephalogram activity in association with sleep-wake states and spontaneous behaviors in the rat. *Neuroscience.* 1997;76(2):541–555.
131. Desmedt JE, Tomberg C. Transient phase-locking of 40 Hz electrical oscillations in prefrontal and parietal human cortex reflects the process of conscious somatic perception. *Neurosci Lett.* 1994; 168(1–2):126–129.
132. Engel AK, Konig P, Kreiter AK, Singer W. Interhemispheric synchronization of oscillatory neuronal responses in cat visual cortex. *Science.* 1991;252(5010):1177–1179.
133. von Stein A, Rappelsberger P, Sarnthein J, Petsche H. Synchronization between temporal and parietal cortex during multimodal object processing in man. *Cereb Cortex.* 1999;9(2): 137–150.
134. von Stein A, Chiang C, Konig P. Top-down processing mediated by interareal synchronization. *Proc Natl Acad Sci U S A.* 2000; 97(26):14748–14753.
135. Munk MH, Roelfsema PR, Konig P, Engel AK, Singer W. Role of reticular activation in the modulation of intracortical synchronization. *Science.* 1996;272(5259):271–274.
136. Sarnthein J, Petsche H, Rappelsberger P, Shaw GL, von Stein A. Synchronization between prefrontal and posterior association cortex during human working memory. *Proc Natl Acad Sci U S A.* 1998;95(12):7092–7096.
137. Melloni L, Molina C, Pena M, Torres D, Singer W, Rodriguez E. Synchronization of neural activity across cortical areas correlates with conscious perception. *J Neurosci.* Mar 14 2007;27(11): 2858–2865.
138. Kulli J, Koch C. Does anesthesia cause loss of consciousness? *Trends Neurosci.* Jan 1991;14(1):6–10.
139. Schwender D, Weninger E, Daunderer M, Klasing S, Poppel E, Peter K. Anesthesia with increasing doses of sufentanil and midlatency auditory evoked potentials in humans. *Anesth Analg.* 1995; 80(3):499–505.
140. Schwender D, Klasing S, Conzen P, Finsterer U, Poppel E, Peter K. Midlatency auditory evoked potentials during anaesthesia with increasing endexpiratory concentrations of desflurane. *Acta Anaesthesiol Scand.* 1996;40(2):171–176.
141. Schwender D, Daunderer M, Mulzer S, Klasing S, Finsterer U, Peter K. Midlatency auditory evoked potentials predict movements during anesthesia with isoflurane or propofol. *Anesth Analg.* 1997;85(1):164–173.
142. Schwender D, Daunderer M, Schnatmann N, Klasing S, Finsterer U, Peter K. Midlatency auditory evoked potentials and motor signs of wakefulness during anaesthesia with midazolam. *Br J Anaesth.* 1997;79(1):53–58.
143. Plourde G, Villemure C. Comparison of the effects of enflurane/N2O on the 40-Hz auditory steady- state response versus the auditory middle-latency response. *Anesth Analg.* 1996;82(1): 75–83.
144. Plourde G, Villemure C, Fiset P, Bonhomme V, Backman SB. Effect of isoflurane on the auditory steady-state response and on consciousness in human volunteers. *Anesthesiology.* 1998;89(4): 844–851.
145. Vanderwolf CH. Are neocortical gamma waves related to consciousness? *Brain Res.* 2000;855(2):217–224.
146. Steriade M. Corticothalamic networks, oscillations, and plasticity. *Adv Neurol.* 1998;77:105–134.
147. Buzsaki G, Leung LW, Vanderwolf CH. Cellular bases of hippocampal EEG in the behaving rat. *Brain Res.* 1983;287(2): 139–171.
148. Kral A, Tillein J, Hartmann R, Klinke R. Monitoring of anaesthesia in neurophysiological experiments. *Neuroreport.* 1999; 10(4):781–787.

149. Fell J, Widman G, Rehberg B, Elger CE, Fernandez G. Human mediotemporal EEG characteristics during propofol anesthesia. *Biol Cybern.* Feb 2005;92(2):92–100.
150. Imas OA, Ropella KM, Wood JD, Hudetz AG. Halothane augments event-related gamma oscillations in rat visual cortex. *Neuroscience.* 2004;123(1):269–278.
151. Imas OA, Ropella KM, Ward BD, Wood JD, Hudetz AG. Volatile anesthetics enhance flash-induced gamma oscillations in rat visual cortex. *Anesthesiology.* May 2005;102(5):937–947.
152. Banoub M, Tetzlaff JE, Schubert A. Pharmacologic and physiologic influences affecting sensory evoked potentials: implications for perioperative monitoring. *Anesthesiology.* Sep 2003;99(3): 716–737.
153. Andrade J, Sapsford DJ, Jeevaratnum D, Pickworth AJ, Jones JG. The coherent frequency in the electroencephalogram as an objective measure of cognitive function during propofol sedation. *Anesth Analg.* 1996;83(6):1279–1284.
154. Bonhomme V, Plourde G, Meuret P, Fiset P, Backman SB. Auditory steady-state response and bispectral index for assessing level of consciousness during propofol sedation and hypnosis. *Anesth Analg.* 2000;91(6):1398–1403.
155. Munglani R, Andrade J, Sapsford DJ, Baddeley A, Jones JG. A measure of consciousness and memory during isoflurane administration: the coherent frequency. *Br J Anaesth.* 1993;71(5): 633–641.
156. Osa M, Ando M, Adachi-Usami E. Human flash visually evoked cortical potentials under different levels of halothane anesthesia [in Japanese]. *Nippon Ganka Gakkai Zasshi.* Feb 1989;93(2): 265–270.
157. Hudetz AG, Vizuete, JA, Pillay S. Differential effects of isoflurane on high-frequency and low-frequency gamma oscillations in the cerebral cortex and hippocampus in freely moving rats. *Anesthesiology* (2011);114(3):588–595.
158. Knight RT. Neuroscience: neural networks debunk phrenology. *Science.* Jun 15 2007;316(5831):1578–1579.
159. John ER, Prichep LS, Kox W, et al. Invariant reversible QEEG effects of anesthetics. *Conscious Cogn.* 2001;10(2):165–183.
160. Mashour GA. Consciousness unbound: toward a paradigm of general anesthesia. *Anesthesiology.* Feb 2004;100(2):428–433.
161. Mashour GA. Cognitive unbinding in sleep and anesthesia. *Science.* Dec 16 2005;310(5755):1768–1769; author reply 1769.
162. Hameroff SR. The entwined mysteries of anesthesia and consciousness: is there a common underlying mechanism? *Anesthesiology.* Aug 2006;105(2):400–412.
163. Imas OA, Ropella KM, Wood JD, Hudetz AG. Isoflurane disrupts anterio-posterior phase synchronization of flash-induced field potentials in the rat. *Neurosci Lett.* Jul 24 2006;402(3):216–221.
164. Koenig T, Prichep L, Lehmann D, et al. Millisecond by millisecond, year by year: normative EEG microstates and developmental stages. *Neuroimage.* May 2002;16(1):41–48.
165. Tononi G. An information integration theory of consciousness. *BMC Neurosci.* Nov 2 2004;5(1):42.
166. Rees G, Kreiman G, Koch C. Neural correlates of consciousness in humans. *Nat Rev Neurosci.* 2002;3(4):261–270.
167. Naghavi HR, Nyberg L. Common fronto-parietal activity in attention, memory, and consciousness: shared demands on integration? *Conscious Cogn.* Jun 2005;14(2):390–425.
168. Jung RE, Haier RJ. The Parieto-Frontal Integration Theory (P-FIT) of intelligence: converging neuroimaging evidence. *Behav Brain Sci.* Apr 2007;30(2):135–154; 154–187.
169. Raichle ME, MacLeod AM, Snyder AZ, Powers WJ, Gusnard DA, Shulman GL. A default mode of brain function. *Proc Natl Acad Sci U S A.* 2001;98(2):676–682.
170. Vincent JL, Patel GH, Fox MD, et al. Intrinsic functional architecture in the anaesthetized monkey brain. *Nature.* May 3 2007; 447(7140):83–86.
171. Peltier SJ, Kerssens C, Hamann SB, Sebel PS, Byas-Smith M, Hu X. Functional connectivity changes with concentration of sevoflurane anesthesia. *Neuroreport.* Feb 28 2005;16(3):285–288.
172. Deshpande G, Kerssens C, Sebel PS, Hu X. Altered local coherence in the default mode network due to sevoflurane anesthesia. *Brain Res.* Mar 8 2010;1318:110–121.
173. Greicius MD, Kiviniemi V, Tervonen O, et al. Persistent default-mode network connectivity during light sedation. *Hum Brain Mapp.* Jul 2008;29(7):839–847.
174. Boly M, Phillips C, Tshibanda L, et al. Intrinsic brain activity in altered states of consciousness: how conscious is the default mode of brain function? *Ann N Y Acad Sci.* 2008;1129:119–129.
175. Honey CJ, Sporns O, Cammoun L, et al. Predicting human resting-state functional connectivity from structural connectivity. *Proc Natl Acad Sci U S A.* Feb 10 2009;106(6):2035–2040.
176. Greicius MD, Supekar K, Menon V, Dougherty RF. Resting-state functional connectivity reflects structural connectivity in the default mode network. *Cereb Cortex.* Jan 2009;19(1):72–78.
177. Imas OA, Ropella KM, Ward BD, Wood JD, Hudetz AG. Volatile anesthetics disrupt frontal-posterior recurrent information transfer at gamma frequencies in rat. *Neurosci Lett.* Oct 28 2005; 387(3):145–150.
178. Lee U, Kim S, Noh GJ, Choi BM, Hwang E, Mashour GA. The directionality and functional organization of frontoparietal connectivity during consciousness and anesthesia in humans. *Conscious Cogn.* Dec 2009;18(4):1069–1078.
179. Lee U, Mashour GA, Kim S, Noh GJ, Choi BM. Propofol induction reduces the capacity for neural information integration: implications for the mechanism of consciousness and general anesthesia. *Conscious Cogn.* Mar 2009;18(1):56–64.
180. Heinke W, Fiebach CJ, Schwarzbauer C, Meyer M, Olthoff D, Alter K. Sequential effects of propofol on functional brain activation induced by auditory language processing: an event-related functional magnetic resonance imaging study. *Br J Anaesth.* May 2004;92(5):641–650.
181. Berg-Johnsen J, Langmoen IA. The effect of isoflurane on unmyelinated and myelinated fibres in the rat brain. *Acta Physiol Scand.* May 1986;127(1):87–93.
182. Swindale NV. Neural synchrony, axonal path lengths, and general anesthesia: a hypothesis. *Neuroscientist.* Dec 2003;9(6):440–445.
183. Wheeler MA, Stuss DT. Remembering and knowing in patients with frontal lobe injuries. *Cortex.* Sep-Dec 2003;39(4–5): 827–846.
184. Stuss DT, Picton TW, Alexander MP. Consciousness, self awareness, and the frontal lobes. In: Salloway S, Malloy P, Duffy JD, eds. *The Frontal Lobes and Neuropsychiatric Illness.* Washington, DC: American Psychiatric Pub.; 2001:101–109.
185. Lipschutz JH, Pascuzzi RM, Bognanno J, Putty T. Bilateral anterior cerebral artery infarction resulting from explosion-type injury to the head and neck. *Stroke.* Jun 1991;22(6):813–815.
186. Vogt BA, Laureys S. Posterior cingulate, precuneal and retrosplenial cortices: cytology and components of the neural network correlates of consciousness. *Prog Brain Res.* 2005;150:205–217.
187. Plourde G, Baribeau J, Bonhomme V. Ketamine increases the amplitude of the 40-Hz auditory steady-state response in humans. *Br J Anaesth.* 1997;78(5):524–529.
188. Crick F, Koch C. A framework for consciousness. *Nat Neurosci.* Feb 2003;6(2):119–126.
189. Laureys S, Pellas F, Van Eeckhout P, et al. The locked-in syndrome: what is it like to be conscious but paralyzed and voiceless? *Prog Brain Res.* 2005;150:495–511.
190. Laureys S, Boly M. What is it like to be vegetative or minimally conscious? *Curr Opin Neurol.* Dec 2007;20(6):609–613.
191. Laureys S, Boly M, Schnakers C, et al. Revelations from the unconscious: studying residual brain function in coma and related states. *Bull Mem Acad R Med Belg.* 2008;163(7–9):381–388; 388–390.

192. Kasmacher H, Petermeyer M, Decker C. Incidence and quality of dreaming during anesthesia with propofol in comparison with enflurane [in German]. *Anaesthesist.* Feb 1996;45(2):146–153.
193. Leslie K, Skrzypek H, Paech MJ, Kurowski I, Whybrow T. Dreaming during anesthesia and anesthetic depth in elective surgery patients: a prospective cohort study. *Anesthesiology.* Jan 2007; 106(1):33–42.
194. Leslie K, Sleigh J, Paech MJ, Voss L, Lim CW, Sleigh C. Dreaming and electroencephalographic changes during anesthesia maintained with propofol or desflurane. *Anesthesiology.* Sep 2009; 111(3):547–555.
195. Strickland RA, Butterworth JF. Sexual dreaming during anesthesia: early case histories (1849–1888) of the phenomenon. *Anesthesiology.* Jun 2007;106(6):1232–1236.
196. Woods JW. Behavior of chronic decerebrate rats. *J Neurophysiol.* Jul 1964;27:635–644.
197. Llinas RR, Pare D. Of dreaming and wakefulness. *Neuroscience.* 1991;44(3):521–535.
198. Llinas R, Ribary U. Coherent 40-Hz oscillation characterizes dream state in humans. *Proc Natl Acad Sci U S A.* 1993;90(5): 2078–2081.
199. Franks NP. General anaesthesia: from molecular targets to neuronal pathways of sleep and arousal. *Nat Rev Neurosci.* May 2008; 9(5):370–386.
200. Villablanca J, Marcus R. Sleep-wakefulness, EEG and behavioral studies of chronic cats without neocortex and striatum: the "diencephalic" cat. *Arch Ital Biol.* Oct 1972;110(3):348–382.
201. Schreckenberger, M., et al., The thalamus as the generator and modulator of EEG alpha rhythm: a combined PET/EEG study with lorazepam challenge in humans. Neuroimage, 2004; 22(2):637–644.
202. Bonhomme, V., et al., The effect of clonidine infusion on distribution of regional cerebral blood flow in volunteers. Anesth Analg. 2008;106(3): 899–909.
203. Nofzinger, E.A., et al., Human regional cerebral glucose metabolism during non-rapid eye movement sleep in relation to waking. Brain. 2002;125(Pt 5):1105–1115.
204. Prielipp, R.C., et al., Dexmedetomidine-induced sedation in volunteers decreases regional and global cerebral blood flow. Anesth Analg. 2002;95(4):1052–1059.
205. Rex, S., et al., Positron emission tomography study of regional cerebral metabolism during general anesthesia with xenon in humans. Anesthesiology. 2006;105(5):936–943.

5

ANESTHETIC MODULATION OF MEMORY PROCESSING IN THE MEDIAL TEMPORAL LOBE

Kane O. Pryor and Robert A. Veselis

The case of H.M., first reported in 1957,[1] stands as one of the most significant milestones in modern neuroscience. In an experimental procedure intended to treat a refractory seizure disorder, portions of his medial temporal lobes—including the hippocampus—were removed bilaterally. The surgery left H.M. completely unable to form new declarative (conscious) memories, a condition known as *anterograde amnesia*. Although he had impaired memory for events occurring in the two years prior to his surgery, more distant memories remained intact, as did his knowledge of the world and most higher executive functions. Further, he possessed intact working memory (the short-term ability to hold information in consciousness, archetypally the ability to hold and recycle a phone number in the present), and was able to acquire new motor skills despite being unable to remember having participated in any learning session. The numerous experiments that H.M. participated in from the time of his surgery until his death in 2008 came to define several of the central tenets that have driven memory research over recent decades: (i) the hippocampus is a necessary structure for the establishment of long-term declarative memory; (ii) established memories are initially dependent on the hippocampus, but become hippocampal-independent over time; and (iii) other forms of memory, including working and procedural memory, as well as the implicit (unconscious) memory demonstrated by successful repetition priming, are subserved by neuromechanistic systems that either do not involve, or are not dependent on the hippocampus.

One of the most remarkable properties of anesthetic drugs is that they possess the ability to create a state of anterograde amnesia that bears striking resemblance to that experienced by H.M. Thus, memory systems theories built on the demonstrated importance of the medial temporal lobe have provided the theoretical and experimental foundation for the study of anesthetic amnesia. *To be clear:* we are not referring to the amnesia that occurs with the state of general anesthesia. As some level of consciousness and attention is a necessary precursor to the establishment of a *conscious* memory, the amnesia of general anesthesia represents a special—and from a memory perspective somewhat trivial—case, as there is simply no conscious percept available to be either remembered or forgotten. Rather, we are referring to phenomena observed at lower brain concentrations of anesthetics, where the majority of complex cognitive functions remain intact, but declarative memory performance is significantly—and thus selectively—impaired. Clinicians encounter this in everyday practice in the patient who is given a small quantity of midazolam and who then participates in a quite normal conversation that they are later unable to recall. Our own research has focused on studying these phenomena in a highly controlled setting, using healthy volunteer subjects, steady-state pharmacokinetic modeling, and sophisticated neuropsychological experimental paradigms—while evaluating regional brain activity via electroencephalography (EEG), positron emission tomography (PET), or functional magnetic resonance imaging (fMRI).

In the following pages we describe a current perspective on anesthetic amnesia. Central to our view is that the phenomenon of greatest interest is memory as humans conventionally think of it and experience it—the complex, hippocampal-dependent declarative memory described above. The extent to which this phenomenon exists in laboratory animals is controversial,[2] and thus while animal and slice studies provide the ability to study biochemistry and neurophysiology in ways that could never be performed in humans, it is exceedingly difficult to define exactly how well rat and mouse models represent the human experience. Thus, we will focus where possible on studies of anesthetic amnesia in humans and attempt to establish a bridge between that body of work and the mechanistic insights derived from animal studies. It is not our intention to discuss the clinical problem of intraoperative awareness or the existence of implicit, nondeclarative memory under anesthesia.

DESCRIBING ANESTHETIC AMNESIA: A TIME-DEPENDENT FUNCTION

On first inspection, the task of identifying which anesthetic actions are necessary and sufficient to cause amnesia appears daunting. It is clear that declarative memory involves a large number of sequential and parallel processes that operate in a hierarchical complexity—ranging from actions defined at the level of the individual synaptic channel, to those involving emergent properties at the level of indefinably complex networks. The theoretical number of mechanistic pathways that could lead to amnesia is enormous. However, the candidates can be narrowed by appreciating that the memory "cascade" is a time-dependent function, and that many of the component processes can be characterized by operating within a specific time domain. Understanding exactly *when* anesthetic amnesia occurs thus powerfully informs and tests mechanistic hypotheses.

PRIMER ON THE TEMPORAL PHASES OF MEMORY

For taxonomic purposes, the temporal course of memory can be divided into four broad phases. A memory must first be *encoded* or *established*, such that a structural or functional change perpetuates some fragment of the conscious percept as a memory trace and separates it from unrelated signal or noise. This initial memory trace is immediate, but is transient and fragile, and must undergo *consolidation* to produce more stable changes in structure and function if it is to be propagated. As we shall later see, phases of consolidation are believed to dominate time domains ranging from a few minutes through to weeks or months after the initial encoding.[3] The consolidated memory then resides in a state of *long-term storage*. It is unclear how long a memory trace that is never reactivated can survive in dormancy, but the fact that adults lose most memories of childhood except for those that are frequently reiterated suggests that the trace signal continuously weakens or is replaced over time. Finally, at some time after encoding, the memory trace is *retrieved*, and reenters awareness by transiently capturing the characteristics of the conscious percept. There is substantial evidence that this retrieval into consciousness reactivates the cascade—a process termed *reconsolidation*.[4] Thus, retrieval renders a memory trace transiently plastic, which allows for augmentation, but also permits contextual shifting and added associations. An important example of this contextual plasticity is the shift in some declarative memories from episodic to semantic. *Episodic* memories possess a personalized spatiotemporal context (for example, my recollections of a vacation in Paris have a distinct sense of personal experience, time, and place). *Semantic* memories describe knowledge of the world that becomes separated from a distinct personalized spatiotemporal context (for example, I know that Paris is the capital city of France). Although at some distant point the acquisition of this knowledge must have had an episodic component—perhaps I came to know it by being told by a particular teacher in a particular class—that spatiotemporal context has long gone, and I now simply remember it as a fact rather than an experience. There is significant evidence that the shift from contextual episodic to noncontextual semantic forms is associated with a memory becoming independent of the hippocampus.[5]

THE ABSENCE OF RETROGRADE AMNESIA IMPLICATES EARLY MEMORY PROCESSES AS THE PRINCIPAL TARGETS OF ANESTHETIC DRUGS

There is no convincing evidence that anesthetics cause retrograde amnesia in humans. The clinician sees this in daily anesthetic practice: patients interviewed postoperatively will frequently recount events right up to the moment when anesthetic drugs are given. Studies on adult patients undergoing general anesthesia have demonstrated normal memory for word lists presented in the holding area,[6] and for visual stimuli presented four minutes prior to the administration of midazolam,[7] while studies of pediatric patients have demonstrated normal memory for pictures presented prior to both propofol[8] and midazolam sedation.[9] In our own laboratory studies using volunteers receiving propofol, midazolam, thiopental, or dexmedetomidine, we have found no evidence of impaired memory for pictures[10] or words[11,12] presented immediately prior to drug administration. Another volunteer study found no effect on memory for cards viewed prior to a full propofol induction.[13]

The failure to cause retrograde amnesia has important mechanistic consequences: it makes it very difficult to rationalize that the key target for anesthetic amnesia is an event that occurs a significant time after encoding. To illustrate, if the target for an anesthetic drug is an arbitrary consolidation process that occurs t_c minutes after the exposure to the stimulus, then at the moment the drug is delivered, that target process is involved in consolidating memory for events that occurred t_c minutes in the past. The behavioral manifestation of inhibiting that process should be weakened memory for events extending t_c minutes prior to the drug administration. The fact that this does not occur strongly suggests that the interval t_c, if it exists, must thus be very short.

MATHEMATICAL MODELING OF ANESTHETIC AMNESIA

Recently, a large study using healthy volunteers provided a detailed characterization of how anesthetic amnesia evolves over time domains by creating a mathematical model of memory decay from experimental data.[12] Just as the technique of Fourier transformation can parse the subcomponents of a complex electroencephalogram waveform, modeling memory decay is based on the principle that discrete mathematical components have mechanistic underpinnings. The basic idea is not new: the knowledge that normal memory undergoes a very rapid initial decline followed by a more gradual loss was established in the late nineteenth century. However, it was almost another century before a rigorous mathematical model was developed.[14] The core structure is a negative power function, which in its most theoretically complete form is complex and beyond the scope of this discussion. However, under typical experimental assumptions it is approximated by the surprisingly simple equation:

$$m_t = \lambda t^{-\psi}$$

where m is the memory strength at time t, λ is a measure of the initial trace strength, and ψ describes the subsequent rate of decay of that trace. The power of the methodology can be appreciated by considering that for any given memory performance m at any given time interval t, there are an infinite number of possible solutions for λ and ψ. Simply measuring the memory effects of anesthetic drugs at a single point in time provides no information about whether the amnesia was characterized by an encoding defect (decrease in λ), a failure of consolidation (increase in ψ), or a combination of both.

The two-parameter power decay function very accurately describes the first 4 hours of memory decay for several intravenous anesthetics (Figure 5.1). More importantly, though, when drugs were compared at equivalent degrees of end-amnesia (i.e., equal values of $m_{4\text{hours}}$), marked differences were identified in the modulation of the individual components. *Dexmedetomidine*—which selectively binds to α_{2A}-adrenoreceptors in the locus coeruleus, decreasing activity in a widespread network of cortical and subcortical noradrenergic pathways associated with arousal and vigilance[15]—is characterized by a dose-dependent decrease in the initial memory strength, but has virtually no effect on memory decay. Thus, memory impairment occurs with dexmedetomidine because items may be weakly encoded, but beyond this they appear to undergo a largely normal consolidation sequence. This characterization—a weakened initial trace followed by minimally altered decay—also largely describes the amnesia caused by *thiopental*, which in contrast has the γ-aminobutyric acid subtype-A receptor ($GABA_A$-R) as a principal target. However, midazolam and propofol, although they share the same principal target ($GABA_A$-R) as thiopental, are able to utilize a different pathway to cause amnesia. When items are presented during an infusion of *midazolam*, the initial pattern is that of a relatively normal initial memory trace that is followed by a markedly accelerated decay—the memory is encoded normally, but then fails to consolidate. As the dose of midazolam is increased, there appears to be a ceiling in the consolidation effect, but memory performance continues to deteriorate because a significant encoding impairment emerges. In the appropriate dose range, *propofol* exerts an even more selective effect on consolidation. Propofol can cause dramatic amnesia even when there is a very robust establishment of the initial memory. Remarkably, at a brain concentration of 0.90 μg mL^{-1}, propofol appears to exhibit a paradoxical phenomenon: the strength of the initial trace is actually augmented, but amnesia rapidly follows because of a profound consolidation collapse leading to highly accelerated decay. Notably, the amnesia caused by *all* of the above anesthetics is dominated by changes occurring within two hours of encoding; beyond this point, the decay slopes are fundamentally indistinguishable from placebo. This is of significance because it falls within the time window of the early, non–protein synthesis phase of long-term potentiation (LTP),[16] which shall be discussed below.

MECHANISTIC INSIGHTS INTO ANESTHETIC AMNESIA

ANESTHETIC EFFECTS ON ENCODING ARE PRINCIPALLY RELATED TO AROUSAL AND ATTENTION

Attention is a necessary feature for the encoding of hippocampal-dependent declarative memory, although the underlying mechanisms are quite poorly understood.[17] Dynamics of attention—through directed selection or shifts in the state of global arousal—are a fundamental characteristic of human cognition, and function as a prime modulator of the degree to which elements of the conscious percept are "captured" into the memory cascade.

Within this framework, there are theoretically three broad pathways for anesthetics to cause memory impairment through loss of encoding processes: (i) decreased arousal, with consequent decrease in attention; (ii) inadequate (divided) attention, independent of arousal; or (iii) mechanisms unrelated to attention or arousal. The approach to the question is hampered by the difficulty in rigorously defining and measuring arousal and attention, but at this time most evidence suggests that the first pathway—decreased attention secondary to the loss of arousal—is the predominant mechanism for the GABAergic agents at amnestic doses. The "dissociative" amnesia caused by the *N*-methyl-D-aspartate receptor (NMDA-R) antagonist ketamine would appear to have qualities similar to divided attention models; however, to date no appropriate studies have been performed. An archetype of the third pathway would be the loss of primary sensory cortical processing. While there is good evidence that anesthetics attenuate cortical sensory processes at concentrations causing unconsciousness, neuroimaging studies at amnestic concentrations demonstrate that early cortical sensory processing remains active.[18–20]

An initial study of propofol, thiopental, and dexmedetomidine using a continuous recognition task demonstrated that the primary acquisition of items into memory—measured by retention at 33 seconds—is related to the level of arousal.[11] That same study also demonstrated

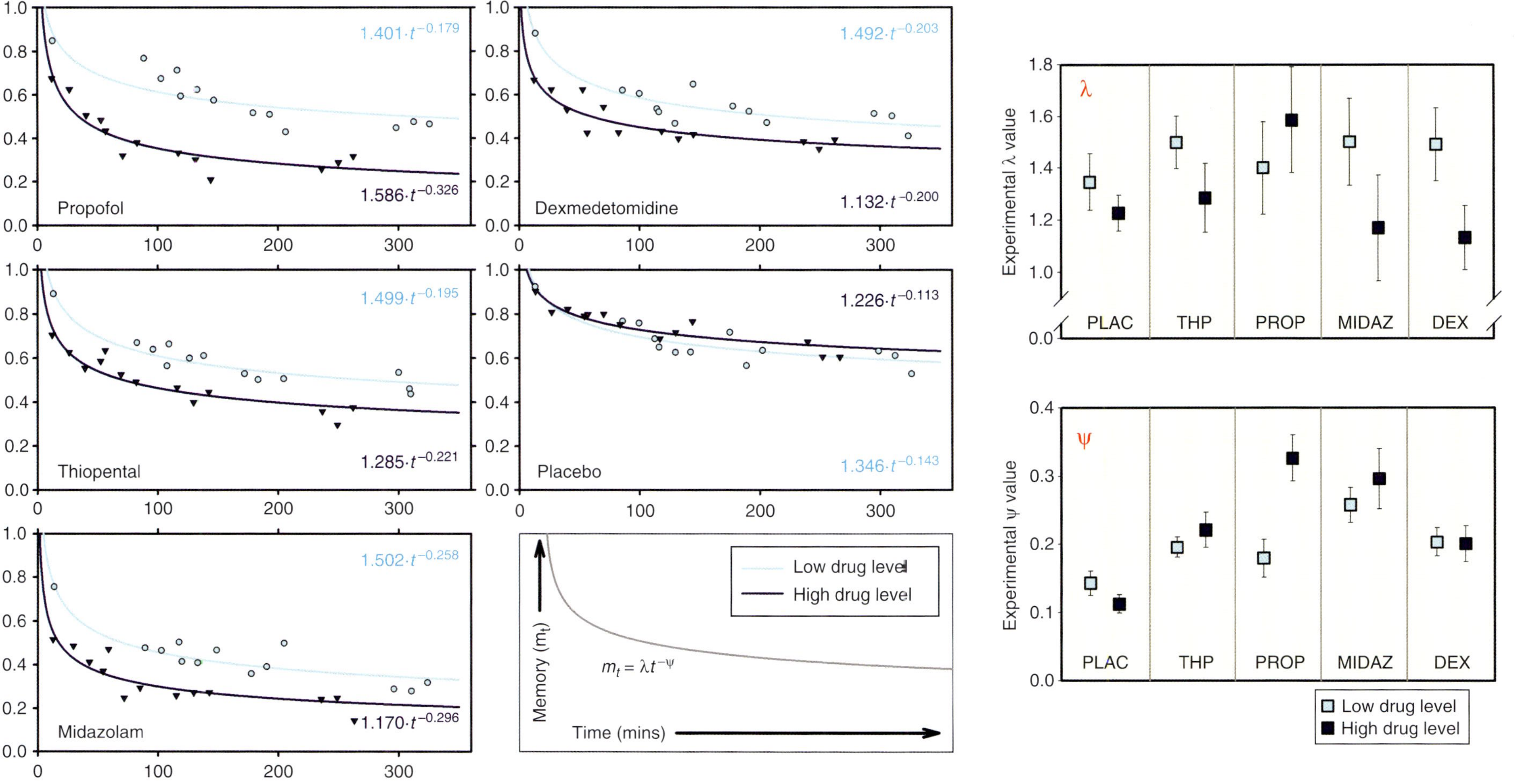

Figure 5.1 *Mathematical Modeling of Anesthetic Effects on Memory.* The panels on the left show decay curves that reflect how the administration of an intravenous anesthetic drug alters the time course of amnesia. In this experiment, healthy subjects received a pharmacokinetically driven steady-state infusion, and then performed a series of encoding tasks using 160 pictures. Memory for these images was probed at different intervals over the course of five hours, enabling a detailed curve to be modeled. The curves for all drugs can be very accurately described by a simple, two-parameter negative power equation, $m_t = \lambda t^{-\psi}$. When drugs are dosed to achieve a similar level of amnesia (m_t), the model reveals marked variability in the modulation of the parameters λ and ψ (right panels). Other elements of the study (not shown) demonstrate that these mathematical descriptors have mechanistic underpinnings. The parameter λ reflects the strength of the initial memory trace (the encoding strength), and is a function of the level of arousal. The parameter ψ measures the decay characteristics of the memory, and thus assesses consolidation; it is extremely closely related to the P2-N2 complex of the event-related potential, and also to reaction time—both of which may be driven by the integrity of coherent neuronal oscillation patterns. Reprinted with permission from Pryor KO, Reinsel RA, Mehta M, Li Y, Wixted JT, Veselis RA. The visual P2-N2 complex and arousal at the time of encoding predict the time domain characteristics of amnesia for multiple intravenous anesthetic drugs in humans. *Anesthesiology*. 2010;113(2):313–326.

that this initial performance is predictive of memory 225 minutes later for thiopental and dexmedetomidine, whereas propofol causes a significantly greater memory loss than can be accounted for by arousal-related effects alone. These findings were confirmed and extended by a subsequent study, which probed memory performance continuously between 6 seconds and 325 minutes to develop a mathematical model of anesthetic amnesia (see above).[12] In that study, tonic arousal predicted the strength of the initial memory trace (λ) for midazolam, thiopental, and dexmedetomidine with remarkable precision and conservation across the drugs. Propofol was again atypical: the model was conserved and predictive at a concentration of 0.45 μg mL $^{-1}$, but when the concentration was raised to 0.90 μg mL $^{-1}$ the strength of the initial trace was greater than would be predicted for the level of sedation. Notably, this concentration is almost identical to that causing paradoxical excitation in neural network models of propofol's effects on $GABA_A$ and intrinsic membrane slow potassium currents. [21] Further, the phenomenon shares similarities to isolated examples of patients with pathologic low-conscious or minimally conscious states whose cognitive function is improved by GABAergic drugs, probably through suppression of inhibitory control signals regulating thalamocortical function.[22]

These neurobehavioral results are supported by findings from positron emission tomography (PET). During an auditory level of processing encoding task, thiopental causes a significant decrease in activity of the left inferior prefrontal cortex (LIPFC)—a region associated with successful auditory encoding function—mirroring the effect seen in placebo subjects when selective attention is challenged by performing the encoding task in parallel with a discrimination task.[23] In contrast, LIPFC function is preserved with propofol at 0.90 μg mL $^{-1}$ (the excitatory dose described above), even though subsequent memory performance at 200 minutes is significantly *worse* than seen with thiopental (Figure 5.2). Earlier investigation of propofol with PET also failed to show decreases in LIPFC activation, but did show a significant decrease in right dorsolateral-prefrontal cortex (DLPFC), a region more associated with working memory than with the encoding of long-term memory.[24] Preserved left prefrontal activation has also been observed with midazolam during an auditory encoding task,[25] although in that study the drug was delivered as a bolus rather than by targeted steady state infusion, making it difficult to attribute the activation pattern to a specific brain concentration.

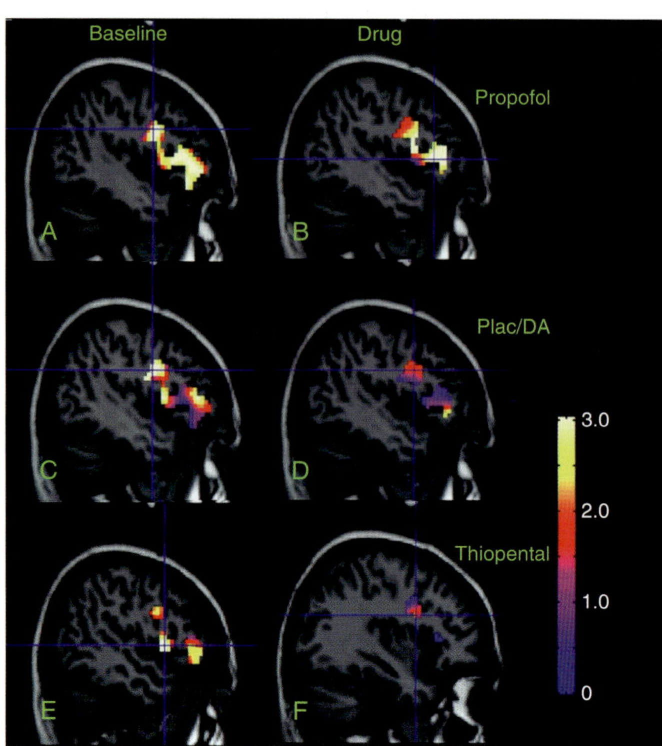

Figure 5.2 *Anesthetic Effects on Encoding Processes in Left Inferior Prefrontal Cortex.* These images depict activation of left inferior prefrontal cortex (LIPFC) in healthy volunteers who were imaged using $H_2{}^{15}O$ positron emission tomography (PET). At baseline, LIPFC is activated during a depth-of-processing auditory memory encoding task in all three study arms (panels A, C, and E). When the task is repeated while subjects receive a steady-state drug infusion, this activation is markedly attenuated in subjects who receive thiopental (panel F) and in subjects who receive placebo but who simultaneously perform a highly distracting task designed to divide attention (panel D). In contrast, LIPFC activation is preserved in subjects receiving propofol (panel B), demonstrating that intact encoding processes occur. Despite the robust encoding, subjects receiving propofol have worse memory performance three hours later, indicating that the memory deficit caused by propofol is a consolidation failure. The crosshairs indicate the voxel of highest activation within the cluster. The scale indicates the statistical T values derived from statistical parametric mapping. Reprinted with permission from Veselis RA, Pryor KO, Reinsel RA, Mehta M, Pan H, Johnson R Jr. Low-dose propofol-induced amnesia is not due to a failure of encoding: left inferior prefrontal cortex is still active. *Anesthesiology.* 2008;109:213–224.

THE AMYGDALA IS AN IMPORTANT SITE FOR ANESTHETIC AMNESIA

Discussion of the medial temporal lobe and anesthetic amnesia necessitates a brief review of a second, but very important medial temporal lobe structure: the amygdala. Activity within the basolateral nucleus of the amygdala is able to modulate the encoding and consolidation of episodic memory in response to emotion, arousal, and stress,[26] and is a critical determinant of the evolutionary dynamic of human memory—the fact that there is some nonrandom purpose in what is remembered and what is forgotten. The effect does not appear to be primarily due to plasticity within the amygdala itself, but rather the result of modulating encoding and consolidation processes in other regions of the brain, most notably in the adjacent hippocampus. It is critically dependent on norepinephrine

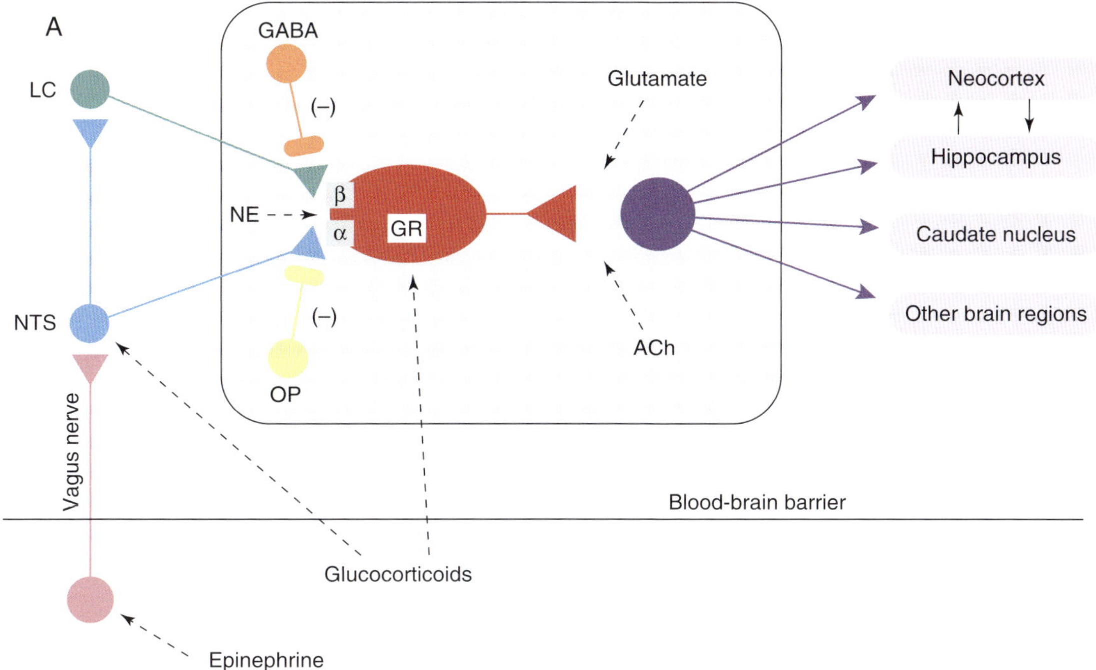

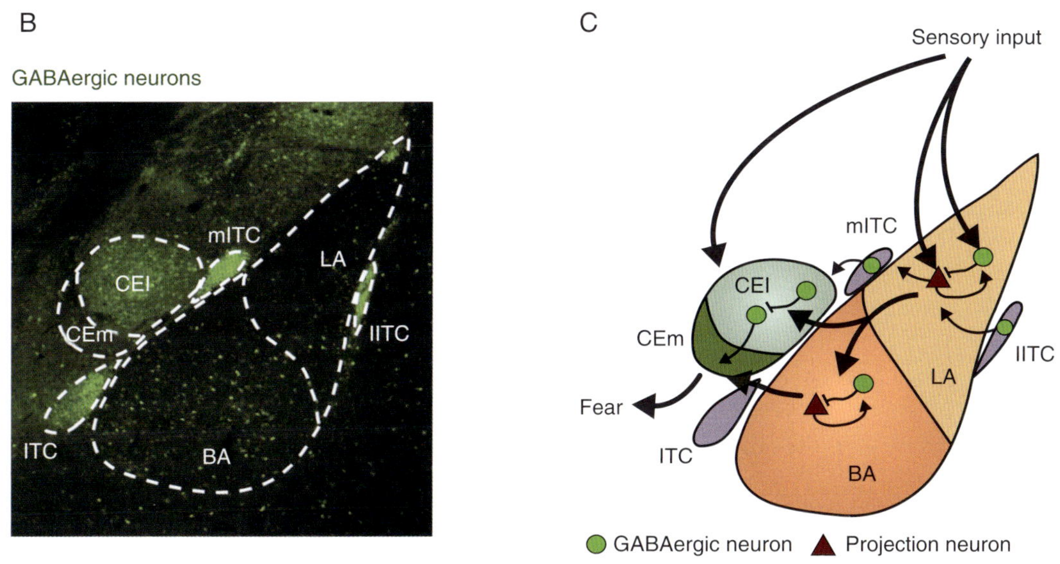

Figure 5.3 *Anesthetic Targets in the Amygdala.* Panel A depicts the basic circuitry underlying amygdala-dependent modulation of declarative memory processes in the hippocampus and other brain regions. Norepinephrine (NE) acts on adrenergic receptors within the basolateral nucleus to modulate downstream processes. The principal target of most anesthetic drugs is likely inhibitory GABA systems that modulate NE release, as do opiates (OP). The system can be activated by systemic influences through the action of epinephrine and glucocorticoids. Epinephrine activates receptors on the ascending vagus nerve projecting to the nucleus of the solitary tract (NTS), which sends noradrenergic projections directly to the BLA, and also indirectly via the locus coeruleus (LC). NE release via the LC can be inhibited by the α_2-adrenergic agonist dexmedetomidine. Panel B illustrates the distribution of GABAergic neurons across the amygdaloid complex in a coronal brain slice stained for the 67 kD isoform of the GABA synthesizing enzyme glutamic acid decarboxylase. Panel C is a schematic of the organization of inhibitory GABAergic interneurons. In the lateral (lITC) and medial (mITC) intercalated cell clusters, a high density of GABAergics neurons relay forward inhibition of the basolateral (BA and LA) and lateral central (lCE) nuclei. Other local interneurons within the BA and LA provide feedforward and feedback inhibition. SOURCES/NOTES: **Panel A:** Reprinted with permission from McGaugh JL. Memory—a century of consolidation. *Science.* 2000; 287:248–51. **Panels B and C:** Reprinted from Ehrlich I, Humeau Y, Grenier F, et al. Amygdala inhibitory circuits and the control of fear memory. *Neuron.* 2009; 62:757–771, with permission from Elsevier.

release, acting at both α and β receptors within the basolateral nucleus,[27] but can also be triggered by systemic epinephrine binding to β-adrenoreceptors in the vagus nerve and projecting to the nucleus of the solitary tract,[28] with downstream modulation of norepinephrine release in the amygdala either directly or via the locus coeruleus (Figure 5.3).

There are several plausible mechanisms by which anesthetic drugs could interfere with episodic memory processes via amygdala-dependent actions. A GABAergic system within the basolateral nucleus and intercalated bundles modulates norepinephrine release, and is characterized by a high density of α_1- and α_2-subunit $GABA_A$-R subtypes, in contrast to the adjacent hippocampus, which is rich in the α_5-subunit subtype.[29] Dexmedetomidine targets α_{2A}-adrenoreceptors in the locus coeruleus to reduce efferent noradrenergic tone, and would thus be expected to attenuate the response of the amygdala to systemic epinephric activation, while cholinergic and glutamatergic drugs modulate memory via effects downstream from the dynamic norepinephrine release.[30]

Nearly twenty years ago it was demonstrated that lesions of the basolateral amygdala blocked diazepam-induced anterograde amnesia for an inhibitory avoidance task in rats.[31] In the last decade, very similar findings have been established for both of the anesthetic agents propofol[32] and sevoflurane.[33] These recent studies provide compelling evidence that the amygdala may be a critically important drug target for anesthetic amnesia in certain contexts. However, some caution in extrapolation is warranted: stimulus-response learning in inhibitory avoidance tasks is highly amygdala-dependent, and it is not known whether the same resistance to anesthetic amnesia occurs with non–fear related contextual memory, which is an essential component of the human experience.

A very limited number of relevant studies in humans have demonstrated that anesthetic drugs have effects on emotional memory modulation that can be dissociated from their global amnestic effects. As the brain concentration of thiopental is slowly increased through the transition zone that is critical for the development of amnesia, images that contain negative/arousing emotional information demonstrate a shifted dose-response dynamic, and are more refractory to the amnestic effects of the drug.[10] The implication is that normal modulatory processes—most likely amygdala-dependent—can remain intact, even while other domains of memory function are collapsing. In contrast, subjects receiving propofol have a starkly different modulatory pattern, and at the critical brain concentration of 0.90 $\mu g\ mL^{-1}$ negative/arousing material loses all demonstrable advantage.[34] The implication is that, in contrast to thiopental, propofol targets emotional modulatory processes with a similar affinity to its effects causing consolidation collapse.

A similar phenomenon is observed with the volatile agent sevoflurane, and has been imaged using PET.[35] When subjects are presented emotionally arousing and neutral images in the presence of 0.1% or 0.2% sevoflurane, a mnemonic advantage for emotionally arousing material is preserved. However, at 0.25% sevoflurane this advantage is absent, representing the loss of emotional modulatory processes. Structural equation modeling of PET data demonstrates that this effect correlates with a loss of right-sided amygdala to hippocampal effective connectivity, with a significant reduction in the influence of the amygdala.

Interest in anesthetic effects on the amygdala are heightened because of its known importance in the neural circuitry of anxiety, phobia, panic disorder, and posttraumatic stress disorder (PTSD),[36,37] which are all characterized by involving amygdala hyperreactivity. The stress response to surgery provides the molecular substrates for an intense activation of the amygdala-dependent fear systems, and there is basis for concern that this intense activation might induce plastic changes that could prime the development of long-term changes in neuropsychological functioning. This is particularly relevant to the high incidence of PTSD following intraoperative awareness[38] and intensive care therapy.[39,40] It is premature to offer recommendations about how anesthetic drugs might be used to prevent or even treat these pathologies, although studies currently in progress promise to offer further insight.

KNOWLEDGE OF IN VIVO HIPPOCAMPAL FUNCTION DURING ANESTHETIC AMNESIA IN HUMANS IS LIMITED

Although the hippocampus is presumed to be a key site for anesthetic amnesia, there are very few neuroimaging or electrophysiologic studies evaluating hippocampal activation during anesthetic amnesia in humans. Because of the deep location of the hippocampus, the techniques have significant challenges. One study used implanted intracranial depth electrodes in epileptic patients to evaluate the effects of propofol on spectral characteristics.[41] At the amnestic concentrations relevant to the present discussion (0.5–1.0 $\mu g\ mL^{-1}$), the hippocampus at rest has a slight increase in spectral power across all frequency bands ranging from δ (1–4 Hz) through γ (32–48 Hz). There is a significant increase in spontaneous coherence between hippocampus and rhinal cortex in the δ band, but a loss of spontaneous coherence in other bands, most notably the θ (4–8 Hz), α (8–12 Hz), and β_1 (12–20 Hz) bands. While hippocampal power and coherence have great mechanistic importance in memory function, the ability to interpret rest data is contextually limited.

Although a number of PET and fMRI studies have been conducted with anesthetic drugs, the emphasis of most has been to study loss of consciousness. Of those evaluating memory, few have been structured to assess hippocampal activity. The task is particularly challenging with PET, as the technique requires the presentation of multiple stimuli in a block, while memory studies optimally assess individual stimuli so that they can be later binned according to whether they were remembered or forgotten. To date, no PET study has convincingly demonstrated changes in hippocampal activation that can be directly correlated with anesthetic amnesia, but this should be interpreted with significant caution because of the limitation just described. In fMRI studies, the benzodiazepine lorazepam and cholinergic antagonist scopolamine cause decreases in hippocampal activation associated with decreased memory for face-name pairs.[42] Sevoflurane at 0.25% reduces hippocampal activation in response to the presentation of simple visual and auditory stimuli,[43] but this has not yet been correlated with subsequent memory performance. In contrast, at rest, sedative doses of propofol, while causing a mild decrease in global cerebral blood flow, may actually cause slight relative increases in hippocampal or perihippocampal regional blood flow.[44,45] Again, the significance of rest-state changes in regional activity offers only very limited insight on how extended networks respond to a specific memory task.

ANESTHETICS AFFECT HIPPOCAMPAL LONG-TERM POTENTIATION IN VITRO

The revelation that the hippocampus is critical for declarative memory has directed intense interest in understanding its intrinsic synaptic plasticity. In its fundamental form, the neural anatomy is described as a trisynaptic circuit: the *perforant path* relays glutamatergic excitatory input from entorhinal cortex to the dentate gyrus; the *mossy fiber* pathway projects from granular cells in the dentate gyrus to CA3 pyramidal neurons; and the *Schaffer collateral* pathway extends excitatory projections from the CA3 to CA1 neurons. CA1 neurons then project widely to the neocortex (Figure 5.4).[46] The most extensively studied form of synaptic plasticity in the circuit is long-term potentiation (LTP), which is a signaling cascade initiated by NMDA-dependent increase in calcium influx, with downstream activation of several kinase pathways and ultimately novel gene expression and protein transcription. Phases of the cascade can be attributed to specific time domains: the kinase-dependent phase is termed *early LTP* and is the dominant form over periods of hours, while the protein

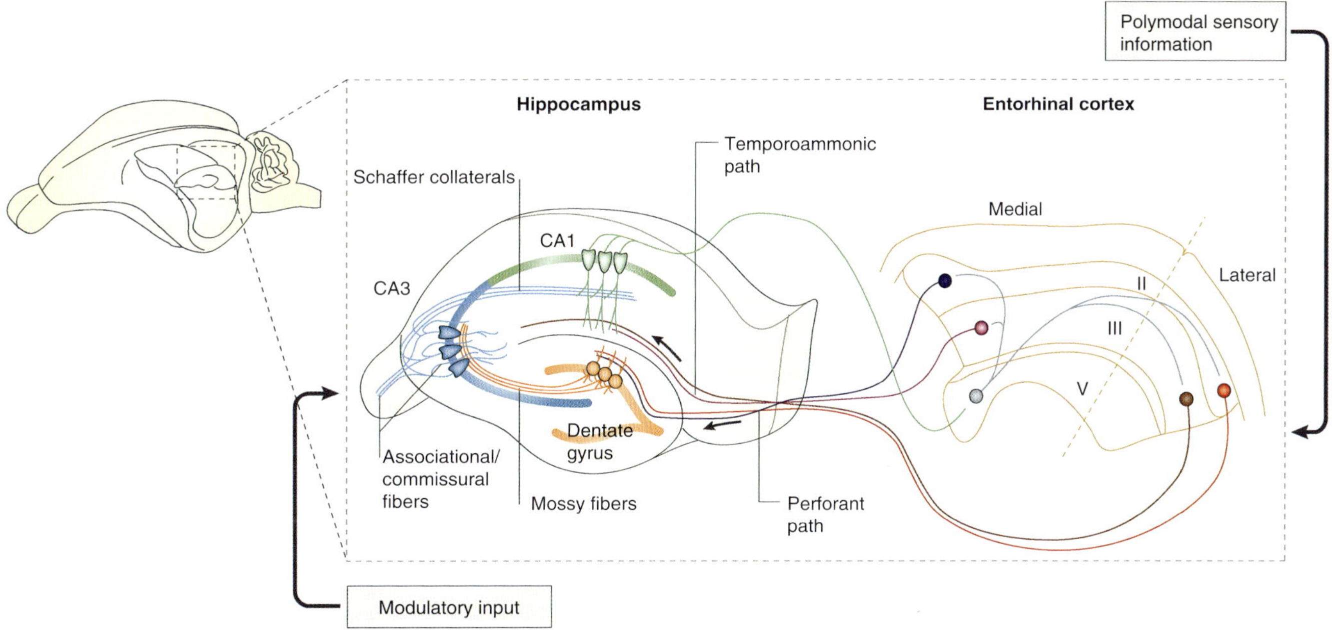

Figure 5.4 *Hippocampal Circuitry.* The hippocampus is traditionally presented as a trisynaptic loop. The major input is the *perforant path*, which conveys sensory information from neurons in layer II of the entorhinal cortex to the dentate gyrus. Perforant path axons make excitatory synaptic contact with the dendrites of granule cells. Granule cells project, through their axons (the *mossy fibers*), to the proximal apical dendrites of CA3 pyramidal cells which, in turn, project to ipsilateral CA1 pyramidal cells through *Schaffer collaterals* and to contralateral CA3 and CA1 pyramidal cells through commissural connections. In addition to the sequential trisynaptic circuit, there is also a dense associative network interconnecting CA3 cells on the same side. Furthermore, there is substantial modulatory input to hippocampal neurons. The hippocampus is home to a rich diversity of inhibitory neurons that are not shown in the figure, including a high density of α_5-subunit containing GABA neurons, which is likely to be one of the main targets for anesthetic amnesia. Reprinted by permission from Macmillan Publishers Ltd: *Nature Reviews Neuroscience*. Neves G, Cooke SF, Bliss TVP. Synaptic plasticity, memory and the hippocampus: a neural network approach to causality. *Nat Rev Neurosci*. 2008;9(1):65–75. Copyright 2008.

synthesis phase is termed *late LTP*, and is responsible for sustained potentiation over days, weeks, or even years.[47] There is considerable evidence that these temporal phases of LTP correspond to dissociable time domains for memory behavior.

GABAergic interneurons—notable for a high density of the α_5-subunit subtype[29]—project both within and across hippocampal subareas,[48] and provide abundant targets for anesthetic action. The volatile anesthetics isoflurane [49] and sevoflurane[50] have been demonstrated to inhibit LTP via effects blocked by the addition of the $GABA_A$ antagonists picrotoxin or bicuculline, suggesting that the underlying mechanism is at least partially GABA-mediated. Similarly, propofol inhibits LTP via GABAergic mechanisms blocked by picrotoxin.[51,52] Recent studies using a α_5-$GABA_A$-knockout mouse model and the selective α_5 antagonist L-655,708 have provided compelling evidence that α_5-$GABA_A$ receptors—most likely extrasynaptic—mediate the amnestic effect of etomidate, but not its other effects.[53,54] While studies have demonstrated effects on LTP subprocesses, including extracellular signal-regulated protein kinase function[55,56] and modulation of hippocampal protein expression,[57] it remains unknown exactly how anesthetics block LTP.

ANESTHETIC EFFECTS ON SYNCHRONOUS NEURONAL OSCILLATIONS IN THE HIPPOCAMPUS

One problematic issue arising from the LTP studies is that the anesthetic concentrations required to elicit the effects in vitro rarely correspond to those required for amnestic effects in vivo. This has given rise to an emerging school of thought that emphasizes the importance and potential susceptibility of synchronous neuronal oscillations. Interaction between the inhibitory GABAergic and excitatory glutamatergic neurons in the hippocampus creates synchronized oscillations across spatially distributed brain areas,[58] and subsets of GABAergic neuron populations can be characterized by their behavior at distinct oscillatory frequencies.[59,60] These oscillatory dynamics are essential for synchronizing neuronal firing across networks, and further appear necessary for the coincident firing that induces synaptic plasticity. The role of neuronal oscillations in transiently "binding" networks has emerged as a fundamental concept in several areas of neuroscience, but none more than in the understanding of memory. Synchronization of both θ and γ oscillations in response to stimuli appears necessary for the induction of LTP in the hippocampus,[61] which converges with findings from cognitive neuroscience demonstrating that hippocampal θ oscillations are phase locked with widely distributed cortical oscillations,[62] and that these correlate with successful memory behavior.[63]

The synchrony-dependent model of anesthetic amnesia suggests that a critical event is the loss of hippocampal-driven integrated synchrony across a distributed network. Loss of synchrony may reduce the coincident firing necessary for LTP induction, and may also have the effect of preventing the effective binding of different elements of the complex dynamic network required for contextually rich declarative memory. The model is largely hypothetical, but is supported by some experimental evidence. Both isoflurane and the nonimmobilizer agent F6—which is characterized by the amnestic but not sedative effects of an anesthetic—modulate θ activity in the CA1 neuronal bundle at amnestic doses.[64] Isoflurane causes slowing of θ oscillations but does not reduce absolute power, while F6 reduces power without slowing; both effects are correlated with amnestic behavior. Halothane dramatically modulates the power of atropine-sensitive type 2 θ oscillations,[65] suggesting that it acts on the circuitry responsible for θ generation. Together these findings suggest that virtually any disruption of normal θ activity may be sufficient to cause amnesia, allowing for drugs to achieve the same endpoint via different pathways.

EVENT-RELATED POTENTIALS PREDICT THE EFFECTS OF ANESTHETICS ON CONSOLIDATION IN HUMANS

The best human evidence that anesthetic amnesia may be related to effects on very early electrophysiologic processes comes from studies using event-related potentials (ERPs). ERPs are perturbations in the EEG that are tightly related to the timing of a cognitive process. The signal of any individual ERP is overwhelmed by other elements of the EEG, but if the cognitive task is repeated multiple times and the sweeps averaged, other elements of the EEG cancel out, and the ERP emerges. It was previously thought that the ERP represented a stimulus-induced increase in the activation of neuronal clusters, leading to an increase in EEG power. More recently, however, consensus has favored the theory that ERPs emerge because of phase resetting of ongoing oscillations.[66] The evolution of this idea converges with the increased interest in the importance of neuronal synchrony in memory cited above.[61]

Curran et al.[67] studied bolus doses of the GABAergic benzodiazepine lorazepam and the cholinergic antagonist scopolamine. Despite targeting entirely different receptors, in a classic oddball paradigm both drugs cause similar changes in components of the ERP associated with declarative memory performance, notably the P3 complex. Both drugs also caused changes in the amplitude of N1 and P2, which are earlier components associated with arousal. By comparing these patterns with those elicited by diphenhydramine, which causes sedation but has little effect on declarative memory, this study demonstrated that drugs used in anesthesia may have amnestic effects quite separate from those caused by sedation, and which further may be evaluated neurophysiologically.

This principle has also formed the basis for a series of studies in our own laboratory. Veselis et al. initially demonstrated that, at equal levels of sedation, midazolam and propofol cause a significantly greater degree of amnesia than does thiopental.[68] Subsequently, these effects were shown to be predicted by significant decreases in the amplitude of P3 and N2-P3 components in the central frontoparietal region.[69] The N2 latency was correlated with reaction time, which was interpreted as a marker of sedation. A later study[70] used a continuous recognition task to examine the *old/new effect*. This is a well-described and robust memory phenomenon, most evident in the parietal region, in which distinct changes in the ERP are evident when an item is correctly remembered as being seen before (i.e., "old"), as compared to when the item is seen for the first time (i.e., "new"). At an interval of 27 seconds, propofol and midazolam attenuate the old/new effect on the ERP, even though subjects respond correctly. Thus, by 27 seconds the memory processes subserving the old/new effect are evidently altered, but the strength of the memory trace remains sufficiently discriminable to support a correct response.

The ERP evidence for the most temporally proximal drug action comes from the mathematical modeling study described above.[12] Examination of the early- and mid-latency parietal complexes demonstrate that the effect of a drug on decay/consolidation, as measured by the coefficient ψ, was tightly correlated with the P2 amplitude and N2 latency *at the time of encoding*. In contrast, no ERP correlates were found for encoding/initial trace strength (λ). The coefficient ψ was also pristinely correlated with reaction time, supporting the N2 $\leftrightarrow$ reaction time relationship established in the earlier study. However, where that study interpreted increased reaction time to be a measure of sedation—a valid assumption in most nondrug experimental paradigms—when the assumption was tested in the mathematical modeling study by looking at other sedation measures, no relationship between sedation and reaction time could be established. This unexpected result might be regarded with some hesitation, were it not for the fact that the reaction time $\leftrightarrow$ consolidation failure (ψ) $\leftrightarrow$ P2-N2 relationships are remarkably consistent across all drugs and dosages—suggesting that each measure is related to and accurately indexes an underlying mechanistic phenomenon.

What is most intriguing about these results is that the P2-N2 complex is known to largely derive from synchronous θ oscillations,[71] which as discussed earlier are critical to the induction of neural plasticity in the hippocampus and elsewhere. Though ERP components cannot be interpreted as direct measures of θ synchrony, the possibility that the memory effects of multiple agents can be closely related to a putative hippocampal-cortical θ network shows great promise for future investigation.

CONCLUSION: AN ENCODING-CONSOLIDATION MODEL OF ANESTHETIC AMNESIA

We propose a systems-level model of anesthetic amnesia in which agents are characterized by their effects on two broad, but dissociable memory functions: encoding and consolidation. *Encoding failure* appears to be largely due to a loss of attentional function, and although top-down, cortically-mediated selectivity processes may be affected, it is likely that the dominant mechanism is simply a decrease in bottom-up levels of tonic arousal. Because memory encoding is a high-level cortical function, and drug effects on arousal are mediated at subcortical sites, it is possible that the effect is largely state-specific rather than pathway-specific—in other words, from a memory perspective, loss of arousal due to inhibitory GABAergic agonism centered in the thalamus may be functionally equivalent to that due to α_2-adrenergic agonism in the locus coeruleus. This question has not been answered. *Consolidation failure* is a far more intriguing and memory-specific drug action. It is mechanistically distinct from the attentionally mediated encoding effects, as is clearly evidenced by several experimental examples of robust encoding followed by profound consolidation collapse. It is archetypally induced by propofol, but is not due to GABAergic activity per se, as the effect is almost completely absent with other GABAergic agents such as thiopental. We hypothesize that the critical event is interference with the dynamic generation of appropriately synchronized neuronal oscillations over a distributed network in response to stimuli. The effect is to dramatically attenuate the induction of the long-term consolidation signaling cascade. Theoretically, the most likely oscillatory network targets are hippocampal θ and γ systems, and while γ remains unexplored, there is now some experimental evidence to implicate θ oscillations. The differences between the GABAergic agents are most likely explained by selectivity variation for specific $GABA_A$ receptor subtypes; a prominent candidate would be the high density of α_5-subunit subtype receptors in the hippocampus, which in combination with glutamatergic neurons appear to be necessary for the generation and regulation of coherent θ rhythms.

The process- and site-specific approach to understanding and studying anesthetic amnesia in humans represents a challenging and intellectually fascinating area of research. Virtually nonexistent fifteen years ago, the emerging field has been largely driven by the increasing availability and affordability of sophisticated technological modalities. Rapid present-day advances in functional neuroimaging promise to provide the ability to appropriately test the theories we have outlined above, and as is the case with any emerging field, it is possible that there will be dramatic changes in our understanding over the coming decade. The results promise to be of interest not only to anesthesiologists, but also to the broader neuroscience community, as a detailed understanding of pharmacologic amnesia is sure to provide a remarkable window into human memory—which remains one of the greatest and most fascinating mysteries in all of science.

REFERENCES

1. Scoville WB, Milner B. Loss of recent memory after bilateral hippocampal lesions. *J Neurol Neurosurg Psychiatry.* Feb 1957;20(1): 11–21.
2. Aggleton JP, Pearce JM. Neural systems underlying episodic memory: insights from animal research. *Philos Trans R Soc Lond B Biol Sci.* Sep 29 2001;356(1413):1467–1482.
3. McGaugh JL. Memory—a century of consolidation. *Science.* Jan 14 2000;287(5451):248–251.
4. Nader K, Hardt O. A single standard for memory: the case for reconsolidation. *Nat Rev Neurosci.* Mar 2009;10(3):224–234.
5. Moscovitch M, Nadel L, Winocur G, Gilboa A, Rosenbaum RS. The cognitive neuroscience of remote episodic, semantic and spatial memory. *Curr Opin Neurobiol.* Apr 2006;16(2):179–190.
6. Ghoneim MM, Block RI. Immediate peri-operative memory. *Acta Anaesthesiol Scand.* Sep 2007;51(8):1054–1061.
7. Bulach R, Myles PS, Russnak M. Double-blind randomized controlled trial to determine extent of amnesia with midazolam given immediately before general anaesthesia. *Br J Anaesth.* Mar 2005; 94(3):300–305.
8. Rich JB, Yaster M, Brandt J. Anterograde and retrograde memory in children anesthetized with propofol. *J Clin Exp Neuropsychol.* Aug 1999;21(4):535–546.
9. Twersky RS, Hartung J, Berger BJ, McClain J, Beaton C. Midazolam enhances anterograde but not retrograde amnesia in pediatric patients. *Anesthesiology.* Jan 1993;78(1):51–55.
10. Pryor KO, Veselis RA, Reinsel RA, Feshchenko VA. Enhanced visual memory effect for negative versus positive emotional content is potentiated at sub-anaesthetic concentrations of thiopental. *Br J Anaesth.* Sep 2004;93(3):348–355.
11. Veselis RA, Reinsel RA, Feshchenko VA, Johnson R Jr. Information loss over time defines the memory defect of propofol: a comparative response with thiopental and dexmedetomidine. *Anesthesiology.* Oct 2004;101(4):831–841.
12. Pryor KO, Reinsel RA, Mehta M, Li Y, Wixted JT, Veselis RA. The visual P2-N2 complex and arousal at the time of encoding predict the time domain characteristics of amnesia for multiple intravenous anesthetic drugs in humans. *Anesthesiology.* 2010;113(2):313–326.
13. Hashimoto K, Okada T, Seo N. Propofol does not induce retrograde amnesia at the hypnotic dose [in Japanese]. *Masui.* Aug 2007; 56(8):920–924.
14. Wickelgren WA. Single-trace fragility theory of memory dynamics. *Mem Cognit.* 1974;2(4):775–780.
15. Nelson LE, Lu J, Guo T, Saper CB, Franks NP, Maze M. The alpha2-adrenoceptor agonist dexmedetomidine converges on an endogenous sleep-promoting pathway to exert its sedative effects. *Anesthesiology.* Feb 2003;98(2):428–436.
16. Vertes RP. Hippocampal theta rhythm: a tag for short-term memory. *Hippocampus.* 2005;15(7):923–935.
17. Muzzio IA, Kentros C, Kandel E. What is remembered? Role of attention on the encoding and retrieval of hippocampal representations. *J Physiol.* Jun 15 2009;587(Pt 12):2837–2854.
18. Veselis RA, Feshchenko VA, Reinsel RA, Beattie B, Akhurst TJ. Propofol and thiopental do not interfere with regional cerebral blood flow response at sedative concentrations. *Anesthesiology.* Jan 2005;102(1):26–34.
19. Plourde G, Belin P, Chartrand D, et al. Cortical processing of complex auditory stimuli during alterations of consciousness with the general anesthetic propofol. *Anesthesiology.* Mar 2006;104(3): 448–457.
20. Dueck MH, Petzke F, Gerbershagen HJ, et al. Propofol attenuates responses of the auditory cortex to acoustic stimulation in a dose-dependent manner: a FMRI study. *Acta Anaesthesiol Scand.* Jul 2005; 49(6):784–791.
21. McCarthy MM, Brown EN, Kopell N. Potential network mechanisms mediating electroencephalographic beta rhythm changes during propofol-induced paradoxical excitation. *J Neurosci.* Dec 10 2008;28(50):13488–13504.
22. Schiff ND, Posner JB. Another "Awakenings." *Ann Neurol.* Jul 2007; 62(1):5–7.
23. Veselis RA, Pryor KO, Reinsel RA, Mehta M, Pan H, Johnson R Jr. Low-dose propofol-induced amnesia is not due to a failure of encoding: left inferior prefrontal cortex is still active. *Anesthesiology.* Aug 2008;109(2):213–224.
24. Veselis RA, Reinsel RA, Feshchenko VA, Dnistrian AM. A neuroanatomical construct for the amnesic effects of propofol. *Anesthesiology.* Aug 2002;97(2):329–337.
25. Bagary M, Fluck E, File SE, Joyce E, Lockwood G, Grasby P. Is benzodiazepine-induced amnesia due to deactivation of the left prefrontal cortex? *Psychopharmacology (Berl).* Jun 2000;150(3): 292–299.
26. McGaugh JL. The amygdala modulates the consolidation of memories of emotionally arousing experiences. *Ann Rev Neurosci.* 2004; 27:1–28.
27. Ferry B, Roozendaal B, McGaugh JL. Basolateral amygdala noradrenergic influences on memory storage are mediated by an interaction between beta- and alpha1-adrenoceptors. *J Neurosci.* Jun 15 1999;19(12):5119–5123.
28. Clayton EC, Williams CL. Noradrenergic receptor blockade of the NTS attenuates the mnemonic effects of epinephrine in an appetitive light-dark discrimination learning task. *Neurobiol Learn Mem.* Sep 2000;74(2):135–145.
29. Sur C, Fresu L, Howell O, McKernan RM, Atack JR. Autoradiographic localization of alpha5 subunit-containing GABAA receptors in rat brain. *Brain Res.* Mar 20 1999;822(1–2): 265–270.
30. Salinas JA, Introini-Collison IB, Dalmaz C, McGaugh JL. Posttraining intraamygdala infusions of oxotremorine and propranolol modulate storage of memory for reductions in reward magnitude. *Neurobiol Learn Mem.* Jul 1997;68(1):51–59.
31. Tomaz C, Dickinson-Anson H, McGaugh JL. Basolateral amygdala lesions block diazepam-induced anterograde amnesia in an inhibitory avoidance task. *Proc Natl Acad Sci U S A.* Apr 15 1992;89(8): 3615–3619.
32. Alkire MT, Vazdarjanova A, Dickinson-Anson H, White NS, Cahill L. Lesions of the basolateral amygdala complex block propofol-induced amnesia for inhibitory avoidance learning in rats. *Anesthesiology.* Sep 2001;95(3):708–715.
33. Alkire MT, Nathan SV. Does the amygdala mediate anesthetic-induced amnesia? Basolateral amygdala lesions block sevoflurane-induced amnesia. *Anesthesiology.* Apr 2005;102(4):754–760.
34. Pryor KO, Murphy E, Reinsel RA, Mehta M, Veselis RA. Heterogeneous effects of intravenous anesthetics on modulatory memory systems in humans. *Anesthesiology.* 2007;107:A1218.
35. Alkire MT, Gruver R, Miller J, McReynolds JR, Hahn EL, Cahill L. Neuroimaging analysis of an anesthetic gas that blocks human emoional memory. *Proc Natl Acad Sci U S A.* Feb 5 2008;105(5): 1722–1727.
36. Protopopescu X, Pan H, Tuescher O, et al. Differential time courses and specificity of amygdala activity in posttraumatic stress disorder subjects and normal control subjects. *Biol Psychiatry.* Mar 1 2005;57(5):464–473.
37. Rauch SL, Whalen PJ, Shin LM, et al. Exaggerated amygdala response to masked facial stimuli in posttraumatic stress disorder: a functional MRI study. *Biol Psychiatry.* May 1 2000;47(9): 769–776.

38. Osterman JE, Hopper J, Heran WJ, Keane TM, van der Kolk BA. Awareness under anesthesia and the development of posttraumatic stress disorder. *Gen Hosp Psychiatry.* Jul-Aug 2001;23(4): 198–204.
39. Schelling G, Stoll C, Haller M, et al. Health-related quality of life and posttraumatic stress disorder in survivors of the acute respiratory distress syndrome. *Crit Care Med.* Apr 1998;26(4):651–659.
40. Schelling G, Richter M, Roozendaal B, et al. Exposure to high stress in the intensive care unit may have negative effects on health-related quality-of-life outcomes after cardiac surgery. *Crit Care Med.* Jul 2003;31(7):1971–1980.
41. Fell J, Widman G, Rehberg B, Elger CE, Fernandez G. Human mediotemporal EEG characteristics during propofol anesthesia. *Biol Cybern.* Feb 2005;92(2):92–100.
42. Sperling R, Greve D, Dale A, et al. Functional MRI detection of pharmacologically induced memory impairment. *Proc Natl Acad Sci U S A.* Jan 8 2002;99(1):455–460.
43. Ramani R, Qiu M, Constable RT. Sevoflurane 0.25 MAC preferentially affects higher order association areas: a functional magnetic resonance imaging study in volunteers. *Anesth Analg.* Sep 2007; 105(3):648–655.
44. Fiset P, Paus T, Daloze T, et al. Brain mechanisms of propofol-induced loss of consciousness in humans: a positron emission tomographic study. *J Neurosci.* Jul 1 1999;19(13):5506–5513.
45. Byas-Smith M, Frolich MA, Votaw JR, Faber TL, Hoffman JM. Cerebral blood flow during propofol induced sedation. *Mol Imaging Biol.* Mar 2002;4(2):139–146.
46. Neves G, Cooke SF, Bliss TVP. Synaptic plasticity, memory and the hippocampus: a neural network approach to causality. *Nat Rev Neurosci.* Jan 2008;9(1):65–75.
47. Malenka RC, Bear MF. LTP and LTD: an embarrassment of riches. *Neuron.* Sep 30 2004;44(1):5–21.
48. Jinno S, Klausberger T, Marton LF, et al. Neuronal diversity in GABAergic long-range projections from the hippocampus. *J Neurosci.* Aug 15 2007;27(33):8790–8804.
49. Simon W, Hapfelmeier G, Kochs E, Zieglgansberger W, Rammes G. Isoflurane blocks synaptic plasticity in the mouse hippocampus. *Anesthesiology.* Jun 2001;94(6):1058–1065.
50. Ishizeki J, Nishikawa K, Kubo K, Saito S, Goto F. Amnestic concentrations of sevoflurane inhibit synaptic plasticity of hippocampal CA1 neurons through gamma-aminobutyric acid-mediated mechanisms. *Anesthesiology.* Mar 2008;108(3):447–456.
51. Takamatsu I, Sekiguchi M, Wada K, Sato T, Ozaki M. Propofol-mediated impairment of CA1 long-term potentiation in mouse hippocampal slices. *Neurosci Lett.* Dec 9 2005;389(3):129–132.
52. Nagashima K, Zorumski CF, Izumi Y. Propofol inhibits long-term potentiation but not long-term depression in rat hippocampal slices. *Anesthesiology.* Aug 2005;103(2):318–326.
53. Cheng VY, Martin LJ, Elliott EM, et al. Alpha5GABAA receptors mediate the amnestic but not sedative-hypnotic effects of the general anesthetic etomidate. *J Neurosci.* Apr 5 2006;26(14):3713–3720.
54. Martin LJ, Oh GH, Orser BA. Etomidate targets alpha5 gamma-aminobutyric acid subtype A receptors to regulate synaptic plasticity and memory blockade. *Anesthesiology.* Nov 2009;111(5): 1025–1035.
55. Fibuch EE, Wang JQ. Inhibition of the MAPK/ERK cascade: a potential transcription-dependent mechanism for the amnesic effect of anesthetic propofol. *Neurosci Bull.* Mar 2007;23(2):119–124.
56. Kozinn J, Mao L, Arora A, Yang L, Fibuch EE, Wang JQ. Inhibition of glutamatergic activation of extracellular signal-regulated protein kinases in hippocampal neurons by the intravenous anesthetic propofol. *Anesthesiology.* Dec 2006;105(6):1182–1191.
57. Ren Y, Zhang FJ, Xue QS, Zhao X, Yu BW. Bilateral inhibition of gamma-aminobutyric acid type A receptor function within the basolateral amygdala blocked propofol-induced amnesia and activity-regulated cytoskeletal protein expression inhibition in the hippocampus. *Anesthesiology.* Nov 2008;109(5):775–781.
58. Mann EO, Paulsen O. Role of GABAergic inhibition in hippocampal network oscillations. *Trends Neurosci.* Jul 2007;30(7): 343–349.
59. Cobb SR, Buhl EH, Halasy K, Paulsen O, Somogyi P. Synchronization of neuronal activity in hippocampus by individual GABAergic interneurons. *Nature.* Nov 2 1995;378(6552):75–78.
60. Klausberger T, Magill PJ, Marton LF, et al. Brain-state- and cell-type-specific firing of hippocampal interneurons in vivo. *Nature.* Feb 20 2003;421(6925):844–848.
61. Axmacher N, Mormann F, Fernandez G, Elger CE, Fell J. Memory formation by neuronal synchronization. *Brain Res Rev.* Aug 30 2006;52(1):170–182.
62. Young CK, McNaughton N. Coupling of theta oscillations between anterior and posterior midline cortex and with the hippocampus in freely behaving rats. *Cereb Cortex.* Jan 2009;19(1):24–40.
63. Summerfield C, Mangels JA. Coherent theta-band EEG activity predicts item-context binding during encoding. *Neuroimage.* Feb 1 2005;24(3):692–703.
64. Perouansky M, Hentschke H, Perkins M, Pearce RA. Amnesic concentrations of the nonimmobilizer 1,2-dichlorohexafluorocyclobutane (F6, 2N) and isoflurane alter hippocampal theta oscillations in vivo. *Anesthesiology.* Jun 2007;106(6):1168–1176.
65. Bland BH, Bland CE, Colom LV, et al. Effect of halothane on type 2 immobility-related hippocampal theta field activity and theta-on/theta-off cell discharges. *Hippocampus.* 2003;13(1): 38–47.
66. Sauseng P, Klimesch W, Gruber WR, Hanslmayr S, Freunberger R, Doppelmayr M. Are event-related potential components generated by phase resetting of brain oscillations? A critical discussion. *Neuroscience.* Jun 8 2007;146(4):1435–1444.
67. Curran HV, Pooviboonsuk P, Dalton JA, Lader MH. Differentiating the effects of centrally acting drugs on arousal and memory: an event-related potential study of scopolamine, lorazepam and diphenhydramine. *Psychopharmacology (Berl).* Jan 1998;135(1):27–36.
68. Veselis RA, Reinsel RA, Feshchenko VA, Wronski M. The comparative amnestic effects of midazolam, propofol, thiopental, and fentanyl at equisedative concentrations. *Anesthesiology.* Oct 1997;87(4): 749–764.
69. Veselis RA, Reinsel RA, Feshchenko VA. Drug-induced amnesia is a separate phenomenon from sedation: electrophysiologic evidence. *Anesthesiology.* Oct 2001;95(4):896–907.
70. Veselis RA, Pryor KO, Reinsel RA, Li Y, Mehta M, Johnson R Jr. Propofol and midazolam inhibit conscious memory processes very soon after encoding: an event-related potential study of familiarity and recollection in volunteers. *Anesthesiology.* Feb 2009;110(2): 295–312.
71. Freunberger R, Klimesch W, Doppelmayr M, Holler Y. Visual P2 component is related to theta phase-locking. *Neurosci Lett.* Oct 22 2007;426(3):181–186.

6

NEUROIMAGING CHANGES ASSOCIATED WITH HUMAN ACUTE AND CHRONIC PAIN

Richard E. Harris, Daniel J. Clauw, and Tobias Schmidt-Wilcke

INTRODUCTION

In the past two decades there has been tremendous progress in our understanding of the spinal and supraspinal mechanisms that are involved in human pain transmission. Some of these insights have occurred because of preclinical studies that can examine the precise cellular and molecular processes and pathways involved in acute pain transmission, and/or animal models of chronic pain. But many of the advances in the pain field have occurred because of the development of our improved ability to study pain mechanisms in humans. In particular, there have been a number of neuroimaging techniques that can probe the functional, structural, and molecular mechanisms involved in pain transmission. Prior to reviewing these imaging modalities and what each has taught us about pain transmission, it is necessary to briefly review some terminology and conceptual advances in the pain field.

Perhaps the biggest clinical advance in the pain field has been to acknowledge the fact that the brain and spinal cord are crucial to pain sensation. This should be obvious, because the brain is the only organ one needs to have pain. It has been known for some time that individuals can experience pain in the absence of the region of the body where the pain is occurring (e.g., phantom limb pain), or because of neurosurgical stimulation of certain brain regions. However, in clinical practice this has been largely ignored until recently. Nearly all diagnostic and therapeutic practices at present presuppose that pain is a direct result of nociception (i.e., the activation of peripheral nociceptors as occurs when there is tissue damage or inflammation). We now understand that there are multiple neurobiological mechanisms leading to more severe acute, or chronic pain, which increase sensory neural activity in the spinal cord and brain. This increase in the "gain" or amplitude of neural activity may play a prominent role in the pathology of chronic pain states. The neuroimaging techniques described herein have been most helpful in elucidating the cortical and subcortical brain regions involved in pain transmission, as well as how damage or dysfunction of these regions (or their projections to the spinal cord) can either increase or decrease pain transmission, in either acute or chronic pain settings.

Figure 6.1 describes at least three different underlying types of chronic pain states: peripheral, neuropathic, and "central" (i.e., spinal cord and brain). Some authors prefer to use the term "neuropathic pain" for pain primarily due to central nervous system dysfunction, but we prefer the term "central pain" because chronic pain due to nerve damage is quite different from that due to hypo- or hyperactivity of brain regions involved in pain processing.

This mechanistic approach to pain is critical because it impacts on the therapies that will work to treat pain. If pain is primarily due to nociceptive peripheral input, as occurs in most acute pain states and some types of chronic pain accompanied by peripheral damage or inflammation, then therapies such as nonsteroidal anti-inflammatory drugs and opioids are generally quite effective, as are procedures or interventions aimed at reducing the peripheral nociceptive input (e.g., replacing a damaged joint). These same therapies are particularly ineffective for "central" chronic pain states such as fibromyalgia, irritable bowel syndrome, interstitial cystitis, tension headaches, etc. In these latter conditions, pain is less responsive (or entirely unresponsive) to nonsteroidal anti-inflammatory drugs, opioids, and surgical procedures, because the pain does not appear to be primarily due to increased peripheral nociceptive input.[1] Instead, drugs that act at spinal or supraspinal levels to inhibit/reduce the activity of neurotransmitters that facilitate pain transmission (e.g., those on the left side of Figure 6.2) or increase the activity of the neurotransmitters that generally inhibit pain transmission (those on the right side of Figure 6.2) tend to be more effective analgesics in these conditions. Moreover, these conditions are consistently characterized by diffuse hyperalgesia (increased pain to normally painful stimuli) and/or allodynia (pain in response to normally nonpainful stimuli), strongly suggesting that augmented central nervous system pain transmission is playing a critical role in these pain states.

Even this figure depicts an oversimplified approach to the underlying mechanisms in chronic pain states, since subsets of individuals with chronic pain states in which

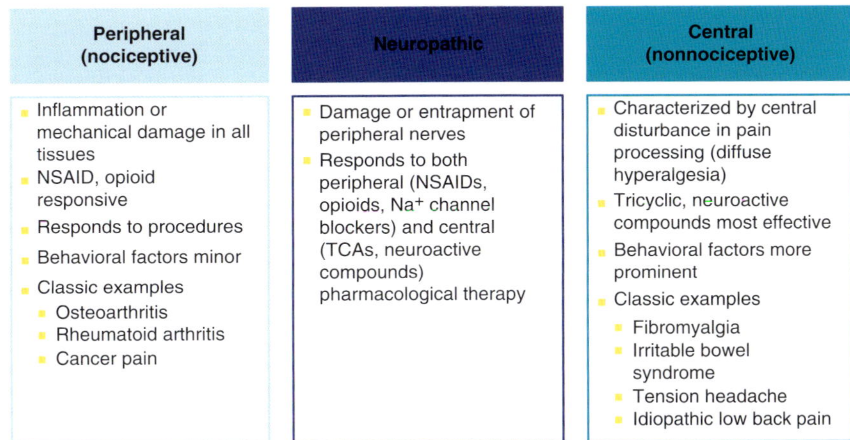

Figure 6.1 Mechanistic characterization of pain. Any combination may be present in a given individual.

there is clearly increased nociceptive input, such as osteoarthritis and rheumatoid arthritis, also display hyperalgesia and/or allodynia, suggesting that superimposed central nervous system (CNS) mechanisms (referred to as central augmentation or sensitization) are increasing pain transmission or sensation.[2–4] Neuropathic pain states seem to have characteristics of both peripheral and central pain states. Many of the above advances in our understanding of the differing underlying mechanisms in acute and chronic pain, and in particular the CNS contributions, have occurred because of the use of neuroimaging techniques.

A variety of neuroimaging techniques have been shown to have utility in giving complementary information regarding the cortical and subcortical processing of pain. In this chapter, we will consider three broad categories of neuroimaging techniques: 1) those that measure changes in regional blood flow, or the degree to which brain regions are activated simultaneously suggesting connectedness of activity, 2) those that examine structural changes that may especially occur in the setting of chronic pain, and 3) those that directly measure the levels of neurotransmitters, the activity of ligands for neurotransmitter receptors, or metabolites thought to be associated with decreased neuronal vitality. For each of the imaging modalities (when available) we review the type of information that can be assessed using these techniques, as well as the strengths and weaknesses of each technique. We then describe studies using these techniques in human pain research in healthy normal individuals receiving experimental pain stimuli, and then review findings in chronic pain states.

TECHNIQUES MEASURING CHANGES IN BLOOD FLOW DURING ACUTE OR CHRONIC PAIN

In the past two decades a variety of *functional* brain imaging techniques in human subjects, including single photon

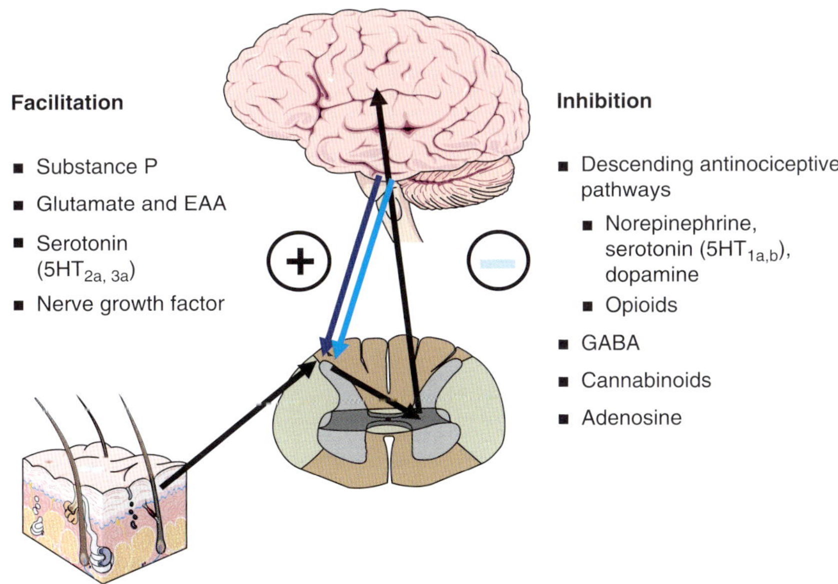

Figure 6.2 Neural influences on pain and sensory processing. EAA = excitatory amino acids.

emission computed tomography (SPECT), positron emission tomography (PET) and functional magnetic resonance imaging (fMRI) have shed light on the way in which the brain reacts to nociceptive stimuli (acute pain) thereby helping to establish the concept of the so-called pain matrix. In addition, these techniques have been used to study differences between patients and controls in regional blood flow, as well as response to therapy, in several chronic pain states.

SINGLE PHOTON EMISSION COMPUTED TOMOGRAPHY (SPECT)

Single photon emission computerized tomography with (99m)Tc can measure blood flow and was arguably the first functional neuroimaging technique used to study central nervous system processing of pain both in healthy humans and in chronic pain states. The principal advantage of SPECT is its widespread availability. Disadvantages include the use of radioisotopes, as well as the poor spatial and temporal resolution of changes in blood flow. Primarily for this reason, fMRI has generally supplanted the use of SPECT in the pain field.

A number of investigators used this technique in the early 1990s to demonstrate that the central nervous system could be activated or deactivated during application of painful stimuli, in brain regions known from animal studies to be involved in pain processing.[5,6] Soon thereafter, investigators used this same technique in a number of enigmatic pain states, such as fibromyalgia, central pain due to spinal cord injury or stroke, restless legs syndrome, phantom limb pain, traumatic brain injury, and headache to show "objective abnormalities" in these conditions. In each instance, these studies showed that although there might not be outward objective abnormalities present on other types of studies, that SPECT showed either hypo- or hyperperfusion of regions now firmly established to be part of the pain matrix.[7–11] Particularly in fibromyalgia and headache, these studies were seminal in the respective fields. In fibromyalgia, these studies helped establish the "central" rather than "peripheral" nature of the pain that was suspected based on other studies, and in headache confirmed that several acute headache states were characterized by changes in cerebral blood flow during the headache period.

More recently, SPECT has been used to examine responsiveness to a variety of chronic pain treatments. Several studies suggest that the technique has utility in this setting, in that the results of SPECT have correlated with clinical findings in studies treating fibromyalgia patients with both ketamine and amitriptyline.[12–15] Another group of investigators showed that responders to treatment can be differentiated from nonresponders among a group of individuals with complex regional pain syndrome type 1 (CRPS 1) treated with multimodal therapy.[16] In addition to studying chronic pain states, SPECT has also been used to study pain as a comorbidity in individuals with depression, by demonstrating differential changes in blood flow in response to antidepressant treatment in brain regions known to be associated with the affective and cognitive processing of pain.[17] This technique has also been used to demonstrate an objective marker of responsiveness to several procedures commonly used to treat chronic pain, including acupuncture, deep brain stimulation, and spinal cord stimulation.[18–20]

PET STUDIES MEASURING BLOOD FLOW

In addition to examining neurotransmitter activity at certain receptors (discussed below) PET can also be used to quantify metabolic activity in the brain. This is typically performed with the 18-fluorodeoxyglucose (FDG) tracer. Studies of migraine patients using FDG-PET show that common pain matrix regions such as the insula and anterior cingulate display reduced metabolism in between attacks.[21] Furthermore the degree of reduced metabolism was correlated with longer disease duration. Since these same structures display hypermetabolism during migraine attacks, a model has been proposed that excessive activity during pain leads to excitotoxicity or inflammation, which in turn may impair metabolic function once the attack subsides. This model is in agreement with the reports of reduced grey matter volume and density in the insula and cingulate of chronic pain patients.

In an elegant study by Kulkarni et al, FDG-PET was performed on knee osteoarthritis patients during either experimental pain or ongoing chronic knee pain.[22] In this study brain areas including the amygdala and the cingulate, which are typically activated more during emotions and fear, displayed greater metabolism during clinical osteoarthritis pain as compared to equally intense experimental heat pain applied to the knee. The authors concluded that clinical arthritic pain involves more activation of the medial pain system as compared to the lateral pain system.

The use of FDG-PET in central or functional pain conditions such as fibromyalgia (FM) has been somewhat limited. Results from these investigations suggest that regional brain metabolic differences between FM patients and controls are minimal, with the possible exception of the retrosplenial cortex.[23–25]

FUNCTIONAL MRI

Functional magnetic resonance imaging (fMRI) has been widely used in neuroscience research, and in particular has had a tremendous impact on the localization and understanding of brain regions involved in pain perception. fMRI is based on measuring and analyzing the so-called BOLD (blood-oxygen-level dependence) effect, described below. fMRI has considerable advantages over using SPECT or PET to assess changes in blood flow in that it does not require the application of a radioactive substance and has a higher spatial resolution compared to these other imaging modalities. Although it has a higher temporal resolution than SPECT and PET, fMRI is not quite as good as electrophysiologic methods such as electroencephalography and magnetoencephalography. On the other hand the exact relationship between neural activity and changes in BOLD signal is still under investigation. As such the BOLD signal is only indirectly linked to neural activity and it remains to be fully elucidated how excitatory and inhibitory neural activity adds up to influence the BOLD signal.

An increase in neural activity leads to a hemodynamic response, which is associated with an increase in regional blood flow and volume resulting in an increase of the oxyhemoglobin–deoxyhemoglobin ratio, which in turn leads to a reduction of local magnetic inhomogeneity. A decrease in magnetic inhomogeneity is associated with slower dephasing of protons, which causes an increase in signal in T_2 weighted images. Activation maps are then created by fitting original data to a model and assessing the quality of the fit. The model is set up by the investigator on the basis of the "on" condition (when a certain stimulus is presented), and an "off" or control condition (rest or when a control stimulus is presented), and a standardized hemodynamic response function, predicting changes in BOLD signal during the time series.

Several meta-analyses of fMRI studies have summarized the brain regions that show activation when experimental pain is applied to human subjects, and these generally agree with SPECT and PET studies noted above. Activation sites across studies vary to some degree, depending on experimental paradigm and pain stimulus (i.e., heat, cold pressure, electric shock, ischemia, etc.). However, the main components of this "pain matrix" are the primary and secondary somatosensory cortex (SI and SII), the insular cortex (IC), the anterior cingulate cortex (ACC), the posterior cingulate cortex, and the thalamus[26,27] Thus, the pain system involves somatosensory, limbic, and associative brain structures. It is more or less true that the medial structures in this matrix (cingulate, insula) respond to the affective dimension of pain (i.e., the emotional valence of pain) whereas the lateral structures (somatosensory cortices) are more involved in the sensory processing of pain (i.e., where it is and how intense it is). There is a wide continuum of how individuals in the general population respond to these painful experimental stimuli (i.e., some individuals are very sensitive and some are very insensitive to pain) and this can be noted on fMRI, where multiple brain regions (especially SII) code for the *perceived* intensity of the stimulus, rather than the objective magnitude of the stimulus.[28] These objective individual differences in pain sensitivity are likely very important in clinical practice.

The two brain sites that fMRI studies have shown to be most consistently activated in response to acute pain stimuli are the ACC and the IC.[26,27] These regions are thought of as multisensory integration sites and have been implicated in various aspects of pain experience and assessment,[29] such as the anticipation[30] and the affective processing of pain and antinociception.[31–33] The motor cortex, supplementary motor areas (SMA),[34,29] and various regions of the frontal cortex, such as the orbitofrontal cortex and the dorsolateral prefrontal cortex (DLPFC), have also been shown to be activated by pain stimuli, but these activations are less reliable, and it is has been suggested that some of them might represent epiphenomena, such as pain-evoked movement suppression. However, there is increasing evidence that different regions in the frontal cortex, such as parts of the orbitofrontal cortex, the DLPFC, and the medial (pre) frontal wall, including the SMA, are critically involved in higher cognitive evaluation of pain stimuli and other cognitive processes (such as distraction) engaged in top-down modulation of the pain system.[35]

fMRI has also been extensively used to determine if a number of chronic pain states are characterized by hyperalgesia (increased pain to normally painful stimuli) in various chronic (clinical) pain states, typically by showing that when a low intensity stimulus is applied experimentally, that individuals have an augmented BOLD response compared to controls. Identifying that hyperalgesia is common to a number of chronic pain states has been a major advance in the pain field and suggests that these chronic pain conditions may have pathophysiological similarities that are also noted in treatment (i.e., individuals with these pain states typically respond to neuroactive drugs). Conditions such as neuropathic pain,[36] including chronic regional pain syndrome (CRPS)[37,38] phantom limb pain,[39,40] chronic back pain, FM,[41–43] various types of headaches[44] and facial pain syndromes,[45] have been studied and are briefly described below.

One of the first studies to investigate changes in cerebral activation in CRPS (formerly called reflex sympathetic dystrophy) was performed by Mainhöfer et al. They showed that pin-prick hyperalgesia, when applied to the affected side, was associated with increased activation in the SI and SII cortices, IC (bilaterally), as well as various parts of the frontal lobe (middle and superior frontal gyrus) and ACC when compared to the activation elicited by the same physical stimulus applied to the nonaffected side.[37] In a subsequent study the same authors could demonstrate that CRPS is associated with motor impairment and that CRPS patients showed a reorganization of motor circuits, with an increased activation of primary and supplementary motor cortices, when performing a finger tapping task, which correlated with the degree of motor impairment.[46] In a longitudinal study investigating pediatric patients with CRPS during disease and after recovery, Lebel et al reported altered cerebral activation associated with cold and mechanical allodynia resembling the pattern previously described in adult patients, with additional sites of increased activation (basal ganglia and parietal lobe).[38] After recovery, patients continued to show an altered pattern of brain activation despite nearly complete elimination of evoked pain. Interestingly, the same stimulus presented to the unaffected side during disease and after recovery would elicit different patterns of brain activation, suggesting that the CRPS brain responds differently to normal stimuli, even when applied to the unaffected regions.

Several studies have also investigated cerebral activation elicited by painful stimuli in chronic low back pain patients.[47] Giesecke et al investigated 11 patients with chronic low back pain and 11 healthy controls (HC), showing that equally painful pressure stimuli applied to the left thumb elicited stronger cerebral activation in the primary and SII in back pain patients as compared to HCs, but less activation in the periaqueductal gray region (PAG) bilaterally. This was interpreted as an indication of generalized hyperactivity of the pain system, even for stimuli that were applied outside the original pain region, together with an impaired descending antinociceptive system.[48] Kobayashi et al applied pressure to the back of six chronic low back pain patients and eight HCs. Pain patients showed increased activation in the right IC, SMA, and posterior cingulate cortex, but not in the somatosensory cortices. Baliki et al, looking at spontaneous fluctuation of pain and contrasting periods of high and low pain intensity, could demonstrate that high sustained pain was associated with increased BOLD signal in the medial prefrontal cortex, including rostral ACC, while periods in which clinical pain increased (dynamic change) elicited an increase in BOLD signal in the IC and SMA.[49] Interestingly, spontaneous activity in the medial prefrontal cortex seemed to correlate with atrophy of the DLPFC.

FM has also been extensively studied using fMRI. Gracely et al reported that in response to mild pressure applied to the thumb, which was perceived as painful by FM patients but not HCs, FM patients revealed a pattern of activation, comparable to that elicited by painful stimulation at nearly twice the pressure in HC,[50] including activation in SI and SII cortices, superior temporal gyrus, IC, putamen, and cerebellum. These findings were subsequently replicated by Pujol et al[43] also using a pressure stimulus, and by Cook et al[42] using a heat stimulus, showing that external pain stimuli often lead to an aberrant and early activation of the human pain system in FM patients.

Pain processing in a variety of types of headache have similarly been studied using fMRI. Investigating 12 migraine patients during the interictal phase and 12 HCs, Moulton et al could show that in response to painful stimuli, migraine patients showed a decreased activation in the nucleus cuneiformis, a brainstem structure involved in descending pain modulation, a finding that was hypothesized to lead to a loss of inhibition or enhanced facilitation of trigeminovascular neurons.[44] Becerra et al used fMRI to investigate neural correlates of brush-evoked allodynia in patients with chronic trigeminal neuropathic pain.[51] Stimulation of the affected side resulted in activation of predominantly frontal region and basal ganglia activation compared to the unaffected side. Differences were also seen in the trigeminal sensory pathway. Due to their ictal pain character, primary headache syndromes such as migraine[52,53] and cluster headache[54,55] have been successfully investigated using brain imaging methods without the application of an external pain stimulus. Interestingly, activations were seen not only in the pain system but also in different brainstem structures, such as the red nucleus and the ipsilateral posterior hypothalamus, which are thought to be regions that possibly trigger the pain attack, rather than being activated in response to an incoming nociceptive stimulus.

SUMMARY OF CHANGES IN BLOOD FLOW DURING ACUTE AND CHRONIC PAIN

A variety of functional neuroimaging techniques demonstrate that administering acutely painful experimental stimuli to healthy individuals reliably leads to increased blood flow (inferred to indicate increased neural activity) in a number of cortical and subcortical structures (sometimes referred to as the pain matrix) involved in pain transmission. Just as there is tremendous interindividual variability in how much pain a given individual experiences from a fixed experimental stimulus, these interindividual differences in pain threshold can also be identified with functional neuroimaging.

In a number of chronic pain states, applying experimental painful stimuli leads to more pain (hyperalgesia) and this can be corroborated by functional neuroimaging techniques. Such studies demonstrate that external pain stimuli often lead to an aberrant and early activation of the human pain system in chronic pain patients and a decreased activity in regions known to be involved in antinociception, thus providing evidence for a hyper(re)active pain system and an impaired antinociceptive system. It is critical to note that so far there is no compelling evidence that examining brain activity in response to experimental pain stimuli can predict brain activity associated with chronic (clinical) pain states. It is becoming increasingly evident that the brain network involved in acute pain perception in healthy subjects differs from that seen in chronic clinical pain conditions[26] and that chronic pain relies, at least to some degree, on brain structures outside the experimentally defined pain system, such as the frontal pole, the superior temporal gyrus and the nucleus accumbens. However, the investigation of persistent (clinical) pain using fMRI is difficult due to the fact that the conventional fMRI approach relies on changes of the BOLD signal, predicted by a model, yielding most reliable results when alternating conditions (i.e., pain and nonpain) are present in the same imaging session. Furthermore, using fMRI to analyze baseline values across subjects or over time is currently not possible.

So far there are only very few studies that have attempted to image spontaneous pain using fMRI,[49] and further research is needed. Investigations of brain activity associated with pain are far from being complete. Stronger magnets, more sophisticated study designs, and new analytical approaches, such as functional and effective connectivity, are used to improve the localization of brain structures involved in pain perception, their connection/interaction, their contribution to different aspects of pain and changes over time and after therapy, which, as stated above, are needed for the exploration of neural correlates of chronic (clinical) pain.

FUNCTIONAL CONNECTIVITY: A TECHNIQUE THAT CAN MEASURE SPONTANEOUS PAIN RATHER THAN EVOKED (EXPERIMENTAL) PAIN

One limitation to standard fMRI techniques is that brain activity occurring when individuals experience spontaneous clinical pain cannot be imaged, because fMRI requires that a stimulus ("on" condition) be compared to a nonstimulated state ("off" condition). Although informative, these analyses only give insights into hyperalgesia and/or allodynia and not ongoing or spontaneous clinical pain. A newer fMRI method has been developed that has the potential to assess brain activity during ongoing spontaneous pain. This technique is called "functional connectivity." In functional connectivity studies researchers are able to assess the degree of correlation (or anticorrelation) between multiple brain regions while the patient is at rest and undergoing spontaneous clinical pain. Analyses of this type of data result in multiple distributed brain regions having temporal correlation of the fMRI signal (i.e., "functional connectivity).[56–58]

One robust brain network that appears to be involved while individuals are at rest, and disturbed in chronic pain conditions, is the default mode network (DMN).[59,60] This network involves brain regions putatively engaged in self-referential cognition that is "deactivated" during a variety of externally focused task conditions.[61] In other words, it is more active at rest than during a task state. Typically, the DMN includes the inferior parietal lobule (IPL) (Brodmann Area [~BA] 40, 39); the posterior cingulate cortex (~BA 30, 23, 31) and precuneus (~BA 7); areas of the inferior, medial, and superior frontal gyri (~BA 8, 9, 10, 47); the hippocampal formation; and the lateral temporal cortex (~BA 21).[32]

While acute experimental pain induces DMN deactivation in healthy control subjects,[62] Baliki et al have shown that chronic low back pain is associated with mitigated DMN deactivation during a visual attention task.[63] This type of finding suggests that DMN activity is altered in chronic pain. Interestingly this result is not limited to the field of pain, as the DMN shows altered activity in other disease states. Decreased DMN connectivity is observed in Alzheimer's disease,[64] while increased DMN connectivity is seen in depression.[65] Resting state connectivity in the DMN has also been shown to change in response to an intervention or task.[66,67]

Fox and Raichle suggest that the functional significance of spontaneous fluctuations in the DMN is fundamental to balancing excitatory and inhibitory inputs to multiple brain networks, thereby setting the "gain" for future task-related response.[68] This type of model is very appealing for pain processing, which could be thought of as a balance between excitatory and inhibitory brain activity. Recently, two papers have independently shown that resting state functional connectivity with the DMN is specifically altered in chronic pain patients. Cauda et al investigated patients with neuropathic pain and found greater DMN connectivity with many pain regions, including the insula.[69] Similarly Napadow et al have found heightened connectivity between the insula and the DMN in FM patients. Moreover, the degree of connectivity was positively correlated with the amount of clinical pain at the time of the scan. The authors propose that this heightened connection between the insula and the DMN may stem from elevated levels of the excitatory neurotransmitter glutamate within the insula itself (see below). These findings have implications for how subjective experiences such as chronic pain arise from a complex interplay of multiple brain networks.

VOLUMETRIC AND STRUCTURAL BRAIN IMAGING IN PAIN

As with functional brain imaging, modern brain morphometry is essentially a statistical approach that compares specified parameters between two or more groups, e.g., a group of patients and a group of HCs, which typically assumes that characteristics distinguishing these groups are associated with the disorder in question. Such parameters may include 1) global: brain volume, brain parenchymal fraction, gray matter volume, gray matter fraction, white matter volume, white matter fraction; 2) regional: variation in size of a lobe or gyrus (e.g., temporal lobe, cingulate gyrus), thickness of the cortex in a predefined region; and 3) voxel-based: values in a three-dimensional entity (i.e., "voxel," in voxel-based morphometry a 1 mm^3 cube), e.g., gray or white matter value, fractional anisotropy, gyrification index, sulcul depth.

Quantitative MRI–based methods can be divided in to MRI-volumetry and MRI-morphometry of the brain. Whereas MRI-volumetry is primarily used to investigate and compare sizes of brain *volumes* (or certain anatomical structures; e.g., lobes, etc.), MRI-morphometry (investigating brain *morphology*) is based on the approach of warping individual brains, which are of different sizes, into a common coordinate system, placing the same anatomical structures across individuals into the same stereotactic position, and making regional units (i.e., voxels) accessible to statistical analysis. Several neurological and psychiatric diseases are associated with an accelerated loss of global and/or regional brain volume, such as Alzheimer's disease,[70] schizophrenia,[71] and multiple sclerosis.[72] Only more recently has altered brain morphology been described in various chronic pain conditions. The three outcome parameters that have been investigated most frequently in chronic pain conditions are 1) regional gray matter density and/or volume as assessed by voxel-based morphometry[73]; 2) cortical thickness and measure of water diffusion, especially fractional anisotropy; and 3) apparent diffusion coefficient, as determined by diffusion tensor imaging (DTI), which is regarded as a marker of white matter integrity.

VOXEL-BASED MORPHOMETRY (VBM) IN CHRONIC PAIN STATES

The number of studies investigating changes in global and/or regional brain volume in chronic pain patients is rapidly expanding. There are two studies that reported decreases in global gray matter volume in pain patients,[74,75] suggesting that pain might be associated with a neurodegenerative process. It must be noted that there are other studies that could not replicate this finding. Furthermore, as with other cross-sectional approaches, it cannot be determined whether pain, in terms of an increased nociceptive input, causes brain atrophy, or whether brain atrophy is a risk factor for the development of chronic pain. Regional brain morphology has been investigated in a variety of chronic pain conditions, including chronic low back pain,[74,76,77] chronic tension-type headache, medication overuse headache,[78] migraine,[79] posttraumatic headache,[80] painful trigeminal neuropathy,[45] atypical facial pain,[81] temporomandibular disorder,[82] FM,[83–86] somatoform pain disorder,[87] phantom limb pain,[88] irritable bowel syndrome,[89] vulvodynia[90] CRPS,[91] and chronic pain associated with recurrent herpes simplex infection.[92] Currently there is only one study in which experimental pain (i.e., not a spontaneously occurring chronic pain state) was used to investigate changes in brain morphology associated with pain. Teutsch et al demonstrated that repeated painful stimulation over several days resulted in an initial increase in gray matter density in several brain regions, including the midcingulate gyrus and somatosensory cortex.[93] These changes receded and were no longer detectable when participants were scanned again after one year. This study indicates that a nociceptive input from a peripheral source leads to an initial increase in gray matter in healthy controls and that gray matter atrophy as often seen in chronic pain patients either reflects a chronic phase (following a prolonged nociceptive input) or a certain preexisting CNS vulnerability of individuals prone to develop a chronic pain syndrome. Some of the above mentioned studies investigating chronic pain will be briefly described in the following section.

Chronic low back pain was the first chronic pain syndrome in which structural changes of the brain could be demonstrated. Apkarian et al investigated 26 patients with chronic back pain (15 patients with musculoskeletal diagnoses, 5 with pure radiculopathy, and 6 with a mixture of musculoskeletal and radicular pain) in comparison with 26 HCs and reported a significant reduction in neocortical gray matter volume in patients compared to controls. Furthermore, VBM analyses revealed a significant gray matter decrease in the DLPFC bilaterally and in the right anterior thalamus. Frontal gray matter decrease and its association with chronic pain were interpreted in the light of a "top-down" role of the DLPFC in regulating orbitofrontal activity, which in turn is critically involved in both perception of negative affect and cognitive modulation of pain. For the thalamic atrophy, the authors stressed the importance of the thalamus as relay between spinal nociceptive input and upstream structures critically involved in pain processing, such as the cingulate cortex. Schmidt-Wilcke et al reported a nonsignificant reduction in whole brain gray matter volume in back pain patients compared to controls (18 patients without acute radiculopathies vs. 18 HCs).[76] VBM revealed a regional increase in gray matter *density* in the posterior part of the putamen bilaterally and the left posterior thalamus, while a decrease in gray matter density was seen in the right somatosensory cortex, the right DLPFC, and in the midbrain. It was suggested that the decrease in gray matter in the brainstem, which projects to/close to the PAG region and was highly correlated with pain intensity, reflected atrophy of a nucleus critically involved in antinociception. This in turn could lead to an nociceptive overflow of upstream structures involved in pain processing, such as the thalamus, the SI and the DLPFC, inducing further structural (mal)adaptive changes.

Kuchinad et al were the first to investigate global and parenchymal volumes in patients suffering from FM (10 FM patients vs. 10 HCs) and reported that FM patients had significantly lower global gray matter and brain parenchymal volumes than HCs. The same study revealed decreased gray matter values in several brain regions, including the midcingulate, left insular, and medial frontal cortices, as well as the left parahippocampal gyrus.[75] Schmidt-Wilcke et al investigated 20 FM patients vs. 22 HCs and found a decrease in gray matter density in the right superior temporal gyrus and the left posterior thalamus, as well as an increase in gray matter density in the left cerebellum, the left orbitofrontal cortex, and in the striatum bilaterally.[86] A subsequent study with a much larger sample size in FM revealed some regions of gray matter loss, but these differences between FM patients and HC disappeared when controlling for psychiatric comorbidity, suggesting that the psychiatric comorbidities that are known to be associated with volume loss need to be considered as potential confounding factors in chronic pain states.[84] The first study to demonstrate changes in a headache syndrome, which was also the first to show decrease gray matter density in the medial pain system (ACC and IC), investigated patients with chronic tension-type headache (CTTH) and with medication-overuse headache, nearly all of whom were migraineurs.[78] CTTH patients showed a significant decrease in gray matter in the dorsal rostral and ventral pons, the perigenual ACC, mid ACC and right posterior cingulate cortex, the anterior and posterior insular cortices bilaterally, the right posterior temporal lobe, the orbitofrontal cortex, the parahippocampus bilaterally, the right cerebellum, and in the midbrain (projecting to the PAG/raphe nuclei). Medication-overuse headache patients showed a nonsignificant decrease in the left orbitofrontal cortex and the right midbrain. A correlation analysis of headache duration in the CTTH group revealed a negative correlation between gray matter values and headache duration in the involved regions. These data suggested that, while both disorders share the feature of chronic headaches, there likely exist fundamental differences in the pathophysiology underlying CTTH and medication-overuse headache. Specifically, regional gray matter decrease in CTTH was interpreted either as the consequence of a prolonged nociceptive input (e.g., from pericranial myofascial tissues), or as an expression of preexisting changes causing central vulnerability to the development of chronic pain. Valfre et al used VBM to investigate patients with chronic migraine.[79] In comparison with HC and episodic migraine patients, chronic migraineurs displayed a regional gray matter decrease in the ACC, left amygdala, left parietal operculum, left middle and inferior frontal gyrus, right inferior gyrus, and the IC bilaterally. Furthermore, there was a significant correlation between frequency of migraine attacks and gray matter reduction in the ACC. The authors suggested that their findings might indicate that migraine is a progressive disorder. In a recently published study, Obermann et al looked at patients who developed and mostly recovered from a posttraumatic headache following mild whiplash injury.[80] Patients developing a chronic headache revealed decreases in gray matter in the ACC and DLPFC after 3 months. These changes resolved after one year, which paralleled the cessation of headache. The same patients showed an increase of gray matter in the midbrain (projecting to the PAG), thalamus bilaterally, and cerebellum one year after the accident. Remarkably, this longitudinal study represented the first demonstration that dynamic gray matter changes in pain patients parallel clinical pain development/improvement. Accordingly, these findings are interpreted in the light of neural plasticity as (mal)adaptive changes in pain processing structures.

DaSilva et al investigated patients with chronic trigeminal neuropathic pain by evaluating cortical thickness and functional brain response during brush-induced allodynia. The authors reported a thinning of cortical gray matter in the sensorimotor cortex bilaterally (projecting to the representational area of the face), the contralateral midcingulate gyrus and ACC, and a thickening in the ipsilateral midcingulate gyrus.[45] Brush-induced allodynia was associated with significantly decreased activation in comparison to HC in the midcingulate gyrus and increased activation in the ACC and sensorimotor cortex. Only recently VBM was used to evaluate patients with persistent idiopathic facial pain (formerly known as atypical facial pain), showing a decrease in gray matter volume in the left ACC and left temporo-insular region, as well as in the left and right sensory-motor area projecting to the representational area of the face. Analyses of laterality index demonstrated an increased asymmetry in the middle-anterior IC in patients in comparison to HCs.[81] Again, these data support previous findings, which show that chronic pain states are associated with changes in brain morphology in brain regions known to be part of the pain system.

DIFFUSION TENSOR IMAGING (DTI) IN CHRONIC PAIN STATES

Currently there are only a limited number of studies that used DTI to investigate patients with chronic pain. In a combined VBM and DTI study, Geha et al investigated cerebral gray and white matter in 21 patients with CRPS and 21 HCs, reporting gray matter atrophy in the right ventromedial prefrontal cortex, right IC, and right nucleus accumbens, as well as a decrease in fractional anisotropy (FA) in the left cingulum-callosal bundle. The authors hypothesize that this decrease in FA might indicate a disconnection between the ACC and the SMA, both regions well known to be involved in different aspects of pain perception. Two studies looked at FA values in FM patients. Sundgren et al described significantly lower FA values in the right thalamus of FM patients as compared to healthy controls.[94] Within the patients' group FA values in the right thalamic region correlated with pain intensity. This finding could be replicated by Lutz et al, who found decreases in FA in the thalamus, in thalamocortical tracts, and in the IC bilaterally.[85] On the other hand, increases in FA were observed in the postcentral gyri, the medial temporal lobes and the medial frontal wall (ACC and superior frontal gyri).

There are few studies that have investigated FA and apparent diffusion coefficient in patients with migraine (with and without aura). DaSilva et al found decreases in FA values in the thalamocortical tracts in patients with migraine; while those with migraine with aura additionally displayed decreased FA values in ventral trigeminothalamic tract, those without aura additionally displayed decreased FA values in the PAG region.[95] Finally, Rocca et al looked specifically at diffusion changes in the visual pathways in patients with migraine and reported decreased FA values in the optic radiation bilaterally in migraine patients.[96]

SUMMARY OF STRUCTURAL CHANGES IN CHRONIC PAIN STATES

The most reproducible finding across pain syndromes is a decrease in gray matter density/volume in the ACC and IC.[97] As such it is possible that initial pain events become associated with a neurodegenerative process that in turn leads to pain chronification. However, most studies that have been performed are cross-sectional and as such it cannot be determined whether structural changes are the consequence of a prolonged nociceptive input to the brain or whether they predispose for the development of chronic pain. On the other hand, studies using a longitudinal approach have begun to shed light on temporal dynamics of structural changes.[80] VBM and DTI cannot disclose the neurobiological basis of morphological differences found, and assumptions regarding the underlying cytoarchitecture remain speculative for now; cross-validation with other imaging methods and postmortem studies are needed to further evaluate histological correlates. DTI creates the possibility of performing tractography, which reconstructs fiber tracts connecting predefined regions, as well as investigating structural connectivity between different parts of a neural system (e.g., pain system). Future approaches combining different imaging methods with the aim to investigate both structural and functional connectivity will be extremely helpful to further improve our understanding of the neurobiological underpinnings of chronic pain.

MEASUREMENT OF NEUROTRANSMITTER SYSTEMS INVOLVED IN PAIN PROCESSING

In addition to providing insights into the temporal and spatial characteristics of neural activity, some functional imaging methods can also provide windows into the molecular underpinnings of pain processing. The two imaging modalities that perform this best are PET, which uses radioactive neurotransmitters or ligands for specific receptors, and proton magnetic resonance spectroscopy (H-MRS). For PET we focus on two pain regulatory transmitters, dopamine and endogenous opioids, as well as glucose metabolism. For H-MRS we focus on glutamate and γ-aminobutyric acid (GABA), the brain's main excitatory and inhibitory neurotransmitters respectively.

USE OF PET TO MEASURE NEUROTRANSMITTER SYSTEMS IN PAIN

PET is a neuroimaging technique that utilizes unstable radionucleotides that have been incorporated into biologically active molecules to infer neuronal function. In the case of the studies below, carbon-11 (^{11}C) is typically incorporated into molecules that bind selectively either to the dopamine 2 receptor (D2) or mu-opioid receptors (MORs). For the D2 receptor, the tracer is ^{11}C-raclopride, whereas for the MORs the tracer is ^{11}C-carfantanil. In PET experiments the binding of these radiotracers is expressed as the binding potential, which is the ratio of the maximal binding over the dissociation constant (i.e., Bmax/Kd). In the case of raclopride and carfentanil, the binding of the tracer to the receptor site can be inhibited by the binding of endogenous ligands at the same receptor site. This reduction in binding potential is typically inferred to be an activation of the receptor system by the endogenous transmitter. However a down-regulation of receptor sites is also plausible.

Although dopamine may be better known as a key player in brain reward mechanisms, the action of this transmitter in the basal ganglia has repeatedly been shown to modulate pain perception. Work in animal models has shown that activation of D2 receptors by agonists can decrease pain nociception, whereas antagonists at this receptor increase pain.[98] The action of dopamine is largely restricted to the basal ganglia, and functional imaging studies in healthy humans have shown that regional cerebral blood flow is increased in the basal ganglia within the striatum during pain. Human pain conditions also show alterations in D2 receptor activity. Conditions such as atypical facial pain and burning mouth pain show increased D2 receptor binding availability, suggesting that there may be either a depletion of dopamine from the synapse or a reduction in receptor density in these patient populations.[99,100] Since diminished levels of dopamine metabolites have also been observed in the cerebrospinal fluid of chronic facial pain patients,[101] this would support the hypothesis of reduced central dopamine concentrations in chronic pain. This is further supported by a PET study in chronic pain patients diagnosed with FM wherein patients exposed to a painful stimulus (hypertonic saline injections) displayed no change in D2 receptor binding potential within the striatum, whereas controls showed reductions in binding potential.[102] These data were interpreted as a disruption in the release of dopamine in the FM patients.

Opioid receptors function to reduce pain by inhibiting synaptic transmission and are positioned strategically in antinociceptive pathways within the central nervous system.[103] There are four types of opioid receptors, the mu, kappa, delta, and opioid receptor-like protein. PET imaging experiments in healthy control participants have defined brain regions where activation of MORs, inferred from a decrease in binding potential, is detected in response to painful stimuli.[104] These regions include the thalamus, insula, hypothalamus, prefrontal cortex, and the amygdala. Three of these regions, the insula, the thalamus, and the amygdala, appear to be involved in chronic pain conditions. PET experiments using [^{11}C]dipreorphine, a nonspecific opioid radiotracer, suggest that patients with either rheumatoid arthritis[105] or neuropathic pain[106] have reduced opioid receptor binding within these structures. Interestingly, both studies found that opioid receptor binding was decreased during pain. This observation is consistent with either activation of antinociceptive pathways (increased release of endogenous opioids) or receptor down-regulation during the pain state. Unfortunately, these experiments cannot distinguish these two possibilities, but changes in receptor occupancy that occur over the course of minutes, as in pain-free control experiments,[104] would favor increased release of endogenous opioids as opposed to a down regulation of MORs, the latter being a complex process that presumably occurs over a longer duration.

Recent data indicate that reduced opioid receptor binding potentialis also present in central pain disorders such as FM. FM patients have reduced MOR binding potential within structures typically observed in imaging studies of experimental pain involving healthy control participants. These structures include the amygdala, the cingulate, and the nucleus accumbens.[107] These regions have previously been noted to play some role in nociception and pain. Opioid activity in the nucleus accumbens and the amygdala has been shown to modulate nociceptive neural transmission in animal models of pain.[108,109] Indeed, endogenous opioids play a central role in analgesia and the perception of painful stimuli.[106] MOR-mediated neurotransmission in the nucleus accumbens and amygdala has also been shown to be modulated by pain in healthy controls reducing the pain experience[104] in a manner consistent with animal data. Since the concentration of endogenous opioids is elevated in the cerebrospinal fluid of FM patients,[110] MORs may be highly occupied by endogenous ligand in an attempt to reduce pain, or down-regulated after prolonged stimulation. Both of these effects could explain the reduced MOR binding potential observed in this study.

Although these data may suggest that reduced opioid receptor availability is a shared feature across chronic pain states, the regional distribution of reduced receptor binding was dissimilar across studies and pain, conditions. In rheumatoid arthritis pain, reduced opioid receptor binding was observed in the cingulate, frontal, and temporal cortices, whereas for central neuropathic pain, reduced opioid receptor availability was detected primarily within the thalamus, somatosensory cortex, cingulate, and insula. In patients with peripheral neuropathic pain, reduced opioid binding potential has been observed bilaterally across brain hemispheres, whereas in central neuropathic pain reductions in binding potential were observed largely isolated to one hemisphere.[111] This heterogeneous pattern of reduced binding may reflect different underlying mechanisms operating in these diverse pain conditions. In the case of FM the reductions in MOR binding potential observed were localized in regions known to be involved in antinociception in animal models,[108,109] as well as pain and emotion regulation (including the affective quality of pain), in humans[104,112,113] (i.e., dorsal anterior cingulate, nucleus accumbens, amygdala).

PROTON MAGNETIC RESONANCE SPECTROSCOPY (H-MRS) TO MEASURE NEUROTRANSMITTERS OR CNS METABOLITES IN CHRONIC PAIN STATES

H-MRS imaging obtains chemical spectra from multiple volume-image elements or voxels within the human brain using radiofrequencies that excite protons.[114] Specific molecules are identified by their characteristic resonance frequency in the spectrum. Once acquired, spectra are analyzed to determine the relative concentrations of different molecules or CNS metabolites within the voxel or field of interest. Typical metabolites identified are: N-acetylaspartate (NAA), choline, and creatine. Abnormalities in the concentrations of these metabolites are associated with various pathological changes in the underlying brain tissue[114] NAA is generally felt to be a marker of cell density or cell viability, whereas choline is a considered a marker of membrane integrity. Creatine reflects adenosine triphosphate metabolism and production and is relatively constant across the brain. More importantly for the exploration of neural processes in pain, concentrations of specific neurotransmitters such as glutamate (Glu) and GABA can also be measured with this technique.

H-MRS methods display multiple features, which are amenable to longitudinal studies. The magnetic fields used in most investigations (i.e., 1.5 or 3 Tesla) have been approved by the U.S. Food and Drug Administration as minimal risk, so (in contrast to PET) individuals can be scanned multiple times without risk of damage to body tissues or organs. In addition, high-resolution anatomical MRI scans can be used to isolate identical brain regions on successive sessions, even weeks apart. Previous H-MRS studies have utilized this aspect to examine changes in the levels of CNS metabolites within individuals over time.[115, 116]

Historically, H-MRS has been used to measure static or basal levels of CNS molecules. However, recently investigators have begun to implement H-MRS technology to assess functional changes in the concentrations of Glu and GABA in response to evoked pain stimuli.[117] Mullins et al have observed that Glu levels increase by as much as 10% in the ACC in response to cold pain applied to the foot. Similarly, Gussew et al found increases of Glu as large as 18% in the anterior insula during heat pain.[118] These changes in Glu have direct implications for neuronal activity, since Glu is a major excitatory neurotransmitter in the brain. However, there are some limitations to these findings. Glu is present in both metabolic and neurotransmitter pools, and the H-MRS technique is unable to differentiate between these two. Furthermore the resonance pattern of Glu overlaps somewhat with glutamine, making it difficult to assign these findings specifically to glutamate. H-MRS detection of GABA, the major inhibitory neurotransmitter in the brain, may circumvent these problems, as GABA is used solely as a neurotransmitter and its resonance spectrum can be differentiated from glutamine. Recently, Kupers et al demonstrated that GABA levels are elevated in the ACC by as much as 15% during heat pain applied to the leg.[119]

Harris et al followed a group of 10 FM patients treated by acupuncture and sham acupuncture and found that clinical pain reduction was highly correlated with the changes in Glu and the combined glutamate + glutamine (Glx) within the posterior insula.[120] Patients with greater reductions in Glu and Glx displayed greater improvements in both clinical and experimental pain. The authors suggested that these neurotransmitters may be a pathological factor in FM. Harris et al have gone on to show that Glu and Glx levels within the posterior insula are significantly elevated in FM and the degree of elevation is associated with pain.[121] Although the precise mechanism(s) for the elevation in Glx and Glu remain to be elucidated, these results imply augmented glutamatergic neurotransmission in chronic pain patients. These individuals may have more Glu within their synaptic vesicles, higher numbers or densities of glutamatergic synapses, or even less uptake of Glu from the synaptic cleft. All of these could result in enhanced excitatory neurotransmission. Indeed, hyperactivity of excitatory neurotransmission has been proposed to be a mechanism of "central sensitization" in functional pain disorders.[122] If true, the pathophysiology of central pain states such as FM may be more akin to conditions such as epilepsy than to the rheumatic disorders with which it has historically been associated. For example, in epilepsy cortical and subcortical neurons appear to be hyperexcitable or "kindled" as a result of elevated concentrations of Glu.[123] These clusters of excited neurons form a locus of heightened activity that can then initiate a spreading wave of activity, which propagates to other connected regions. FM and other central pain disorders may simply represent a condition where glutamatergic "kindling" occurs within brain regions devoted to processing and modulating pain (i.e., the "pain matrix"). This hypothesis is consistent with the fact that one of the U.S. Food and Drug Administration approved medications for FM is pregabalin, a drug whose action is thought to involve inhibition of presynaptic Glu release.[124] The role of GABA in chronic pain is currently unexplored and may be a fruitful area of research on the horizon.

Measurement of CNS metabolites using H-MRS has been only minimally used in chronic pain. Grachev et al were the first to discover that the level of NAA[125,126] was lower within the DLPFC of individuals with chronic low back pain as compared to healthy controls.[127] This suggests that the pathology of this condition may involve reduced neuronal viability in this brain region. Recent work in functional pain syndromes such as FM also shows abnormalities in the DLPFC. Petrou et al found that choline levels were highly variable in the DLPFC of FM patients and that these levels were positively correlated with chronic pain report.[128] Although these findings are significant, the precise roles of choline and NAA in brain function, as measured with H-MRS, are somewhat uncertain.

SUMMARY

A number of functional and structural neuroimaging techniques have been extremely helpful in understanding of the mechanisms that underlie acute and chronic pain transmission in humans. Perhaps the most important discovery is that there are large interindividual differences in pain sensitivity and that some of the same CNS changes that increase an individual's acute pain sensitivity also put them at higher risk for developing chronic pain. It is important that the field of anesthesiology understands these CNS mechanisms because they are clearly important in the perioperative setting and beyond, and will likely lead to "personalized analgesia" in the future.

REFERENCES

1. Williams DA, Clauw DJ. Understanding fibromyalgia: lessons from the broader pain research community. *J Pain.* 2009;10: 777–791.
2. Gwilym SE, Keltner JR, Warnaby CE, et al. Psychophysical and functional imaging evidence supporting the presence of central sensitization in a cohort of osteoarthritis patients. *Arthritis Rheum.* 2009;61:1226–1234.
3. Clauw DJ, Witter J. Pain and rheumatology: thinking outside the joint. *Arthritis Rheum.* 2009;60:321–324.
4. Lee YC, Chibnik LB, Lu B, et al. The relationship between disease activity, sleep, psychiatric distress and pain sensitivity in rheumatoid arthritis: a cross-sectional study. *Arthritis Res Ther.* 2009;11:R160.
5. Apkarian AV, Stea RA, Manglos SH, Szeverenyi NM, King RB, Thomas FD. Persistent pain inhibits contralateral somatosensory cortical activity in humans. *Neurosci Lett.* 1992;140:141–147.
6. Di Piero V, Ferracuti S, Sabatini U, Pantano P, Cruccu G, Lenzi GL. A cerebral blood flow study on tonic pain activation in man. *Pain.* 1994;56:167–173.
7. Mountz JM, Bradley LA, Modell JG, et al. Fibromyalgia in women: abnormalities of regional cerebral blood flow in the thalamus and the caudate nucleus are associated with low pain threshold levels. *Arthritis Rheum.* 1995;38:926–938.
8. Soriani S, Feggi L, Battistella PA, Arnaldi C, De CL, Stipa S. Interictal and ictal phase study with Tc 99m HMPAO brain SPECT in juvenile migraine with aura. *Headache.* 1997;37:31–36.
9. Abdel-Dayem HM, Abu-Judeh H, Kumar M, et al. SPECT brain perfusion abnormalities in mild or moderate traumatic brain injury. *Clin Nucl Med.* 1998;23:309–317.
10. Di Piero V, Fiacco F, Tombari D, Pantano P. Tonic pain: A SPET study in normal subjects and cluster headache patients. *Pain.* 1997;70: 185–191.
11. De BG, Ferrari Da PC, Granata G, Lorenzetti A. CBF changes during headache-free periods and spontaneous/induced attacks in migraine with and without aura: a TCD and SPECT comparison study. *J Neurosurg Sci.* 1999;43:141–146.
12. Guedj E, Taieb D, Cammilleri S, et al. 99mTc-ECD brain perfusion SPECT in hyperalgesic fibromyalgia. *Eur J Nucl Med Mol Imaging.* 2007;34:130–134.
13. Guedj E, Cammilleri S, Niboyet J, et al. Clinical correlate of brain SPECT perfusion abnormalities in fibromyalgia. *J Nucl Med.* 2008; 49(11):1798.
14. Guedj E, Cammilleri S, Colavolpe C, Laforte C, Niboyet J, Mundler O. Follow-up of pain processing recovery after ketamine in hyperalgesic fibromyalgia patients using brain perfusion ECD-SPECT. *Eur J Nucl Med Mol Imaging.* 2007;34:2115–2119.
15. Guedj E, Cammilleri S, Colavolpe C, et al. Predictive value of brain perfusion SPECT for ketamine response in hyperalgesic fibromyalgia. *Eur J Nucl Med Mol Imaging.* 2007;34:1274–1279.
16. Wu CT, Fan YM, Sun CM, et al. Correlation between changes in regional cerebral blood flow and pain relief in complex regional pain syndrome type 1. *Clin Nucl Med.* 2006;31:317–320.

17. Graff-Guerrero A, Pellicer F, Mendoza-Espinosa Y, Martinez-Medina P, Romero-Romo J, Fuente-Sandoval C. Cerebral blood flow changes associated with experimental pain stimulation in patients with major depression. *J Affect Disord.* 2008;107:161–168.
18. Pereira EA, Green AL, Bradley KM, et al. Regional cerebral perfusion differences between periventricular grey, thalamic and dual target deep brain stimulation for chronic neuropathic pain. *Stereotact Funct Neurosurg.* 2007;85:175–183.
19. Newberg AB, Lariccia PJ, Lee BY, Farrar JT, Lee L, Alavi A. Cerebral blood flow effects of pain and acupuncture: a preliminary single-photon emission computed tomography imaging study. *J Neuroimaging.* 2005;15:43–49.
20. Nagamachi S, Fujita S, Nishii R, et al. Alteration of regional cerebral blood flow in patients with chronic pain—evaluation before and after epidural spinal cord stimulation. *Ann Nucl Med.* 2006;20: 303–310.
21. Kim J, Kim S, Suh SI, Koh SB, Park KW, Oh K. Interictal metabolic changes in episodic migraine: a voxel-based FDG-PET study. *Cephalalgia.* 2010;30(1):53–61.
22. Kulkarni B, Bentley DE, Elliott R, et al. Arthritic pain is processed in brain areas concerned with emotions and fear. *Arthritis Rheum.* 2007;56:1345–1354.
23. Wik G, Fischer H, Bragee B, Finer B, Fredrikson M. Functional anatomy of hypnotic analgesia: A PET study of patients with fibromyalgia. *Eur J Pain.* 1999;3:7–12.
24. Wik G, Fischer H, Bragee B, Kristianson M, Fredrikson M. Retrosplenial cortical activation in the fibromyalgia syndrome. *Neuroreport.* 2003;14;619–621.
25. Yunus MB, Young CS, Saeed SA, Mountz JM, Aldag JC. Positron emission tomography in patients with fibromyalgia syndrome and healthy controls. *Arthritis Rheum.* 2004;51:513–518.
26. Apkarian AV, Bushnell MC, Treede RD, Zubieta JK. Human brain mechanisms of pain perception and regulation in health and disease. *Eur J Pain.* 2005;9:463–484.
27. Peyron R, Laurent B, Garcia-Larrea L. Functional imaging of brain responses to pain. A review and meta-analysis (2000). *Neurophysiol Clin.* 2000;30:263–288.
28. Coghill RC, McHaffie JG, Yen YF. Neural correlates of interindividual differences in the subjective experience of pain. *Proc Natl Acad Sci U S A.* 2003;100:8538–8542.
29. Buchel C, Bornhovd K, Quante M, Glauche V, Bromm B, Weiller C. Dissociable neural responses related to pain intensity, stimulus intensity, and stimulus awareness within the anterior cingulate cortex: a parametric single-trial laser functional magnetic resonance imaging study. *J Neurosci.* 2002;22:970–976.
30. Ploghaus A, Tracey I, Gati JS, et al. Dissociating pain from its anticipation in the human brain. *Science.* 1999;284:1979–1981.
31. Petrovic P, Kalso E, Petersson KM, Ingvar M. Placebo and opioid analgesia—imaging a shared neuronal network. *Science.* 2002;295: 1737–1740.
32. Bingel U, Schoell E, Herken W, Buchel C, May A. Habituation to painful stimulation involves the antinociceptive system. *Pain.* 2007;131:21–30.
33. Bingel U, Lorenz J, Schoell E, Weiller C, Buchel C. Mechanisms of placebo analgesia: rACC recruitment of a subcortical antinociceptive network. *Pain.* 2006;120:8–15.
34. Arienzo D, Babiloni C, Ferretti A, et al. Somatotopy of anterior cingulate cortex (ACC) and supplementary motor area (SMA) for electric stimulation of the median and tibial nerves: an fMRI study. *Neuroimage.* 2006;33:700–705.
35. Lorenz J, Minoshima S, Casey KL. Keeping pain out of mind: the role of the dorsolateral prefrontal cortex in pain modulation. *Brain.* 2003;126:1079–1091.
36. Maihofner C, Handwerker HO, Birklein F. Functional imaging of allodynia in complex regional pain syndrome. *Neurology.* 2006;66: 711–717.
37. Maihofner C, Forster C, Birklein F, Neundorfer B, Handwerker HO. Brain processing during mechanical hyperalgesia in complex regional pain syndrome: a functional MRI study. *Pain.* 2005;114: 93–103.
38. Lebel A, Becerra L, Wallin D, et al. fMRI reveals distinct CNS processing during symptomatic and recovered complex regional pain syndrome in children. *Brain.* 2008;131:1854–1879.
39. Lotze M, Flor H, Grodd W, Larbig W, Birbaumer N. Phantom movements and pain: an fMRI study in upper limb amputees. *Brain.* 2001;124:2268–2277.
40. MacIver K, Lloyd DM, Kelly S, Roberts N, Nurmikko T. Phantom limb pain, cortical reorganization and the therapeutic effect of mental imagery. *Brain.* 2008;131:2181–2191.
41. Derbyshire SW, Jones AK, Creed F, et al. Cerebral responses to noxious thermal stimulation in chronic low back pain patients and normal controls. *Neuroimage.* 2002;16:158–168.
42. Cook DB, Lange G, Ciccone DS, Liu WC, Steffener J, Natelson BH. Functional imaging of pain in patients with primary fibromyalgia. *J Rheumatol.* 2004;31:364–378.
43. Pujol J, Lopez-Sola M, Ortiz H, et al. Mapping brain response to pain in fibromyalgia patients using temporal analysis of FMRI. *PLoS ONE.* 2009;4:e5224.
44. Moulton EA, Burstein R, Tully S, Hargreaves R, Becerra L, Borsook D. Interictal dysfunction of a brainstem descending modulatory center in migraine patients. *PLoS ONE.* 2008;3:e3799.
45. DaSilva AF, Becerra L, Pendse G, Chizh B, Tully S, Borsook D. Colocalized structural and functional changes in the cortex of patients with trigeminal neuropathic pain. *PLoS ONE.* 2008;3:e3396.
46. Maihofner C, Baron R, DeCol R, et al. The motor system shows adaptive changes in complex regional pain syndrome. *Brain.* 2007; 130:2671–2687.
47. Kobayashi Y, Kurata J, Sekiguchi M, et al. Augmented cerebral activation by lumbar mechanical stimulus in chronic low back pain patients: an FMRI study. *Spine.* 2009;34:2431–2436.
48. Giesecke T, Gracely RH, Clauw DJ, et al. Central pain processing in chronic low back pain. Evidence for reduced pain inhibition [in German]. *Schmerz.* 2006;20:411–4, 6–7.
49. Baliki MN, Chialvo DR, Geha PY, et al. Chronic pain and the emotional brain: specific brain activity associated with spontaneous fluctuations of intensity of chronic back pain. *J Neurosci.* 2006;26: 12165–12173.
50. Gracely RH, Petzke F, Wolf JM, Clauw DJ. Functional magnetic resonance imaging evidence of augmented pain processing in fibromyalgia. *Arthritis Rheum.* 2002;46:1333–1343.
51. Becerra L, Morris S, Bazes S, et al. Trigeminal neuropathic pain alters responses in CNS circuits to mechanical (brush) and thermal (cold and heat) stimuli. *J Neurosci.* 2006;26:10646–10657.
52. Weiller C, May A, Limmroth V, et al. Brain stem activation in spontaneous human migraine attacks. *Nat Med.* 1995;1:658–660.
53. Cao Y, Aurora SK, Nagesh V, Patel SC, Welch KM. Functional MRI-BOLD of brainstem structures during visually triggered migraine. *Neurology.* 2002;59:72–78.
54. May A, Bahra A, Büchel C, Frackowiak RSJ, Goadsby PJ. Hypothalamic activation in cluster headache attacks. *Lancet.* 1998; 352:275–278.
55. Morelli N, Pesaresi I, Cafforio G, et al. Functional magnetic resonance imaging in episodic cluster headache. *J Headache Pain.* 2009;10:11–14.
56. Biswal B, Yetkin FZ, Haughton VM, Hyde JS. Functional connectivity in the motor cortex of resting human brain using echo-planar MRI. *Magn Reson Med.* 1995;34:537–541.
57. De LM, Beckmann CF, De SN, Matthews PM, Smith SM. fMRI resting state networks define distinct modes of long-distance interactions in the human brain. *Neuroimage.* 2006;29:1359–1367.
58. Fransson P. Spontaneous low-frequency BOLD signal fluctuations: an fMRI investigation of the resting-state default mode of brain function hypothesis. *Hum Brain Mapp.* 2005;26:15–29.
59. Greicius MD, Krasnow B, Reiss AL, Menon V. Functional connectivity in the resting brain: a network analysis of the default mode hypothesis. *Proc Natl Acad Sci U S A.* 2003;100:253–258.

60. Vincent JL, Patel GH, Fox MD, et al. Intrinsic functional architecture in the anaesthetized monkey brain. *Nature.* 2007;447:83–86.
61. Gusnard DA, Raichle ME. Searching for a baseline: functional imaging and the resting human brain. *Nat Rev Neurosci.* 2001;2: 685–694.
62. Seminowicz DA, Davis KD. Interactions of pain intensity and cognitive load: the brain stays on task. *Cereb Cortex.* 2007;17:1412–1422.
63. Baliki MN, Geha PY, Apkarian AV, Chialvo DR. Beyond feeling: chronic pain hurts the brain, disrupting the default-mode network dynamics. *J Neurosci.* 2008;28:1398–1403.
64. Greicius MD, Srivastava G, Reiss AL, Menon V. Default-mode network activity distinguishes Alzheimer's disease from healthy aging: evidence from functional MRI. *Proc Natl Acad Sci U S A.* 2004;101:4637–4642.
65. Greicius MD, Flores BH, Menon V, et al. Resting-state functional connectivity in major depression: abnormally increased contributions from subgenual cingulate cortex and thalamus. *Biol Psychiatry.* 2007;62:429–437.
66. Dhond R, Yeh K, Park K, Kettner N, Napadow V. Acupuncture modulates resting state connectivity in default and sensorimotor brain networks. *Pain.* 2008;136(3):407–418.
67. Waites AB, Stanislavsky A, Abbott DF, Jackson GD. Effect of prior cognitive state on resting state networks measured with functional connectivity. *Hum Brain Mapp.* 2005;24:59–68.
68. Fox MD, Raichle ME. Spontaneous fluctuations in brain activity observed with functional magnetic resonance imaging. *Nat Rev Neurosci.* 2007;8:700–711.
69. Cauda F, Sacco K, Duca S, et al. Altered resting state in diabetic neuropathic pain. *PLoS One.* 2009;4:e4542.
70. Chetelat G, Desgranges B, de la Sayette V, et al. Dissociating atrophy and hypometabolism impact on episodic memory in mild cognitive impairment. *Brain.* 2003;126:1955–1967.
71. Hazlett-Stevens H, Craske MG, Mayer EA, Chang L, Naliboff BD. Prevalence of irritable bowel syndrome among university students: the roles of worry, neuroticism, anxiety sensitivity and visceral anxiety. *J Psychosom Res.* 2003;55:501–505.
72. Sastre-Garriga J, Ingle GT, Chard DT, et al. Grey and white matter volume changes in early primary progressive multiple sclerosis: a longitudinal study. *Brain.* 2005;128:1454–1460.
73. Ashburner J, Friston KJ. Voxel-based morphometry—the methods. *Neuroimage.* 2000;11:805–821.
74. Apkarian AV, Sosa Y, Sonty S, et al. Chronic back pain is associated with decreased prefrontal and thalamic gray matter density. *J Neurosci.* 2004;24:10410–10415.
75. Kuchinad A, Schweinhardt P, Seminowicz DA, Wood PB, Chizh BA, Bushnell MC. Accelerated brain gray matter loss in fibromyalgia patients: premature aging of the brain? *J Neurosci.* 2007;27: 4004–4007.
76. Schmidt-Wilcke T, Leinisch E, Ganssbauer S, et al. Affective components and intensity of pain correlate with structural differences in gray matter in chronic back pain patients. *Pain.* 2006;125:89–97.
77. Buckalew N, Haut MW, Morrow L, Weiner D. Chronic pain is associated with brain volume loss in older adults: preliminary evidence. *Pain Med.* 2008;9:240–248.
78. Schmidt-Wilcke T, Leinisch E, Straube A, et al. Gray matter decrease in patients with chronic tension type headache. *Neurology.* 2005;65: 1483–1486.
79. Valfre W, Rainero I, Bergui M, Pinessi L. Voxel-based morphometry reveals gray matter abnormalities in migraine. *Headache.* 2008;48: 109–117.
80. Obermann M, Nebel K, Schumann C, et al. Gray matter changes related to chronic posttraumatic headache. *Neurology.* 2009;73:978–983.
81. Schmidt-Wilcke T, Hierlmeier S, Leinisch E. Altered regional brain morphology in patients with chronic facial pain. *Headache.* 2010; 50(8):1278–1285.
82. Younger JW, Shen YF, Goddard G, Mackey SC. Chronic myofascial temporomandibular pain is associated with neural abnormalities in the trigeminal and limbic systems. *Pain.* 2010;149(2):222.
83. Burgmer M, Gaubitz M, Konrad C, et al. Decreased gray matter volumes in the cingulo-frontal cortex and the amygdala in patients with fibromyalgia. *Psychosom Med.* 2009;71:566–573.
84. Hsu MC, Harris RE, Sundgren PC, et al. No consistent difference in gray matter volume between individuals with fibromyalgia and age-matched healthy subjects when controlling for affective disorder. *Pain.* 2009;143:262–267.
85. Lutz J, Jager L, de Quervain D, et al. White and gray matter abnormalities in the brain of patients with fibromyalgia: a diffusion-tensor and volumetric imaging study. *Arthritis Rheum.* 2008; 58:3960–3969.
86. Schmidt-Wilcke T, Luerding R, Weigand T, et al. Striatal grey matter increase in patients suffering from fibromyalgia—a voxel-based morphometry study. *Pain.* 2007;132(Suppl 1):S109–116.
87. Valet M, Gundel H, Sprenger T, et al. Patients with pain disorder show gray-matter loss in pain-processing structures: a voxel-based morphometric study. *Psychosom Med.* 2009;71:49–56.
88. Draganski B, Moser T, Lummel N, et al. Decrease of thalamic gray matter following limb amputation. *Neuroimage.* 2006;31:951–957.
89. Davis KD, Pope G, Chen J, Kwan CL, Crawley AP, Diamant NE. Cortical thinning in IBS: implications for homeostatic, attention, and pain processing. *Neurology.* 2008;70:153–154.
90. Schweinhardt P, Kuchinad A, Pukall CF, Bushnell MC. Increased gray matter density in young women with chronic vulvar pain. *Pain.* 2008;140:411–419.
91. Geha PY, Baliki MN, Harden RN, Bauer WR, Parrish TB, Apkarian AV. The brain in chronic CRPS pain: abnormal gray-white matter interactions in emotional and autonomic regions. *Neuron.* 2008;60:570–581.
92. Vartiainen N, Kallio-Laine K, Hlushchuk Y, et al. Changes in brain function and morphology in patients with recurring herpes simplex virus infections and chronic pain. *Pain.* 2009;144:200–208.
93. Teutsch S, Herken W, Bingel U, Schoell E, May A. Changes in brain gray matter due to repetitive painful stimulation. *Neuroimage.* 2008;42:845–849.
94. Sundgren PC, Petrou M, Harris RE, et al. Diffusion-weighted and diffusion tensor imaging in fibromyalgia patients: a prospective study of whole brain diffusivity, apparent diffusion coefficient, and fraction anisotropy in different regions of the brain and correlation with symptom severity. *Acad Radiol.* 2007;14:839–846.
95. DaSilva AF, Granziera C, Tuch DS, Snyder J, Vincent M, Hadjikhani N. Interictal alterations of the trigeminal somatosensory pathway and periaqueductal gray matter in migraine. *Neuroreport.* 2007;18:301–305.
96. Rocca MA, Pagani E, Colombo B, et al. Selective diffusion changes of the visual pathways in patients with migraine: a 3-T tractography study. *Cephalalgia.* 2008;28:1061–1068.
97. May A. Chronic pain may change the structure of the brain. *Pain.* 2008;137:7–15.
98. Hagelberg N, Jaaskelainen SK, Martikainen IK, et al. Striatal dopamine D2 receptors in modulation of pain in humans: a review. *Eur J Pharmacol.* 2004;500:187–192.
99. Hagelberg N, Forssell H, Aalto S, et al. Altered dopamine D2 receptor binding in atypical facial pain. *Pain.* 2003;106:43–48.
100. Hagelberg N, Forssell H, Rinne JO, et al. Striatal dopamine D1 and D2 receptors in burning mouth syndrome. *Pain.* 2003;101: 149–154.
101. Bouckoms AJ, Sweet WH, Poletti C, et al. Monoamines in the brain cerebrospinal fluid of facial pain patients. *Anesth Prog.* 1992;39:201–208.
102. Wood PB, Schweinhardt P, Jaeger E, et al. Fibromyalgia patients show an abnormal dopamine response to pain. *Eur J Neurosci.* 2007;25:3576–3582.
103. Fields H. State-dependent opioid control of pain. *Nat Rev Neurosci.* 2004;5:565–575.
104. Zubieta JK, Smith YR, Bueller JA, et al. Regional mu opioid receptor regulation of sensory and affective dimensions of pain. *Science.* 2001;293:311–315.

105. Jones AK, Cunningham VJ, Ha-Kawa S, et al. Changes in central opioid receptor binding in relation to inflammation and pain in patients with rheumatoid arthritis. *Br J Rheumatol.* 1994;33: 909–916.
106. Jones AK, Watabe H, Cunningham VJ, Jones T. Cerebral decreases in opioid receptor binding in patients with central neuropathic pain measured by [11C]diprenorphine binding and PET. *Eur J Pain.* 2004;8:479–485.
107. Harris RE, Clauw DJ, Scott DJ, McLean SA, Gracely RH, Zubieta JK. Decreased central mu-opioid receptor availability in fibromyalgia. *J Neurosci.* 2007;27:10000–10006.
108. Gear RW, Levine JD. Antinociception produced by an ascending spino-supraspinal pathway. *J Neurosci.* 1995;15:3154–3161.
109. Manning BH. A lateralized deficit in morphine antinociception after unilateral inactivation of the central amygdala. *J Neurosci.* 1998;18:9453–9470.
110. Baraniuk JN, Whalen G, Cunningham J, Clauw DJ. Cerebrospinal fluid levels of opioid peptides in fibromyalgia and chronic low back pain. *BMC Musculoskelet Disord.* 2004;5:48.
111. Maarrawi J, Peyron R, Mertens P, et al. Differential brain opioid receptor availability in central and peripheral neuropathic pain. *Pain.* 2007;127:183–194.
112. Rainville P, Duncan GH, Price DD, Carrier B, Bushnell MC. Pain affect encoded in human anterior cingulate but not somatosensory cortex. *Science.* 1997;277:968–971.
113. Zubieta JK, Ketter TA, Bueller JA, et al. Regulation of human affective responses by anterior cingulate and limbic mu-opioid neurotransmission. *Arch Gen Psychiatry.* 2003;60:1145–1153.
114. Ross AJ, Sachdev PS. Magnetic resonance spectroscopy in cognitive research. *Brain Res Rev.* 2004;44:83–102.
115. Hammen T, Stadlbauer A, Tomandl B, et al. Short TE single-voxel 1H-MR spectroscopy of hippocampal structures in healthy adults at 1.5 Tesla—how reproducible are the results? *NMR Biomed.* 2005;18:195–201.
116. Geurts JJ, Barkhof F, Castelijns JA, Uitdehaag BM, Polman CH, Pouwels PJ. Quantitative 1H-MRS of healthy human cortex, hippocampus, and thalamus: metabolite concentrations, quantification precision, and reproducibility. *J Magn Reson Imaging.* 2004;20:366–371.
117. Mullins PG, Rowland LM, Jung RE, Sibbitt WL Jr. A novel technique to study the brain's response to pain: proton magnetic resonance spectroscopy. *Neuroimage.* 2005;26:642–646.
118. Gussew A, Rzanny R, Erdtel M, et al. Time-resolved functional 1H MR spectroscopic detection of glutamate concentration changes in the brain during acute heat pain stimulation. *Neuroimage.* 2010;49:1895–1902.
119. Kupers R, Danielsen ER, Kehlet H, Christensen R, Thomsen C. Painful tonic heat stimulation induces GABA accumulation in the prefrontal cortex in man. *Pain.* 2009;142:89–93.
120. Harris RE, Sundgren PC, Pang Y, et al. Dynamic levels of glutamate within the insula are associated with improvements in multiple pain domains in fibromyalgia. *Arthritis Rheum.* 2008;58:903–907.
121. Harris RE, Sundgren PC, Craig AD, et al. Elevated insular glutamate (Glu) in fibromyalgia (FM) is associated with experimental pain. *Arthritis Rheum.* 2009;60:3146–3152.
122. Zhuo M. Cortical excitation and chronic pain. *Trends Neurosci.* 2008;31:199–207.
123. Helms G, Ciumas C, Kyaga S, Savic I. Increased thalamus levels of glutamate and glutamine (Glx) in patients with idiopathic generalised epilepsy. *J Neurol Neurosurg Psychiatry.* 2006;77:489–494.
124. Crofford LJ, Rowbotham MC, Mease PJ, et al. Pregabalin for the treatment of fibromyalgia syndrome: results of a randomized, double-blind, placebo-controlled trial. *Arthritis Rheum.* 2005;52: 1264–1273.
125. Nakano M, Ueda H, Li JY, Matsumoto M, Yanagihara T. Measurement of regional N-acetylaspartate after transient global ischemia in gerbils with and without ischemic tolerance: an index of neuronal survival. *Ann Neurol.* 1998;44:334–340.
126. Sager TN, Topp S, Torup L, Hanson LG, Egestad B, Moller A. Evaluation of CA1 damage using single-voxel 1H-MRS and un-biased stereology: Can non-invasive measures of N-acetyl-asparate following global ischemia be used as a reliable measure of neuronal damage? *Brain Res.* 2001;892:166–175.
127. Grachev ID, Fredrickson BE, Apkarian AV. Abnormal brain chemistry in chronic back pain: an in vivo proton magnetic resonance spectroscopy study. *Pain.* 2000;89:7–18.
128. Petrou M, Harris RE, Foerster BR, et al. Proton MR spectroscopy in the evaluation of cerebral metabolism in patients with fibromyalgia: comparison with healthy controls and correlation with symptom severity. *Am J Neuroradiol.* 2008;29(5):913–918.

PART III

SPINAL CORD

7

SPINAL CORD TARGETS OF RELEVANCE TO THE ANESTHESIOLOGIST

Dhananjay Namjoshi, Sanja Vukicevic,

Raul Sanoja, and Peter J. Soja

Classical characteristic features of the anesthetic state include analgesia, immobility, unconsciousness, a loss of autonomic integrity, and amnesia.[1–4] While Section II of this volume deals with anesthetic actions on the higher brain centers, this chapter will provide an overview of the known anatomical targets within the spinal cord that serve as a foundation for how anesthetic agents contribute to a reduction in somatosensory, somatomotor, and autonomic outflow. Where appropriate, various anesthetic agents are mentioned with respect to their principal mechanism of action on such targets. Emphasis is placed on studies performed in in vivo preparations.

ANATOMICAL OVERVIEW OF THE SPINAL CORD

The human spinal cord is composed of 31 segments, which are divided into five groups, namely, eight cervical, twelve thoracic, five lumbar, five sacral, and one coccygeal. Each spinal segment innervates peripheral organs via a pair of mixed (sensory and motor) spinal nerves. The sensory nerves enter the dorsal horn of the spinal cord via the dorsal roots. The cell bodies of the spinal sensory neurons are pseudo-unipolar and located in the dorsal root ganglia. The axon of the dorsal root ganglion cell bifurcates into the peripheral and central branches. The peripheral branch innervates skin, muscle, joints, or other tissues as a free nociceptive nerve ending or in association with sensory (Pacinian and Meissner's corpuscles, Ruffini endings, Golgi tendon organ, muscle spindles) receptors. The central branch relays input to the spinal cord gray matter. Different somatic sensory modalities are processed by distinct populations of primary afferents. Thus, nonmyelinated, slow-conducting C fibers and myelinated Aδ fibers principally convey nociceptive input to the spinal cord. Fast-conducting, myelinated group Ia and Ib afferents from the muscle spindles and Golgi tendon organs, respectively, transmit proprioceptive information.

A cross section of the spinal cord reveals two distinct regions, the inner, butterfly wing–shaped gray matter and the surrounding outer white matter (Figure 7.1). The gray matter consists of the dorsal and ventral horns. Rexed[5] identified ten layers of gray matter in the spinal cord based on the differences in neuronal cytoarchitecture. These layers or laminae are numbered I to X, starting from the dorsal horn. Primary afferent neurons carrying different sensory modalities show lamina-specific synaptic connections. The primary afferent fibers of mechanoreceptors tend to make synapses with the neurons in the deeper laminae (III-VI) of the dorsal horn, while small-diameter afferents from nociceptors and thermoreceptors enter more laterally to terminate in more superficial laminae I-II. Neurons in the laminae VIII and IX are located in the ventral horn and provide motor output. Lamina X corresponds to the neurons encircling the central canal. The target neurons of primary afferent fibers can be neurons of ascending spinal tracts, interneurons, or motoneurons. For example, the C fibers and Aδ primary afferents synapse on the ascending tract neurons that transmit information to supraspinal structures (Figure 7.1).

The second-order spinal tracts convey sensory input from the primary afferents to supraspinal structures. Examples of important spinal sensory tracts include the spinothalamic tract (STT; Figure 7.1), spinoreticular tract (SRT; Figure 7.1), dorsal spinocerebellar tract (DSCT; Figure 7.1), and spinomesencephalic tract. Cell bodies of the STT are located mainly in the Rexed laminae I and IV-VI. Axons of the majority of the STT neurons decussate to the opposite side of the spinal cord, ascend through the anterolateral quadrant, and terminate in the sensory nuclei of the thalamus.[6] The SRT originates in the deep dorsal horn and laminae VII and VIII of the ventral horn and terminates in the contralateral reticular formation.[7] On the other hand, the axons of the DSCT neurons (Figure 7.1) originate in Clarke's column in the lamina X and ascend ipsilaterally providing proprioceptive and exteroceptive input to the cerebellum[8–9] and thalamus.[10]

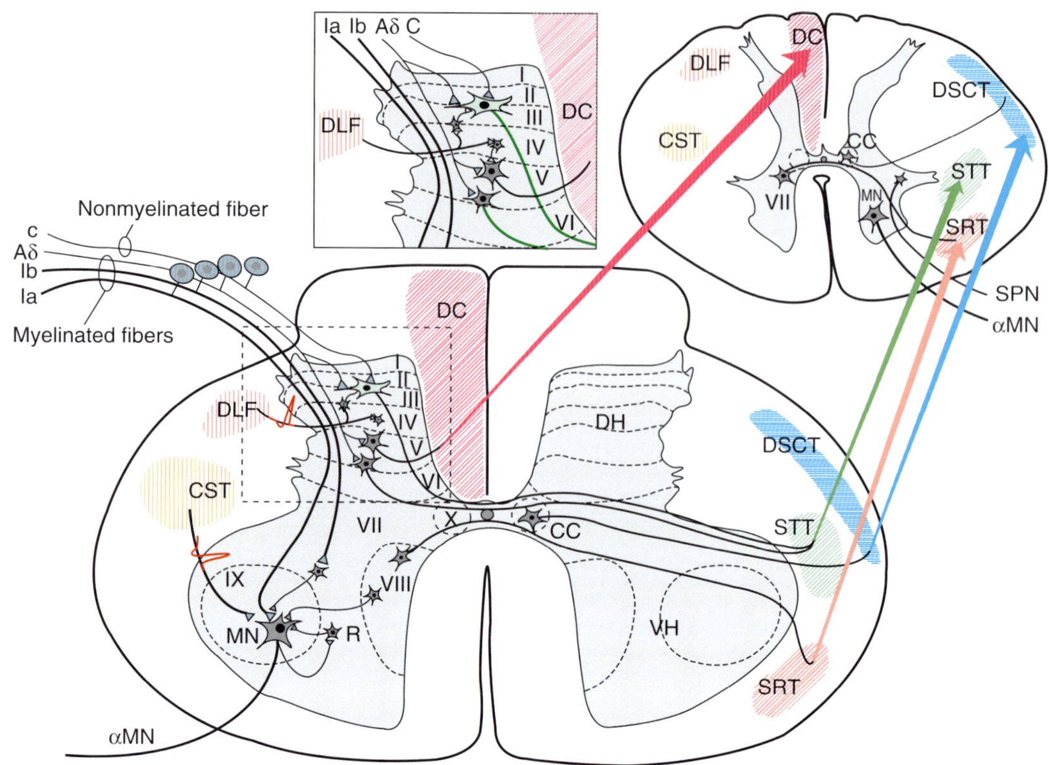

Figure 7.1 *Anatomy of the spinal cord.* This figure depicts a general overview of spinal cord anatomy and neural connectivities important from an anesthesiologist's perspective. At spinal cord level, general anesthetics can affect afferent neurons (from periphery and from supraspinal structures) and/or spinal efferent neurons. The central spinal gray matter is divided into ten Rexed's laminae (I to X) containing different populations of spinal neurons. In general, the spinal sensory neurons are located in the dorsal horn, while motor neurons are located in the ventral horn. The spinal neurons receive peripheral input via primary afferents, which include the fast-conducting, myelinated Ia and Ib spindle afferents as well as Aδ and slow-conducting and nonmyelinated C fibers. In addition the spinal neurons also receive input from supraspinal structures. For example, as shown in the figure, corticospinal tract (CST) provides major supraspinal input to motoneurons in the spinal cord. The spinal efferents include ascending sensory tract neurons, motoneurons, preganglionic neurons of the autonomic nervous system, and interneurons. The axons of the spinal sensory neurons ascend through the spinal gray matter to the ipsilateral or contralateral supraspinal structures. The figure shows three important spinal sensory tracts, namely, the spinothalamic tract (originates in the superficial dorsal horn), spinoreticular tract (originates in the deep dorsal horn) and dorsal spinocerebellar tract (originates in the Clarke's column). Cell bodies of spinal motoneurons are located in the ventral horn and send their axons that emerge through ventral roots. The axons of spinal interneurons may terminate within the same spinal segment (e.g., Renshaw cell) or may ascend or descend through several spinal segments. The cells of spinal preganglionic neurons (SPN) are located in the intermediolateral columns. The axons of SPNs emerge from ventral roots and terminate in the ganglia located outside the cerebrospinal axis. Abbreviations: αMN–alpha motor neuron, CC–Clarke's column, CST–corticospinal tract, DC–dorsal columns, DH–dorsal horn, DLF–dorsolateral funiculus, DSCT–dorsal spinocerebellar tract, R–Renshaw cell, SPN–spinal preganglionic neuron, SRT–spinoreticular tract, STT–spinothalamic tract, VH–ventral horn.

The group Ib and Ia afferents from the Golgi tendon organ and muscle spindles, respectively, form direct or indirect (through inhibitory interneurons) connectivities with the α-motor neurons, which exit the spinal cord through the ventral roots (Figure 7.1).

The sensory and motor neuron pools in the spinal cord also receive descending projections from supraspinal structures, which can modulate the output from the spinal neurons. The corticospinal tract (CST; Figure 7.1) for example provides important descending input to the motoneurons in the ventral horn. On the other hand, sensory neurons in the dorsal horn receive descending inputs from the brainstem periaqueductal gray via the Raphe nuclei.[11]

From an anesthesiologist's viewpoint, various elements of spinal cord white and gray matter form quintessential targets of anesthetic agents, namely, primary afferent neurons, segmental and intersegmental interneurons, second-order sensory tract neurons, preganglionic neurons, and somatic motoneurons. Further, descending modulatory influences impinging on each of these spinal cord elements constitute additional targets for anesthetic actions. Although literature on site-specific actions of currently used anesthetics such as sevoflurane and desflurane is very limited, evidence is available for older, traditional anesthetics such as halothane and barbiturates. The following sections give a brief overview of the actions of various anesthetic agents on each of these spinal elements.

GENERAL ANESTHETIC ACTIONS ON PERIPHERAL TERMINALS OF PRIMARY AFFERENT FIBERS

Primary afferent fibers transmit information from sensory receptors to the dorsal and ventral horn gray matter of the spinal cord. Different classes of primary afferent neurons convey different sensory modalities. The fast-conducting group Ia, Ib, and II sensory fibers transmit proprioceptive information, group II and III conduct mechanoceptive information, while the slowest conducting unmyelinated fibers transmit nociceptive information to the spinal cord. Inhalational anesthetics (e.g., halothane, isoflurane, enflurane, and possibly sevoflurane) have differential actions on sensory receptors including excitatory or inhibitory actions. These effects seem to occur at peripheral nerve endings.[12–16] Over the last decade, evidence has also accrued that peripheral $NMDA_{2B}$ receptors play a key role in sensitizing nociceptive afferent fibers in the periphery especially in neuropathic pain patients and animals with chronic nerve lesions.[17–18] Anesthetics that act via NMDA receptor antagonism, such as ketamine, may exert their analgesic action by a peripheral site of action on nociceptive afferent finer endings.[17]

GENERAL ANESTHETIC ACTIONS ON CENTRAL TERMINALS OF PRIMARY AFFERENT FIBERS

General anesthetics also exert profound effects on the neurotransmitter release from central terminals of primary afferent fibers in the dorsal and ventral horn. A classic index of spinal presynaptic inhibition is the process of primary afferent depolarization (PAD; Figure 7.2). The phenomenon of PAD has been inferred from earlier in vivo experimental paradigms assessing changes in the magnitude or time course of dorsal root reflexes, dorsal root potentials, and the excitability of the central terminals of primary afferents.[19] For example, the time course of dorsal root potentials evoked by stimulation of adjacent dorsal roots is enhanced by pentobarbital (PB), suggesting that barbiturates enhance presynaptic inhibition of transmitter release from primary afferents.[20–23] Older benzodiazepines (e.g., diazepam, midazolam), the more currently used induction agent propofol, and inhalational agent sevoflurane also increase presynaptic inhibition in the spinal cord via an enhancement of GABA-mediated (axoaxonic PAD) presynaptic inhibition.[24–27,28] In addition, GABAmimetic-mediated

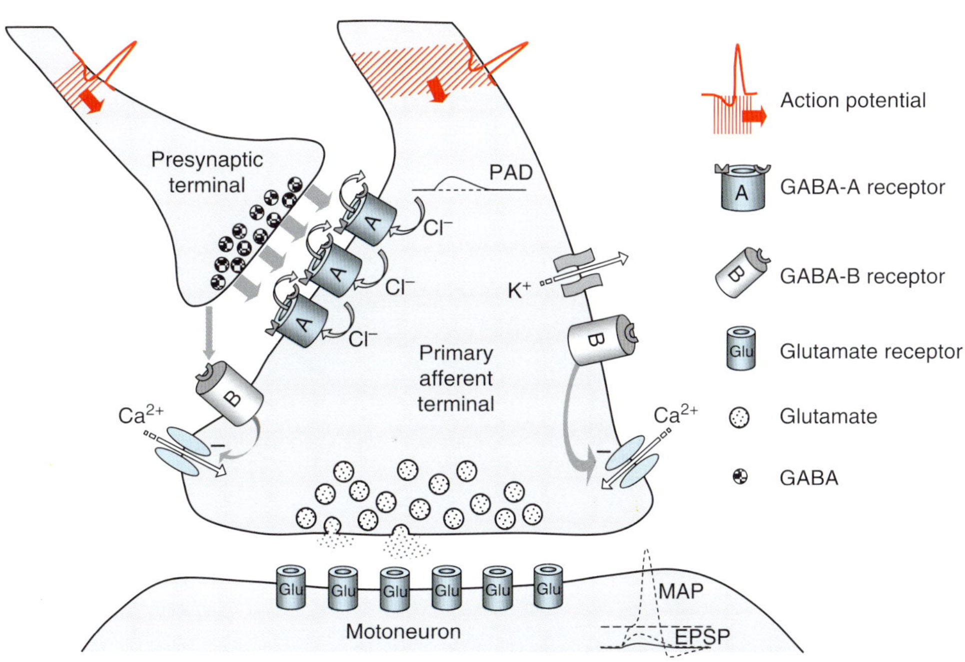

Figure 7.2 *Schematic diagram of axoaxonic, GABAergic primary afferent depolarization (PAD) for Ia-motoneuron synapse.* Presynaptic inhibition of (Ia) primary afferent fibers is mediated by the release of GABA at axoaxonic synapses. In the mammalian spinal cord, $GABA_A$ and $GABA_B$ receptors exist on primary afferent terminals. Presynaptic inhibition may result from GABA's action at either receptor. $GABA_A$ receptor activation increases chloride (Cl^-) conductance such that Cl^- normally moves down its concentration gradient (in this case out of the nerve terminal) when the GABA-gated Cl^- channels are in their open state thus depolarizing the terminal (PAD). As a result, the amplitude and duration of the incoming action potential are reduced, which, in turn, decreases the Ca^{++} influx into the terminal and neurotransmitter (glutamate) release. $GABA_B$ agonists (e.g., baclofen) also suppress Ca^{++} influx thereby reducing neurotransmitter release. PAD can also occur by drug-induced increases in outward K^+ conductance(s). This is reflected postsynaptically by a lower-amplitude monosynaptic excitatory potential (EPSP, solid trace). Benzodiazepines and barbiturates are known to enhance PAD. For further details, see Redman.[169]

increases in presynaptic inhibition can also occur via local anesthetic effects, e.g., via a blockade of impulse invasion into the central terminals of afferent fibers[29–30] and/or a blockade of depolarization-induced Ca^{++} entry into the presynaptic terminals.[31–32]

Another issue that markedly complicates this viewpoint of barbiturate anesthetics, and for that matter, all other anesthetic agents affecting presynaptic inhibition, is the phenomenon of "differential PAD," which can be measured simultaneously from different populations of presynaptic inputs.[33] More recently, this idea was investigated for two intraspinal collaterals of the same muscle spindle afferent, which are also subjected to opposing supraspinal influences[34–36] (see also reviews by Rudomin[37–39]). Differential PAD may simply represent presynaptic inhibition which, at each terminal locus, varies in magnitude due to supraspinal influences. This may partly explain how sensorimotor commands are sculpted during various movements, (e.g., sitting, standing, walking, etc.). From an experimental viewpoint, the actions of anesthetics may be useful in further defining the phenomenon of differential PAD and its underlying neural circuitry within the spinal cord. From an anesthesiologist's viewpoint, the anesthetic depression of the spinal cord may render the phenomenon of differential PAD insignificant. Nevertheless, future studies are warranted to delineate this aspect of anesthetic action on presynaptic controls.

In vitro studies have also been performed to assess the presynaptic actions of anesthetics. Earlier assessments of nociceptive neurotransmission in the spinal cord included the measurement of slow ventral root potentials, which were suppressed by volatile anesthetics.[40–41] Although these potentials were recorded from motoneurons, they are nevertheless considered "nociceptive" in nature.[42–44]

Sensory neurons in the superficial laminae of the dorsal horn, namely the substantia gelatinosa, were driven synaptically by nociceptive inputs. When these neurons were studied using whole-cell patch-clamp recording methods, the volatile anesthetic isoflurane reversibly depressed spontaneous and miniature excitatory postsynaptic currents as well as those evoked by dorsal root stimulation.[45] Neither the resting potential nor input resistance of the recorded neurons was affected by isoflurane. These findings suggest that volatile anesthetics may act presynaptically to depress neurotransmitter release from nociceptive afferent fibers which, in turn, may partly underlie the analgesia of the anesthetic state.[45]

Ketamine, a "dissociative" anesthetic, induces marked analgesia and is therefore employed in a variety of surgical procedures.[46] Ketamine has been shown to exert a variety of effects in the spinal cord through its antagonist actions on NMDA receptors. NMDA receptors are known to partly underlie dorsal horn spinal plasticity mechanisms.[47–50] Presynaptic NMDA autoreceptors that label positively for glutamate are located on primary afferent terminals.[51] Thus, ketamine may directly decrease NMDA autoreceptor-mediated transmitter release from presynaptic terminals[51] or through indirect mechanisms. Ketamine's action at these receptors could reflect a presynaptic inhibitory control of nociceptive transmitter release. Curtis et al and others have shown that the excitability of primary afferent terminals, as reflected by a relative decrease in the threshold for antidromic activation, is increased by acidic amino acids such as NMDA and glutamate.[52] Clearly, NMDA mechanisms contribute to various indices of presynaptic inhibition that might contribute to the analgesic actions of ketamine.

Hence, as briefly surveyed here, there is substantial evidence that agents used for general anesthesia target primary afferent input into the spinal cord and lead to a reduction in transmitter release. Depending on the postsynaptic targets of primary afferent fibers, i.e., sensory tract neuron, or motoneuron, the reduction in transmitter release could partially account for a given agent's analgesic and/or myorelaxant properties.

GENERAL ANESTHETIC ACTION ON SPINAL NEURONS

Spinal neurons essentially fall into four main groups, namely, ascending sensory tract neurons, interneurons, somatic motoneurons, and preganglionic autonomic neurons. Inhalational and intravenous anesthetics act within the spinal cord to exert their actions on each of these elements. The remaining portions of this chapter will focus on each of these targets.

Over the past 50 years, acute in vivo electrophysiological studies have provided a vast wealth of knowledge regarding the (non)nociceptive coding properties of spinal sensory neurons. However, it should be noted that such experiments performed by different investigative teams vary enormously from each other in terms of the procedures used to deal with the identity of the recorded neurons under study. In some studies, the neurons are painstakingly identified precisely using classical antidromic stimulation and/or intracellular staining[53–54] procedures. Neurons comprising the spinothalamic tract (STT), spinoreticular tract (SRT), or postsynaptic dorsal column pathway[53,55–57] have been successfully and unequivocally identified using these procedures.

Ideally, some investigators who identified the axonal projections of their neurons also characterized their cell populations further by their response profile to natural (non)noxious receptive field stimulation and/or electrical stimulation of peripheral nerves. This combined approach of cellular identification and characterization has provided a wealth of foundational information on these classical sensory tract pathways. Many other investigators described their recorded sensory neurons only in terms of one of various classification schemes that have emerged over the years,[58–63] which has led to some confusion in the literature on whether the same neurons were being investigated among the different laboratories.

Perhaps a more important concern that is endemic to all acute in vivo studies is that the excitability of spinal neurons prior to investigating the actions of anesthetics is distorted by invasive surgery, neural ablation, e.g., decerebration, denervation caused by neuromuscular blockers, and last but not least, background anesthesia used during surgery and recording.[64] Recording spinal sensory neuron activity from chronic intact animals that have recovered from recent surgery would circumvent these concerns and provide near-natural conditions for examining anesthetic action on sensory neurons. Unfortunately, this is technically difficult and, as such, has discouraged investigators from attempting such studies to understand how and to what extent spinal neurons, especially STT, SRT, and other tract neurons, are suppressed by clinically used anesthetics.[65]

These caveats notwithstanding, the action of anesthetics on sensory neurons will be discussed below according to the type of experimental preparation used and whether the neurons were identified or not.

ANESTHETIC ACTIONS ON NON-IDENTIFIED SPINAL SENSORY NEURONS—ACUTE PREPARATION

A vast majority of the in vivo studies have been conducted using extracellular recording techniques to investigate anesthetic mechanisms on spinal sensory neurons. Many of these studies were performed in acute animal preparations where the axonal projections of the recorded neurons were not identified and the recorded cells were characterized using various classification schemes mentioned previously.[58–63] Dose-related depressant actions on low-threshold (nonnociceptive) and wide-dynamic-range (WDR)-type neurons have been reported for isoflurane and halothane,[66–72] nitrous oxide,[73–77] thiopental[76,78] and propofol.[66,79–80] Further details of these agents on spinal sensory neurons can be found in more extensive reviews[4,81–82] and also in Chapter 8 in this volume.

ANESTHETIC ACTIONS ON IDENTIFIED SPINAL ASCENDING SENSORY TRACT NEURONS—ACUTE PREPARATION

Surprisingly, after one half century, only one in vivo study reported the actions of an injectable anesthetic on *identified* sensory tract cells without the distortion introduced by a preparative anesthetic itself.[83] In the study of Hori and colleagues,[83] lumbar STT-like neurons recorded in "midcollicular" decerebrate primates were "backfired" from the contralateral upper ventral cervical spinal white matter, and their excitability, i.e., spontaneous spike activity, natural stimulus, and peripheral nerve-evoked responses, were assessed following low (1–5mg/kg, *i.v.*) and higher (10–15mg/kg, *i.v.*) doses of PB. The excitability of STT-like neurons was slightly increased and decreased by the low and high doses of the barbiturate, respectively. The decerebration procedure effectively provided a drug-free unconscious state but also lowered the STT neuron excitability compared to STT neurons recorded in intact animals prepared under α-chloralose anesthesia. The lower baseline firing rate was attributed to a greater degree of tonic supraspinal inhibition in the decerebrate state, while the increased responsiveness exerted by low doses of PB was interpreted as a lifting of "tonic supraspinal inhibition." To this day, tonic supraspinal inhibition remains as an enigmatic unconfirmed property of STT neurons that has been reported repeatedly for other sensory tract neurons (e.g., SCT, postsynaptic dorsal column neurons) and unidentified nociceptive neurons following reversible cold block spinalization in acute preparations.[58]

ANESTHETIC ACTIONS ON IDENTIFIED SPINAL ASCENDING SENSORY TRACT NEURONS—CHRONIC PREPARATION

Only one study to date has reported the actions of the barbiturate anesthetic thiopental on identified spinal sensory neurons in the chronically instrumented awake cat preparation.[84] This preparation was developed[85] to examine how sensory inflow through identified ascending sensory tracts is modulated during sleep compared to wakefulness.[65] Proprioceptive and nociceptive neurons comprising the DSCT and SRT, respectively, were recorded along with cortical electroencephalogram (EEG), electro-oculogram (EOG), and neck electromyogram (EMG) activities. EEG, EOG, and EMG activities are classical physiological parameters used to distinguish sleep-wake states[65,85–86] and were particularly advantageous in this study for distinguishing the relative duration of action of an intravenous barbiturate on spinal sensory neurons, motoneurons and cortical neurons.

During quiet wakefulness, DSCT and SRT neurons in this preparation displayed robust ongoing activity together with moderate tone in the EMG and cortical EEG desynchronization. Following the intravenous injection of the rapid-acting barbiturate thiopental, "fast," desynchronized cortical EEG activity was replaced by "slow," synchronized, sleeplike "spindle" oscillations. Furthermore, EMG activity was also abolished, indicating atonia. The DSCT and SRT neuron spontaneous spike activities were concomitantly depressed (>50%), as were their spike activities driven by microiontophoretic, juxtacellular glutamate ejections or low-intensity sciatic nerve stimulation.[84]

For ethical reasons and to exert precise experimental control, "pulsatile" juxtacellular glutamate excitations of these cells was preferred over manually applied nonnoxious, noxious thermal, or mechanical stimulation of receptive fields. The finding that thiopental suppressed glutamate-evoked excitations by ~42% indicates that the recorded DSCT and SRT neurons were subject to a process of somatic hyperpolarization[87] during thiopental anesthesia.[84] The barbiturate-induced depression of cortical neuron activity recovered within 10 minutes, whereas DSCT and SRT neuron excitability gradually recovered within 15–17 minutes as the animal emerged from thiopental anesthesia. Suppression of spinal motoneuron activity, however, lasted ~10 minutes longer than sensory neuron activity.[84] This study provides information in an intact drug-free mammalian system regarding the extent of anesthetic depression of lumbar sensory (proprioceptive and nociceptive) tract neurons and motoneurons under near-natural conditions. It also partly explained how "hangover" effects of barbiturate anesthetics in humans may be due to drug actions on sensorimotor processing.[84]

ANESTHETIC ACTIONS ON NONIDENTIFIED SPINAL SENSORY NEURONS—CHRONIC PREPARATION

In earlier work conducted in awake cats by Collins and coworkers, spinal sensory neurons were characterized as being of the "low-threshold" or WDR type by their response profile to hair/skin brushing and pinch/noxious heating of the cells' peripheral receptive fields. WDR neurons were rather seldom encountered in awake cats compared to acute anesthetized preparations. Collins and Ren[88] concluded that barbiturate anesthesia (20 mg/kg, *i.v.*) reduces tonic inhibitory influences because dorsal horn units that are characterized as being "low-threshold" exhibit WDR-like characteristics following administration of barbiturates in chronic cats.

Herrero and Headley reported on the excitability of populations of characterized dorsal and ventral horn neurons recorded in awake sheep vs. halothane-anesthetized sheep.[89] They reported that the ongoing firing rate of low-threshold, WDR neurons and other neurons characterized as "high-threshold mechanoreceptive" were not markedly different whether they were recorded in awake or halothane-anesthetized (1.5–2.5%) animals. However, mean mechanical thresholds were significantly higher for only WDR neurons recorded in halothane-anesthetized sheep.[89]

Collins and coworkers also assessed certain inhalational and injectable anesthetics on "low-threshold" or wide-dynamic-range (WDR) type dorsal horn neurons in chronic awake cats.[90–92] These investigators found that halothane (1.3%) exerted a marked (~48%) depression of brush-induced responses in nearly all the low-threshold-type neurons tested. One WDR neuron responding to noxious heat was claimed to be reduced by 30%.[91] Intravenously administered ketamine (20 mg/kg) did not alter the response of low-threshold dorsal horn neurons to low-intensity sensory stimulation but did suppress noxiously evoked activity of the two WDR neurons.[90] Propofol (10mg/kg, *i.v.*) inhibited by ~64% all low-threshold neurons evoked by hair-mechanoreceptor activation.[92]

Studies reviewed above that were performed in chronic, intact drug-free animal preparations suggest that inhalational and injectable anesthetics suppress nonidentified low-threshold and WDR neurons to varying degrees. Claims have been made that halothane and pentobarbital reduce tonic supraspinal inhibition impinging on sensory neurons but, unfortunately, tonic supraspinal inhibition was never directly quantified before or after anesthetic administration.[88–89] Comparable studies assessing the actions of modern agents such as sevoflurane and desflurane have not yet been reported. It is also unfortunate that the axonal projection sites of the neurons recorded in all of the studies by Collins and coworkers and Herrero and Headley were not identified. This made it difficult to conclude if the recorded units were classical spinal interneurons intercalated in various sensorimotor reflex arcs or whether the information they encoded was predominantly transmitted upstream to higher brain centers.

To determine to what extent lumbar sensory inflow to higher brain centers is attenuated by anesthetic drugs, every effort must be made when conducting neurophysiological recording studies in chronic animals to identify the neurons as projection neurons. In addition, monitoring EMG, cortical EEG, and EOG activities can provide additional indirect insights on how anesthetics alter somatic motoneurons and cortical pyramidal cells in comparison to natural sleep states.[65,93–95] Additional studies using drug-free intact preparations are certainly needed to identify neurons accurately, with considerable attention paid to the experimental design in order to minimize stress to the animal.

ANESTHETIC ACTIONS ON IDENTIFIED SPINAL INTERNEURONS

The preceding sections deal with anesthetic action on sensory inflow by neurons whose axons are antidromically identified from thalamus or pontomedullary reticular sites, as well as unidentified neurons that were characterized by their response profile to nonnociceptive afferent inputs. An important factor to consider here is the latter studies employing classification schemes alone to characterize "sensory neurons" may have likely included a substantial number of interneurons whose axons are confined entirely to the spinal segments and are involved exclusively in sensorimotor coordination. Indeed, an enormous wealth of information exists on the organization of spinal interneurons involved in sensorimotor integration. Practically all of these studies again are derived from acute in vivo experiments in which invasive preparatory surgery under inhalational or intravenous anesthesia was administered (see reviews by Jankowska[96,97]). The primary goal of these impressive studies was to understand the neural circuitry and their role in generating coordinated excitation, mostly presynaptic and postsynaptic inhibition of their target motoneurons and their control by higher brain centers. Virtually no studies exist where individual Ia or Ib or other identified spinal interneurons such as those driven by flexor reflex afferents were examined before and after the administration of a general anesthetic agent. From the anesthesiologist's viewpoint, this would not provide much useful information given the depressant actions of most agents on most spinal cord neurons. However, such neurons do likely display state-dependent activities during the myoclonia and atonia of rapid eye movement (REM) sleep or locomotion during wakefulness. Further studies designed to investigate these issues are sorely needed.

GENERAL ANESTHETIC ACTION ON SPINAL MOTONEURONS

The earliest in vivo studies employing intracellular recording techniques on spinal motoneurons revealed that reflex depression produced by thiopental and diethyl ether was due to these agents' ability to reduce the magnitude of the monosynaptic excitatory postsynaptic potential (EPSP) without exerting any obvious effect on motoneuron membrane potential.[98] Such an action may be due to remote inhibition[99] and or presynaptic inhibition as mentioned earlier.[37–39] Only one intracellular recording study performed in awake cats has investigated the actions of halothane (5%) or PB (35 mg/kg, *i.v.*) on spinal motoneuron activity.[100] Both PB and halothane hyperpolarized motoneurons by up to 5 mV. The PB and halothane-induced hyperpolarizations were accompanied by a reduction in spontaneous excitatory synaptic activity influencing the recorded neurons. Input resistance tended to be decreased by each agent. The reduction in the unitary EPSP frequencies by these agents was thought to contribute to the hyperpolarization of motoneurons from the transition into the anesthetic state.[100]

Electrophysiological studies gradually shifted from in vivo to in vitro approaches with the introduction of the neonatal rat spinal cord preparation[101] that have further advanced to measuring the actions of whole-cell currents.[102] With these approaches, the inhalational anesthetic halothane hyperpolarized motoneurons via an increased outward K^+ conductance mechanism.[103] Further details of the anesthetic actions on motoneurons, as revealed from reduced preparations, have been presented by Kendig.[81, 104–106] More recent studies have shown that inhalational anesthetics such as isoflurane enhance K^+ currents regulated by TASK-1 and/or TASK-3 subunits. Such actions may partially account for anesthetic-activated background K^+ currents in motoneurons.[107–108] The suppression of motoneuron excitability afforded by all clinically used anesthetic agents would partially explain the myorelaxant properties of these agents. However, the susceptibility of motoneurons vs. other spinal neurons to various individual agents is quite variable.[109] While privation of senses and atonia are consequential to the unconscious state caused by most intravenous and inhalational anesthetic drugs per se, it should be remembered that analgesia and motor atonia during surgery are usually controlled with additional analgesics and neuromuscular blocking agents, respectively. Another primary concern of the anesthesiologist for the patient during general anesthesia is to maintain stable homeostatic autonomic function. The actions of anesthetics on spinal cord targets involved in autonomic function are presented below.

ANESTHETIC ACTIONS ON SPINAL PREGANGLIONIC AUTONOMIC NEURONS

The autonomic nervous system (ANS) is involved in maintaining unconscious internal homeostasis, including organ-specific control under nonstressful conditions, the "fight or flight" response, and "rest and digest" functions[110–111] (see Chapters 13 and 14 in this volume). General anesthesia produced by classic intravenous GABAmimetic agents such as propofol and barbiturates can be expected to "shut down" the ANS to affect physiological parameters, such as heart rate and blood pressure. Spinal neurons comprising the ANS constitute important targets of anesthetic drugs. Specifically, from a spinal cord perspective, the preganglionic neuron is a key target of anesthetic agents. In addition, visceral afferents, descending fibers from brainstem nuclei and/or forebrain structures, and axon collaterals of intrasegmental spinal neurons that provide input to preganglionic neurons are targeted by systemic anesthetics.[112–113] The following is a brief overview of important actions of various anesthetic drugs on the spinal neurons comprising the ANS.

SPECIFIC ANESTHETIC EFFECTS ON SYMPATHETIC PREGANGLIONIC NEURONS

The cell bodies of the sympathetic spinal preganglionic neurons (sSPN) are located in the intermediolateral column of the spinal gray matter from the first thoracic to third lumbar segments and project their axons to peripheral ganglia (refer to Figure 7.1 for details and Chapters 13 and 14 in this volume). The sSPN is a well-known site of action for anesthetic agents and specific mechanisms have been researched using various preparations.

Acute In Vivo Studies

Studies exploring the excitability of individual sSPNs in vivo under anesthetic-free conditions are virtually nonexistent. Most of what is known about the in vivo activity of these neurons is derived from studies performed in acute anesthetized animals using anesthetic agents such as α-chloralose and halothane. Often, the excitability of a population of sSPNs is indirectly assessed by integrating and recording efferent activity from sympathetic nerves. Decreases in efferent discharge have been reported in most of these studies[46,114–116] and may be due to systemic effects of test anesthetic agents such as halothane and short-acting barbiturates. In particular, barbiturates have been shown to indirectly inhibit sSPNs by reducing activity of medullary presympathetic descending neurons that impinge on sSPNs. This would lead to disfacilitation-induced depression of sSPN neuron activity.[115] A direct spinal action of barbiturates, that may involve direct sSPN inhibition, is also possible.[46]

Ketamine has been reported to increase,[117–118] decrease,[119–120] cause a biphasic effect,[121] or exert no net effect on sympathetic outflow.[116] It is unclear from in vivo studies whether ketamine acts directly on sSPNs. Ketamine's in vitro actions are discussed below.

There are also single unit recording studies that have described the input/output characteristics of identified sSPNs using α-chloralose as a preparatory anesthetic.[122–123] Unfortunately, the actions of test anesthetic agents have not been reported with single neuron recording methods for sSPNs.

In Vitro Studies

An alternative approach is the use of anesthetic-free in vitro slice or neonatal rat preparations, which allow precise control of the external and internal milieu. A major disadvantage of this approach is the obvious lack of feedback compensatory loops of afferent and/or descending origins that exist in an intact preparation. Moreover, caution should be taken in extrapolating results from neonatal rats to clinical observations due to developmental differences in the immature nervous system. Nevertheless, several studies have examined the cellular actions of various anesthetics on sSPNs in vitro and provide a foundation for understanding the overall effect of anesthetics on autonomic outflow in intact systems.

Specifically, the actions of anesthetics, and other agents used adjacently during anesthesia, such as alphaxalone, ketamine, propofol, and midazolam on sSPNs have been analyzed using in vitro techniques. Saffan, a steroid anesthetic combination containing alphaxalone and alphadolone, was found to reduce the frequency of spontaneous firing, abolish spontaneous membrane potential oscillations, and decrease the input resistance of sSPNs, observed by whole-cell patch-clamp recordings of rat spinal cord splices.[124] It was noted that responses to Saffan were blocked by the $GABA_A$ receptor antagonists bicuculline and picrotoxin and unaffected by strychnine, a glycine antagonist.[124] Thus, one potential site of action of steroid anesthetics such as Saffan on sSPNs is the $GABA_A$ receptor.[124–126]

Propofol is a widely used intravenous induction agent that is administered prior to achieving a balanced, surgical plane of anesthesia. Midazolam, a benzodiazepine, can be used as a sedative. Propofol and midazolam at high concentrations have been shown to reduce sSPN activity in the in vitro neonatal splanchnic nerve–spinal cord preparation.[127] Given that the sympathetic nervous system, on demand, increases blood pressure, propofol's inhibitory actions on sSPN activity may be partly responsible for its hypotensive effect during induction of unconsciousness and anesthesia.[127] A likely mechanism of action of propofol and midazolam on sSPN neurons involves enhancement of GABAergic inhibition through actions at the $GABA_A$ receptor.[127–129] Other lines of evidence suggest that spinal $GABA_B$ receptors and adenosine A_1 receptors may contribute to the depressant actions of propofol and midazolam on spinal sympathetic outflow.[130–131]

Ketamine is of particular interest as, when given systemically, it is thought to have "sympathomimetic" effects resulting in elevated arterial blood pressure and heart rate with an inconsistent effect on sympathetic outflow.[116–121,132–133] Ho and colleagues directly investigated whether the unusual effects of ketamine, such as blood pressure and heart rate elevation, are due solely to its actions on sSPNs by utilizing an in vitro splanchnic nerve-spinal cord preparation. Activity in the splanchnic nerve (with the exception of pelvic splanchnic nerve) reflects spike activity of individual sSPNs. In a concentration-dependent manner, ketamine reduced the splanchnic nerve activity emerging from sSPNs in the intermediolateral cell column, suggesting that the increase in blood pressure and heart rate following systemic ketamine administration is not due to the drug's actions on sSPNs but rather to extraspinal factors, including, but not limited to, baroreceptor feedback neural networks and descending modulatory influences.[132–133]

SPECIFIC ANESTHETIC EFFECTS ON PARASYMPATHETIC PREGANGLIONIC NEURONS

Neurons of the parasympathetic nervous system originate in the brainstem, as well as the sacral spinal cord segments. The latter therefore constitute additional spinal cord targets of anesthetic agents. Specifically, the cell bodies of parasympathetic spinal preganglionic neurons (pSPN) are located in the sacral gray matter and project to peripheral ganglia near end organs. Sacral pSPNs ultimately provide autonomic outflow to sexual organs, the bladder, and the rectum (see Chapters 13 and 14). The majority of the evidence investigating the effects of intravenous anesthetics, such as propofol and ketamine, and inhalational anesthetics on the sacral portion of the spinal cord is centered around nociceptive inflow[134] and motor outflow pathways.[135] Although a paucity of information exists regarding anesthetic actions on sacral pSPNs, physiological studies do show that these neurons are postsynaptically inhibited by GABAergic and glycinergic input.[136–138] Accordingly, anesthetic agents may target GABAergic and glycinergic receptors located postsynaptically, resulting in reduced sacral preganglionic parasympathetic outflow.

LOCAL SPINAL AND EPIDURAL ANESTHESIA

An analysis of spinal cord sites of action of anesthetics would not be complete without the mention of central neuraxial block, that is, spinal and epidural anesthesia. In spinal anesthesia, also known as subarachnoid block, the local anesthetic is injected into the subarachnoid or intrathecal space in the lumbar region below the termination of the spinal cord. Robust sensory and motor blockade results. Anesthetics used in short-duration spinal anesthesia include lidocaine, mepivacaine, and procaine, while long-duration spinal anesthesia is effectively achieved with bupivacaine, tetracaine, and ropivacaine.[139] Epidural anesthesia involves the injection of local anesthetic into the space outside of the dura mater, but within the vertebral canal. Although it has a slower onset, epidural anesthesia allows for greater control over the intensity of sensory and motor block and is associated with a lower incidence of systemic hypotension compared to spinal anesthesia.[139] The aforementioned local anesthetics, lidocaine, bupivacaine, ropivacaine, as well as chloroprocaine and levobupivacaine, are commonly used in epidural anesthesia.[139]

The primary action of local anesthetic agents is to block the production and axonal propagation of action potentials in all spinal neurons and their axons.[140–142] The transient increase in Na^+ permeability due to initial membrane depolarization is blocked from the inner surface of the neuronal membrane by anesthetics directly interacting with voltage-gated Na^+ channels.[140–141,143] Conduction blockade may depend on the type of neuron involved and its previous "history."[142–143] For example, autonomic and small-diameter (un)myelinated fibers are blocked before large-diameter myelinated fibers, explaining why sympathetic nervous system innervation and nociception are interrupted first during local anesthesia.[144–145] Furthermore, local anesthetics cause a greater degree of neuronal blockade in spinal neurons that are frequently stimulated as neuronal stimulation allows the anesthetic to access its site of action inside the Na^+ channel.[142–143] The extent to which spinal elements are targeted by a local anesthetic depends partly on the technique (i.e., intrathecal versus epidural) and the anesthetic agent used.

SUPRASPINAL NEURAL NETWORKS INTERACTING WITH SPINAL NEURONS AS ANESTHETIC SITES OF ACTION

As surveyed in the preceding portions of this chapter, inhalational and injectable agents exert diverse actions on spinal cord targets. Systemically administered anesthetic agents act at a multitude of supraspinal sites; possibly, their combined actions at spinal and supraspinal sites will ultimately culminate in the state of general anesthesia. In recent years, the notion emerged that neural networks that control sleep-wake cycles may also mediate key characteristics of general anesthesia. Few studies have addressed this issue utilizing focal microinjections of general anesthetics to identify brain areas involved in induction of unconsciousness, antinociception, and motor atonia.[146–149]

In the pioneering study by Devor and Zalkind,[146] the authors injected nanoliter volumes of PB, into the brainstem of conscious rats and assessed the drug's ability to evoke key characteristics of the anesthetic state. When PB was microinjected into the mesopontine tegmentum located near the periaqueductal gray nucleus and the pedunculopontine tegmentum, reversible marked anesthesia occurred. Cortical suppression, as reflected by shift to slow EEG bandwidths (1 4 Hz), occurred along with behavioral attributes, notably antinociception and immobility. Devor and Zalkind[146] designated this specific brain site as the mesopontine tegmentum anesthesia area (MPTA). The aforementioned changes also occurred following *systemic* administration of PB in awake animals, supporting the idea that pentobarbital-induced anesthesia is at least partly due to a "barbiturate-sensitive switch" in the MPTA that controls cortical and spinal activity.[146]

Not surprisingly, not all anesthetics exert the same "state" when microinjected into the MPTA as described by Devor and Zalkind.[146] For example, propofol evoked antinociceptive effects, while thiopentone, a fast-acting barbiturate, affected both nociception and posture and resulted in a behavioral state resembling moderate to deep anesthesia.[149] Cortical excitability was not affected by the focal microinjection of either anesthetic. Possible explanations for the differing effects of propofol and thiopentone include, but are not limited to, structural dissimilarities of the drugs and interactions with different $GABA_A$ receptor isoforms. Since anesthesia did not occur after microinjection of propofol into the MPTA[149] it is likely that propofol, when given systemically, induces anesthesia by its actions at other CNS sites. However, the MPTA may play a key role in antinociception. The above studies do not provide mechanistic details on how this may occur.[146,149]

The antinociception, reported by Devor and Zalkind[146] as "analgesia," was based on standard rodent behavioral tests and may be consequential to a number of network processes, including a brain stem–mediated reduction of spinal sensory inflow via classical ascending spinal sensory pathways and/or spinal motor outflow. Antinociception scores in the studies of Devor and Zalkind[146] may also be the consequence of atonia alone. We recently addressed this issue by examining the excitability of identified STT neurons in the acute, isoflurane-anesthetized rat before and after the microinjection of PB into the MPTA (Figure 7.3).[150]

Excitability was assessed by quantifying the spontaneous spike activity, magnitude of peripheral nerve-evoked responses, and the antidromic firing index (FI) of STT

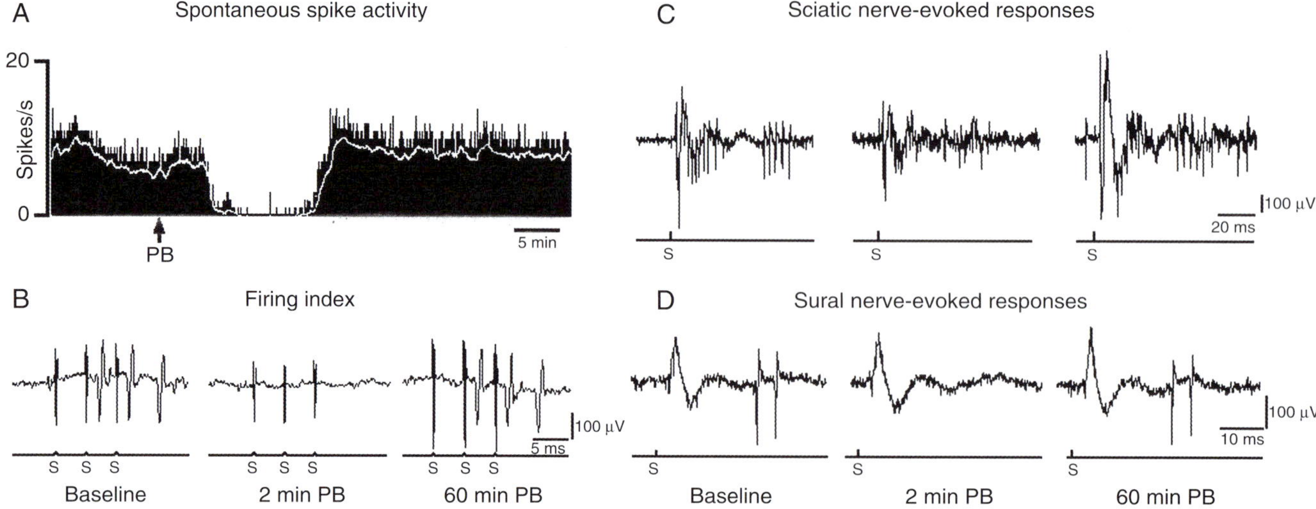

Figure 7.3 *Microinjections of PB into rat mesopontine tegmentum suppress activity of spinothalamic tract (STT) neurons.* The above figure depicts spontaneous spike activity (A, spikes/s), antidromic firing index (B), sciatic (C), and sural (D) nerve-evoked responses of an identified lumbar STT neuron before and after microinjections of PB into the rat mesopontine tegmentum. PB microinjections rapidly abolished the spike activity of this particular STT neuron (A) followed by return of the spike activity to baseline within 30 min of microinjections. PB also suppressed firing index (B), sciatic (C) and sural (D) nerve-evoked responses of the STT neuron within 2 min followed by recovery within 60 min. For further details, see Namjoshi et al.[150]

neurons (Figure 7.3). The FI is a particularly sensitive index that has been used to infer changes in somatic conductance.[54] PB, but not vehicle microinjections into the MPTA, exerted profound depressant actions on each of these parameters over the same time course as the behavioral nociception reported by Devor and Zalkind.[146] These findings indicate that the antinociception following PB microinjections into the MPTA are due, in part, to a reduction in sensory inflow via "second-order" STT neurons.[150] The immediate reduction in antidromic responsiveness, i.e., FI, of STT neurons following MPTA microinjections of PB suggests that a supraspinal neural network was engaged to suppress STT neurons directly, even during the presence of background isoflurane anesthesia.[150]

More recent analyses of cortical EEG activity were conducted in the same experiments where STT neuron excitability was assessed during background isoflurane anesthesia.[151] Total power values within classical delta, theta, alpha, and beta bandwidths were quantified using "fast Fourier transformation" during the same time epochs that STT neuron activities were assessed. None of the EEG bandwidths changed significantly in terms of total power following PB microinjections vs. the premicroinjection.[151] These findings indicate that PB depresses sensory inflow via the STT but not cortical EEG activity. Whether background isoflurane anesthesia used to record STT neurons masks PB-induced cortical suppression and/or uncouples the network(s) driving cortical suppression observed in conscious animals is not clear and warrants future studies using a chronic preparation to differentiate definitively between these possibilities.[146–149,151]

Anatomical studies conducted by Devor's group have confirmed that the axons of MPTA neurons project to and arborize in spinal dorsal and ventral gray matter where STT neurons and motoneurons are located, respectively.[152–154] That CNS depressant agents such as PB or muscimol can promote anesthesia begs the question: what functional purpose does the MPTA serve with respect to nociceptive modulation, per se, during the awake state? One intriguing possibility from the findings of Devor and Zalkind[146] and Namjoshi et al[150] is that MPTA neurons may, under normal circumstances, facilitate sensory inflow tonically through the STT during wakefulness; a concept that directly opposes the classical notion that STT neurons are subjected to tonic descending inhibition[83] akin to that originally discovered by Wall.[155] Indeed, other investigators have claimed that tonic supraspinal inhibition is depressed by barbiturates and halothane.[88–89]

The action of anesthetic agents on tonic supraspinal modulation of STT neurons is critical here in that few experimental studies have actually determined how tonic supraspinal controls affect inflow through identified ascending sensory pathways, in particular, the STT.[83,156] Additionally, little is known about whether different anesthetics exert distinct actions on neural networks mediating tonic supraspinal controls.[149] We have discovered that extracellularly recorded STT neurons are subject to tonic supraspinal *facilitation* under isoflurane anesthesia (Figure 7.4).[157]

Interestingly, when isoflurane is slowly withdrawn and carefully replaced by the *i.v.* administration of PB, tonic supraspinal facilitation influencing the same recorded STT neuron converts to tonic descending *inhibition* (Figure 7.4).

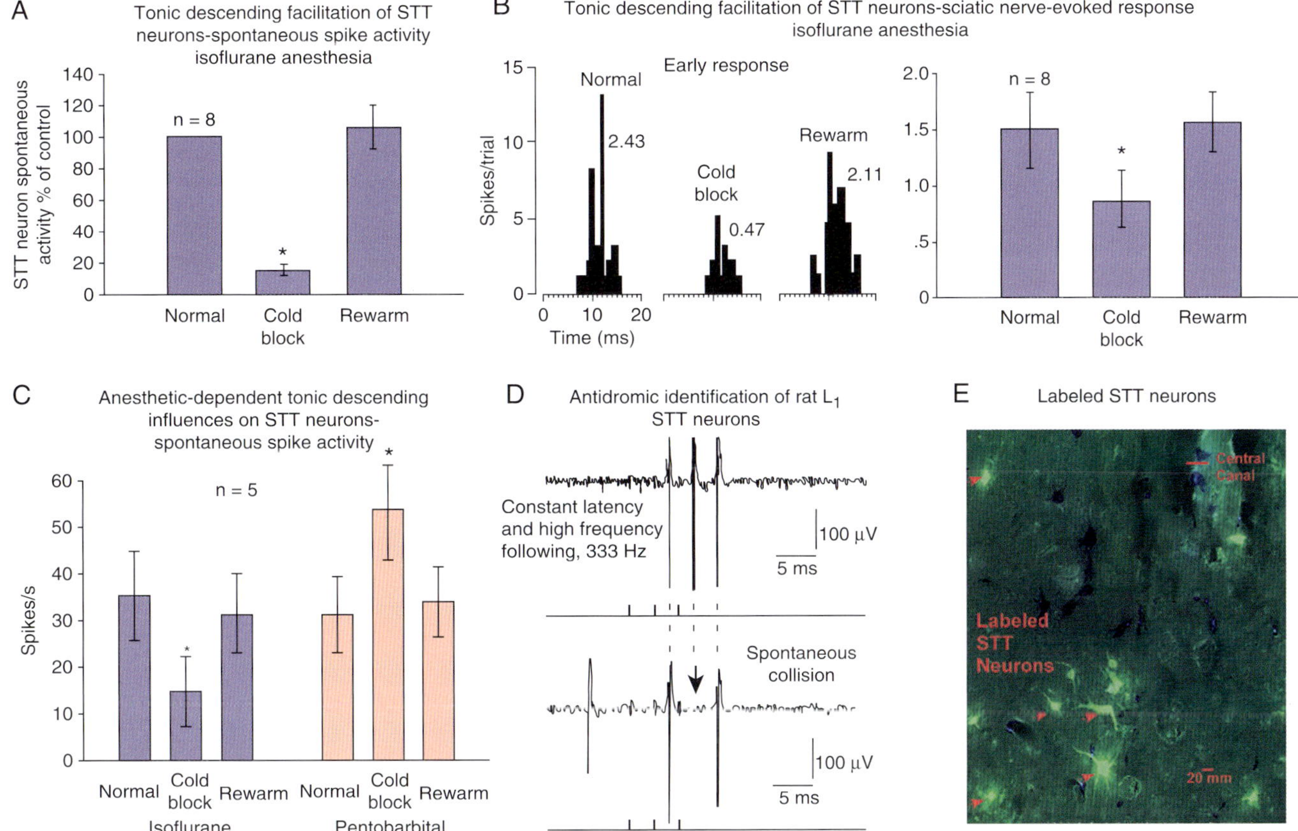

Figure 7.4 Tonic facilitation of L1 STT neuron activity in the isoflurane (ISO)-anesthetized (1.7%) rat revealed by reversible T_9 cold block spinalization (CB). **(A)** Relative change in spontaneous firing rate, (n = 8), tonic facilitation-normal vs. cold block state of the spinal cord. **(B)** Histogram responses of STT neurons (n = 8) to 100 consecutive sciatic nerve stimuli (0.2 ms, 100µA, 1.0 Hz) before, during, and after CB. **(C)** Conversion of tonic facilitation under ISO to tonic inhibition (orange bars) following ISO withdrawal and replacement with PB (PB, Induction: 3.0 mg/kg/min, maintenance: 0.003 mg/kg/min) anesthesia *in the same STT neurons* (n = 5, *, $p < 0.05$, ANOVA, repeated measures, Tukey test). **(D)** Antidromic spikes failed during CB. **(E)** Labeled STT neurons (see orange arrowheads) following HRP injections into the contralateral "VPL" nucleus. The data suggest that the nature of tonic descending controls influencing STT neurons in conventional "acute" anesthetized animal preparations may depend on the type of anesthetic used. A determination of which anesthetic's (i.e., ISO or PB) "spinal" action is greater is confounded by the inherent lack of control, drug-free responses.[156–157] This is a critical problem that is endemic to this type of experimental design.

Hence, different anesthetics may be expected to exert markedly different actions on supraspinal networks involved in the descending control of spinal cord sensory activity. This issue is further confounded by the difficulty in determining isoflurane vs. PB's actions (Figure 7.4C) on the same STT neurons in the absence of supraspinal influences, i.e., during the "spinal" cold block state *without* corresponding drug-free control data for comparison. Our findings presented above warrant concern for the notion that tonic supraspinal *inhibition*, per se, is indeed a fundamental property of spinal cord sensory neurons when recorded in vivo especially when many published studies in the literature utilized intravenous agents that are never used in human anesthesia (e.g., α-chloralose, urethane, etc.).[156–157] Hence, future electrophysiological studies addressing anesthetic actions on tonic supraspinal modulatory control of spinal sensory tract neurons will be faced with the conundrum of proper experimental design that provides a sound drug-free control of the phenomenon under study. These areas are clearly understudied and the findings above serve as a compelling provenance for future work.

SUMMARY

This chapter summarizes our current understanding regarding spinal cord targets of anesthetic agents. From an anesthesiologist's viewpoint, most current intravenous $GABA_A$ mimetic agents, i.e., propofol and thiopental, depress the CNS. The spinal cord is markedly depressed by these drugs and this depression will result in useful properties associated with the state of general anesthesia, namely myorelaxation, a reduced sensory inflow to higher brain centers, and reduced autonomic outflow. An enormous wealth of knowledge has been obtained from in vivo studies over the past 50 years regarding the anatomical and physiological aspects of spinal sensorimotor integration. However, most of the information was derived, by necessity, using anesthesia to actually perform such experiments. Where do we go from here? What does the future hold for anesthesia research and associated spinal cord targets? The avenues are many, but one tempting direction is to focus on in vitro preparations of extrasynaptic $GABA_A$ receptors that mediate sustained tonic inhibition, which may turn out to be useful targets for the action of a number of anesthetics, and hypnotics.[158–161]

Another approach is to exploit how the spinal cord is dampened down under natural conditions, such as that which occurs during naturally occurring REM sleep, where diminished sensory inflow and atonia are hallmark features.[94,162–164] Here, glycine is the principal neurotransmitter that contributes mainly to postsynaptic inhibition of sensory tract neurons and motoneurons leading to reduced sensory inflow and atonia. Future research in anesthesia might also include drug development programs aimed at glycine-based drugs that would effectively inhibit (non) nociceptive sensory inflow and/or motor outflow.[165–166] Such agents may be designed to selectively activate extrasynaptic receptors causing a tonic leak conductance that effectively shunts spike genesis. Drugs similar in chemical structure to glycine and GABA, e.g., isovaline, which agonize $GABA_B$ receptors may also be designed and found effective for targeting spinal nociceptive tract neurons exclusively.[167–168] Such future agents may allow the anesthesiologist additional means to provide their patients effective and selective analgesia, or myorelaxation.

ACKNOWLEDGMENTS

The author's (PJS) work was supported by National Institutes of Health Grants GM58277, NS32306, NS34716, NS41921, and the Canadian Institutes of Health Research (CIHR MOP 89909). We thank Dr. Niwat Taepavarapruk for outstanding artwork.

REFERENCES

1. Campagna JA, Miller KW, Forman SA. Mechanisms of actions of inhaled anesthetics. *N Engl J Med.* May 22 2003;348(21):2110–2124.
2. Orser BA. Lifting the fog around anesthesia. *Sci Am.* Jun 2007; 296(6):54–61.
3. Urban BW. Current assessment of targets and theories of anaesthesia. *Br J Anaesth.* Jul 2002;89(1):167–183.
4. Collins JG, Kendig JJ, Mason P. Anesthetic actions within the spinal cord: contributions to the state of general anesthesia. *Trends Neurosci.* Dec 1995;18(12):549–553.
5. Dinges DF, Pack F, Williams K, et al. Cumulative sleepiness, mood disturbance, and psychomotor vigilance performance decrements during a week of sleep restricted to 4–5 hours per night. *Sleep.* Apr 1997;20(4):267–277.
6. Hodge CJ, Jr., Apkarian AV. The spinothalamic tract. *Crit Rev Neurobiol.* 1990;5(4):363–397.
7. Soja PJ, Pang W, Taepavarapruk N, McErlane SA. Spontaneous spike activity of spinoreticular tract neurons during sleep and wakefulness. *Sleep.* Feb 1 2001;24(1):18–25.
8. Bosco G, Poppele RE. Proprioception from a spinocerebellar perspective. *Physiol Rev.* Apr 2001;81(2):539–568.
9. Walmsley B. Central synaptic transmission: studies at the connection between primary afferent fibres and dorsal spinocerebellar tract (DSCT) neurones in Clarke's column of the spinal cord. *Prog Neurobiol.* 1991;36(5):391–423.
10. Johansson H, Silfvenius H. Axon-collateral activation by dorsal spinocerebellar tract fibres of group I relay cells of nucleus Z in the cat medulla oblongata. *J Physiol.* Feb 1977;265(2):341–369.
11. Millan MJ. Descending control of pain. *Prog Neurobiol.* Apr 2002;66(6):355–474.
12. Campbell JN, Raja SN, Meyer RA. Halothane sensitizes cutaneous nociceptors in monkeys. *J Neurophysiol.* Oct 1984;52(4):762–770.
13. MacIver MB, Tanelian DL. Volatile anesthetics excite mammalian nociceptor afferents recorded in vitro. *Anesthesiology.* Jun 1990; 72(6):1022–1030.
14. MacIver MB, Roth SH. Anesthetics produce differential actions on membrane responses of the crayfish stretch receptor neuron. *Eur J Pharmacol.* Sep 2 1987;141(1):67–77.
15. MacIver MB, Roth SH. Anesthetics produce differential actions on the discharge activity of a single neuron. *Eur J Pharmacol.* Jul 2 1987;139(1):43–52.
16. Butterworth JFt, Raymond SA, Roscoe RF. Effects of halothane and enflurane on firing threshold of frog myelinated axons. *J Physiol.* Apr 1989;411:493–516.
17. Carlton SM. Peripheral NMDA receptors revisited—hope floats. *Pain.* Nov 2009;146(1–2):1–2.
18. Carlton SM, Coggeshall RE. Inflammation-induced changes in peripheral glutamate receptor populations. *Brain Res.* Feb 27 1999; 820(1–2):63–70.
19. Barron DH, Matthews BH. The interpretation of potential changes in the spinal cord. *J Physiol.* Apr 14 1938;92(3):276–321.
20. Richens A. The action of general anaesthetic agents on root responses of the frog isolated spinal cord. *Br J Pharmacol.* Jun 1969;36(2):294–311.
21. Levy RA. The role of GABA in primary afferent depolarization. *Prog Neurobiol.* 1977;9(4):211–267.
22. Lloyd DP. Electrotonus in dorsal nerve roots. *Cold Spring Harb Symp Quant Biol.* 1952;17:203–219.
23. Eccles JC, Schmidt R, Willis WD. Pharmacological studies on presynaptic inhibition. *J Physiol.* Oct 1963;168:500–530.
24. Schmidt RF, Vogel ME, Zimmermann M. [Effect of diazepam on presynaptic inhibition and other spinal reflexes]. *Naunyn Schmiedebergs Arch Exp Pathol Pharmakol.* 1967;258(1):69–82.
25. Leah JD, Malik R, Curtis DR. Actions of midazolam in the spinal cord of the cat. *Neuropharmacology.* Dec 1983;22(12A): 1349–1356.
26. Shimizu M, Yamakura T, Tobita T, et al. Propofol enhances GABA(A) receptor-mediated presynaptic inhibition in human spinal cord. *Neuroreport.* Mar 4 2002;13(3):357–360.
27. Baars JH, von Dincklage F, Reiche J, Rehberg B. Propofol increases presynaptic inhibition of ia afferents in the intact human spinal cord. *Anesthesiology.* Apr 2006;104(4):798–804.
28. Baars JH, Benzke M, von Dincklage F, Reiche J, Schlattmann P, Rehberg B. Presynaptic and postsynaptic effects of the anesthetics sevoflurane and nitrous oxide in the human spinal cord. *Anesthesiology.* Oct 2007;107(4):553–562.
29. Loyning Y, Oshima T, Yokota T. Site of action of thiamylal sodium on the monosynaptic spinal reflex pathway in cats. *J Neurophysiol.* May 1964;27:408–428.
30. Somjen G. Effects of anesthetics on spinal cord of mammals. *Anesthesiology.* Jan-Feb 1967;28(1):135–143.
31. Blaustein MP. Barbiturates block calcium uptake by stimulated and potassium-depolarized rat sympathetic ganglia. *J Pharmacol Exp Ther.* Jan 1976;196(1):80–86.
32. Haycock JW, Levy WB, Cotman CW. Pentobarbital depression of stimulus-secretion coupling in brain—selective inhibition of depolarization-induced calcium-dependent release. *Biochem Pharmacol.* Jan 15 1977;26(2):159–161.

33. Selzer M, Spencer WA. Interactions between visceral and cutaneous afferents in the spinal cord: reciprocal primary afferent fiber depolarization. *Brain Res.* Jul 1969;14(2):349–366.
34. Lomeli J, Quevedo J, Linares P, Rudomin P. Local control of information flow in segmental and ascending collaterals of single afferents. *Nature.* Oct 8 1998;395(6702):600–604.
35. Eguibar JR, Quevedo J, Jimenez I, Rudomin P. Selective cortical control of information flow through different intraspinal collaterals of the same muscle afferent fiber. *Brain Res.* Apr 18 1994;643(1–2): 328–333.
36. Eguibar JR, Quevedo J, Rudomin P. Selective cortical and segmen-tal control of primary afferent depolarization of single muscle afferents in the cat spinal cord. *Exp Brain Res.* Mar 1997;113(3):411–430.
37. Rudomin P. Selectivity of presynaptic inhibition: a mechanism for independent control of information flow through individual collaterals of single muscle spindle afferents. *Prog Brain Res.* 1999;123: 109–117.
38. Rudomin P. Presynaptic selection of afferent inflow in the spinal cord. *J Physiol Paris.* Sep-Oct 1999;93(4):329–347.
39. Rudomin P. Selectivity of the central control of sensory information in the mammalian spinal cord. *Adv Exp Med Biol.* 2002;508:157–170.
40. Savola MK, Woodley SJ, Kendig JJ. Isoflurane depresses both glutamate- and peptide-mediated slow synaptic transmission in neonatal rat spinal cord. *Ann N Y Acad Sci.* 1991;625:281–282.
41. Savola MK, Woodley SJ, Maze M, Kendig JJ. Isoflurane and an alpha 2-adrenoceptor agonist suppress nociceptive neurotransmission in neonatal rat spinal cord. *Anesthesiology.* Sep 1991;75(3):489–498.
42. Yanagisawa M, Otsuka M, Konishi S, Akagi H, Folkers K, Rosell S. A substance P antagonist inhibits a slow reflex response in the spinal cord of the newborn rat. *Acta Physiol Scand.* Sep 1982;116(1): 109–112.
43. Yanagisawa M, Murakoshi T, Tamai S, Otsuka M. Tail-pinch method in vitro and the effects of some antinociceptive compounds. *Eur J Pharmacol.* Nov 13 1984;106(2):231–239.
44. Akagi H, Konishi S, Otsuka M, Yanagisawa M. The role of substance P as a neurotransmitter in the reflexes of slow time courses in the neonatal rat spinal cord. *Br J Pharmacol.* Mar 1985;84(3):663–673.
45. Haseneder R, Kurz J, Dodt HU, et al. Isoflurane reduces glutamatergic transmission in neurons in the spinal cord superficial dorsal horn: evidence for a presynaptic site of an analgesic action. *Anesth Analg.* Jun 2004;98(6):1718–1723, table of contents.
46. Millar RA, Warden JC, Cooperman LH, Price HL. Further studies of sympathetic actions of anaesthetics in intact and spinal animals. *Br J Anaesth.* May 1970;42(5):366–378.
47. Herrero JF, Laird JM, Lopez-Garcia JA. Wind-up of spinal cord neurones and pain sensation: much ado about something? *Prog Neurobiol.* Jun 2000;61(2):169–203.
48. Liu XG, Sandkuhler J. Long-term potentiation of C-fiber-evoked potentials in the rat spinal dorsal horn is prevented by spinal N-methyl-D-aspartic acid receptor blockage. *Neurosci Lett.* May 19 1995;191(1–2):43–46.
49. Svendsen F, Tjolsen A, Hole K. AMPA and NMDA receptor-dependent spinal LTP after nociceptive tetanic stimulation. *Neuroreport.* Apr 20 1998;9(6):1185–1190.
50. Willis WD. Role of neurotransmitters in sensitization of pain responses. *Ann N Y Acad Sci.* Mar 2001;933:142–156.
51. Liu H, Wang H, Sheng M, Jan LY, Jan YN, Basbaum AI. Evidence for presynaptic N-methyl-D-aspartate autoreceptors in the spinal cord dorsal horn. *Proc Natl Acad Sci U S A.* Aug 30 1994;91(18): 8383–8387.
52. Curtis DR, Headley PM, Lodge D. Depolarization of feline primary afferent fibres by acidic amino acids. *J Physiol.* Jun 1984;351: 461–472.
53. Brown AG. *Organization in the Spinal Cord: The Anatomy and Physiology of Identified Neurones.* Berlin; New York: Springer-Verlag; 1981.
54. Lipski J. Antidromic activation of neurones as an analytic tool in the study of the central nervous system. *J Neurosci Methods.* Jun 1981; 4(1):1–32.
55. Willis WD. *The Pain System: The Neural Basis of Nociceptive Transmission in the Mammalian Nervous System.* Basel; New York: Karger; 1985.
56. Willis WD, Coggeshall RE. *Sensory Mechanisms of the Spinal Cord.* 2nd ed. New York: Plenum Press; 1991.
57. Brown AG, Rose PK, Snow PJ. The morphology of spinocervical tract neurones revealed by intracellular injection of horseradish peroxidase. *J Physiol.* Sep 1977;270(3):747–764.
58. Wall PD. The laminar organization of dorsal horn and effects of descending impulses. *J Physiol.* Feb 1967;188(3):403–423.
59. Kolmodin GM, Skoglund CR. Analysis of spinal interneurons activated by tactile and nociceptive stimulation. *Acta Physiol Scand.* Dec 30 1960;50:337–355.
60. Tapper DN, Brown PB, Moraff H. Functional organization of the cat's dorsal horn: connectivity of myelinated fiber systems of hairy skin. *J Neurophysiol.* Sep 1973;36(5):817–826.
61. Gregor M, Zimmermann M. Characteristics of spinal neurones responding to cutaneous myelinated and unmyelinated fibres. *J Physiol.* Mar 1972;221(3):555–576.
62. Menetrey D, Giesler GJ Jr., Besson JM. An analysis of response properties of spinal cord dorsal horn neurones to nonnoxious and noxious stimuli in the spinal rat. *Exp Brain Res.* Jan 18 1977;27(1): 15–33.
63. Cervero F, Iggo A. Reciprocal sensory interaction in the spinal cord [proceedings]. *J Physiol.* Nov 1978;284:84P–85P.
64. Li HS, Monhemius R, Simpson BA, Roberts MH. Supraspinal inhibition of nociceptive dorsal horn neurones in the anaesthetized rat: tonic or dynamic? *J Physiol.* Jan 15 1998;506(Pt 2):459–469.
65. Soja P. Modulation of prethalamic sensory inflow during sleep versus wakefulness. In: *Sleep and Pain*: International Association for the Study of Pain (IASP) book series; 2007:45–76.
66. Barter LS, Mark LO, Jinks SL, Carstens EE, Antognini JF. Immobilizing doses of halothane, isoflurane or propofol, do not preferentially depress noxious heat-evoked responses of rat lumbar dorsal horn neurons with ascending projections. *Anesth Analg.* Mar 2008;106(3):985–990, table of contents.
67. Cuellar JM, Dutton RC, Antognini JF, Carstens E. Differential effects of halothane and isoflurane on lumbar dorsal horn neuronal windup and excitability. *Br J Anaesth.* May 2005;94(5):617–625.
68. De Jong RH, Robles R, Heavner JE. Suppression of impulse transmission in the cat's dorsal horn by inhalation anesthetics. *Anesthesiology.* May 1970;32(5):440–445.
69. De Jong RH, Robles R, Morikawa KI. Actions of halothane and nitrous oxide on dorsal horn neurons ("The Spinal Gate"). *Anesthesiology.* Sep 1969;31(3):205–212.
70. De Jong RH, Wagman IH. Block of afferent impulses in the dorsal horn of monkey: a possible mechanism of anesthesia. *Exp Neurol.* Mar 1968;20(3):352–358.
71. Jinks S, Antognini JF, Carstens E, Buzin V, Simons C. Isoflurane can indirectly depress lumbar dorsal horn activity in the goat via action within the brain. *Br J Anaesth.* Feb 1999;82(2):244–249.
72. Kim J, Yao A, Atherley R, Carstens E, Jinks SL, Antognini JF. Neurons in the ventral spinal cord are more depressed by isoflurane, halothane, and propofol than are neurons in the dorsal spinal cord. *Anesth Analg.* Oct 2007;105(4):1020–1026, table of contents.
73. Antognini JF, Atherley RJ, Dutton RC, Laster MJ, Eger EI 2nd, Carstens E. The excitatory and inhibitory effects of nitrous oxide on spinal neuronal responses to noxious stimulation. *Anesth Analg.* Apr 2007;104(4):829–835.
74. Antognini JF, Atherley RJ, Laster MJ, Carstens E, Dutton RC, Eger EI 2nd. A method for recording single unit activity in lumbar spinal cord in rats anesthetized with nitrous oxide in a hyperbaric chamber. *J Neurosci Methods.* Mar 15 2007;160(2):215–222.
75. Antognini JF, Chen XG, Sudo M, Sudo S, Carstens E. Variable effects of nitrous oxide at multiple levels of the central nervous system in goats. *Vet Res Commun.* Oct 2001;25(7):523–538.
76. Kitahata LM, Ghazi-Saidi K, Yamashita M, Kosaka Y, Bonikos C, Taub A. The depressant effect of halothane and sodium thiopental

on the spontaneous and evoked activity of dorsal horn cells: lamina specificity, time course and dose dependence. *J Pharmacol Exp Ther.* Dec 1975;195(3):515–521.

77. Taub HA, Eisenberg L. A comparison of memory under three methods of anaesthesia with nitrous oxide and curare. *Can Anaesth Soc J.* May 1975;22(3):298–306.
78. Sudo M, Sudo S, Chen XG, Piercy M, Carstens E, Antognini JF. Thiopental directly depresses lumbar dorsal horn neuronal responses to noxious mechanical stimulation in goats. *Acta Anaesthesiol Scand.* Aug 2001;45(7):823–829.
79. Antognini JF, Wang XW, Piercy M, Carstens E. Propofol directly depresses lumbar dorsal horn neuronal responses to noxious stimulation in goats. *Can J Anaesth.* Mar 2000;47(3):273–279.
80. Ng KP, Antognini JF. Isoflurane and propofol have similar effects on spinal neuronal windup at concentrations that block movement. *Anesth Analg.* Dec 2006;103(6):1453–1458.
81. Sonner JM, Antognini JF, Dutton RC, et al. Inhaled anesthetics and immobility: mechanisms, mysteries, and minimum alveolar anesthetic concentration. *Anesth Analg.* Sep 2003;97(3):718–740.
82. Antognini JF, Carstens E. Anesthesia, the spinal cord and motor responses to noxious stimulation. In: Antognini JF, Carstens E, eds. *Neural Mechanisms of Anesthesia*. Totowa: Humana Press; 2003: 183–204.
83. Hori Y, Lee KH, Chung JM, Endo K, Willis WD. The effects of small doses of barbiturate on the activity of primate nociceptive tract cells. *Brain Res.* Jul 30 1984;307(1–2):9–15.
84. Soja PJ, Taepavarapruk N, Pang W, Cairns BE, McErlane SA, Fragoso MC. Transmission through the dorsal spinocerebellar and spinoreticular tracts: wakefulness versus thiopental anesthesia. *Anesthesiology.* Nov 2002;97(5):1178–1188.
85. Soja PJ, Fragoso MC, Cairns BE, Oka JI. Dorsal spinocerebellar tract neuronal activity in the intact chronic cat. *J Neurosci Methods.* Aug 1995;60(1–2):227–239.
86. Soja PJ, Fragoso MC, Cairns BE, Jia WG. Dorsal spinocerebellar tract neurons in the chronic intact cat during wakefulness and sleep: analysis of spontaneous spike activity. *J Neurosci.* Feb 1 1996; 16(3):1260–1272.
87. Soja PJ, Pang W, Taepavarapruk N, Cairns BE, McErlane SA. On the reduction of spontaneous and glutamate-driven spinocerebellar and spinoreticular tract neuronal activity during active sleep. *Neuroscience.* 2001;104(1):199–206.
88. Collins JG, Ren K. WDR response profiles of spinal dorsal horn neurons may be unmasked by barbiturate anesthesia. *Pain.* Mar 1987;28(3):369–378.
89. Herrero JF, Headley PM. Cutaneous responsiveness of lumbar spinal neurons in awake and halothane-anesthetized sheep. *J Neurophysiol.* Oct 1995;74(4):1549–1562.
90. Collins JG. Effects of ketamine on low intensity tactile sensory input are not dependent upon a spinal site of action. *Anesth Analg.* Nov 1986;65(11):1123–1129.
91. Ota K, Yanagidani T, Kishikawa K, Yamamori Y, Collins JG. Cutaneous responsiveness of lumbar spinal dorsal horn neurons is reduced by general anesthesia, an effect dependent in part on GABAA mechanisms. *J Neurophysiol.* Sep 1998;80(3):1383–1390.
92. Uchida H, Kishikawa K, Collins JG. Effect of propofol on spinal dorsal horn neurons. Comparison with lack of ketamine effects. *Anesthesiology.* Dec 1995;83(6):1312–1322.
93. Chase MH. Confirmation of the consensus that glycinergic postsynaptic inhibition is responsible for the atonia of REM sleep. *Sleep.* Nov 1 2008;31(11):1487–1491.
94. Chase MH, Morales FR. The atonia and myoclonia of active (REM) sleep. *Annu Rev Psychol.* 1990;41:557–584.
95. Xi MC, Morales FR, Chase MH. Interactions between GABAergic and cholinergic processes in the nucleus pontis oralis: neuronal mechanisms controlling active (rapid eye movement) sleep and wakefulness. *J Neurosci.* Nov 24 2004;24(47):10670–10678.
96. Jankowska E. Spinal interneuronal networks in the cat: elementary components. *Brain Res Rev.* Jan 2008;57(1):46–55.
97. Jankowska E, Hammar I. Spinal interneurones; how can studies in animals contribute to the understanding of spinal interneuronal systems in man? *Brain Res Rev.* Oct 2002;40(1–3):19–28.
98. Somjen GG, Gill M. The mechanism of the blockade of synaptic transmission in the mammalian spinal cord by diethyl ether and by thiopental. *J Pharmacol Exp Ther.* Apr 1963;140:19–30.
99. Frank K, Fuortes MGF. Presynaptic and postsynaptic inhibition of monosynaptic reflexes. *Federation Proceedings.* 1957;16:39–40.
100. Whitney JF, Glenn LL. Pentobarbital and halothane hyperpolarize cat alpha-motoneurons. *Brain Res.* Aug 27 1986;381(1):199–203.
101. Otsuka M, Konishi S. Electrophysiology of mammalian spinal cord in vitro. *Nature.* Dec 20 1974;252(5485):733–734.
102. Takahashi T. Membrane currents in visually identified motoneurones of neonatal rat spinal cord. *J Physiol.* Apr 1990;423:27–46.
103. Takenoshita M, Takahashi T. Mechanisms of halothane action on synaptic transmission in motoneurons of the newborn rat spinal cord in vitro. *Brain Res.* Feb 3 1987;402(2):303–310.
104. Cheng G, Kendig JJ. Enflurane decreases glutamate neurotransmission to spinal cord motor neurons by both pre- and postsynaptic actions. *Anesth Analg.* May 2003;96(5):1354–1359, table of contents.
105. Eger EI 2nd, Zhang Y, Laster M, Flood P, Kendig JJ, Sonner JM. Acetylcholine receptors do not mediate the immobilization produced by inhaled anesthetics. *Anesth Analg.* Jun 2002;94(6): 1500–1504, table of contents.
106. Kendig JJ. Spinal Cord. In: Antognini JF, Carstens E, Raines DE, eds. *Neural Mechanisms of Anesthesia*. Totowa: Humana Press; 2003:215–230.
107. Lazarenko RM, Willcox SC, Shu S, et al. Motoneuronal TASK channels contribute to immobilizing effects of inhalational general anesthetics. *J Neurosci.* Jun 2 2010;30(22):7691–7704.
108. Sirois JE, Lei Q, Talley EM, Lynch C 3rd, Bayliss DA. The TASK-1 two-pore domain K^+ channel is a molecular substrate for neuronal effects of inhalation anesthetics. *J Neurosci.* Sep 1 2000;20(17): 6347–6354.
109. Barter LS, Mark LO, Antognini JF. Proprioceptive function is more sensitive than motor function to desflurane anesthesia. *Anesth Analg.* Mar 2009;108(3):867–872.
110. Richerson G. The autonomic nervous system. In: Boron W, Boulpaep E, eds. *Medical Physiology: A Cellular and Molecular Approach*. Updated ed. Philadelphia: Elsevier Saunders; 2005: 378–398.
111. Moss J, Glick D. The autonomic nervous system. In: Miller R, ed. *Miller's Anesthesia*. Philadelphia: Churchill-Livingstone, Inc.; 2005:617–677.
112. Andreson M, Kunze D. Nucleus tractus solitarius—gateway to neural circulatory control. *Annu Rev Physiol.* 1994;56:93–116.
113. Jansen AS, Nguyen XV, Karpitskiy V, Mettenleiter TC, Loewy AD. Central command neurons of the sympathetic nervous system: basis of the fight-or-flight response. *Science.* Oct 27 1995;270(5236):644–646.
114. Skovsted P, Price ML, Price HL. The effects of short-acting barbiturates on arterial pressure, preganglionic sympathetic activity and barostatic reflexes. *Anesthesiology.* Jul 1970;33(1):10–18.
115. Skovsted P, Price ML, Price HL. Effects of basal anesthesia on the response of sympathetic nervous activity and barostatic reflexes to a subsequent administration of halothane. *J Pharmacol Exp Ther.* Oct 1970;175(1):183–188.
116. Yamamura T, Kimura T, Furukawa K. Effects of halothane, thiamylal, and ketamine on central sympathetic and vagal tone. *Anesth Analg.* Feb 1983;62(2):129–134.
117. Okamoto H, Hoka S, Kawasaki T, Okuyama T, Takahashi S. L-arginine attenuates ketamine-induced increase in renal sympathetic nerve activity. *Anesthesiology.* Jul 1994;81(1):137–146.
118. Akine A, Suzuka H, Hayashida Y, Kato Y. Effects of ketamine and propofol on autonomic cardiovascular function in chronically instrumented rats. *Auton Neurosci.* Mar 23 2001;87(2–3): 201–208.

119. Kienbaum P, Heuter T, Michel MC, Peters J. Racemic ketamine decreases muscle sympathetic activity but maintains the neural response to hypotensive challenges in humans. *Anesthesiology.* Jan 2000;92(1):94–101.
120. McGrath JC, MacKenzie JE, Millar RA. Effects of ketamine on central sympathetic discharge and the baroreceptor reflex during mechanical ventilation. *Br J Anaesth.* Nov 1975;47(11):1141–1147.
121. Shirahata M, Okada Y, Ninomiya I. Effects of ketamine on renal nerve activity, arterial pressure and heart rate in rats. *Jpn J Physiol.* 1983;33(3):391–401.
122. Dembowsky K, Lackner K, Czachurski J, Seller H. Tonic catecholaminergic inhibition of the spinal somato-sympathetic reflexes originating in the ventrolateral medulla oblongata. *J Auton Nerv Syst.* Apr 1981;3(2–4):277–290.
123. Dembowsky K, McAllen RM. Baroreceptor inhibition of subretrofacial neurons: evidence from intracellular recordings in the cat. *Neurosci Lett.* Mar 26 1990;111(1–2):139–143.
124. Nolan MF, Gibson IC, Logan SD. Actions of the anaesthetic Saffan on rat sympathetic preganglionic neurones in vitro. *Br J Pharmacol.* May 1997;121(2):324–330.
125. Barker JL, Harrison NL, Lange GD, Owen DG. Potentiation of gamma-aminobutyric-acid-activated chloride conductance by a steroid anaesthetic in cultured rat spinal neurones. *J Physiol.* May 1987;386:485–501.
126. Cottrell GA, Lambert JJ, Peters JA. Modulation of GABAA receptor activity by alphaxalone. *Br J Pharmacol.* Mar 1987;90(3):491–500.
127. Ho CM, Tarng GW, Su CK. Comparison of effects of propofol and midazolam at sedative concentrations on sympathetic tone generation in the isolated spinal cord of neonatal rats. *Acta Anaesthesiol Scand.* Jul 2007;51(6):708–713.
128. Tanelian DL, Kosek P, Mody I, MacIver MB. The role of the GABAA receptor/chloride channel complex in anesthesia. *Anesthesiology.* Apr 1993;78(4):757–776.
129. Inokuchi H, Yoshimura M, Trzebski A, Polosa C, Nishi S. Fast inhibitory postsynaptic potentials and responses to inhibitory amino acids of sympathetic preganglionic neurons in the adult cat. *J Auton Nerv Syst.* Nov 1992;41(1–2):53–59.
130. Cheng YW, Ku MC, Ho CM, Chai CY, Su CK. GABAB-receptor-mediated suppression of sympathetic outflow from the spinal cord of neonatal rats. *J Appl Physiol.* Nov 2005;99(5):1658–1667.
131. Peng SC, Ho CM, Ho ST, Tsai SK, Su CK. The role of intraspinal adenosine A1 receptors in sympathetic regulation. *Eur J Pharmacol.* May 10 2004;492(1):49–55.
132. Ho CM, Su CK. Ketamine attenuates sympathetic activity through mechanisms not mediated by N-methyl-D-aspartate receptors in the isolated spinal cord of neonatal rats. *Anesth Analg.* Mar 2006; 102(3):806–810.
133. Wang WZ, Rong WF, Wang JJ, Yuan WJ. Effect of ketamine on presympathetic neurons in rostral ventrolateral medulla of rats. *Acta Pharmacol Sin.* Feb 2001;22(2):97–102.
134. Dutton RC, Cuellar JM, Eger EI, 2nd, Antognini JF, Carstens E. Temporal and spatial determinants of sacral dorsal horn neuronal windup in relation to isoflurane-induced immobility. *Anesth Analg.* Dec 2007;105(6):1665–1674, table of contents.
135. Jinks SL, Antognini JF, Martin JT, Jung S, Carstens E, Atherley R. Isoflurane, but not halothane, depresses c-fos expression in rat spinal cord at concentrations that suppress reflex movement after supramaximal noxious stimulation. *Anesth Analg.* Dec 2002;95(6): 1622–1628, table of contents.
136. Araki I. Inhibitory postsynaptic currents and the effects of GABA on visually identified sacral parasympathetic preganglionic neurons in neonatal rats. *J Neurophysiol.* Dec 1994;72(6):2903–2910.
137. De Groat WC. The effects of glycine, GABA and strychnine on sacral parasympathetic preganglionic neurones. *Brain Res.* Mar 17 1970;18(3):542–544.
138. De Groat WC, Ryall RW. Recurrent inhibition in sacral parasympathetic pathways to the bladder. *J Physiol.* Jun 1968;196(3): 579–591.
139. Drasner K, Larson MD. Spinal and epidural anesthesia. In: Stoelting RK, Miller RD, eds. *Basics of Anesthesia.* 5th ed. Philadelphia: Churchill Livingstone Elsevier; 2007:241–271.
140. Strichartz GR, Ritchie JM. The action of local anesthetics on ion channels of excitable tissues. In: Strichartz GR, ed. *Local Anesthetics: Handbook of Experimental Pharmacology.* Vol. 81. Berlin: Springer-Verlag; 1987:21–53.
141. Catterall WA. From ionic currents to molecular mechanisms: the structure and function of voltage-gated sodium channels. *Neuron.* Apr 2000;26(1):13–25.
142. Butterworth JF, Strichartz GR. Molecular mechanisms of local anesthesia: a review. *Anesthesiology.* Apr 1990;72(4):711–734.
143. Courtney KR, Strichartz GR. Structural elements which determine local anesthetic activity. In: Strichartz GR, ed. *Local Anesthetics: Handbook of Experimental Pharmacology.* Vol. 81. Berlin: Springer-Verlag; 1987:53–94.
144. Huang JH, Thalhammer JG, Raymond SA, Strichartz GR. Susceptibility to lidocaine of impulses in different somatosensory afferent fibers of rat sciatic nerve. *J Pharmacol Exp Ther.* Aug 1997;282(2):802–811.
145. Raymond SA, Steffensen SC, Gugino LD, Strichartz GR. The role of length of nerve exposed to local anesthetics in impulse blocking action. *Anesth Analg.* May 1989;68(5):563–570.
146. Devor M, Zalkind V. Reversible analgesia, atonia, and loss of consciousness on bilateral intracerebral microinjection of pentobarbital. *Pain.* Oct 2001;94(1):101–112.
147. Mendelson WB. Sleep induction by microinjection of pentobarbital into the medial preoptic area in rats. *Life Sci.* 1996;59(22): 1821–1828.
148. Nelson LE, Guo TZ, Lu J, Saper CB, Franks NP, Maze M. The sedative component of anesthesia is mediated by GABA(A) receptors in an endogenous sleep pathway. *Nat Neurosci.* Oct 2002;5(10):979–984.
149. Voss LJ, Young BJ, Barnards JP, Sleigh J. Differential anaesthetic effects following microinjection of thiopentone and propofol into the pons of adult rats: a pilot study. *Anaesth Intensive Care.* Jun 2005;33(3):373–380.
150. Namjoshi DR, McErlane SA, Taepavarapruk N, Soja PJ. Network actions of pentobarbital in the rat mesopontine tegmentum on sensory inflow through the spinothalamic tract. *J Neurophysiol.* Aug 2009;102(2):700–713.
151. Namjoshi D, Lin S-W, Soja P. Cortical EEG activity does not change during suppression of spinothalamic tract neuron excitability induced by pentobarbital microinjections into the mesopontine tegmental anesthesia area. In: Miller KW, Roth SH, Orser B, eds. *MAC 2010: 8th International Conference on Mechanisms of Anesthesia.* Toronto, Canada: University of Toronto; 2010:70.
152. Reiner K, Sukhotinsky I, Devor M. Mesopontine tegmental anesthesia area projects independently to the rostromedial medulla and to the spinal cord. *Neuroscience.* May 25 2007;146(3): 1355–1370.
153. Sukhotinsky I, Hopkins DA, Lu J, Saper CB, Devor M. Movement suppression during anesthesia: neural projections from the mesopontine tegmentum to areas involved in motor control. *J Comp Neurol.* Sep 5 2005;489(4):425–448.
154. Sukhotinsky I, Reiner K, Govrin-Lippmann R, et al. Projections from the mesopontine tegmental anesthesia area to regions involved in pain modulation. *J Chem Neuroanat.* Dec 2006; 32(2–4):159–178.
155. Wall PD. Neurophysiological studies on the mechanism of anesthesia. *Anesthesiology.* Sep-Oct 1967;28(5):799–800.
156. Soja P. Anesthetic actions on tonic descending control of the spinothalamic tract. In: Vesce, G. ed. *Proceedings of the Naples Pain Conference: Research and Therapy for Human and Animal Suffering.* Naples, Italy: University of Napoli Federico II Press; 2010: 217–222.
157. Xhu X, McErlane S, Soja P. Tonic supraspinal and segmental influences on rat spinothalamic tract (STT) neurons. *Society for*

Neuroscience Abstract Viewer/Itinerary Planner. 2005; Program No. 623.22.
158. Belelli D, Peden DR, Rosahl TW, Wafford KA, Lambert JJ. Extrasynaptic GABAA receptors of thalamocortical neurons: a molecular target for hypnotics. *J Neurosci.* Dec 14 2005; 25(50):11513–11520.
159. Cope DW, Hughes SW, Crunelli V. GABAA receptor-mediated tonic inhibition in thalamic neurons. *J Neurosci.* Dec 14 2005;25(50):11553–11563.
160. Herd MB, Belelli D, Lambert JJ. Neurosteroid modulation of synaptic and extrasynaptic GABA(A) receptors. *Pharmacol Ther.* Oct 2007;116(1):20–34.
161. Stell BM, Brickley SG, Tang CY, Farrant M, Mody I. Neuroactive steroids reduce neuronal excitability by selectively enhancing tonic inhibition mediated by delta subunit-containing GABAA receptors. *Proc Natl Acad Sci U S A.* Nov 25 2003;100(24):14439–14444.
162. Soja PJ. Modulation of prethalamic sensory inflow during sleep versus wakefulness. In: Lavigne G, Sessle BJ, Choiniere M, Soja PJ, eds. *Sleep and Pain*. Seattle: IASP Press; 2007:45–76.
163. Taepavarapruk N, Taepavarapruk P, John J, et al. State-dependent changes in glutamate, glycine, GABA, and dopamine levels in cat lumbar spinal cord. *J Neurophysiol.* Aug 2008;100(2):598–608.
164. Soja PJ. Glycine-mediated postsynaptic inhibition is responsible for REM sleep atonia. *Sleep.* Nov 1 2008;31(11):1483–1486.
165. Nishikawa Y, Sasaki A, Kuraishi Y. Blockade of glycine transporter (GlyT) 2, but not GlyT1, ameliorates dynamic and static mechanical allodynia in mice with herpetic or postherpetic pain. *J Pharmacol Sci.* Mar 19 2010;112(3):352–360.
166. Centeno MV, Mutso A, Millecamps M, Apkarian AV. Prefrontal cortex and spinal cord mediated anti-neuropathy and analgesia induced by sarcosine, a glycine-T1 transporter inhibitor. *Pain.* Sep 2009;145(1–2):176–183.
167. Cooke JE, Mathers DA, Puil E. Isovaline causes inhibition by increasing potassium conductance in thalamic neurons. *Neuroscience.* Dec 15 2009;164(3):1235–1243.
168. MacLeod BA, Wang JT, Chung CC, Ries CR, Schwarz SK, Puil E. Analgesic properties of the novel amino acid, isovaline. *Anesth Analg.* Apr 1 2010;110(4):1206–1214.
169. Redman SJ. The relative contributions of GABA-A and GABA-B receptors to presynaptic inhibition of group Ia EPSPs. In: Rudomin P, Ranulfo R, Mendell LM, eds. *Presynaptic Inhibition and Neural Control.* New York: Oxford University Press; 1998: 162–177.

8

ANESTHETIC-INDUCED IMMOBILITY

Steven L. Jinks and Joseph F. Antognini

Immobility is one of the key hallmarks and goals of anesthesia. Immobility, along with amnesia and unconsciousness, are the three endpoints that qualify the state of general anesthesia. The neural substrates and molecular mechanisms of anesthetics remain poorly understood—particularly for inhaled anesthetics, which are known to modulate a multitude of neuronal ion channels, receptors, and intracellular signaling processes.[1] Some of these effects appear to be more important to anesthetic-induced immobility than others. It also appears that anesthetic effects at one site in a sensorimotor circuit are more important than effects at another site in that pathway. Therefore, understanding how anesthetics produce immobility requires delineation of relevant anesthetic effects, and how these effects play out in relevant sites of the nervous system. In this scenario, understanding *where* anesthetics act is paramount to understanding *how* they act, and thus we believe a deductive, or "top down" approach is warranted, especially for anesthetics that produce a myriad of effects. This approach has served us well in homing in on the sites and mechanisms of anesthetics, although there is much to learn before we begin to develop safer anesthetics using a priori knowledge.

In this chapter we will describe the studies that have been performed to elucidate the mechanisms by which anesthetics produce immobility. We first begin with a historical perspective, followed by anatomical and physiological information that is the basis for understanding anesthetic-induced immobility. We end with discussion of recent models used to investigate anesthetic-induced immobility, and studies that have advanced our understanding of this important area.

HISTORICAL PERSPECTIVE ON THE SITES OF ANESTHETIC IMMOBILIZING ACTION

Soon after the introduction of anesthesia, immobility was recognized as a sine qua non of general anesthesia. Early experimentation with nitrous oxide demonstrated that although patients did not experience pain, or had vague recollections, movement during surgical procedures indicated inadequate anesthesia. Before the development of muscle relaxants such as curare, there was no other way to pharmacologically produce immobility except with anesthetics. While nitrous oxide could be used for minor procedures such as tooth extraction, extensive procedures could not be performed without the patient moving uncontrollably, an indication of nitrous oxide's weak potency. Ether and chloroform, the earliest anesthetics, produced immobility and permitted more extensive operations, including intra-abdominal, intrathoracic, and intracranial procedures.

The rapid spread of the use of ether anesthesia naturally led to investigations about ether's properties and how it produced anesthesia. Claude Bernard, one of the preeminent scientists of the 19th century, was interested in how anesthesia occurred. Although he had few tools to probe this nascent area of research, his simple but elegant experiments shed abundant light on anatomical sites important to anesthetic action. Bernard performed studies using frogs to demonstrate that the central nervous system, including the spinal cord, was the site where chloroform produced immobility.[2] He used a glass jar filled with water to which he had added chloroform in a 1:200 mixture. The jar was covered with a rubber membrane that had a small hole in the center, through which he could immerse part of a frog's body into the solution, with the remainder of the body sticking out of the jar. He used frogs as the experimental model because frogs respire in part through their skin.

In one experiment, Bernard placed ligatures around the frog's tissue (including aorta), separating the rostral part of the frog's body from the caudal part (i.e., the hindlimbs) but left the spinal cord intact. In this manner he was able to prevent circulation to the hindlimbs and thereby prevented the anesthetic from entering. The nervous system communication was still intact, and he found that when only the rostral portion of the frog was placed into the jar, the hindlimbs became anesthetized. He concluded that the anesthetic must have acted on the central nervous system because the anesthetic was prevented from entering directly into the hindlimbs. When the caudal portion of the frog was placed into the jar, anesthesia did not develop in any part of the frog, suggesting that the anesthetic was not acting on peripheral sites.

In further experiments Bernard severed the spinal cord above the segments controlling the hindlimbs, but left the tissue/aorta nonoccluded. The frogs still exhibited spinal reflexes (i.e., they did not develop spinal shock). When the frogs were placed into the chloroform solution, anesthesia occurred throughout the frog's body whether the rostral portion or the caudal portion was immersed into the solution. He concluded that the anesthetic need not first act on the brain and then transmit that action to the spinal cord, as the latter was severed.

Bernard's studies were instructive but largely ignored for nearly a century. The question of whether results from amphibians could be extrapolated to mammalian species remained elusive. Despite these limitations, Bernard must be credited as the first to discover the main anatomic site where anesthetics produce immobility—the spinal cord.

CONCEPT OF MINIMUM ALVEOLAR CONCENTRATION

For many years studies of anesthetic action languished in an intellectual quagmire because a standard of anesthetic potency was lacking. One could not satisfactorily compare two or more anesthetics because these anesthetics had different potencies, and, without a common pharmacological endpoint, interpretation of these differences was limited. The introduction of "minimum alveolar concentration" (MAC) permitted such comparisons,[3,4] as investigators could now determine differences between anesthetics using equipotent concentrations. The endpoint (or yardstick) that was used to determine potency was abolition of movement in response to a supramaximal noxious stimulus. The latter was determined by showing that increased stimulation did not increase the concentration needed to prevent movement. MAC determination, the standard method for testing anesthetic immobilizing potency, is performed by measuring the minimum alveolar anesthetic concentration necessary to prevent movement in the face of supramaximal noxious stimulation (surgical incision, or clamping an animal's tail) in 50% of subjects. Furthermore, in MAC testing "gross purposeful" (multisegmentally mediated) movement is assessed. Eger and colleagues arbitrarily chose "gross, purposeful" movement as the endpoint.[3,4] This consisted of a pawing or running motion, or turning of the head toward the stimulus. They excluded stiffening, coughing, and swallowing, and we and others excluded simple reflex withdrawal response. Although some may argue that such movements (indeed any movements) should be included, it is fortuitous that Eger and others focused on purposeful movements, as it forced a closer examination of spinal cord sites (e.g., locomotor networks) that otherwise might have been overlooked. We have found that tail clamping in rodents primarily produces locomotor-type responses, resembling a repetitive "galloping" pattern.[5] Therefore it appears that supramaximal noxious stimulation strongly activates locomotor networks. But, do anesthetics produce immobility by acting

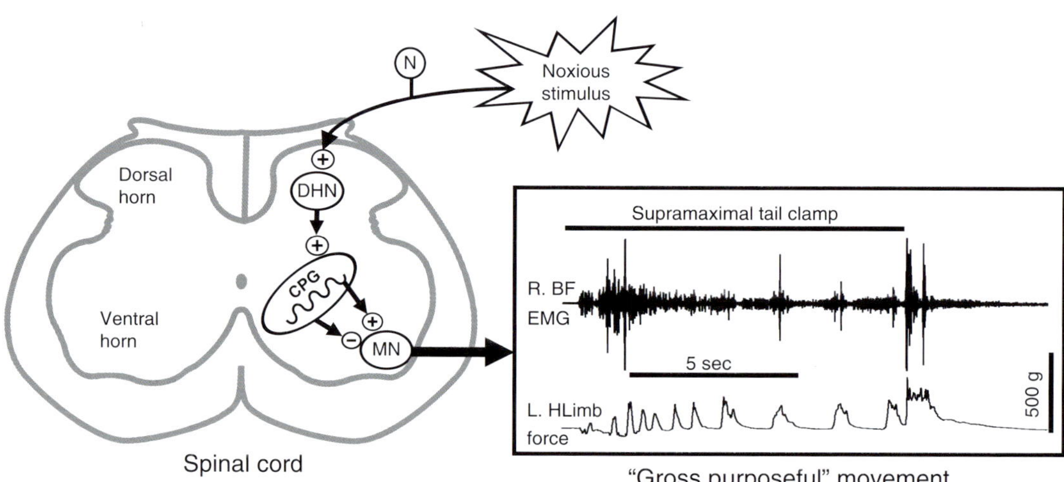

Figure 8.1 Components of a nociceptive sensorimotor transformation. A noxious stimulus in the periphery is transduced into action potentials in primary afferent nociceptors (N), which are either thinly myelinated (Aδ) or unmyelinated (C) nerve fibers with cell bodies located in the dorsal root ganglia (DRG). Nociceptors terminate centrally in the spinal dorsal horn, where they synapse with dorsal horn neurons (DHN). Nociceptor activity excites dorsal horn neurons. Intense excitation of dorsal horn neurons by a supramaximal noxious stimulus activates the central pattern generator (CPG), a network of excitatory and inhibitory interneurons that establishes rhythmic neural activity underlying locomotion. CPG activity imparts rhythmic excitation and inhibition of motoneurons (MN), which represent the final common pathway for muscle activation leading to overt motor behavior. Rhythmic motoneuron activation by the CPG leads to an organized locomotor escape reaction to a supramaximal stimulus. The tracings to the right of the spinal cord schematic were taken from a rat responding to noxious tail clamp under 0.6 MAC halothane anesthesia. The rat had one freely moving hindlimb, from which biceps femoris electromyogram (BF EMG) activity was recorded (top trace). The opposite limb was extended and tethered to a strain gauge to record isometric limb force (bottom trace). The tracings show "gross, purposeful movement," an organized rhythmic motor response of both hindlimbs to a 10-second tail clamp.

uniformly across all neuronal classes in this sensorimotor transformation, including primary afferent nociceptors, dorsal horn neurons, locomotor interneurons (comprising the "CPG" or central pattern generator), and motoneurons, (see Figure 8.1), or do they preferentially disrupt a certain component?

PERTINENT ANATOMY AND PHYSIOLOGY OF THE SPINAL CORD

Although spinal cord anatomy and physiology are covered elsewhere in this book we review important concepts relevant to anesthetic-induced immobility. Noxious stimulation in the periphery will excite nociceptors and initiate impulse propagation along axons, proximally toward the spinal cord (Figure 8.1). The central axons of nociceptors synapse onto dorsal horn neurons, or "second-order neurons." Nociceptors activate dorsal horn neurons via glutamate and excitatory neuropeptides such as substance P and CGRP (calcitonin gene-related peptide). Dorsal horn neurons may possess ascending projections to higher centers in the brain (e.g., spinoreticular or spinothalamic neurons). In return, spinal circuits are subject to descending projections from the brain, which can modulate both dorsal horn (sensory) or ventral horn (motor) processing. If the dorsal horn neuron is part of a withdrawal reflex circuit, it projects to local reflex interneurons, which in turn synapse on motoneurons. A motoneuron sends an axonal projection that exits the spinal cord via a ventral root, courses through peripheral nerves, and synapses onto muscle fibers. When a noxious stimulus activates this reflex arc, motoneuron activation engages muscle groups that move the afflicted body part away from the offending stimulus, thus avoiding tissue damage. Supramaximal activation of nociceptive pathways may activate spinal networks involved in locomotion, termed "central pattern generators" (CPG), to initiate organized escape responses. The CPG is a network of inhibitory and excitatory interneurons that imparts rhythmic activation (and inhibition) of motoneurons to produce rhythmic locomotor behavior. Figure 8.1 depicts the proposed pathway by which a supramaximal noxious stimulus elicits organized movement.

THE ISOLATED SPINAL CORD GENERATES COMPLEX MOVEMENTS

That anesthetics act in the spinal cord to prevent gross, purposeful movement invites the question, what type of movement can the spinal cord generate? Surprisingly, the spinal cord can generate complex movements well beyond a simple withdrawal reflex.

Frogs demonstrate what is termed the wiping reflex, wherein if a noxious stimulus is placed on the torso or a forelimb, the hindlimb will reach to the stimulus to wipe it away.[6] This wiping reflex is present even if the frog has had its spinal cord severed at a high cervical segment. In fact, if the forelimb is moved to a different location, the hindlimb "knows" where the forelimb is in space, and is able to wipe away the offending stimulus.[6] Thus, the amphibian spinal cord is able to determine limb location using proprioception, entirely without input from the brain.

Mammals are also capable of complex movements that are solely spinal cord–generated. Modern neuroscience has strong foundations that include the work of Charles Sherrington and colleagues, including Thomas Graham Brown, who in the early part of the last century established that spinally transected cats or guinea pigs exhibit hindlimb "walking." Stepping behavior continues even in the absence of sensory input from the periphery. Rats decerebrated at the precollicular level can survive, and after recovery display normal behaviors, including feeding, grooming, licking, and climbing.[7] Lastly, brain-dead humans can have complex movements[8,9] referred to as "Lazarus sign" after the biblical individual who was raised from the dead. These patients can cross their arms over their chests, sit up in bed, and also turn their heads, in response to noxious stimulation, but sometimes spontaneously.

More recently, isolated spinal cord preparations have been developed using the lamprey, a jawless fish, and neonatal rodents. A section of spinal cord at least several segments in length is excised and placed in oxygenated Ringer's solution. When excitatory agents (e.g., glutamate receptor agonists) are added to the bath, the spinal cord will generate "fictive locomotion." "Fictive" because the spinal cord is freed from all musculature and locomotion must be monitored by recording neural activity from the ventral roots (motoneuron axons). The pattern of locomotion encoded in bursts of ventral root activity is nearly identical to that seen in an intact animal. Taken together, these examples clearly show that the spinal cord is capable of generating organized movements that, in a MAC study, would be considered "gross and purposeful."

THE SPINAL CORD AND ANESTHETIC-INDUCED IMMOBILITY

The limitations of Bernard's work (e.g., an amphibian animal model) along with theories that anesthetics primarily acted in gray matter of the cerebral cortex raised the question of where anesthetics produce immobility in mammals.[4] Studies by Ira Rampil, along with our work, revived the preeminence of the spinal cord as a vital site of anesthetic action.

Rampil showed that rats anesthetized with isoflurane did not have any specific electroencephalographic pattern that could consistently identify whether a rat would move or not move in response to a noxious stimulus.[10] Indeed, he reported that, in some rats, movement occurred despite burst suppression on the electroencephalogram. This begged an obvious question: if the brain was so depressed in the face of stimulus-induced movement, was the brain needed at all as a site of anesthetic action? This intriguing question was in part answered in a study by Rampil et al,[11] which demonstrated that precollicular decerebration did not change isoflurane MAC. It was therefore concluded that anesthetic-induced immobility in the face of noxious stimulation did not require forebrain structures.

Our group investigated this area using a preparation in which we could selectively deliver anesthetics to the in vivo brain.[12,13] We used a goat model because of its unique cerebral circulation. The arterial blood supply to the brain of the goat consists almost exclusively of the external carotid system. The internal carotid arteries are of minimal to no significance, as is the vertebral/basilar arterial system. One need only tie off the occipital arteries (which otherwise link the carotid system with the vertebral arteries) and isolate the carotid arteries to be able to control the blood supply to the brain. The venous blood returns via the external jugular veins, although there is some return via other venous collaterals (including epidural veins). By draining the venous blood into an oxygenator, and infusing the oxygenated blood into a carotid artery, selective delivery of anesthetics is possible. This preparation separates the arterial blood supply to the central nervous system at the level of the caudal medulla and upper cervical spinal cord.

When isoflurane was selectively delivered to just the brain (with a low concentration to the torso) nearly threefold normal immobilizing concentrations were needed in the brain to prevent movement.[12] We repeated this study using halothane and thiopental, and obtained similar results.[13] Conversely, we found that anesthetic immobilizing concentrations were actually *decreased* by 30% when isoflurane was selectively delivered to the torso (spinal cord) while maintaining low brain isoflurane concentrations. These data strongly suggested that anesthetics act in the spinal cord to prevent movement.

BRAINSTEM MODULATION PAINTS THE FULL PICTURE

It should be noted that while many anesthetics produce immobility primarily by a direct spinal action, supraspinal actions can modulate anesthetic immobilizing requirements, and the magnitude or pattern of noxious stimulus–evoked movement that may occur in an anesthetized patient or animal.[14–16] These supraspinal actions reside in the brainstem, because Rampil's study and confirmation by our groups demonstrate that precollicular decerebration does not change MAC. As mentioned, selective delivery of isoflurane to the goat spinal cord (with very low cranial concentration) produces a 30% decrease in MAC. Furthermore, we found that spinally transected rats exhibited at least 40% decrease in MAC.[17] This was true whether the rat received an acute but nondamaging and reversible "transection" by spinal cooling, or whether the rat had received a chronic surgical transection and was MAC-tested long after the animal had recovered from "spinal shock." In these animals, MAC values from forelimb stimulation (above the transection level) remained unchanged. These data suggest that while immobility results from a direct spinal action, facilitation from the brainstem counteracts spinal depression and elevates anesthetic requirements. We recently investigated what areas mediated the brainstem effect on MAC.[14] Of particular importance was the midbrain locomotor region (MLR), which encompasses the cuneiform and pedunculopontine nuclei. Electrical or chemical MLR stimulation activates the CPG locomotor interneurons[18] and produces robust locomotion (we elaborate more on the MLR and locomotor networks in the next section). Selective lidocaine inactivation or surgical removal of the MLR leads to a 30–40% decrease in MAC.[14] At isoflurane concentrations permitting movement, removal of the MLR leads to a reduction in the number and magnitude of movements evoked by noxious tail clamp. Furthermore, MLR neuronal responses to tail clamp are profoundly depressed by peri-MAC isoflurane. We propose that once MLR neurons are depressed at MAC, spinal depression prevails and the animal becomes immobile. Therefore, supraspinal actions must be considered to *fully* explain normal anesthetic immobilizing requirements, and the MLR is a key area involved in elevating MAC and promoting robust, repetitive movement to noxious stimuli under anesthesia.

WHERE IN THE SPINAL CORD?

The preceding studies clearly support the important role that the spinal cord has in anesthetic-induced immobility—but where in the spinal cord might this action occur? Is anesthetic action uniform across classes of spinal neurons, or is it selective for a particular class? For many decades research has been focused on the dorsal horn of the spinal cord, as this is the "gate" though which impulses are transmitted to the spinal cord and supraspinal sites. Kitahata, Collins, and others showed that numerous anesthetics and analgesics depress neuronal responses to noxious stimulation.[19,20] These studies had limitations, however, including the fact that the stimuli were not often standardized and that the anesthetic concentrations were not rigorously controlled (i.e., equilibration time was not used and large concentration ranges were studied).

Recent evidence has diminished the relevance of dorsal horn neurons to anesthetic-induced immobility.[21–24] We previously found that 0.8–1.4 MAC isoflurane did not suppress dorsal horn neurons.[23] Another group[24] found that naloxone completely reversed the halothane-induced depression of dorsal horn neurons, but did not reverse motor unit depression. The mismatch between inhaled anesthetic effects on motor output and dorsal horn activity implies that inhaled anesthetics acted more potently on ventrally located spinal neurons, such as motoneurons, or late-order interneurons, which participate in both spinal reflexes and locomotion.[25–29]

We then sought to determine how anesthetics affected neuronal responses to noxious stimulation in the dorsal horn versus those in the ventral horn. We used an in vivo rat model, often with decerebration, the latter procedure permitting us to obtain data in the anesthetic-free control condition. We found that neurons in the ventral horn were more sensitive to various anesthetics than neurons in the dorsal horn. The results were consistent across a broad range of anesthetics, including isoflurane, halothane, propofol, and nitrous oxide (the latter was studied using a hyperbaric chamber).[30,31] Thus, it appears that neurons in the ventral spinal cord are, as a class, more sensitive to anesthetics and are likely to be an important site of anesthetic action.

Still, there are problems with interpretations that discount the role of dorsal horn neurons in anesthetic-induced immobility. For one, it is difficult and often impossible to identify the true nature of a neuron in terms of its projection pattern as well as its role and "weight" in sensorimotor function or ascending pain transmission. Therefore, a particular subclass of dorsal horn neurons important to noxious stimulus-induced movement might be especially sensitive to anesthetics while many others are not. In fact, we found that nociceptive specific dorsal horn neurons show greater sensitivity to depression by anesthetics than wide-dynamic-range neurons.[32] Furthermore, a small dorsal horn effect could culminate in a larger depression of ventral neurons as activity progresses through nociceptive sensorimotor transformations, known to be polysynaptic. These hypotheses could become prohibitively laborious to unequivocally support or refute.

We recently obviated these caveats by using MLR stimulation in rats to behaviorally dissect dorsal vs. ventral horn anesthetic effects[33] (Figure 8.2). Electrical or chemical MLR stimulation activates the CPG locomotor interneurons[18] (and produces locomotion) while it inhibits dorsal horn sensory neurons.[34,35] Therefore, one can test anesthetic immobilizing effects on MLR-elicited movement that bypasses the dorsal horn, and compare this with immobilizing effects on movement that *requires* dorsal horn activation, i.e., tail clamp–elicited "locomotion," as in a typical MAC determination. We measured isoflurane and halothane requirements to block MLR-elicited movement and found that they were only 10% greater than MAC for isoflurane and 20% greater for halothane. The slightly greater halothane requirements for suppressing MLR-elicited movement is consistent with halothane's modest depression of dorsal horn neurons in the peri-MAC range.[23,24] Thus, it appears that anesthetic action in the dorsal horn contributes but a small fraction of the immobilizing effect. The dominant anesthetic action in the immediate peri-MAC range was the abolition of stepping behavior. This finding

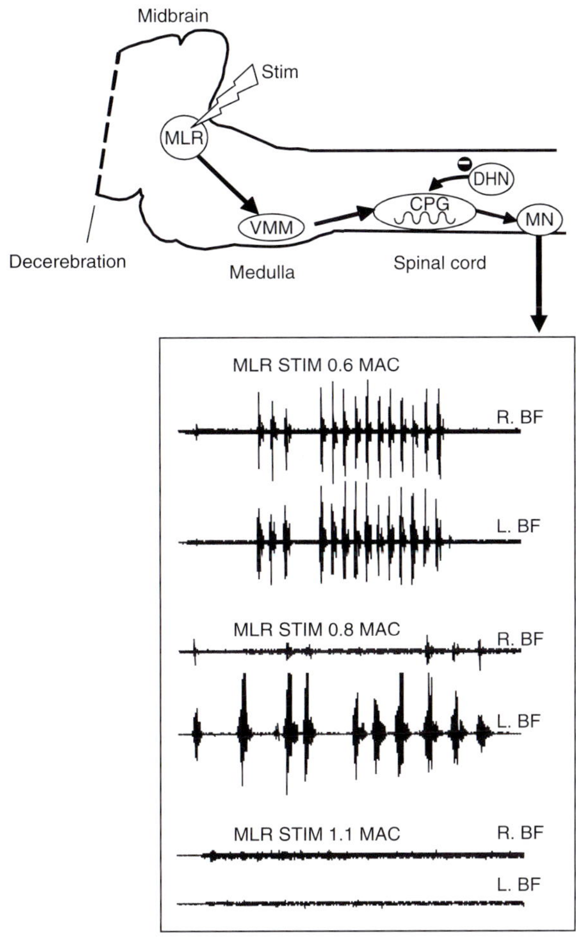

Figure 8.2 Schematic diagram depicting movement pathways from the mesencephalic locomotor region (MLR). Animals are decerebrated (dashed line) at the rostral edge of the superior colliculus. Electrical stimulation of the MLR elicits coordinated locomotion in all limbs. Projections from the MLR in the cuneiform and pedunculopontine nuclei synapse on reticulospinal neurons in the ventromedial medulla (VMM), which in turn project to the spinal cord to activate ventrally located central pattern generating (CPG) networks that produce rhythmic locomotor activity in motoneurons (MN). By comparing anesthetic requirements to block MLR-elicited movement (that is independent of dorsal horn activation) with those for noxious stimulus–evoked movement (resulting from dorsal horn activation), it is possible to dissect the relative importance of dorsal and ventral spinal cord sites in producing immobility. The tracings below the diagram show biceps femoris electromyogram responses to electrical microstimulation of the MLR at 2.0 times threshold for locomotion under different MAC concentrations of isoflurane anesthesia. MAC was determined with a tail clamp before and during data collection. In this animal the isoflurane requirement to block MLR-elicited movement was identical to isoflurane requirement to block movement to tail clamp. Because MLR-elicited movement excludes dorsal horn activation, the data demonstrate on a behavioral level that isoflurane does not produce significant immobilizing effects by action dorsal horn neurons. The data rather suggest that isoflurane's primary immobilizing effect occurs in the ventral horn, consistent with electrophysiological data.

implicates CPG locomotor interneurons as the main immobilizing target of inhaled anesthetic action in the spinal cord. However, due to the fact that locomotor interneurons and motoneurons are anatomically intermingled in the spinal cord, and interneurons are difficult to identify, it is inherently difficult to segregate anesthetic effects on interneurons from those on motoneurons using in vivo preparations. In the next section we propose methods to obviate these problems using isolated spinal cord preparations.

Others have shown that anesthetics depress motoneurons. Rampil and others used the F-wave as an indirect means to investigate anesthetic actions on the motoneuron.[36,37] The F-wave is measured from muscle and can be elicited by stimulation of a peripheral nerve. The resulting impulses travel antidromically to the motoneuron, which causes the motoneuron to be excited and produce depolarization of the motoneuron. This depolarization sends impulses back down the motor nerve to the muscle, causing muscle depolarization that is recorded on the electromyogram. The F-wave is thought to reflect motoneuron excitability. Various anesthetics depress the F-wave, consistent with the hypothesis that anesthetics depress motoneurons, possibly by hyperpolarizing them. It should be noted that F-wave measurements are indirect, and motoneuron excitability can be modulated by interneuronal activity presynaptic to a motoneuron. Using rodent spinal cord slice preparations, Kendig and colleagues have recorded from motoneurons using patch clamp methods, and they have demonstrated directly a depression of motoneurons by some inhaled anesthetics.[38] However, there is motor depression and then there is immobility. We have found that between 0.4 and 0.6 MAC, isoflurane produces nearly 50% decrease in hindlimb force elicited by MLR stimulation,[33] yet clinically speaking these animals are still moving quite vigorously to noxious stimulation at 0.6 MAC. We do not know if any depression of motoneurons is sufficient to produce immobility at MAC, but our recent data in the following sections suggest it is not.

Some evidence indicates that anesthetic effects on motoneurons do not explain immobility. Single-limb withdrawals are well known to persist above MAC, suggesting that motoneurons have enough excitability to move the limbs. Furthermore, from 0.6 to 0.9 MAC, inhaled anesthetics reduce the number, but not the force, of movements evoked by a noxious stimulus,[5] indicative of CPG (rhythm generation) depression rather than motoneuron depression. Furthermore, selective delivery of isoflurane to the mid-region of the lamprey spinal cord leads to a two-fold increase in immobilizing requirements in that region compared to whole-cord immobilizing concentrations,[39,40] a finding not consistent with a predominantly direct motoneuron immobilizing effect. Because, under normal circumstances, CPG neurons are intimately linked to motoneurons, the relative importance of these neuronal classes to anesthetic-induced immobilizing properties remains elusive. Using isolated spinal cord preparations as described below, we can tease apart the effects of inhaled anesthetics on each of these circuit components.

In summary, recent evidence indicates that primary immobilizing effects of inhaled anesthetics occur in the spinal ventral (anterior) horn, with dorsal horn effects making a lesser contribution. The ventral horn houses interneuronal networks mediating locomotion, and motoneurons, the final common pathway for motor output. Regarding immobility, the relative importance of effects on locomotor interneurons versus effects on motoneurons is not known. We are currently resolving this problem, and recent data suggest that anesthetic-induced immobility results primarily by disrupting interneuronal spinal locomotor networks (i.e., the CPG).

CENTRAL PATTERN GENERATORS

Locomotor interneurons are critical to movement, as they receive both peripheral sensory and descending motor commands [41,42] and rhythmically activate motoneurons.[43,44] Of particular importance is the role of central pattern generators (CPG), which is a multisegmental ("distributed") network of rhythmogenic interneurons. In mammals the CPG is located in the ventromedial aspect of the spinal cord but distributed across several segments.[45] CPG circuitry is not fully understood, especially in mammals. However, it is known that CPGs establish the locomotor rhythm that is then transmitted to motoneurons. The CPG also coordinates this rhythmic activity such that intralimb flexion-extension and interlimb alternations is timed appropriately. In the simpler lamprey these rostrocaudal, left-right alternating rhythms underlie the ability of the lamprey to swim forward, while in higher species the CPGs mandate walking and running. Because anesthetics depress these complex organized movements, understanding the physiology and anatomy of CPGs is important to understanding anesthetic-induced immobility.

Spinal CPG networks contain all the circuitry necessary for producing locomotor rhythms such as swimming and walking.[46,47] Basic mammalian and lamprey CPG circuits are surprisingly conserved across vertebrate evolution, with similar functional and neurochemical organization.[48] These consist of rhythmic-bursting glutamatergic excitatory interneurons with ipsilateral projections to motoneurons,[49–51] and commissural pathways that produce glycinergic inhibition of motoneurons, resulting in left-right alternation of motor output.[52,53]

CPG organization in the lamprey is the best understood vertebrate locomotor system, and has been used extensively as a "simple" model for vertebrate locomotion. Bath-applied glutamate agonists produce "fictive" swimming, a coordinated pattern of activity among ventral roots that closely matches the in vivo swimming pattern, and remains stable for many hours.[54] The spinal cord is only 200 μm thick, and avascular, as the exchange of physiologic gases and nutrients occurs through cerebrospinal fluid diffusion,[55] allowing for rapid drug equilibration. Another advantage is that different subclasses of CPG interneurons have been identified.[56] The two main classes of CPG neurons responsible for locomotor rhythm generation are glutamatergic excitatory interneurons, with ipsilateral axons; and glycinergic inhibitory neurons, with long descending commissural (contralateral) axons (Figure 8.3). The detailed knowledge of lamprey spinal networks permits us to conduct detailed studies of anesthetic effects on CPG neurons and their rhythmic excitatory (glutamatergic) and inhibitory (glycinergic) output to motoneurons. Bath separation with vaseline makes it possible to selectively activate specific spinal regions, thereby functionally isolating CPG activity from that of motoneurons.[57] Bath separation additionally permits selective anesthetic delivery to specific spinal regions.

Figure 8.4A shows a lamprey isolated spinal cord experimental set-up, in which we used bath separation to selectively activate fictive swimming in the rostral cord ("active bath"). A motoneuron is recorded intracellulary in the inactive caudal bath ("passive bath"). Motoneurons in the caudal passive bath are driven from the active CPG in the rostral bath, and exhibit locomotor related oscillations consisting of alternating glutamatergic depolarization and glycinergic hyperpolarization. Therefore the caudal bath motoneuron oscillations act as a "readout" of the rostral bath CPG activity. When we delivered inhaled anesthetic (isoflurane or desflurane) selectively to the rostral bath, anesthetic concentrations that produced immobility in the rostral bath were associated with the abolition of CPG-driven motoneuron oscillations in the anesthetic-free caudal bath (Figure 8.4B). These data strongly indicate that immobility results from severe disruption of the CPG network.

We recently found in the lamprey that isoflurane requirements to block D-glutamate-induced fictive locomotion were the same as requirements to block motor output elicited by noxious tail stimulation in tail-attached preparations.[40] Sensory neurons are necessarily activated by tail pinch but are not active during fictive locomotion.[58] Therefore, as in mammals, sensory neurons do not appear to play a major role in mediating inhaled anesthetic-induced immobility in lampreys. Furthermore, the data justify the use of pharmacologic activation of the CPG as relevant to studying anesthetic effects on motor responses activated by noxious peripheral stimulation. Our preliminary data in the isolated neonatal rat spinal cord similarly support the use of pharmacologically induced locomotor activity to understand inhaled anesthetic immobilizing mechanisms. Therefore, pharmacologic activation of locomotor networks (producing a regular, well-defined motor pattern) appears to be a clinically relevant yet a convenient, powerful way to explore network mechanisms of inhaled anesthetics.

Although the basic functional and neurochemical organization of the CPG is conserved among vertebrates, relatively little detail is known in mammals, which have complex neural CPG architecture necessary for controlling intra- and interlimb coordination, and typically multiple motor repertoires (walking, galloping, climbing). The isolated neonatal

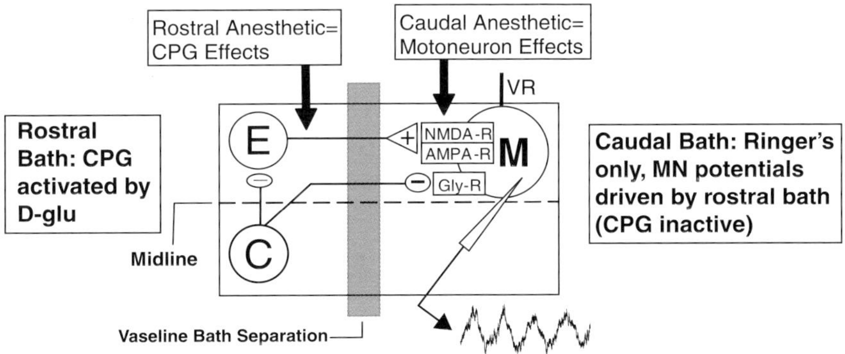

Figure 8.3 Lamprey CPG organization and the use of bath separation to dissect CPG vs. motoneurons effects. In the lamprey spinal cord it is possible to identify specific classes of CPG interneurons. Two important classes of CPG neurons in the lamprey spinal cord are glutamatergic excitatory interneurons (E) with ipsilateral monosynaptic projections to motoneurons (MN), and glycinergic inhibitory commissural interneurons (C) with crossed monosynaptic projections to E neurons and motoneurons. E neurons excite motoneurons via NMDA and AMPA type glutamate receptors. C neurons inhibit E neurons and motoneurons via glycine receptors. The two populations burst in alternation, producing rhythmic oscillations in motoneurons during swimming. The trace below the diagram is an intracellular recording of a lamprey motoneuron exhibiting locomotor oscillations in membrane potential during fictive swimming, which was induced by D-glutamate. Bath separation (shaded bar) dissociates CPG and motoneuron components when CPG networks are only activated in the rostral bath (by adding D-glutamate only to the rostral bath) to drive caudal-bath motoneurons. Anesthetics are then applied to the rostral or caudal bath to test direct effects on CPG or motoneurons independently. VR = ventral root. Dashed line indicates midline.

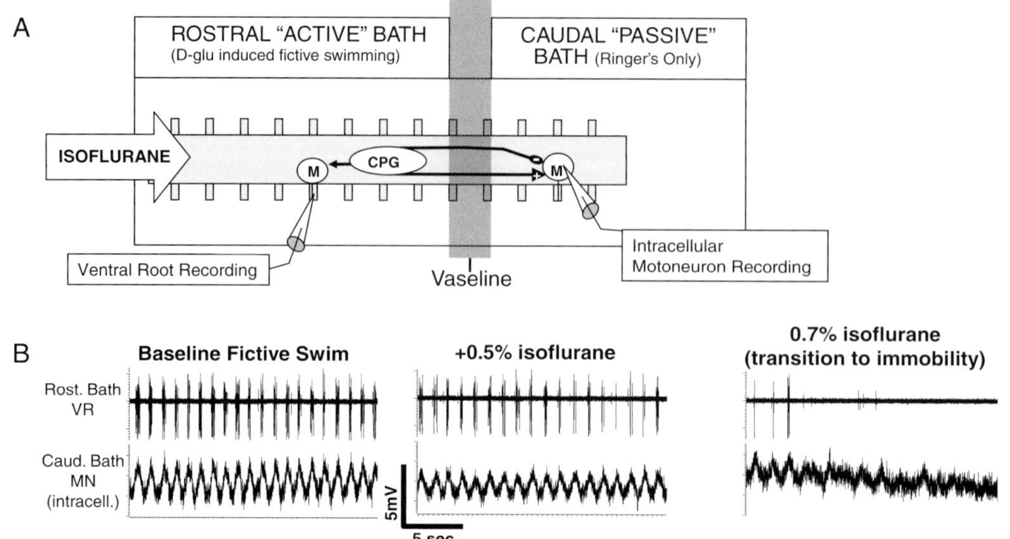

Figure 8.4 Isoflurane (ISO) induced immobility is associated with the abolishment of CPG drive to motoneurons in the lamprey isolated spinal cord. An individual example, in which isoflurane was selectively delivered to the rostral bath in a split-bath design as depicted in Figure 8.3. (A) Experimental preparation and design. D-glutamate-induced fictive swimming is selectively activated in the rostral bath, where fictive swimming (or anesthetic-induced immobility) is monitored via a ventral root recording. An intracellular recording is taken from a motoneuron in the caudal bath, where the CPG is inactive due to lack of D-glutamate. (B) During baseline fictive swimming (left traces), the CPG network activated in the rostral bath drives caudal-bath motoneuron oscillations (bottom traces). Isoflurane delivered selectively to the rostral bath at a subimmobilizing concentration caused depression of fictive swimming (reduced ventral root bursting), which was associated with a reduction in the amplitude of locomotor-related motoneuron oscillations (middle traces). Immobility occurred during isoflurane equilibration from 0.5% to 0.7% isoflurane, and motoneuron oscillations (again, driven by the rostral bath CPG) were abolished (right traces). These data suggest that immobility results from a direct isoflurane disruption of the spinal CPG network in the lamprey.

rodent spinal cord is viable in vitro from neonates up to five days old. The cord is unmyelinated and lacks a blood-brain barrier, permitting direct access of pharmacologic agents to their neural substrates.[59] Prolonged, stable fictive locomotion is induced by bath application of excitatory amino acids and 5-hydroxytryptamine (5-HT), or by activation of descending or sensory inputs.[60] In mammals, the CPG network is distributed, but not uniformly as in the lamprey.

In quadrupedal vertebrates, there exists a CPG excitability gradient, with the predominant rhythm-generating components located rostrally in the lower thoracic and upper lumbar segments.[45,61–63] In the rodent neonatal isolated spinal cord we can exploit this rostrocaudal gradient of rhythmogenic capacity, using bath separation techniques to distinguish CPG vs. motoneuron inhaled anesthetic effects. Cazalets et al. used vaseline barriers to selectively deliver drugs to the upper lumbar (T13-L2) or lower lumbosacral segments. When NMDA/5-HT was administered to the rostral bath, it elicited rhythmic locomotor activity in L1–2 ventral roots and drove rhythmic oscillations and left-right alternation in L5 motoneurons located in the caudal bath, but NMDA/5HT applied to the caudal bath produced only tonic ventral root firing.[63] Prior studies have taken advantage of this CPG gradient, using bath separation to assess roles of ligand- and voltage-gated ion channels in CPG vs. motoneurons.[57,63] We have begun using similar methods to distinguish effects of inhaled anesthetics on the CPG from those on motoneurons.

Figure 8.5 shows a neonatal rat isolated spinal cord experimental set-up, in which we used bath separation to dissect anesthetic effects on the CPG from motoneurons. We recorded from L2 and L5 ventral roots to monitor fictive walking induced by bath-applied NMDA and 5HT. The spinal cord is bath-separated by vaseline at the L3 level. Clinical anesthetic concentrations applied only to the rostral bath (CPG) severely depress locomotor bursts and finally produce immobility. The caudal bath also becomes inactive despite being anesthetic-free and containing the same concentrations of agonists as the rostral bath, supporting prior evidence that rostral segments provide the vast majority of rhythmogenicity. However, anesthetic delivery to only the caudal bath (motoneuron pools) shows strikingly different effects. Caudal bath delivery of clinical isoflurane concentrations (~1.3 MAC) only marginally affects caudal bath ventral root activity, and has no effect on rostral bath activity. At maximum isoflurane vaporizer output (~4 MAC) caudal ventral root bursting is depressed but motoneuron bursting continues. Rostral bursting (L2)

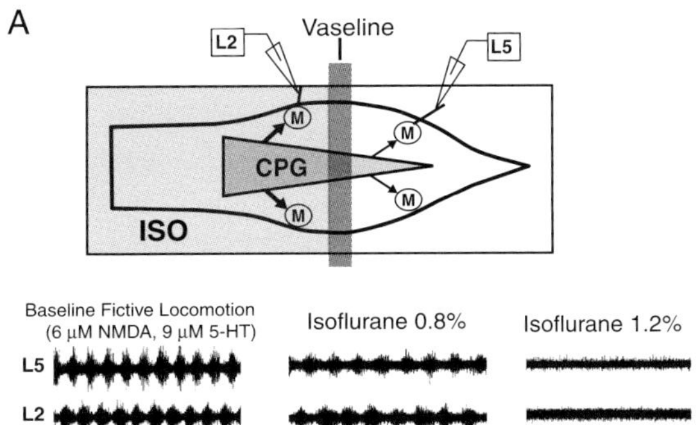

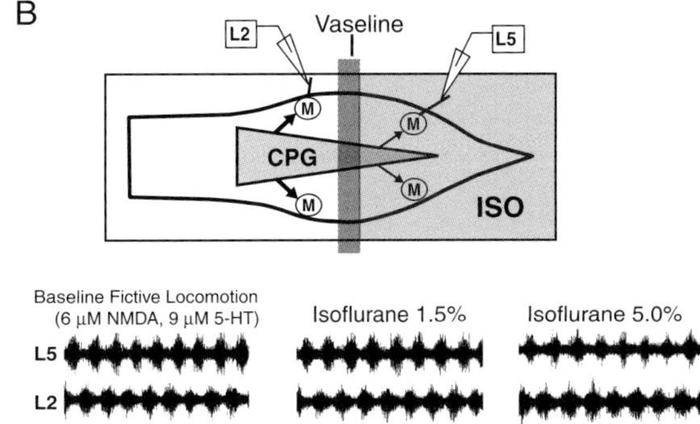

Figure 8.5 CPG organization in rodents and individual example of a split bath experiment, demonstrating that isoflurane acts selectively on the CPG to produce immobility in the neonatal rat spinal cord. The CPG controlling the hind limbs in mammals possesses a rostrocaudal gradient of rhythmogenic capacity, which is greatest in lower thoracic/upper lumbar segments (triangle represents CPG rhythm-generating capability). As in lampreys, alternating phases of glycinergic and glutamatergic CPG output produce motoneuron oscillations. A bath separation at L3/4 segregates the main CPG component from L5/6 motoneuron pools. Using pharmacologic, brainstem, or sensory activation of fictive locomotion, we can then test anesthetic effects on the CPG and motoneurons separately. The traces are ventral root activity recorded during a split bath experiment in a neonatal rat spinal cord, showing isoflurane (ISO) effects on NMDA/5HT-induced fictive locomotion. (A) Clinical concentrations of isoflurane applied to the rostral lumbar cord abolished both rostral (L2) and caudal (L5) ventral root activity. Immobilizing isoflurane concentrations are similar for whole-cord anesthetic delivery (data not shown). Note that the caudal L5 rhythm was abolished despite agonists present in the bath, but no anesthetic. This convincingly demonstrates that the rostral CPG is driving the caudal rhythm at agonist concentrations that fail to elicit locomotion in the caudal cord alone. (B) Isoflurane delivered to the caudal bath did not stop locomotion in caudal segments when isoflurane was approximately four times the normal immobilizing concentration. Caudal bath isoflurane application failed to affect rostral bath (L2) ventral root activity, again demonstrating that the rostral segments establish locomotion.

remains unaffected, again suggesting that the majority of CPG network is located in rostral hindlimb segments.

LIGAND-GATED ION CHANNELS AND IMMOBILITY

A large body of evidence shows that inhaled anesthetics modulate different ligand-gated ion channels. They can potentiate $GABA_A$ and glycine receptor function but suppress NMDA glutamate receptor function. It is still unclear to what degree inhaled anesthetics might cause immobility through enhancement of inhibitory synaptic transmission versus depression of excitatory synaptic transmission. There is evidence that anesthetics could produce immobility by modulating channels regulating intrinsic excitability or presynaptic transmitter release, possibly by enhancing conductances of two-pore potassium leak channels, or by inhibiting voltage-gated sodium (Nav) channels.[65–70] Still, little is known of the relative importance of all of these effects to anesthetic-induced immobility.

Eger and colleagues, as well as Rudolph and coworkers, have made major contributions to our understanding of what receptors and ion-channels are important to anesthesia and immobility.[71–73] Using a model in which rats receive intrathecal infusions, intracerebroventricular infusions, or both, of various ion-channel agonists and antagonists, Eger et al have found that $GABA_A$ receptors, glycine receptors, and NMDA receptors are involved, to varying degrees, in anesthetic-induced immobility. For example, for inhaled anesthetics, the $GABA_A$ receptor appears to be minimally involved, while the NMDA receptor is more important for ketamine. With regard to inhaled anesthetics, most studies suggest that no specific receptor is of paramount importance.[73]

The $GABA_A$ receptor has been shown to be critical to the action of propofol and etomidate. In a pioneering study, Rudolph and colleagues produced mice that had a mutation of the beta-3 subunit of the $GABA_A$ receptor. These mice were resistant to the actions of etomidate and propofol, but had only minimal increased requirements for inhaled anesthetics.[71,72] Sonner et al found that intravenous administration of the $GABA_A$ antagonist picrotoxin increased propofol requirements much more than isoflurane or ketamine requirements,[74] consistent with the work of Jurd et al.[71]

To understand the molecular mechanisms of anesthetic-induced immobility, we need to examine which, and to what degree, agents affect processes most essential to CPG and motoneuron function. The related hypotheses are able to be tested most directly in isolated spinal cord of lampreys and neonatal rodents, for which we have the most detailed understanding. Bath application of drugs to the isolated neonatal rodent or lamprey spinal cord, or intrathecal application of antagonists during stimulation of the MLR in adult cats,[75] demonstrate that both NMDA- and AMPA-type glutamate receptors are critical to locomotion throughout mammalian development and across vertebrate evolution. Because glutamate receptor antagonism in neonates blocks locomotor activity induced by other agonist drugs such as 5-HT, glutamatergic transmission appears essential to function within the CPG kernel, rather than merely providing extrinsic drive to this network.[76] Effects of clinically relevant concentrations of inhaled anesthetics on AMPA receptors are weak, and effects on NMDA receptors are modest.[1,77] It is not known if the magnitude of these effects on glutamatergic transmission in the spinal cord is sufficient to produce immobility.

Isoflurane reduces spontaneous activity of ventral horn neurons in cultured embryonic spinal cord slices through GABAergic and glycinergic mechanisms.[78] However, studies assessing effects of $GABA_A$ and glycine receptor antagonists on MAC suggest that inhaled anesthetic effects on $GABA_A$ receptors play little role in inhaled anesthetic-induced immobilization,[74,79] while actions at glycine receptors appear to play a partial role.[80,81] The limited role of inhibitory receptors in immobility suggests that inhaled anesthetics have important effects on intrinsic excitability of glutamatergic interneurons or their synaptic transmission. As mentioned, glycine receptors mediate left-right alternation in the neonatal rodent and lamprey spinal cord, and underlie the main component of rhythmic inhibition that motoneurons receive from the CPG. Studies of anesthetic effects on glycinergic and glutamatergic transmission to motoneurons in rodent spinal cord slice preparations indicate that anesthetic effects on interconnected inhibitory and excitatory neurons can, not surprisingly, be complex. For example, inhaled anesthetics can cause presynaptic suppression of glycine release, which counteracts postsynaptic enhancement of glycine-mediated currents, resulting in a net unchanged charge transfer.[80] Yet because excitatory currents are reduced, the *relative* amount of net inhibition on motoneurons is increased, which may explain why glycine receptors appear to play a partial but limited role in immobility. As mentioned, $GABA_A$ receptors play little role in inhaled anesthetic immobilizing effects despite a demonstrated significant enhancement of postsynaptic $GABA_A$ receptor currents by inhaled anesthetics. This inconsistency could be because inhaled anesthetics suppress presynaptic GABA release more so than glycine release, but more importantly it demonstrates that an isolated receptor effect may not necessarily extrapolate to an important role within an intact network.

Inhaled anesthetics also affect ion channels that modulate intrinsic neuronal excitability and/or transmitter release. There is debate surrounding the role of two-pore potassium channels in anesthetic action, and the evidence supporting or refuting this role will not be discussed here. Another channel of recent intense interest concerning inhaled anesthetic action is the voltage-gated sodium (Nav) channel. At present, there is little data regarding inhaled anesthetic effects on Nav currents in the spinal cord. However, intrathecal infusion of increased Na^+ concentrations in rats modestly increases isoflurane MAC.[82] Recently the persistent sodium current (INaP), mediated by Nav channels, was shown to be critical for locomotor rhythm generation in isolated rodent spinal cords.[83,84] In these studies, the ability of low micromolar concentrations of riluzole (3–10 μM) to abolish locomotor activity was attributed to inhibition of a tetrodotoxin-sensitive INaP. Because Nav channels are a plausible inhaled anesthetic target, and INaP mediated via Nav channels is so critical to locomotor rhythm generation, anesthetic effects on INaP is one plausible mechanism by which inhaled anesthetics produce immobility. However, investigations providing direct evidence of inhaled anesthetic effects on INaP in spinal neurons (and elsewhere in the central nervous system) are lacking. INaP plays an important role in rhythm generation for networks throughout the nervous system—in the spinal cord as well as in hippocampal and thalamocortical networks.[85–88] Therefore inhaled anesthetic effects on INaP could represent one mechanism common to several anesthetic endpoints (immobility, amnesia, unconsciousness).

SUMMARY

The spinal cord remains the key site where anesthetics, in particular inhaled anesthetics, produce immobility. However brainstem modulation must factor into our understanding of the complete picture of anesthetic-induced immobility. Understanding sites of anesthetic effects on different components of spinal sensorimotor circuits is important to understanding the mechanisms of anesthetic-induced immobility. Such knowledge becomes vital when considering the multitude of inhaled anesthetic effects that must be considered. We propose that immobility produced by inhaled anesthetics results primarily by disruption of the spinal locomotor network (CPG), more so than impeding local segmental sensory input or motor output. This primary immobilizing effect of CPG disruption appears to be conserved throughout vertebrate evolution—from lampreys to mammals. Lamprey and rodent isolated spinal cord preparations, while not having significant clinical relevance, complement one another by simplicity, and both represent powerful tools for exploring sites and mechanisms of anesthetics. Because the CPG is comprised of interacting excitatory and inhibitory neurons, it is necessary to understand how anesthetic effects on different receptors/channels play out in dynamic, operating networks. For many of these neuronal signaling processes it is unclear how important each effect is to producing immobility. However, the task of piecing this together becomes somewhat less daunting now that progress is being made toward understanding the sites of anesthetic action, and which factors are critical to normal function at these sites.

ACKNOWLEDGMENTS

We thank Dr. James T. Buchanan (Professor of Biological Sciences, Marquette University, Milwaukee, WI) for his advice, expertise, and training regarding lamprey intracellular spinal cord recordings.

REFERENCES

1. Krasowski MD, Harrison NL. General anaesthetic actions on ligand-gated ion channels. *Cell Mol Life Sci.* 1999; 55:1278–1303.
2. Bernard C: Lectures on Anesthetics and on Asphyxia. Medical study courses of the college De France 1875.
3. Merkel G, Eger EI. A comparative study of halothane and halopropane anesthesia: including a method for determining equipotency. *Anesthesiology.* 1963;24:346–357.
4. Quasha AL, Eger EI, Tinker JH. Determination and applications of MAC. *Anesthesiology.* 1980;53:315–334.
5. Antognini JF, Wang XW, Carstens E. Quantitative and qualitative effects of isoflurane on movement occurring after noxious stimulation. *Anesthesiology.* 1999;91:1064–1071.
6. Fukson OI, Berkinblit MB, Feldman AG. The spinal frog takes into account the scheme of its body during the wiping reflex. *Science.* 1980;209:1261–1263.
7. Woods JW. Behavior of chronic decerebrate rats. *J Neurophysiol.* 1964;27:635–644.
8. Heytens L, Verlooy J, Gheuens J, Bossaert L. Lazarus sign and extensor posturing in a brain-dead patient: Case report. *J Neurosurg.* 1989;71:449–451.
9. Christie JM, O'Lenic TD, Cane RD. Head turning in brain death. *J Clin Anesth.* 1996;8:141–143.
10. Rampil IJ, Laster MJ. No correlation between quantitative electroencephalographic measurements and movement response to noxious stimuli during isoflurane anesthesia in rats. *Anesthesiology.* 1992; 77:920–925.
11. Rampil IJ, Mason P, Singh H. Anesthetic potency (MAC) is independent of forebrain structures in the rat. *Anesthesiology.* 1993;78:707–712.
12. Antognini JF, Schwartz K. Exaggerated anesthetic requirements in the preferentially anesthetized brain. *Anesthesiology.* 1993;79:1244–1249.
13. Antognini JF, Carstens E, Atherley R. Does the immobilizing effect of thiopental in brain exceed that of halothane? *Anesthesiology.* 2002;96:980–986.
14. Jinks SL, Bravo M, Satter O, Chan YM. Brainstem regions affecting minimum alveolar concentration and movement pattern during isoflurane anesthesia. *Anesthesiology.* 2010;112:316–324.
15. Kingery WS, Agashe GS, Guo TZ, et al. Isoflurane and nociception: Spinal alpha2A adrenoceptors mediate antinociception while supraspinal alpha1 adrenoceptors mediate pronociception. *Anesthesiology.* 2002;96:367–374.
16. Devor M, Zalkind V: Reversible analgesia, atonia, and loss of consciousness on bilateral intracerebral microinjection of pentobarbital. Pain 2001;94:101–112.
17. Jinks SL, Dominguez CL, Antognini JF. Drastic decrease in isoflurane minimum alveolar concentration and limb movement forces after thoracic spinal cooling and chronic spinal transection in rats. *Anesthesiology.* 2005;102:624–632.
18. Whelan PJ. Control of locomotion in the decerebrate cat. *Prog Neurobiol.* 1996;49:481–515.
19. Kitahata LM, Ghazi-Saidi K, Yamashita M, Kosaka Y, Bonikos C, Taub A. The depressant effect of halothane and sodium thiopental on the spontaneous and evoked activity of dorsal horn cells: lamina specificity, time course and dose dependence. *J Pharmacol Exp Ther.* 1975;195:515–521.
20. Kitahata LM, Kosaka Y, Taub A, Bonikos K, Hoffert M. Lamina-specific suppression of dorsal-horn unit activity by morphine sulfate. *Anesthesiology.* 1974;41:39–48.
21. Antognini JF, Carstens E. Increasing isoflurane from 0.9 to 1.1 minimum alveolar concentration minimally affects dorsal horn cell responses to noxious stimulation. *Anesthesiology.* 1999;90: 208–214.
22. Jinks SL, Antognini JF, Carstens E. Isoflurane depresses diffuse noxious inhibitory controls in rats between 0.8 and 1.2 minimum alveolar anesthetic concentration. *Anesth Analg.* 2003;97:111–116, table of contents.
23. Jinks SL, Martin JT, Carstens E, Jung SW, Antognini JF. Peri-MAC depression of a nociceptive withdrawal reflex is accompanied by reduced dorsal horn activity with halothane but not isoflurane. *Anesthesiology.* 2003;98:1128–1138.
24. You HJ, Colpaert FC, Arendt-Nielsen L. Nociceptive spinal withdrawal reflexes but not spinal dorsal horn wide-dynamic range neuron activities are specifically inhibited by halothane anaesthesia in spinalized rats. *Eur J Neurosci.* 2005;22:354–360.
25. Burke RE, Degtyarenko AM, Simon ES. Patterns of locomotor drive to motoneurons and last-order interneurons: clues to the structure of the CPG. *J Neurophysiol.* 2001;86:447–462.
26. Degtyarenko AM, Simon ES, Norden-Krichmar T, Burke RE. Modulation of oligosynaptic cutaneous and muscle afferent reflex pathways during fictive locomotion and scratching in the cat. *J Neurophysiol.* 1998;79:447–463.
27. Moschovakis AK, Solodkin M, Burke RE. Anatomical and physiological study of interneurons in an oligosynaptic cutaneous reflex pathway in the cat hindlimb. *Brain Res.* 1992;586:311–318.
28. McCrea DA. Neuronal basis of afferent-evoked enhancement of locomotor activity. *Ann N Y Acad Sci.* 1998;860:216–225.
29. Jankowska E. Spinal interneuronal systems: identification, multifunctional character and reconfigurations in mammals. *J Physiol.* 2001;533:31–40.
30. Kim J, Yao A, Atherely RJ, Carstens E, Jinks SL, Antognini JF. Neurons in the ventral spinal cord are more depressed by isoflurane, halothane and propofol than are neurons in the dorsal spinal cord. *Anesth Analg.* 2007;105:1020–1026, table of contents.
31. Antognini JF, Atherley RJ, Dutton RC, Laster MJ, Eger EI, Carstens E. The excitatory and inhibitory effects of nitrous oxide on spinal neuronal responses to noxious stimulation. *Anesth Analg.* 2007;104:829–835.
32. Barter LS, Carstens EE, Jinks SL, Antognini JF. Rat dorsal horn nociceptive-specific neurons are more sensitive than wide dynamic range neurons to depression by immobilizing doses of volatile anesthetics: an effect partially reversed by the opioid receptor antagonist naloxone. *Anesth Analg.* 2009;109:641–647.
33. Jinks SL, Bravo M, Hayes SG. Volatile anesthetic effects on midbrain-elicited locomotion suggest that the locomotor network in the ventral spinal cord is the primary site for immobility. *Anesthesiology.* 2008;108:1016–1024.
34. Degtyarenko AM, Kaufman MP. Fictive locomotion and scratching inhibit dorsal horn neurons receiving thin fiber afferent input. *Am J Physiol Regul Integr Comp Physiol.* 2000;279:R394–R403.
35. Carstens E, Klumpp D, Zimmermann M. Differential inhibitory effects of medial and lateral midbrain stimulation on spinal neuronal discharges to noxious skin heating in the cat. *J Neurophysiol.* 1980;43:332–342.
36. Rampil IJ, King BS. Volatile anesthetics depress spinal motor neurons. *Anesthesiology.* 1996;85:129–134.
37. Zhou HH, Mehta M, Leis AA. Spinal cord motoneuron excitability during isoflurane and nitrous oxide anesthesia. *Anesthesiology.* 1997;86:302–307.
38. Cheng G, Kendig JJ. Enflurane directly depresses glutamate AMPA and NMDA currents in mouse spinal cord motor neurons independent of actions on GABAA or glycine receptors. *Anesthesiology.* 2000;93:1075–1084.

39. Jinks SL, Atherley RJ, Dominguez CL, Sigvardt KA, Antognini JF. Isoflurane disrupts central pattern generator activity and coordination in the lamprey isolated spinal cord. *Anesthesiology.* 2005;103: 567–575.
40. Jinks, SL: Volatile anesthetic immobilizing action in the lamprey isolated spinal cord: validation and pharmacology. *Society for Neuroscience Abstracts* 2007; Program No. 288.7.
41. Paggett KC, Jackson AW, McClellan AD. Organization of higher-order brain areas that initiate locomotor activity in larval lamprey. *Neuroscience.* 2004;125:25–33.
42. Edgley SA, Jankowska E, Shefchyk S. Evidence that mid-lumbar neurones in reflex pathways from group II afferents are involved in locomotion in the cat. *J Physiol.(Lond).* 1988;403:57–71.
43. Hagevik A, McClellan AD. Coordination of locomotor activity in the lamprey: role of descending drive to oscillators along the spinal cord. *Exp Brain Res.* 1999;128:481–490.
44. Butt SJ, Kiehn O. Functional identification of interneurons responsible for left-right coordination of hindlimbs in mammals. *Neuron.* 2003;38:953–963.
45. Kjaerulff O, Kiehn O. Distribution of networks generating and coordinating locomotor activity in the neonatal rat spinal cord in vitro: a lesion study. *J Neurosci.* 1996;16:5777–5794.
46. Barbeau H, McCrea DA, O'Donovan MJ, Rossignol S, Grill WM, Lemay MA. Tapping into spinal circuits to restore motor function. *Brain Res Rev.* 1999;30:27–51.
47. Fulton JF, Sherrington CS. State of the flexor reflex in paraplegic dog and monkey respectively. *J Physiol.* 1932;17–22.
48. Alford S, Schwartz E, Viana di Prisco G: The pharmacology of vertebrate spinal central pattern generators. *Neuroscientist.* 2003;9: 217–228.
49. Whelan P, Bonnot A, O'Donovan MJ. Properties of rhythmic activity generated by the isolated spinal cord of the neonatal mouse. *J Neurophysiol.* 2000;84:2821–2833.
50. Hinckley CA, Hartley R, Wu L, Todd A, Ziskind-Conhaim L. Locomotor-like rhythms in a genetically distinct cluster of interneurons in the mammalian spinal cord. *J Neurophysiol.* 2005;93: 1439–1449.
51. Buchanan JT, Grillner S. Newly identified "glutamate interneurons" and their role in locomotion in the lamprey spinal cord. *Science.* 1987;236:312–314.
52. Butt SJ, Lebret JM, Kiehn O. Organization of left-right coordination in the mammalian locomotor network. *Brain Res Rev.* 2002;40: 107–117.
53. Buchanan JT. Commissural interneurons in rhythm generation and intersegmental coupling in the lamprey spinal cord. *J Neurophysiol.* 1999;81:2037–2045.
54. Wallen P, Williams TL. Fictive locomotion in the lamprey spinal cord in vitro compared with swimming in the intact and spinal animal. *J Physiol.* 1984;347:225–239.
55. Rovainen CM. Neurobiology of lampreys. *Physiol Rev.* 1979; 59:1007–1077.
56. Buchanan JT. The roles of spinal interneurons and motoneurons in the lamprey locomotor network. *Prog Brain Res.* 1999;123:| 311–321.
57. Dale N. Excitatory synaptic drive for swimming mediated by amino acid receptors in the lamprey. *J Neurosci.* 1986;6:2662–2675.
58. Buchanan JT, Cohen AH: Activities of identified interneurons, motoneurons, and muscle fibers during fictive swimming in the lamprey and effects of reticulospinal and dorsal cell stimulation. *J Neurophysiol.* 1982;47:948–960.
59. Clarac F, Pearlstein E, Pflieger JF, Vinay L. The in vitro neonatal rat spinal cord preparation: a new insight into mammalian locomotor mechanisms. *J Comp Physiol A Neuroethol Sens Neural Behav Physiol.* 2004;190:343–357.
60. Zaporozhets E, Cowley KC, Schmidt BJ. A reliable technique for the induction of locomotor-like activity in the in vitro neonatal rat spinal cord using brainstem electrical stimulation. *J Neurosci Methods.* 2004;139:33–41.
61. Mortin LI, Stein PS. Spinal cord segments containing key elements of the central pattern generators for three forms of scratch reflex in the turtle. *J Neurosci.* 1989;9:2285–2296.
62. Deliagina TG, Orlovsky GN, Pavlova GA. The capacity for generation of rhythmic oscillations is distributed in the lumbosacral spinal cord of the cat. *Exp Brain Res.* 1983;53:81–90.
63. Cazalets JR, Borde M, Clarac F. Localization and organization of the central pattern generator for hindlimb locomotion in newborn rat. *J Neurosci.* 1995;15:4943–4951.
64. Hemmings HC, Jr., Akabas MH, Goldstein PA, Trudell JR, Orser BA, Harrison NL: Emerging molecular mechanisms of general anesthetic action. *Trends Pharmacol Sci.* 2005; 26: 503–510.
65. Ouyang W, Wang G, Hemmings HC Jr. Isoflurane and propofol inhibit voltage-gated sodium channels in isolated rat neurohypophysial nerve terminals. *Mol Pharmacol.* 2003;64:373–381.
66. Franks NP, Lieb WR. Volatile general anaesthetics activate a novel neuronal K^+ current. *Nature.* 1988;333:662–664.
67. Yost CS. Update on tandem pore (2P) domain K^+ channels. *Curr Drug Targets.* 2003;4:347–351.
68. Wu XS, Sun JY, Evers AS, Crowder M, Wu LG. Isoflurane inhibits transmitter release and the presynaptic action potential. *Anesthesiology.* 2004;100:663–670.
69. Ying SW, Abbas SY, Harrison NL, Goldstein PA: Propofol block of I(h) contributes to the suppression of neuronal excitability and rhythmic burst firing in thalamocortical neurons. *Eur J Neurosci.* 2006;23:465–480.
70. Chen X, Sirois JE, Lei Q, Talley EM, Lynch C, 3rd, Bayliss DA: HCN subunit-specific and cAMP-modulated effects of anesthetics on neuronal pacemaker currents. J Neurosci. 2005;25:5803–5814.
71. Jurd R, Arras M, Lambert S, Drexler B, Siegwart R, Crestani F, Zaugg M, Vogt KE, Ledermann B, Antkowiak B, Rudolph U. General anesthetic actions in vivo strongly attenuated by a point mutation in the GABA(A) receptor beta3 subunit. *FASEB J.* 2003;17:250–252.
72. Liao M, Sonner JM, Jurd R, Rudolph U, Borghese CM, Harris RA, Laster MJ, Eger EI. Beta3-containing gamma-aminobutyric acidA receptors are not major targets for the amnesic and immobilizing actions of isoflurane. *Anesth Analg.* 2005;101:412–418, table of contents.
73. Eger EI, 2nd, Raines DE, Shafer SL, Hemmings HC Jr., Sonner JM. Is a new paradigm needed to explain how inhaled anesthetics produce immobility? *Anesth Analg.* 2008;107:832–48.
74. Sonner JM, Zhang Y, Stabernack C, Abaigar W, Xing Y, Laster MJ. GABA(A) receptor blockade antagonizes the immobilizing action of propofol but not ketamine or isoflurane in a dose-related manner. *Anesth Analg.* 2003;96:706–712, table.
75. Douglas JR, Noga BR, Dai X, Jordan LM. The effects of intrathecal administration of excitatory amino acid agonists and antagonists on the initiation of locomotion in the adult cat. *J Neurosci.* 1993;13:990–1000.
76. Kiehn O. Locomotor circuits in the mammalian spinal cord. *Annu Rev Neurosci.* 2006;29:279–306.
77. Hollmann MW, Liu HT, Hoenemann CW, Liu WH, Durieux ME. Modulation of NMDA receptor function by ketamine and magnesium, Part II: interactions with volatile anesthetics. *Anesth Analg.* 2001;92:1182–1191.
78. Grasshoff C, Antkowiak B. Effects of isoflurane and enflurane on GABAA and glycine receptors contribute equally to depressant actions on spinal ventral horn neurones in rats. *Br J Anaesth.* 2006;97:687–694.
79. Zhang Y, Sonner JM, Eger EI, 2nd, Stabernack CR, Laster MJ, Raines DE, Harris RA. Gamma-aminobutyric acidA receptors do not mediate the immobility produced by isoflurane. *Anesth Analg.* 2004;99:85–90.

80. Cheng G, Kendig JJ. Pre- and postsynaptic volatile anaesthetic actions on glycinergic transmission to spinal cord motor neurons. *Br J Pharmacol.* 2002;136: 673–684.
81. Zhang Y, Laster MJ, Hara K, Harris RA, Eger EI, 2nd, Stabernack CR, Sonner JM. Glycine receptors mediate part of the immobility produced by inhaled anesthetics. *Anesth Analg.* 2003;96:97–101, table of contents.
82. Laster MJ, Zhang Y, Eger EI, 2nd, Shnayderman D, Sonner JM. Alterations in spinal, but not cerebral, cerebrospinal fluid Na^+ concentrations affect the isoflurane minimum alveolar concentration in rats. *Anesth Analg.* 2007;105:661–665.
83. Tazerart S, Viemari JC, Darbon P, Vinay L, Brocard F. Contribution of persistent sodium current to locomotor pattern generation in neonatal rats. *J Neurophysiol.* 2007;98:613–628.
84. Zhong G, Masino MA, Harris-Warrick RM. Persistent sodium currents participate in fictive locomotion generation in neonatal mouse spinal cord. *J Neurosci.* 2007;27:4507–4518.
85. French CR, Sah P, Buckett KJ, Gage PW. A voltage-dependent persistent sodium current in mammalian hippocampal neurons. *J Gen Physiol.* 1990;95:1139–1157.
86. Martella G, De Persis C, Bonsi P, Natoli S, Cuomo D, Bernardi G, Calabresi P, Pisani A. Inhibition of persistent sodium current fraction and voltage-gated L-type calcium current by propofol in cortical neurons: implications for its antiepileptic activity. *Epilepsia.* 2005;46:624–635.
87. Stafstrom CE, Schwindt PC, Crill WE. Negative slope conductance due to a persistent subthreshold sodium current in cat neocortical neurons in vitro. *Brain Res.* 1982;236:221–226.
88. Timofeev I, Grenier F, Steriade M. Impact of intrinsic properties and synaptic factors on the activity of neocortical networks in vivo. *J Physiol Paris.* 2000;94:343–355.

9

MECHANISMS OF SPINAL ANALGESIA

Adam J. Carinci, Mihir M. Kamdar,

Smith C. Manion, and Jianren Mao

INTRODUCTION

Intraspinal drug delivery is used extensively for a variety of pain conditions including both malignant and nonmalignant etiologies. The first report on the clinical use of spinal analgesia was described in 1899 by Dr. August Bier, who published a series of six cases of orthopedic surgery under spinal anesthesia with cocaine.[1] To date, preservative free morphine and ziconotide are the only drugs approved by the Food and Drug Administration (FDA) for intraspinal delivery for chronic pain management.[2] Baclofen is also FDA-approved, but only for the specific indication of spasticity. There are, however, a number of agents that have been used safely and successfully to provide analgesia via the intraspinal route. Current therapies can be broadly divided into seven general categories of compounds based on their common mechanisms of action: opioids, local anesthetics, α_2-adrenergic agonists, N-type voltage-sensitive calcium channel blockers, GABA agonists, NMDA antagonists, and others. (See Table 9.1) Herein we describe these various compounds, with particular attention to their mechanisms of action.

SPINAL NEURAL ANATOMY

The spinal cord begins at the base of the brainstem and typically terminates at the L1-L2 level in the adult as the conus medullaris. Variation does exist however, as the spinal cord may end at T12 in 30% of individuals and at L3 in 10% of individuals.[4] The spinal cord gives rise to 31 pairs of spinal nerves, each composed of an anterior motor root and a posterior sensory root. Each nerve root is composed of multiple rootlets. A cord segment is the portion of the spinal cord that gives rise to all of the rootlets of a single spinal nerve. Each spinal nerve exits through the intervertebral foramen to divide into the posterior primary ramus and the anterior primary ramus. (Figure 9.1). A dermatome describes the skin area innervated by a given spinal nerve and its corresponding cord segment. Dermatome levels are important in accessing the height of a given intraspinal block.

Numerous variables have been explored as potential determinants of block height (Table 9.2). The single most significant physiologic factor related to block height is cerebrospinal fluid (CSF) volume, whereas the principle variables that can be manipulated to alter block height are baricity, drug dose, and patient positioning.

INTRATHECAL OPIOIDS

While the use of spinally administered opioid analgesia may have begun over a century ago, our knowledge of the mechanism by which intrathecal opioids mediate antinociception has evolved significantly over the past quarter century. Morphine was used intrathecally as early as 1901 by the Japanese surgeon Otojiro Kitagawa,[6] though it was not until the early 1970s that opioid receptors were first proposed[7] and described in the central nervous system.[8] In 1976, the existence of multiple classes of opioid receptors was proposed,[9] and in the same year the first demonstration of analgesia from intrathecal administration of opioids in an animal model was demonstrated.[10] Soon thereafter, Wang and colleagues reported analgesia from intrathecal delivery of morphine in humans with cancer pain in 1979.[11] Over the past 30 years, spinally delivered opioid therapy has become a standard means of analgesia for treating acute and chronic forms of both malignant and nonmalignant pain.

CELLULAR MECHANISMS OF SPINAL OPIOID ANALGESIA

Intense noxious stimuli has been shown to cause activation of second-order neurons within the spinal cord dorsal horn mediated through release of substance P, glutamate, and calcitonin gene-related peptide (CGRP) from presynaptic terminals of peripheral nociceptors within laminae I and II.[12–13] Likewise, noxious stimuli have also been shown to cause release of endogenous opioid peptides, such as endorphins and enkephalins, into the spinal cord dorsal horn, causing activation of opioid receptor–mediated analgesic pathways.[14–17] Hence the transmission of pain from

Table 9.1 INTRATHECAL DRUGS OVERVIEW[3]

DRUG CLASS	DRUG(S)
Opioids:	Morphine, Hydromorphone, Fentanyl, Sufentanil, Meperidine, Methadone
Local Anesthetics	Common: Bupivacaine, Ropivacaine, Tetracaine Less Common: Lidocaine, Procaine, Mepivacaine
α_2-Adrenergic Agonists	Clonidine/Tizanidine
N-Type Voltage-Sensitive Calcium Channel Blockers	Ziconotide
GABA Agonists	Baclofen/Midazolam
NMDA Antagonists	Ketamine
Others:	Adenosine, Aspirin, Droperidol, Gabapentin, Ketorolac, Neostigmine, Octreotide

the periphery to the cortex relies on a complex balance between both excitation of the nociceptive pathways and inhibition by antinociceptive spinal opioid pathways.

Studies have demonstrated the presence of multiple distinct sites of opioid action. First, opioid receptors have been demonstrated to exist in the periphery, which attenuate the excitability of primary afferent nociceptors. However, while peripheral opioid receptors exist, the primary sites of opioid-induced antinociception appear to occur within the central nervous system. In particular, these effects occur in the superficial layers of the substantia gelatinosa of the dorsal horn in the spinal cord, where primary afferent Aδ and C-fibers terminate. Within the dorsal horn, opioid receptors exist on the presynaptic terminals of these primary afferent nociceptors, as well as on the postsynaptic membranes of second-order neurons in the dorsal horn.[18] Supraspinal opioid receptors have been found in the brainstem, thalamus, and cortex.[18] The above sites of opioid receptors belong to what is referred to as the *ascending pain pathway*. Opioid receptors have also been discovered in the midbrain periaqueductal gray (PAG), rostral ventral medulla, and nucleus raphe magnus, which activate descending inhibitory pathways.[18] All of the above sites of opioid receptors except for peripherally located receptors, play a significant role in spinally mediated opioid analgesia.

A major step in the understanding of opioid antinociception came in the early 1990s, when molecular cloning yielded discovery of three distinct genes encoding mu, kappa, and delta opioid receptors (MORs, KORs, and DORs, respectively).[19–22] Furthermore, numerous subclasses of opioid receptors such as mu_{1-2}, delta_{1-2}, and kappa_{1-4} have been described.[23–24]

Regardless of classes and subclasses, all opioid receptors belong to the rhodopsin G-protein coupled receptor superfamily. When exogenous or endogenous opioid ligands bind to the G-protein coupled opioid receptor, a conformational change occurs in the receptor, activating a cascade of events that result in either adenyl cyclase inhibition, inhibition of voltage-gated calcium channels, activation of potassium channels, or a combination of these events to cause inhibition of neuronal activation.

In particular, activation of the MOR on the presynaptic terminals of primary afferent nociceptors in the dorsal horn causes activation of the $G\alpha_I$ subunit of the opioid receptor, which binds to adenylyl cyclase and hence inhibits production of cyclic adenosine monophosphate (cAMP). Decreased cyclic AMP levels indirectly resulting in inhibition of presynaptic voltage-gated calcium channels play an important

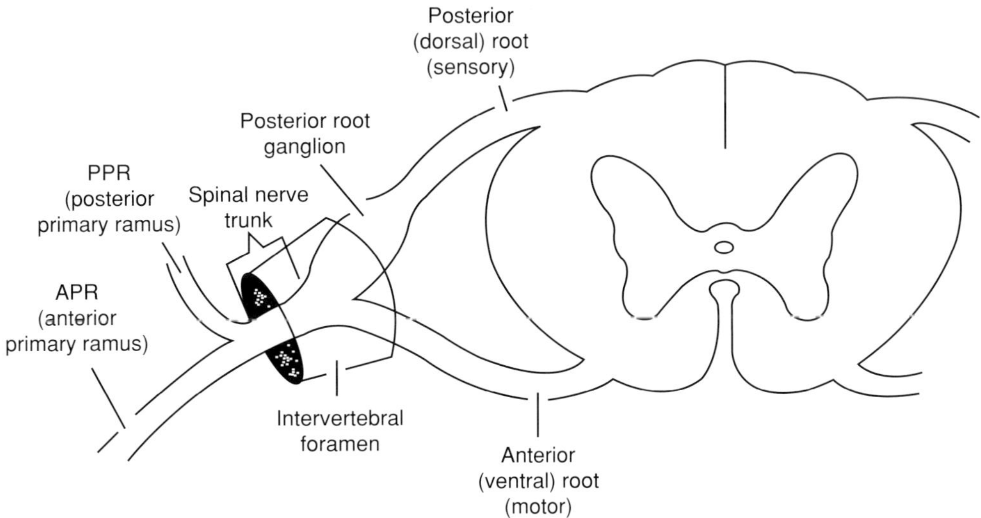

Figure 9.1 Spinal cord and spinal nerve.

Table 9.2 **DETERMINANTS OF BLOCK HEIGHT**[5]

Patient Characteristics
Age
Height
Weight
Gender
Intra-abdominal Pressure
Characteristics of Injectate
Baricity
Dose
Concentration
Volume
Temperature
Technical Variations
Patient Positioning
Site of Injection
Speed of Injection
Direction of Bevel
Barbotage
CSF Characteristics
Volume
Density
Velocity, Circulation

role in release of nociception-related pain neurotransmitters such as substance P, glutamate, and CGRP from the presynaptic terminal of afferent nociceptors. Hence through this mechanism, activation of opioid receptors indirectly causes suppression of nociceptive pain transmission by inhibiting neurotransmitter release from the terminals of afferent nociceptors within the spinal cord dorsal horn.

Opioid receptor activation also results in direct effects on both presynaptic and postsynaptic potassium channels. Agonist binding to the MOR and DOR activates the $G\beta\gamma$ subunit of the opioid receptor, which directly opens membrane G-protein inward rectifying potassium (GIRK) channels within the spinal cord dorsal horn, allowing potassium ions to flow down their transcellular concentration gradient. This efflux of potassium ions results in hyperpolarization of the neurons, which plays an important role in the postsynaptic suppression of second-order neurons and subsequent inhibition of ascending pain transmission.[25]

Descending modulatory pathways also serve an important role in the mechanism by which opioids cause analgesia within the spinal cord.[18,26] These pathways originate in the supraspinal regions but mediate their inhibitory effects within the spinal cord. Opioid receptors exist within the descending modulatory pathways beginning in the PAG region of the midbrain. Neurons of PAG origin synapse in the medullary reticular formation and locus coeruleus, likely through a process of disinhibition of active interneurons. The medullary reticular formation and locus coeruleus then project to the spinal cord dorsal horn via the dorsolateral funiculus. The terminal targets of the dorsolateral funiculus include primary afferent nociceptors, second-order neurons (projection neurons), and spinal interneurons. It is believed that this descending modulatory system exerts its effects via two mechanisms: 1) local release of endogenous opioids from interneurons within the spinal cord dorsal horn, and 2) release of norepinephrine and serotonin, which both serve to inhibit release of neurotransmitters from the presynaptic terminal and to suppress the activation of postsynaptic second-order neurons.

Furthermore, intrathecal opioids may contribute to analgesia by means of spinal adenosine release and adenosine receptor activation. Similar to opioid receptors, adenosine receptors have been found in high concentration within the dorsal horn of the spinal cord. Intrathecal opioids have been shown to cause increased levels of adenosine within the CSF.[27] This increase in spinal adenosine was not seen with intravenous opioids, possibly suggesting a role in spinally mediated opioid analgesia.

INTRATHECAL OPIOID PHARMACOKINETICS

Once administered into the intrathecal space, the lipophilicity of individual opioids dictates their distribution, and the differences in dispersion often predict their varying clinical effects.

The pharmacologic distribution and clearance kinetics of intrathecal opioids is a complex phenomenon, as Ummenhofer demonstrated in 2000.[28] Upon delivery into the intrathecal space, opioids concurrently 1) enter the spinal cord to bind to opioid receptors in the dorsal horn as well as to nonspecific sites in the white matter, 2) travel cephalad toward supraspinal regions within the CSF, and 3) move across the dura mater into the epidural space and distribute into the epidural fat (Figure 9.2). Opioids within the spinal cord and epidural space are eventually cleared into the systemic plasma compartment via venous uptake.

It is the sum of these routes of distribution that dictate the pharmacologic profile of intrathecal opioids, including the time of onset, duration of action, and extent of rostral travel. In fact, the potency of various intrathecal opioids has been shown to be inversely proportional to their respective

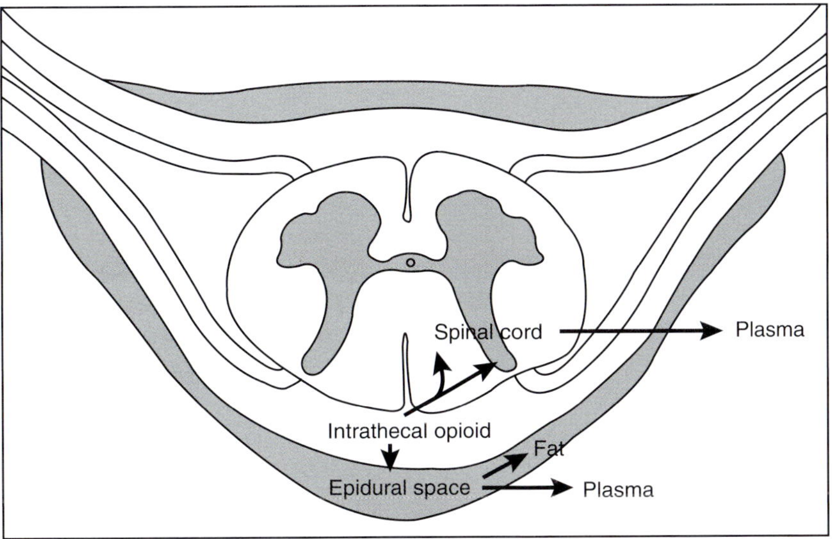

Figure 9.2 Disposition of opioid after intrathecal administration.

lipophilicity. Lipophilic opioids, such as fentanyl and SL Sufentanıl, traverse rapidly into the spinal cord and bind to opioid receptors within the spinal cord dorsal horn, prior to entering the plasma compartment. Lipophilic opioids also diffuse quickly across the dura into the epidural fat and are hence rapidly cleared into the systemic circulation. Furthermore, lipophilic opioids have limited cephalad spread given their rapidity of distribution. The aggregate of these characteristics results in lipophilic opioids having a quicker onset of analgesic action, a briefer duration of action, a narrower band of effect at the injection site, and earlier respiratory depression as compared to hydrophilic opioids.

Conversely, hydrophilic opioids, such as morphine and hydromorphone, travel more slowly into the spinal cord, with less affinity for nonspecific binding in the white matter and more specificity for opioid receptors in the dorsal horn, resulting in slower clearance into the venous system. Hydrophilic opioids cross the dura more slowly into the epidural space, where they bind less to the epidural fat and have slower uptake into the plasma compartment. For these reasons, hydrophilic opioids tend to have a greater reservoir within the CSF, and hence have a slower onset of action, a longer duration of action, and a higher degree of cephalad spread, yielding a wider band of effect at the site of injection and delayed respiratory depression.

MORPHINE

Morphine is a prototypic mu-opioid receptor agonist and also the most hydrophilic of the commonly used intrathecal opioids, which is reflected in its clinical characteristics as a spinal analgesic. Intrathecal morphine has a relatively slow onset due to its slower diffusion to opioid receptors in the dorsal horn as compared to its more lipophilic counterparts. Likewise, the hydrophilic nature of morphine yields a smaller intrathecal volume of distribution and slower spinal clearance, as evidenced by data demonstrating that morphine is not detectable in the systemic circulation for two hours following intrathecal administration.[29] Slow clearance of intrathecal morphine yields a higher relative concentration within the CSF, resulting in a long duration of action and increased rostral spread. Increased rostral spread causes a wider band of analgesia for intrathecal morphine as compared to other opioids, and also carries a higher risk of the potential for delayed respiratory depression. The relative potency of intrathecal morphine is felt to be approximately 10 times that of epidural morphine, and approximately 100 times that of intravenous morphine.[30]

As aforementioned, intrathecal opioid clearance to the systemic circulation occurs via venous uptake by the spinal vasculature. Nonetheless with transient administration of morphine, it appears there is limited metabolism within the CSF as demonstrated by the similarity in terms of duration of action of intrathecal morphine and its rate of clearance to the plasma circulation.[31] Morphine-6-glucuronide (M6G) and morphine-3-glucuronide (M3G) are the two primary active metabolites of morphine. M6G is felt to generate analgesic properties of morphine,[32] but also contributes to side effect of morphine-related respiratory depression.[33] Unlike M6G, M3G does not appear to have analgesic properties, but demonstrates neuro-excitatory effects when administered directly into the CNS.[34] Intrathecal potency of M6G has been shown to be between 10 and 45 times greater than that of morphine.[35]

Morphine is perhaps the most commonly used neuraxial opioid in the clinical setting and is the only opioid that has been approved by the FDA for intrathecal use. Furthermore, polyanalgesic consensus guidelines regarding the management of pain by intrathecal drug delivery have recommended morphine as a first-line agent.[36]

HYDROMORPHONE

Hydromorphone is a semisynthetic ketone of morphine and, like morphine, is considered to be relatively hydrophilic, though not quite to the same degree. Because of its slightly more lipophilic nature, hydromorphone has a faster onset of action and shorter duration than morphine. Furthermore, intrathecal potency of hydromorphone is approximately five times that of morphine, with an equivalent or more favorable side effect profile perhaps due to fewer active metabolites than morphine and smaller volume of distribution.[36–38] The effects of hydromorphone appear to be mediated by mu- as well as delta- and kappa-opioid receptors, unlike morphine, which is a prototypic mu-opioid receptor agonist.[39] Hydromorphone has been suggested as an alternative first-line intrathecal analgesic agent to morphine according to recent polyanalgesic consensus guidelines.[36]

FENTANYL

Fentanyl is a highly lipophilic anilidopiperidine opioid with a partition coefficient (octanol:water) 100 times greater than morphine.[40] Due to its lipophilicity, fentanyl has a rapid onset of action, limited duration of effect, restricted segmental area of analgesia, and limited cephalad spread. Given its rapid clearance from the CSF to the plasma compartment, there has been some thought that the effects of intrathecal fentanyl may be mediated though systemic effects; however when administered intrathecally, fentanyl is 10 times more potent than intravenous fentanyl, suggesting there is a greater local effect at the spinal level when delivered directly into the CSF.[38]

SUFENTANIL

Sufentanil is the 4-anilidopiperadine thienyl analog of fentanyl, a selective mu-opioid receptor agonist and frequently studied intrathecal analgesic.[41] However, sufentanil is even more lipophilic than fentanyl, with a partition coefficient (octanol:water) 1000 times greater than morphine.[40] ecause of its highly lipophilic nature, sufentanil has an extremely rapid onset of action, limited duration of effect, restricted segmental area of analgesia, and limited cephalad spread. Furthermore, it requires binding to fewer opioid receptors than morphine to yield equianalgesia. It is even more potent than fentanyl with a comparative 4.5 times greater potency when administered intrathecally in obstetric patients.[42]

METHADONE

Methadone is a unique opioid in that the commonly used clinical form is a racemic mixture of D- and L-isomers, each of which carry different properties. The L-isomer mediates the majority of the opioid properties of methadone. The D-isomer is a weak opioid that has low-affinity for the N-methyl-D-aspartate (NMDA) glutamate receptor. The NMDA receptor has been shown to play a role in neuropathic pain, central sensitization, and hyperalgesia.[43–44] An animal study isolating the antinociceptive and antihyperalgesia effects of each of the methadone isomers demonstrated that D-methadone decreased morphine-induced hyperalgesia and enhanced antinociception.[45] Hence, methadone may have potential added clinical benefit in situations of neuropathic pain and hyperalgesia as compared to other opioids. Methadone is considered a lipophilic opioid, and has been shown to have rapid clearance from the CSF and limited rostral spread as compared to morphine when administered intrathecally, predicting a rapid onset of action and more segmental effect similar to other lipophilic opioids.[46]

MEPERIDINE

Meperidine is a synthetic phenylpiperidine opioid with local anesthetic-like properties through its effects on sodium channels.[47] Furthermore, meperidine has intermediate lipophilicity, with a quicker onset, more rapid clearance, and less cephalad spread than morphine.[48] These properties make meperidine a good potential candidate for the treatment of neuropathic and postsurgical pain. However, meperidine and its active metabolite, normeperidine, have been shown to cause neuro-excitatory effects when administered intrathecally.[49] Furthermore, meperidine has been associated with frequent nausea and vomiting.[38] For these reasons, meperidine has not gained significant popularity as an intrathecal analgesic.

LOCAL ANESTHETICS

Clinically useful and spinally administered local anesthetics include bupivacaine, ropivacaine, and tetracaine, although the use of lidocaine, procaine, and mepivacaine has also been reported. Bupivacaine has a long track record for its safety and efficacy[50] and is the most common local anesthetic administered when a long duration of anesthetic block is required. All local anesthetics share the same basic structure, consisting of a lipophilic aromatic ring linked to a hydrophilic amino group via an intermediate alkyl chain consisting of either an amide or ester linkage. The nature of this linkage is the basis for classifying local anesthetics as either esters or amides. Local anesthetics in solution are weak bases that exist in equilibrium between the lipid-soluble neutral form and the charged hydrophilic form. The charged form appears to be the predominantly active form responsible for the pharmacologic mechanism of action.[51]

Local anesthetics, given intrathecally, exert a profound neuronal block by virtue of their sodium channel blocking properties. The failure of Na^+ ion channel permeability to increase slows the rate of cell membrane depolarization so that the threshold potential is not reached and thus an action potential is not propagated. Local anesthetics render neurons less excitable by directly binding to and inhibiting the ability of voltage-gated Na^+ channels to conduct Na^+ currents.[51–52] This action essentially prevents a conformational change in the Na^+ channel itself, thereby inhibiting the propagation of the action potential and thus the nerve conduction. Local anesthetics administered within the subarachnoid space act on the superficial layers of the spinal cord, but the principal site of action is the preganglionic fibers as they leave the spinal cord in the anterior rami. Multiple studies have shown that following intrathecal administration of local anesthetics, somatosensory evoked potentials from the tibial nerve (peripheral nervous system) are abolished, whereas direct spinal cord stimulation remains unchanged.[53–54] This is consistent with the theory that the spinal nerve rootlets are the primary site of action of intrathecally administered local anesthetics, not the spinal cord per se.[5]

α-2 ADRENERGIC AGONISTS (CLONIDINE/TIZANIDINE)

The analgesic effect of spinally administered α-2 agonists has been observed in numerous species including the mouse, rat, cat, dog, sheep, goat, and primate. Bulbospinal noradrenergic pathways project via the lateral funiculi to the dorsal and ventral gray matter, where α-2 agonists appear to regulate antinociceptive processes. Further, the antinociceptive effects of α-2-agonist have been shown to be blocked by spinal administration of α-2 antagonists such as yohimbine. However, the exact mechanism of action of the α-2 agonists remains incompletely understood.

The two most commonly used α-2 adrenoreceptor agonist drugs are clonidine and tizanidine, although dexmetotomidine has been used intravenously. Clonidine and tizanidine are highly lipid soluble and rapidly absorbed and eliminated from the CSF. Their antinociceptive mechanism appears to correlate with binding to the α-2 receptor in the superficial layers of the spinal cord dorsal horn as opposed to the ventral horn of the spinal cord. α-2 adrenoreceptor agonists are thought to mediate presynaptic inhibition of neurotransmitter release from C-afferent fibers, such as substance P and CGRP and also mediate a postsynaptic effect on spinal cord dorsal horn transmission neurons. Activation of α-2 adrenergic receptors (so-called autoreceptors) can block the opening of voltage-sensitive calcium channels and hyperpolarize neurons by a G_i-coupled potassium conductance.[55] The rapid onset of antinociceptive action when α-2 agonists are given intrathecally provides a strong argument that the major pharmacologic effects occur at the segmental spinal level. However, sedation and analgesia from α-2 adrenergic agonists occur by actions within a small group of neurons in the locus coeruleus of the brainstem. Thus, a supraspinal mechanism cannot be excluded, as may be seen with rapid drug absorption and systemic redistribution.[56] Intraspinal clonidine and tizanidine do not demonstrate evidence of local neurotoxicity.[57]

N-TYPE VOLTAGE-SENSITIVE CALCIUM CHANNEL BLOCKERS (ZICONOTIDE)

Ziconotide (also known as SNX-111) is a synthetic version of the omega-conotoxin MVIIA originally isolated from the venom of the predatory marine snail *Conus magnus*. In animals, it has been shown to be a selective and reversible blocker of the N-type voltage-sensitive calcium channels, although its mechanism of action in humans remains to be determined.[58] Neuronal N-type voltage-sensitive calcium channels are highly expressed in the superficial laminae (I and II) of the spinal cord dorsal horn and are also found in presynaptic nerve terminals, where they permit the calcium influx necessary for depolarization-induced neurotransmitter release from both central and peripheral nerves. By blocking the N-type voltage-sensitive calcium channels, ziconotide inhibits release of excitatory transmitters such as glutamate, CGRP, and substance P involved in neuronal excitability and neurotransmission from nociceptive afferents (A-δ and C-fibers) that terminate in the spinal cord dorsal horn. Ziconotide has been shown to diminish heat hyperalgesia and mechanical allodynia in animal models and continues to be studied in both neuropathic and cancer-related pain states in humans.[59–60] Despite its narrow therapeutic window and associated adverse effects, it remains the only other agent along with morphine that is FDA-approved for intrathecal administration.

GABA AGONISTS (BACLOFEN/MIDAZOLAM)

BACLOFEN

Numerous studies have evaluated the antinociceptive and antispasmodic properties of baclofen when administered via the intrathecal route. Baclofen is a gamma-aminobutyric acid (GABA) receptor$_B$ agonist that has poor lipid solubility and does not readily cross the blood-brain barrier when administered orally. The excessive systemic effects of high-dose oral baclofen can be minimized when administered directly into the cerebrospinal fluid.

The $GABA_B$ receptor is G_i/G_o-protein-coupled with mixed effects on adenylate cyclase activity. Baclofen binds the $GABA_B$ receptor and inhibits neurotransmitter release onto spinal cord motor neurons. Baclofen largely acts presynaptically on small diameter primary afferent terminals, as it binds to presynaptic receptors at lower concentrations than it does at postsynaptic receptors. Presynaptic activation decreases the evoked release of sensory neurotransmitters such as substance P and glutamate by suppressing neuronal calcium conductance. Baclofen also binds to postsynaptic $GABA_B$ receptors where activation produces an increase in membrane potassium conductance and associated neuronal hyperpolarization.[61] $GABA_B$ receptor agonists have also been shown to inhibit the expression of neurokinin-1 receptor mRNA.[62] The highest density of $GABA_B$ binding sites is in the thalamic nuclei, cerebellum, cerebral cortex, interpeduncular nucleus, and the dorsal horn of the spinal cord. Thus the sites of action are expected to be both spinally and supraspinally mediated. The antinociceptive effects of baclofen are not reversed by naloxone, suggesting that baclofen does not provide analgesia via release of endogenous opiates. The effects of long-term administration of baclofen on neuronal growth and synaptic plasticity remain to be elucidated.

MIDAZOLAM

Midazolam is a water-soluble benzodiazepine that has been shown to produce segmental spinal-mediated analgesia when administered intrathecally in rats.[63] Benzodiazepines have been linked with the GABA-chloride-channel complex in the central nervous system, and midazolam appears to be a $GABA_A$ receptor agonist. Midazolam potentiates GABA to open chloride channels on neuronal surfaces to produce hyperpolarization and inhibition of neuronal transmission. Regulation of calcium channel activity and possible increased potassium conductance has also been speculated. Midazolam may even regulate adenosine release in the spinal cord and depress cerebral cortical neurons.[64] Overall, intrathecal midazolam appears to produce a segmental nociceptive effect in the spinal cord dorsal horn and potentiates the antinociceptive effects of opioid medications. Intrathecal midazolam may even suppress the morphine withdrawal response by regulating nitric oxide synthase. These effects were not suppressed by naloxone but were reversed by the benzodiazepine antagonist flumazenil. However, some studies have demonstrated neurotoxic effects of intrathecal midazolam in animals, and thus further research appears to be warranted before recommending clinical use.[65]

NMDA ANTAGONISTS (KETAMINE)

Ketamine is a highly lipid soluble drug that mediates spinal analgesia primarily through its antagonism of the NMDA receptor. NMDA receptors are ionotropic glutamate receptor-channel complexes with several allosteric regulatory sites. Glycine is an important coactivator.[66] NMDA receptors are abundantly expressed in spinal cord dorsal horn neurons but also on astrocytes and oligodendrocytes.[67] Activation of the NMDA receptor primarily allows the voltage-dependent influx of Ca^{++} ions into the cell. This voltage-dependent activation is normally blocked by extracellular Mg^{++}. The intracellular calcium flux following activation of the NMDA receptor is thought to play a pivotal role in the spinal cord dorsal horn nociceptive processing after tissue and nerve injury as well as in synaptic plasticity.[68]

Ketamine noncompetitively blocks the NMDA receptor-coupled calcium channel, thereby preventing inflow of Ca^{++} into the cell and the subsequent release of excitatory neurotransmitters involved in nociceptive transmission. Ketamine is a racemic drug of R- and S-stereoisomers, where the S-enantiomer appears to have greater analgesic effects and less psychotropic effects than the R-enantiomer. S-ketamine is undergoing trials as a possible replacement for the racemic mixture. However, there is some evidence of neurotoxic effects with intrathecal ketamine administration in animals, and thus further investigation into the safety of intrathecal NMDA receptor antagonists appears indicated.[69]

OTHERS (ADENOSINE, ASPIRIN, DROPERIDOL, GABAPENTIN, KETOROLAC, NEOSTIGMINE, OCTREOTIDE)

ADENOSINE

Adenosine is a purine that is felt to be an endogenous analgesic ligand with effects noted at both the periphery and central nervous system.[70] Of particular importance to intrathecal analgesia, adenosine receptors have been found in high concentration within the dorsal horn of the spinal cord.[70–71] At least four types of adenosine receptor are involved in spinally mediated analgesia: A1, A2A, A2B, and A3.[72–74] Similar to opioid receptors, adenosine A1 receptors are shown to exert their effects at laminae I and II of the dorsal horn.[75] While the precise spinal mechanism of action is unclear, neuraxial administration of adenosine A1 receptor agonists have been shown to yield analgesic effects in animal models of acute, inflammatory, and neuropathic pain.[71]

In one small study of humans with neuropathic pain, intrathecal adenosine was noted to have no antinociceptive effects on chemical or thermal pain, but did reduce allodynia and mechanical hyperalgesia.[76] Intrathecal opioids have been shown to cause increased levels of adenosine within the CSF; however, no significant increase in spinal adenosine concentration was noted with intravenous opioids, implying a possible role for adenosine in spinally mediated opioid analgesia.[76] Furthermore, adenosine receptor antagonism has been demonstrated to reduce the efficacy of intrathecal and systemic morphine.[76] Another small, open label study of patients with chronic neuropathic pain who underwent intrathecal adenosine administration found significant decreases in spontaneous and evoked pain, as well as tactile hyperalgesia and allodynia.[77] Intrathecal adenosine demonstrated reduced mechanical hyperalgesia and allodynia but no significant reduction in pain as compared to intravenous adenosine in a small randomized study of patients with chronic neuropathic pain.[76] More data are needed to clearly delineate the role of intrathecal adenosine as an antinociceptive agent, but data thus far suggest it may have a potential role in the treatment of neuropathic pain.

ASPIRIN

Acetylsalicylic acid, or aspirin, is an irreversible inhibitor of cyclo-oxygenase-1 and 2 (COX-1 and 2) enzymes by means of acetylation. COX-1 and 2 generate prostaglandin E2 (PGE2) and have been shown to play a role in neuropathic pain states.[78] PGE2 may mediate nociception by its effects on two sites in the spinal cord dorsal horn, acting on presynaptic primary afferent nociceptors to increase release of glutamate and on postsynaptic second-order pain neurons by activating nonselective cation channels.[79–81] Prostaglandins may also inhibit endogenous opioid analgesic pathways by blocking spinal noradrenergic transmission within the descending pain modulation system.[82] These prostaglandin E2 effects appear to play a role in central sensitization and hyperalgesia, as intrathecal delivery of nonsteroidal anti-inflammatory drugs have been shown to block release of PGE2 and development of hyperalgesia.[79,83] Several studies have demonstrated analgesia with intrathecal administration of aspirin in animal models, and two human studies have demonstrated improved analgesia in patients with chronic pain that underwent intrathecal aspirin delivery.[84–85] The only significant side effect from intrathecal delivery of aspirin in humans appears to be fatigue.[84]

DROPERIDOL

Droperidol is a butyrophenone dopamine D2-receptor antagonist that has been used neuraxially as a potential antinociceptive agent. The exact mechanism by which droperidol may exert an antinociceptive effect is not entirely clear, but may be due to the presence of D2 receptors in the descending dopaminergic tracts within the spinal cord dorsal horn.[86] Activation of D2 receptors in the spinal cord shave been shown to inhibit calcium channels and augment potassium efflux via G-protein receptor mediated pathways, which may serve to suppress nociceptive transmission.[26]

Epidural droperidol has been shown to potentiate the analgesic effects of epidural morphine.[87–88] Droperidol was also shown to decrease the time of onset and lengthen the analgesic effect of epidural tramadol.[89] However, droperidol was shown to shorten the duration of effect with epidural sufentanil, although it did decrease opioid-related side effects.[90] A retrospective study of patients with chronic pain demonstrated that epidural droperidol yielded decreased opioid requirements and improved pain control when added to epidural opioids.[87] While there has been some suggestion that droperidol may have antinociceptive effects when administered epidurally, animal models of droperidol used intrathecally demonstrated no intrinsic analgesic activity nor any added antinociceptive effect when used in combination with intrathecal morphine.[91]

While droperidol may have benefits in terms of decreasing side effects of nausea, vomiting, and pruritis when used with neuraxial opioids, its exact mechanisms and potential as a spinal analgesic agent remain to be fully elucidated.[92–93]

GABAPENTIN

Gabapentin is an anticonvulsant that was synthesized as a structural analog[94] to GABA but does not interact with either the $GABA_A$ or $GABA_B$ receptors. Gabapentin has been shown to possess analgesic properties in a wide range of chronic pain models. Intrathecal or systemic administration of gabapentin diminishes hyperalgesia in tissue injury rat pain models.[95–96] Gabapentin binds with high affinity to the $\alpha_2\delta$ subunit of voltage-gated calcium channels, which modulate the release of excitatory amino acids such as glutamate at the level of the spinal dorsal horn.[97] It is believed that gabapentin produces analgesia in part by activating descending noradrenergic spinal inhibitory pathways.[98]

KETOROLAC

Ketorolac, a potent water-soluble nonsteroidal anti-inflammatory drug, inhibits both COX-1 and 2.[99] COX is the rate-limiting enzyme in arachidonic acid metabolism and thus in the production of prostaglandins.[100] Prostaglandins stimulate and enhance evoked release of excitatory neurotransmitters in the spinal cord, directly excite dorsal horn neurons, and elicit nociceptive behavior in animals when administered intrathecally. Intrathecal administration of ketorolac has a significant antinociceptive effect in rats.[101–102] Additionally, intrathecal administration of ketorolac in dogs leads to suppression of prostaglandin synthesis in the CSF.[103] A phase I clinical trial of intrathecal ketorolac has shown that this has an analgesic effect without inducing any significant neuropathological changes.[104] Ketorolac does not readily cross the blood-brain barrier because of its poor lipophilicity.[100] The mechanism of the central action of ketorolac has not been fully clarified, but the expression of COX isoforms in the rat spinal cord suggests a central COX inhibitory effect.

NEOSTIGMINE

Neostigmine is an anticholinesterase that inhibits the enzyme acetylcholinesterase, which is normally responsible for the rapid hydrolysis of the neurotransmitter acetylcholine to choline and acetic acid. The inhibition of acetylcholine hydrolysis results in the greater availability of acetylcholine at its site of actions, namely, preganglionic sympathetic and parasympathetic nerve endings. Spinal administration of neostigmine produces antinociception in animal and human studies.[105–106] Cholinesterase inhibitors such as neostigmine have pharmacologic actions on both spinal muscarinic and nicotinic receptors, and both receptors are thought to contribute to the mechanism of analgesia produced by cholinesterase inhibitors.[107] It is thought that intrathecal neostigmine inhibits the metabolism of spinally released acetylcholine while increasing the CSF concentration of acetylcholine.[108] Intrathecal neostigmine inhibits the activity of cholinesterase present in the spinal cord,[109] thereby increasing the concentration of CSF acetylcholine, which in turn likely acts on spinal muscarinic and nicotinic receptors causing the antinociceptive effect.

OCTREOTIDE

Octreotide is a synthetic octapeptide derivative of the growth hormone somatostatin. Somatostatin is a polypeptide present in many human tissues including the nervous system, gastrointestinal system, and the substantia gelatinosa of the spinal cord dorsal horn, where it is thought to mitigate nociception. Somatostatin has been found specifically in lamina II of the dorsal horn, where it is present in small-diameter afferents and intrinsic neurons and in the dorsal root ganglia associated with C-fiber afferents.[110] Its functional role is not well understood, since both inhibitory and excitatory effects have been reported. The analgesic effect of somatostatin in various types of pain has been reported in both animal and human studies[111–112] as has the analgesic effect of octreotide in both nociceptive and neuropathic pain states.[113] While the exact mechanism of action of somatostatin and octreotide are unknown, various possibilities have been postulated including a role in an endogenous antinociceptive system that links substance P with somatostatin-mediated nociceptive transmission in the spinal cord[113] as well as other nonopioid analgesic peptide mechanisms.

REFERENCES

1. Bier AKG, Von Esmarch JFA. Versuche uber cocainisiring des Ruckenmarkes. *Deutsche Zeitschrift fur Chirurgie.* 1899;51:361–369.
2. Smith HS, et al. Intrathecal drug delivery. *Pain Physician.* 2008; 11(2 Suppl):S89–S104.
3. Ahmed S. Intrathecal drug delivery for chronic pain management. In: Mao J, ed. *Translational pain research.* New York: Nova Science Publishers, Inc.; 2006. pp 383–402.
4. Reiman A, Anson B. Vertebral level of termination of the spinal cord with report of a case of sacral cord. *Anat Rec.* 1944;88:127.
5. Warren DT, Liu SS, eds. Neuraxial anesthesia. In: Benzon HT, et al, eds. *Raj's Practical Management of Pain.* Philadelphia: Elsevier; 2008. pp 927–943.
6. Matsuki A. Nothing new under the sun—a Japanese pioneer in the clinical use of intrathecal morphine. *Anesthesiology.* 1983;58(3): 289–290.
7. Goldstein A, Lowney LI, Pal BK. Stereospecific and nonspecific interactions of the morphine congener levorphanol in subcellular fractions of mouse brain. *Proc Natl Acad Sci U S A.* 1971;68(8):1742–1747.
8. Pert CB, Snyder SH. Opiate receptor: demonstration in nervous tissue. *Science.* 1973;179(77):1011–1014.
9. Martin WR, et al. The effects of morphine- and nalorphine- like drugs in the nondependent and morphine-dependent chronic spinal dog. *J Pharmacol Exp Ther.* 1976;197(3):517–532.
10. Yaksh TL, Rudy TA. Analgesia mediated by a direct spinal action of narcotics. *Science.* 1976;192(4246):1357–1358.
11. Wang JK, Nauss LA, Thomas JE. Pain relief by intrathecally applied morphine in man. *Anesthesiology.* 1979;50(2):149–151.
12. Smullin DH, Skilling SR, Larson AA. Interactions between substance P, calcitonin gene-related peptide, taurine and excitatory amino acids in the spinal cord. *Pain.* 1990;42(1):93–101.
13. Riedel W, Neeck G. Nociception, pain, and antinociception: current concepts. *Z Rheumatol.* 2001;60(6):404–415.
14. Yaksh TL, Elde RP. Factors governing release of methionine enkephalin-like immunoreactivity from mesencephalon and spinal cord of the cat in vivo. *J Neurophysiol.* 1981;46(5):1056–1075.
15. Basbaum AI, Fields HL. Endogenous pain control systems: brainstem spinal pathways and endorphin circuitry. *Annu Rev Neurosci.* 1984;7:309–338.
16. Iadarola MJ, et al. Analgesic activity and release of [MET5]enkephalin-Arg6-Gly7-Leu8 from rat spinal cord in vivo. *Eur J Pharmacol.* 1986; 121(1):39–48.
17. Song B, Marvizon JC. Dorsal horn neurons firing at high frequency, but not primary afferents, release opioid peptides that produce micro-opioid receptor internalization in the rat spinal cord. *J Neurosci.* 2003;23(27):9171–9184.
18. Vanderah TW. Pathophysiology of pain. *Med Clin North Am.* 2007;91(1):1–12.
19. Evans CJ, et al. Cloning of a delta opioid receptor by functional expression. *Science.* 1992;258(5090):1952–1955.
20. Kieffer BL, et al. The delta-opioid receptor: isolation of a cDNA by expression cloning and pharmacological characterization. *Proc Natl Acad Sci U S A.* 1992;89(24):12048–12052.
21. Yasuda K, et al. Cloning and functional comparison of kappa and delta opioid receptors from mouse brain. *Proc Natl Acad Sci U S A.* 1993;90(14):6736–6740.
22. Chen Y, et al. Molecular cloning and functional expression of a mu-opioid receptor from rat brain. *Mol Pharmacol.* 1993;44(1):8–12.
23. Pasternak GW, Pharmacological mechanisms of opioid analgesics. *Clin Neuropharmacol.* 1993;16(1):1–18.
24. Jiang Q, et al. Differential antagonism of opioid delta antinociception by [D-Ala2,Leu5,Cys6]enkephalin and naltrindole 5'-isothiocyanate: evidence for delta receptor subtypes. *J Pharmacol Exp Ther.* 1991; 257(3):1069–1075.
25. Marker CL, et al. Spinal G-protein-gated potassium channels contribute in a dose-dependent manner to the analgesic effect of mu- and delta- but not kappa-opioids. *J Neurosci.* 2005;25(14): 3551–3559.
26. Millan MJ. Descending control of pain. *Prog Neurobiol.* 2002; 66(6):355–474.
27. Eisenach JC, Hood DD, Curry R. Preliminary efficacy assessment of intrathecal injection of an American formulation of adenosine in humans. *Anesthesiology.* 2002;96(1):29–34.
28. Ummenhofer WC, et al. Comparative spinal distribution and clearance kinetics of intrathecally administered morphine, fentanyl, alfentanil, and sufentanil. *Anesthesiology.* 2000;92(3):739–753.
29. Nordberg G Pharmacokinetic aspects of spinal morphine analgesia. *Acta Anaesthesiol Scand Suppl.* 1984;79:1–38.
30. Krames ES. Intraspinal opioid therapy for chronic nonmalignant pain: current practice and clinical guidelines. *J Pain Symptom Manage.* 1996;11(6):333–352.

31. Sandouk P, Scherrmann JM, Chauvin M. Rate-limiting diffusion processes following intrathecal administration of morphine. *Eur J Clin Pharmacol.* 1986;30(5):575–579.
32. Portenoy RK, et al. The metabolite morphine-6-glucuronide contributes to the analgesia produced by morphine infusion in patients with pain and normal renal function. *Clin Pharmacol Ther.* 1992;51(4):422–431.
33. Tiseo PJ, et al. Morphine-6-glucuronide concentrations and opioid-related side effects: a survey in cancer patients. *Pain.* 1995;61(1): 47–54.
34. Smith MT. Neuroexcitatory effects of morphine and hydromorphone: evidence implicating the 3-glucuronide metabolites. *Clin Exp Pharmacol Physiol.* 2000;27(7):524–528.
35. Bennett G, et al. Clinical guidelines for intraspinal infusion: report of an expert panel. PolyAnalgesic Consensus Conference 2000. *J Pain Symptom Manage.* 2000;20(2):S37–43.
36. Deer T. Polyanalgesic Consensus Conference 2007: recommendations for the management of pain by intrathecal (intraspinal) drug delivery: report of an interdisciplinary expert panel. *Neuromodulation.* 2007;10(4):300–328.
37. Anderson VC, Burchiel KJ. A prospective study of long-term intrathecal morphine in the management of chronic nonmalignant pain. *Neurosurgery.* 1999;44(2):289–300; discussion 300–301.
38. Rathmell JP, Lair TR, Nauman B. The role of intrathecal drugs in the treatment of acute pain. *Anesth Analg.* 2005;101(5 Suppl):S30–43.
39. Johansen MJ, et al. Continuous intrathecal infusion of hydromorphone: safety in the sheep model and clinical implications. *Pain Med.* 2004;5(1):14–25.
40. Waara-Wolleat KL, Hildebrand KR, Stewart GR. A review of intrathecal fentanyl and sufentanil for the treatment of chronic pain. *Pain Med.* 2006;7(3):251–259.
41. Monk JP, Beresford R, Ward A. Sufentanil: a review of its pharmacological properties and therapeutic use. *Drugs.* 1988;36(3): 286–313.
42. D'Angelo R, et al. Epidural fentanyl produces labor analgesia by a spinal mechanism. *Anesthesiology.* 1998;88(6):1519–1523.
43. Bennett GJ. Update on the neurophysiology of pain transmission and modulation: focus on the NMDA-receptor. *J Pain Symptom Manage.* 2000;19(1 Suppl):S2–6.
44. Davis AM, Inturrisi CE. d-Methadone blocks morphine tolerance and N-methyl-D-aspartate-induced hyperalgesia. *J Pharmacol Exp Ther.* 1999;289(2):1048–1053.
45. Holtman JR Jr., Wala EP. Characterization of the antinociceptive and pronociceptive effects of methadone in rats. *Anesthesiology.* 2007;106(3):563–571.
46. Payne R, Inturrisi CE. CSF distribution of morphine, methadone and sucrose after intrathecal injection. *Life Sci.* 1985;37(12):1137–1144.
47. Wagner LE 2nd, et al. Meperidine and lidocaine block of recombinant voltage-dependent Na^+ channels: evidence that meperidine is a local anesthetic. *Anesthesiology.* 1999;91(5):1481–1490.
48. Sjostrom S, et al. Pharmacokinetics of intrathecal morphine and meperidine in humans. *Anesthesiology.* 1987;67(6):889–895.
49. Vranken JH, et al. Plasma concentrations of meperidine and normeperidine following continuous intrathecal meperidine in patients with neuropathic cancer pain. *Acta Anaesthesiol Scand.* 2005;49(5): 665–670.
50. Bennett G, et al. Evidence-based review of the literature on intrathecal delivery of pain medication. *J Pain Symptom Manage.* 2000;20:S12 S36.
51. Butterworth JF, Strichartz GR. Molecular mechanisms of local anesthetics: A review. *Anesthesiology.* 1990;72:711–734.
52. Catterall WA. Form ionic currents to molecular mechanisms: the structure and function of voltage-gated sodium channels. *Neuron.* 2000;26:13–25.
53. Boswell MV, Iacono RP, Guthkelch AN. Sites of action of subarachnoid lidocaine and tetracaine: observations with evoked potential monitoring during spinal cord stimulator implantation. *Reg Anesth.* 1992;17(1):37–42.
54. Lang E, Krainick JU, Gerbershagen HU. Spinal cord transmission of impulses during high spinal anesthesia as measured by cortical evoked potentials. *Anesth Analg.* 1989;69(1):15–20.
55. Kroin JS, et al. Continuous intrathecal clonidine and tizanidine in conscious dogs: analgesic and hemodynamic effects. *Anesth Analg.* 2003;96(3):776–782, table of contents.
56. Eisenach JC. Overview: first international symposium on alpha 2-adrenergic mechanisms of spinal anesthesia. *Reg Anesth.* 1993; 18(4):207–212.
57. Yaksh TL, et al. Chronically infused intrathecal morphine in dogs. *Anesthesiology.* 2003;99(1):174–187.
58. Rauck RL, et al. Intrathecal ziconotide for neuropathic pain: a review. *Pain Pract.* 2009;9(5):327–337.
59. Wang YX, et al. Effects of intrathecal administration of ziconotide, a selective neuronal N-type calcium channel blocker, on mechanical allodynia and heat hyperalgesia in a rat model of postoperative pain. *Pain.* 2000;84(2–3):151–158.
60. Staats PS, et al. Intrathecal ziconotide in the treatment of refractory pain in patients with cancer or AIDS: a randomized controlled trial. *JAMA.* 2004;291(1):63–70.
61. Bowery NG, et al. International union of pharmacology, XXXIII: mammalian gamma-aminobutyric acid(B) receptors: structure and function. *Pharmacol Rev.* 2002;54(2):247–264.
62. Brennan PM, Whittle IR. Intrathecal baclofen therapy for neurological disorders: a sound knowledge base but many challenges remain. *Br J Neurosurg.* 2008;22(4):508–519.
63. Serrao JM, et al. Intrathecal midazolam and fentanyl in the rat: evidence for different spinal antinociceptive effects. *Anesthesiology.* 1989;70(5):780–786.
64. Carlen PL, Gurevich N, Polc P. Low-dose benzodiazepine neuronal inhibition: enhanced $Ca2^+$-mediated K^+-conductance. *Brain Res.* 1983;271(2):358–364.
65. Edwards M, et al. On the mechanism by which midazolam causes spinally mediated analgesia. *Anesthesiology.* 1990;73(2):273–777.
66. Mao J, et al. Differential roles of NMDA and non-NMDA receptor activation in induction and maintenance of thermal hyperalgesia in rats with painful peripheral mononeuropathy. *Brain Res.* 1992;598(1–2): 271–278.
67. Matute C. Oligodendrocyte NMDA receptors: a novel therapeutic target. *Trends Mol Med.* 2006;12(7):289–292.
68. Dingledine R, et al. The glutamate receptor ion channels. *Pharmacol Rev.* 1999;51(1):7–61.
69. Yaksh TL, et al. Toxicology profile of N-methyl-D-aspartate antagonists delivered by intrathecal infusion in the canine model. *Anesthesiology.* 2008;108(5):938–949.
70. Kekesi G, et al. The antinociceptive potencies and interactions of endogenous ligands during continuous intrathecal administration: adenosine, agmatine, and endomorphin-1. *Anesth Analg.* 2004;98(2): 420–426, table of contents.
71. Sawynok J. Adenosine receptor activation and nociception. *Eur J Pharmacol.* 1998;347(1):1–11.
72. Yoon MH, Bae HB, Choi JI. Antinociception of intrathecal adenosine receptor subtype agonists in rat formalin test. *Anesth Analg.* 2005;101(5):1417–1421.
73. Yoon MH, et al. Roles of adenosine receptor subtypes in the antinociceptive effect of intrathecal adenosine in a rat formalin test. *Pharmacology.* 2006;78(1):21–26.
74. Yoon MH, et al. Analysis of interactions between serotonin and gabapentin or adenosine in the spinal cord of rats. *Pharmacology.* 2005;74(1):15–22.
75. Poon A, Sawynok J. Antinociception by adenosine analogs and inhibitors of adenosine metabolism in an inflammatory thermal hyperalgesia model in the rat. *Pain.* 1998;74(2–3):235–245.
76. Eisenach JC, et al. Intrathecal but not intravenous opioids release adenosine from the spinal cord. *J Pain.* 2004;5(1):64–68.
77. Belfrage M, et al. The safety and efficacy of intrathecal adenosine in patients with chronic neuropathic pain. *Anesth Analg.* 1999;89(1): 136–142.

78. Lashbrook JM, et al. Synergistic antiallodynic effects of spinal morphine with ketorolac and selective COX1- and COX2-inhibitors in nerve-injured rats. *Pain*. 1999;82(1):65–72.
79. Malmberg AB, Yaksh TL. Cyclooxygenase inhibition and the spinal release of prostaglandin E2 and amino acids evoked by paw formalin injection: a microdialysis study in unanesthetized rats. *J Neurosci*. 1995;15(4):2768–2776.
80. Ferreira SH, Lorenzetti BB. Intrathecal administration of prostaglandin E2 causes sensitization of the primary afferent neuron via the spinal release of glutamate. *Inflamm Res*. 1996;45(10):499–502.
81. Benzon H, et al. *Raj's Practical Management of Pain*. 4th ed. Philadelphia: Mosby Elsevier; 2008.
82. Taiwo YO, Levine JD. Prostaglandins inhibit endogenous pain control mechanisms by blocking transmission at spinal noradrenergic synapses. *J Neurosci*. 1988;8(4):1346–1349.
83. Malmberg AB, Yaksh TL. Hyperalgesia mediated by spinal glutamate or substance P receptor blocked by spinal cyclooxygenase inhibition. *Science*. 1992;257(5074):1276–1279.
84. Pellerin M, et al. Chronic refractory pain in cancer patients: value of the spinal injection of lysine acetylsalicylate; 60 cases [in French]. *Presse Med*. 1987;16(30):1465–1468.
85. Devoghel JC. Small intrathecal doses of lysine-acetylsalicylate relieve intractable pain in man. *J Int Med Res*. 1983;11(2):90–91.
86. Gao X, Zhang Y, Wu G. Effects of dopaminergic agents on carrageenan hyperalgesia after intrathecal administration to rats. *Eur J Pharmacol*. 2001;418(1–2):73–77.
87. Bach V, et al. Potentiation of epidural opioids with epidural droperidol: a one year retrospective study. *Anaesthesia*. 1986; 41(11):1116–1119.
88. Naji P, et al. Epidural droperidol and morphine for postoperative pain. *Anesth Analg*. 1990;70(6):583–588.
89. Gurses E, et al. The addition of droperidol or clonidine to epidural tramadol shortens onset time and increases duration of postoperative analgesia. *Can J Anaesth*. 2003;50(2):147–152.
90. Wilder-Smith CH, et al. Epidural droperidol reduces the side effects and duration of analgesia of epidural sufentanil. *Anesth Analg*. 1994;79(1):98–104.
91. Grip G, et al. Histopathology and evaluation of potentiation of morphine-induced antinociception by intrathecal droperidol in the rat. *Acta Anaesthesiol Scand*. 1992;36(2):145–152.
92. Szarvas S, Harmon D, Murphy D. Neuraxial opioid-induced pruritus: a review. *J Clin Anesth*. 2003;15(3):234–239.
93. Lee IH, Lee IO. The antipruritic and antiemetic effects of epidural droperidol: a study of three methods of administration. *Anesth Analg*. 2007;105(1):251–255.
94. Taylor CP, et al. A summary of mechanistic hypothesis of gabapentin pharmacology. *Epilepsy Res*. 1998;29:233–249.
95. Yoon MH, Yaksh TL. The effect of intrathecal gabapentin on pain behavior and hemodynamics on the formalin test in the rat. *Anesth Analg*.1999;89:434–439.
96. Yoon MH, Yaksh TL. Evaluation of interaction between gabapentin and ibuprofen on the formalin test in rats. *Anesthesiology*. 1999; 91:1006–1013.
97. Gee NS, et al. The novel anticonvulsant drug, gabapentin (Neurontin), binds to the alpha2delta subunit of a calcium channel. *J Biol Chem*. 1996;27:5768–5776.
98. Hayashida K, et al. Gabapentin activates spinal noradrenergic activity in rats and humans and reduces hypersensitivity after surgery. *Anesthesiology*. 2007;106:557–562.
99. Hsieh YC, et al. Protective effect of intrathecal ketorolac in spinal cord ischemia in rats: a microdialysis study. *Acta Anaesthesiol Scand*. 2007;51:410–414.
100. Jett MF, et al. Characterization of the analgesic and anti-inflammatory activities of ketorolac and its enantiomers in the rat. *J Pharmacol Exp Ther*. 1999;288(3):1288–97.
101. Conklin DR, Eisenach JC. Intrathecal ketorolac enhances antinociception from clonidine. *Anesth Analg*. 2003;96(1):191–194.
102. Ma W, Du W, Eisenach JC. Intrathecal lidocaine reverses tactile allodynia caused by nerve injuries and potentiates the antiallodynic effect of the COX inhibitor ketorolac. *Anesthesiology*. 2003;98(1): 203–208.
103. Yaksh TL, et al. Intrathecal ketorolac in dogs and rats. *Toxicol Sci*. 2004;80(2):322–334.
104. Eisenach JC, et al. Phase I safety assessment of intrathecal ketorolac. *Pain*. 2002;99(3):599–604.
105. Hwang JH, et al. The antiallodynic effects of intrathecal cholinesterase inhibitors in a rat model of neuropathic pain. *Anesthesiology*. 1999;90(2):492–499.
106. Naguib M, Yaksh TL. Antinociceptive effects of spinal cholinesterase inhibition and isobolographic analysis of the interaction with mu and alpha 2 receptor systems. *Anesthesiology*. 1994;80(6): 1338–1348.
107. Yoon MH, Choi JI, Jeong SW. Antinociception of intrathecal cholinesterase inhibitors and cholinergic receptors in rats. *Acta Anaesthesiol Scand*. 2003;47(9):1079–1084.
108. Shafer SL, et al. Cerebrospinal fluid pharmacokinetics and pharmacodynamics of intrathecal neostigmine methylsulfate in humans. *Anesthesiology*. 1998;89(5):1074–1088.
109. Ummenhofer WC, Brown SM, Bernards CM. Acetylcholinesterase and butyrylcholinesterase are expressed in the spinal meninges of monkeys and pigs. *Anesthesiology*. 1998;88(5):1259–1265.
110. Gaumann DM, et al. Intrathecal somatostatin, somatostatin analogs, substance P analog and dynorphin A cause comparable neurotoxicity in rats. *Neuroscience*. 1990;39(3):761–774.
111. Chapman V, Dickenson AH. The effects of sandostatin and somatostatin on nociceptive transmission in the dorsal horn of the rat spinal cord. *Neuropeptides*. 1992;23(3):147–152.
112. Chrubasik J, et al. The effect of epidural somatostatin on postoperative pain. *Anesth Analg*. 1985;64(11):1085–1088.
113. Tsai YC, et al. Effect of intrathecal octreotide on thermal hyperalgesia and evoked spinal c-Fos expression in rats with sciatic constriction injury. *Pain*. 2002;99(3):407–413.

PART IV

PERIPHERAL NERVOUS SYSTEM

10

PERIPHERAL NERVOUS SYSTEM

ANATOMY AND FUNCTION

Marnie B. Welch and Chad M. Brummett

INTRODUCTION

The peripheral nervous system (PNS) consists of neural tissue outside of the brain and spinal cord and is derived embryologically from the neural crest. Its primary function is to transmit sensory information from the periphery and motor information from the brain and spinal cord. The autonomic and enteric nervous systems[1] are also subdivisions of the PNS. For the anesthesiologist, blockade of the PNS for anesthesia and analgesia, as well as appropriate padding and positioning to avoid nerve injury, is of great clinical importance. This chapter will focus on the basics of the anatomy and physiology of the PNS and provide some clinical correlation for the anesthesiologist.

BASICS OF ANATOMY AND FUNCTION

Neurons consist of a cell body, a dendrite, and an axon. In the PNS, neurons are grouped into "ganglia," as opposed to the "nuclei" of the brain. In each neuron, the nucleus resides in the cell body, and its cytoplasm is the axoplasm. This cytoplasm also flows within and around a system of microtubules and neurofilaments, within the axon. Dendrites are typically short branching processes that receive signals from other neurons, while axons typically conduct impulses away from the cell body. Some neurons, however, have no axon, and dendrites conduct signals in both directions.

Peripheral axons are accompanied by Schwann cells—the glia of the PNS—which separate them from the endoneurial space with their basement membrane. Together, Schwann cells and axons constitute a nerve fiber. Peripheral axons are classified as either myelinated or unmyelinated. Myelin is a lipoproteinaceous membrane laid down by Schwann cells in the PNS; these cells are tubular and ensheathe all axons in the peripheral nervous system. In myelinated nerve fibers, one single axon is associated with a string of longitudinally arranged Schwann cells.[1] In nonmyelinated axons, the arrangement differs; the axons are located in large numbers in the cytoplasm of the surrounding Schwann cell.

First discovered in the late 19th century, the Nodes of Ranvier are interruptions in the myelin that serve as junctions between regions created by one Schwann cell. The conduction of ions occurs along theses nodes on myelinated axons. The action potential jumping from one node to the next is known as saltatory conduction, as first described by Huxley in 1949.[2] Myelin serves several functions, including increasing the conduction velocity, providing insulation to prevent disruption of action potentials, and potentially repairing the axon when injury occurs. Signaling is much faster in myelinated nerves than those that are unmyelinated. This discontinuity in the myelin sheath allows for one individual axon to extend the entire length of the body, from the cell body in the lumbar dorsal root ganglion to a synaptic terminal in the foot. In all mammals, the length of PNS axons varies greatly, from 1 cm to several meters.[1]

ORGANIZATION OF NERVE FIBERS

In addition to the presence of myelin, a larger diameter fiber increases conduction velocity. The nerve fiber types were organized by Erlanger in the 1930s as follows: The **group A fibers are myelinated fibers and have higher conduction velocities.** The A-alpha motor fibers are the largest (12–20 micrometer external diameter) and fastest (70–120 m/s). These fibers innervate skeletal muscle fibers and larger sized sensory fibers. The A-beta, A-delta, and A-gamma are sensory fibers, which range from 3 to 8 micrometers in external diameter and have a conduction velocity of 10–80 m/s. The A-beta fibers transmit sensations of light touch or muscle movement, while the A-gamma sense pressure and touch. The only myelinated pain fibers are the small A-delta fibers. **The group B fibers are myelinated but smaller; they are either preganglionic or autonomic fibers.** They have an external diameter of 1–3 micrometers and a 5–15 m/s conduction velocity. Finally, **the group C fibers are nonmyelinated visceral and somatic pain fibers.** These have the smallest external diameter (0.2 to 1.2 micrometers) with slower conduction velocities or 0.5–2.5 m/s.[3]

AXONAL TRANSPORT

The distance between a cell body and the axon terminal can be very long and requires a special system known as axonal transport for the neuron to communicate and transport substances.[4] Most substances needed for transport are synthesized in the nerve cell body and are usually transported to the terminal parts (anterograde axonal transport) for use. Neurotransmitter precursors are among the substances transported away from the cell body, specifically to the end plate. Transport in the opposite direction (retrograde axonal transport), can either be from the terminals to the cell body, or the periphery to the cell body. Axonal transport can be classified as either slow (0.1–30 mm/day) or fast (410 mm/day) and serves to dispose of materials and transport growth factors. The bidirectional flow is evident because a nerve will swell both distally and proximally from the point of direct pressure. Various toxic substances and deprivation of blood flow will slow or block this transport.[5] Overall, the axonal transport system demonstrates that the axon is very reliant on the periphery, mainly the surrounding Schwann cells, to maintain its survival and growth.

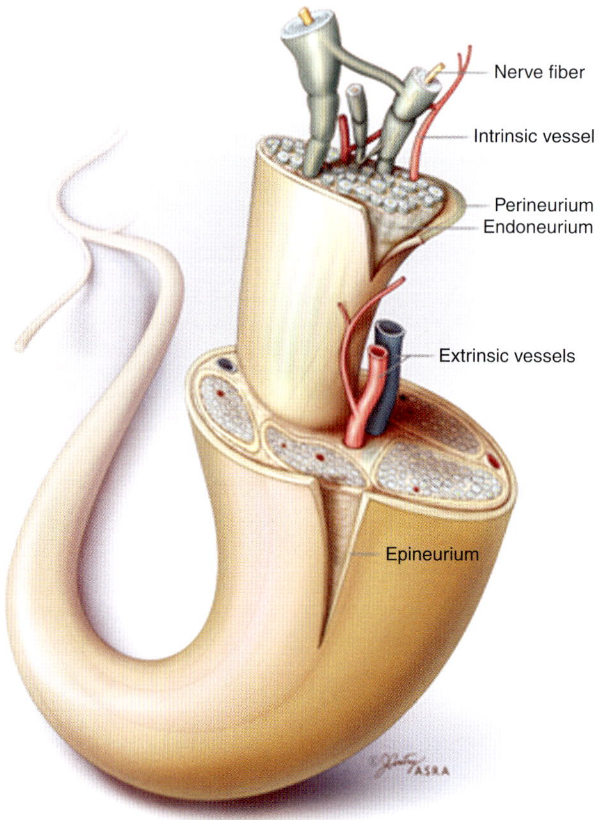

Figure 10.1 *Peripheral nerve anatomy* There are three layers of connective tissue surrounding a nerve fiber: the inner layer (*endoneurium*), the middle layer (*perineurium*), and the outermost encasing layering (*epineurium*). The intrinsic and extrinsic blood supply is also depicted within these layers of tissue. (From the American Society of Regional Anesthesia and Pain Medicine, with permission)

PERIPHERAL NERVOUS SYSTEM FIBERS AND SURROUNDING TISSUES

ENDONEURIUM

The most proximal part of the PNS is made up of both myelinated and unmyelinated neurons, bundled into spinal and cranial nerve roots. These roots exit from the subarachnoid space and are bathed in cerebrospinal fluid. Roots consist of multiple nerve fibers that, except for the smallest among them, are bundled into particular layers of connective tissue, as observed clearly by electron microscopy.[6] Nerve fibers are encased in a network of fibroblasts, Schwann cells, and collagen, called the endoneurium (Figure 10.1). They are encased with a slight undulation within the endoneurial tubules, allowing for some degree of stretch. However, the endoneurium contains no lymphatic channels, which implies that any change in pressure, as can occur with edema, could interfere with conduction and axoplasmic flow.

PERINEURIUM

The next encasing layer is known as the perineurium. The multiple aforementioned nerve fibers are bundled together in a fascicle. Each fascicle is surrounded by a connective tissue layer, or layers, of fibroblasts and collagen fibers, composed of flattened cells presenting basement membranes on both sides, called the "perineurium epithelium."[7] There is no basal lamina between perineurial cells and the cells overlap to form "tight junctions." Lundborg outlined the role of the perineurium: 1) Protects the contents of the endoneurial tubes, 2) Acts as a mechanical barrier to external forces, 3) Serves as a diffusion barrier, keeping certain substances out of the internal environment.[8] The perineurium serves in particular as the connective tissue barrier that surrounds individual nerve fascicles and protects them from the external milieu, including neurotoxic drugs and foreign bodies such as needles or catheters. In fact, the connective tissue comprises 50–66% of the nerve's cross-sectional area, providing further protection.[9] Many of the collagen fibers run parallel to the direction of the nerve fiber. However, there are circular and oblique bundles that may protect the nerve from kinking when it takes an acute angle.

EPINEURIUM

Surrounding a group of fascicles is a dense connective tissue sheath called the epineurium. This grouping also contains numerous blood vessels and a few fat cells, which fill the space in between the fascicles. This layer serves to surround,

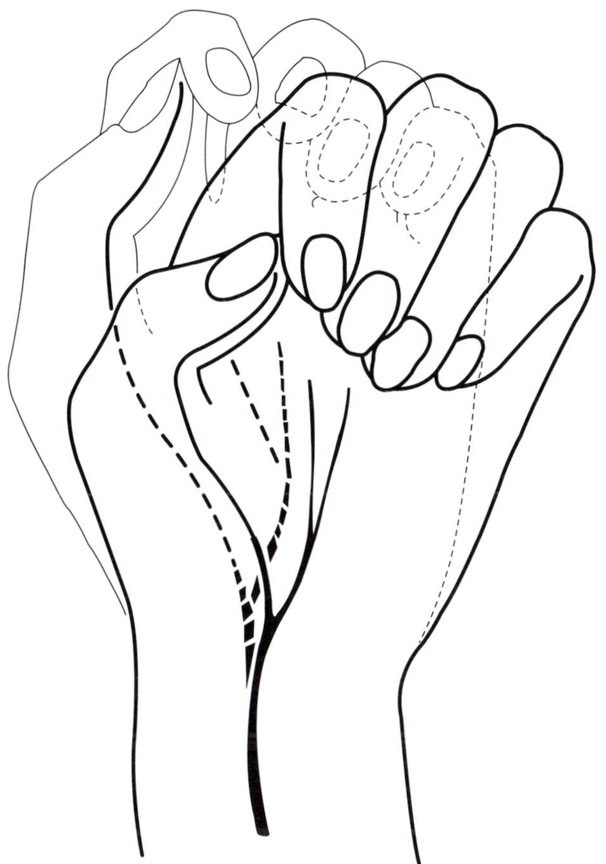

Figure 10.2 Median nerve excursion from wrist extension and motion, illustrating the amount of movement in nerve fibers. This figure was published in Wilgis EF, Murphy R. The significance of longitudinal excursion in peripheral nerves. *Hand Clin*. 1986;2:761–766. Copyright Elsevier 1986.

protect, and cushion the fascicle. It consists of both collagen and elastic fibers, mainly arranged longitudinally to the perineurium. The amount of epineurium varies significantly among nerves and level. For example, there is more epineurium where more gliding needs to occur, such as nerve trunks crossing joints or in tunnel areas, such as the carpal tunnel. The epineurial collagen fibers also have some undulations, allowing for stretching of the nerve that comes with flexion and other movement. A considerable range of motion in the nerve trunk is allowed. It is, however, anchored to the surrounding tissues at various points.

NERVE MOVEMENT

On the outside of a nerve trunk is a conjunctiva-like adventitia that allows a certain amount of moment, or excursions, of the nerve trunk within this covering. Within the nerve trunk, smaller divisions of nerves can also glide against each other. Millesi calculated that the bed of the median nerve is 18% longer from wrist and elbow flexion to wrist and elbow extension.[10] Wilgris showed that the brachial plexus can move about 15 mm with the abduction-adduction of the shoulder.[11] Near the elbow, the median and ulnar nerve can glide 7.3 mm and 9.8 mm (Figure 10.2), respectively, while near the carpal tunnel the same nerves can glide more, at 14.5 mm and 13.8 mm. The nerves must be adaptable in order to conduct impulses during these movements. This ability to glide can be compromised with fibrosis. The inability of the nerves to move can induce edema, inflammation, and further fibrosis, leading to irritation, inflammation, and clinical symptoms.

The PNS, from its origin, undergoes multiple divisions into multiple plexuses. The PNS comes into contact with a variety of structures[12] that can be hard, such as bone (for example, the radial nerve in the spiral groove of the humerus), or soft, such as tissue. Thus, the spectrum varies from osseous structures, to fibro-osseous structures, to soft tissue. The type of structure the nervous system is adjacent to can directly affect the nature and extent of injury.

INTRANEURAL CIRCULATION

ANATOMY OF CIRCULATION

The nerves in the PNS are densely supplied with blood vessels. A dual blood supply exists in an extrinsic and intrinsic system.[13] The **extrinsic system** receives a mainly nonnutritive blood supply and is predominately under adrenergic control (Figure 10.3). This supply starts as feeder arteries to the nerve. From there, a well developed microvascular system provides nutrients to all layers of the nerve. Arteries enter, then traverse and anastomose in the epineurium to form a network called the vasa nervorum. From this network, smaller arteries penetrate the perineurium and connect with the **intrinsic system**, forming a network of arterioles, capillaries, and venules in the endoneurium. The distribution of vessels with adrenergic innervation is limited to the larger blood vessels in the epineurium,[14] thus the intrinsic system is not under adrenergic control.

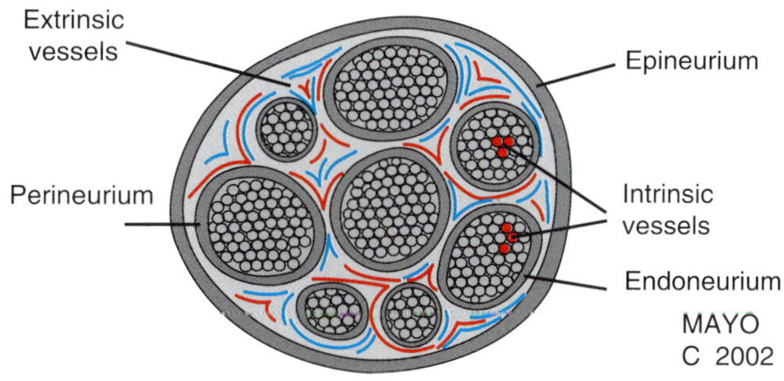

Figure 10.3 *Blood supply of the peripheral nerve* The dual extrinsic (under adrenergic control) and intrinsic blood supply are shown. Extrinsic vessels are located within the epineurium and perineurium, while intrinsic vessels are located within the endoneurium. Reprinted with permission from Neal JM. Effects of epinephrine in local anesthetics on the central and peripheral nervous systems: neurotoxicity and neural blood flow. *Reg Anesth Pain Med*. 2003;28:124–134.

The structure of the system appears to be organized to ensure blood supply to the nerve, because when an extrinsic, main feeder artery is stripped, the intrinsic system is still in place.[15] However, in the intrinsic structure of the endoneurium, the vessels have thin walls and rudimentary elastic laminae, making them vulnerable to collapse from pressure.[16]

Overall, the blood vessels and connective tissue arrangement around the nerves provide mechanical and nutritional support for the peripheral nerves, and serve as a barrier against entry of macromolecules and microorganisms. At the level of the perineurium, the perineurial cells are joined by tight junctions. The permeability of this barrier varies by age (greater in prenatal and perinatal period) and location (greater at neuromuscular junction). Thus, when edema forms rapidly in the epineurium, either from trauma, irritation, or compression injury, the diffusion barrier in the perineurial sheath will not allow it to penetrate into the fascicles, thus protecting the nerve fibers.[17] The second barrier is the extrinsic blood vessels, as they have a fenestrated endothelium. This forms an effective, but not an absolute, blood-nerve barrier, analogous to the blood-brain barrier. However, insults such as ischemia that lead to edema will increase the endoneurial fluid pressure. If the pressure is increased enough from within, it will consequently close the barrier.[8] This blood-nerve barrier is more permeable in some parts of the PNS, such as the nerve roots and ganglia.

FUNCTION OF CIRCULATION

The nervous system (central and peripheral) consumes 20% of the available oxygen in the blood yet only represents 2% of the body mass.[18] Neurons, when compared to other cells, have high metabolic demand and thus are especially sensitive to alterations in blood flow. Although peripheral nerves are less sensitive to ischemia than the brain or spinal cord, alterations in blood flow will eventually lead to damage. The vasa nervorum represents the blood supply to the nerves and can still be affected by interruptions in metabolic demands from alterations in blood flow.[12] Its function depends on uninterrupted flow, regardless of the position of the nerve in relation to surrounding tissue. However, low-grade compression, as well as elongation of 12% or more, is sufficient to cause alterations of action potential and the nerve shows minimal recovery.[19] Elongation of 11% also showed circulatory disturbance, inhibiting retrograde transport.[20] These changes include reduced circulation, resulting in nerve ischemia, endoneurial edema, suppression of axonal transport, and altered conduction characteristics. These events can stem from the multiple etiologies that are responsible for nerve injury. Besides the aforementioned compression and elongation, direct needle or catheter related mechanism damage, ischemia, and drug-related neurotoxicity can lead to temporary or permanent nerve damage. Regarding compression, any slight change in blood supply, whether from direct compression or increase in tissue pressures above certain critical levels, can lead to varying levels of neurological dysfunction. Two established anatomical sites where this occurs due to space limitations are the cubital tunnel and carpal tunnel.[21] Blood supply can also be disrupted by substances such as epinephrine, particularly in the PNS due to its α-1-adrenergic agonist properties, which can be a concern when using it as an additive in peripheral nerve block solution.[22] Irritation and inflammation, either preexisting from chronic medical conditions or acutely from neurotoxic drugs, in conjunction with disruption of blood supply, can be especially damaging.

SOMATIC AND AUTONOMIC NERVOUS SYSTEMS

Three kinds of nerve fibers are carried in the peripheral nerve—motor, sensory, and autonomic. Traditionally, the PNS is divided into two parts, the somatic and the autonomic. The somatic system consists of both cranial and spinal nerves. They are distinct from the autonomic system, as the somatic system is involved in sensory and motor function, while the autonomic system regulates body functions that can proceed independently from voluntary control.

SOMATIC NERVOUS SYSTEM

The somatic nervous system can further be divided into the somatic efferent (motor) and the somatic afferent (sensory) nerves. The efferent neurons originate within the spinal cord and brainstem. Their cell bodies are in the ventral gray horns of the spinal cord and motor nuclei of the cranial nerves; their axons traverse the ventral roots and spinal nerves and terminate in the motor end plates of the skeletal muscle fibers.

The afferent, or sensory neurons, receive sensory information from the periphery. These general sensory endings are scattered profusely throughout the body and transport information to the central nervous system (CNS). The afferent nerve's cell body is located outside the CNS in either the dorsal root ganglia of the spinal cord or an equivalent cranial nerve ganglion. Spinal ganglia contain the cell bodies of primary sensory neurons and are located on the dorsal roots of the spinal nerves, in the intervertebral foramina. These spinal ganglia contain both the dorsal root ganglia and the ganglia of the cranial nerves. Upon entering the CNS, the dorsal root fibers divide into the ascending and descending branches and are distributed into either reflex responses or transmission of sensory data to the brain.

The largest neurons in the sensory ganglia are proprioception and discriminative touch. Those of intermediate size mediate light touch, pressure, pain, and temperature, and the smallest neurons transmit impulses for pain and temperature as well. Each cell body, as previously discussed, has a supportive layer of a Schwann cell sheath, and external to this is connective tissue, collagen fibers, and blood vessels.

AUTONOMIC NERVOUS SYSTEM

The autonomic nervous system comprises a third class of sensory endings, known as the interoceptors, in the viscera. The autonomic nervous system can be further divided into two parts, the sympathetic and parasympathetic. The visceral efferents carry information from the internal organs regarding pain or functional regulation of internal organs; thus, they serve as another pathway for pain information besides the sensory efferents. For autonomic receptors involved in pain or functional regulation of internal organs, the sensory axon reaches the sympathetic trunk through a white communicating ramus and continues to a viscus in the branch of the sympathetic trunk. Some have their cell bodies in cranial nerve ganglia and are connected centrally within the brainstem. The visceral efferents of the autonomic nervous system transmit messages from the CNS to smooth muscle cells, cardiac muscle cells, or secretory cells. The autonomic nervous system is discussed more extensively in Chapters 13 and 14.

ANATOMY AND FUNCTION OF THE SYNAPSE AND ACTION POTENTIALS

In 1952, Hodgkin and Huxley proposed a scientific model to explain how action potentials are initiated and propagated in neurons and cardiac myocytes.[23] These equations approximated, for the first time, electrical characteristics of these cells, using a squid giant axon. The surface of the neuron is where the initiation and transmission of signals occur, on the plasma membrane. This membrane contains transmembrane proteins that provide hydrophilic channels through which inorganic ions can enter and leave by diffusion. Other channels are specific for different ions such as Na^+, K^+, Cl^-, and Ca^{2+}, as well as mixed channels that allow multiple ions to enter and exit. Some of these channels are voltage gated, meaning they open and close in response to an electrical potential change. Others are ligand-gated responsive, meaning they respond to certain neurotransmitters.

The most abundant ions in the extracellular fluid are the Na^+ and Cl^-, while inside the cell K^+ is most abundant. The extracellular fluid and cytoplasm are neutral, and the inside is negative (−70 mV) with respect to the outside when the neuron is not conducting a signal. Thus, this resting membrane potential opposes the outward movement of K^+ ions and the inward movement of Cl^- ions. The membrane is not very permeable to Na^+ because the voltage-gated channels for this ion stay closed with a negative resting membrane potential. When an axon is stimulated, the signal carried by the neuron changes the potential difference across the plasma membrane to +40 mV. This reversal, or action potential, is an all-or-none phenomenon, meaning a sufficient signal is generated leading to an impulse, or not.

Action potentials transmit across the axon to a point of functional contact between two neurons called a synapse. The term "synapse," meaning a conjunction or connection, was introduced by Sherrington in 1897. In the 1950s, the advent of the electron microscope confirmed this idea, showing that the synapse consists of the axonal ending (presynaptic side), the dendritic side (postsynaptic side), and the cleft in between. At this location, the electrical impulse from one cell to another is transmitted. There are two main types of synapse, chemical and electrical. Most of the synapses in the mammalian PNS are chemical.

When a membrane potential of a presynaptic neuron is reversed by the arrival of an action potential, calcium channels are opened and Ca^{2+} ions diffuse into the cell, as they are present at a higher concentration in the extracellular fluid than in the cytoplasm. This calcium entry leads to the release of neurotransmitters and neuromodulators into the synaptic cleft. They diffuse across the cleft and then bind to a specific receptor. Classic neurotransmitters either stimulate or inhibit the postsynaptic cell. Thus, the transmission can depolarize the membrane potential, making it more positive, or hyperpolarize it, making it more negative. Neuromodulators have other actions, including modifying the responsiveness to the transmitters. Some of theses neurotransmitters and modulators act rapidly, within milliseconds, by combining with the ionotropic receptors. Others, such as peptides, take seconds, minutes, and even hours to act.

FUNCTION OF SOMATIC AFFERENTS, RECEPTORS, AND FIBERS

The sensory neurons are biological transducers, in which physical or chemical stimuli create action potentials in nerve endings. The resulting nerve impulse, upon reaching the CNS, produces a reflex response, awareness of the stimuli, or both. Exteroceptors are located on the skin and respond to pain, temperature, touch, and pressure. Examples of these receptors are Meissner's corpuscles, Pacinian corpuscles, or free nerve endings called nociceptors. Proprioceptors are in the muscles, tendons, and joints and allow for awareness of position and movement, as well as reflex adjustments of muscle actions. Pain—triggered by physical injury, local inflammation or ischemia—can also originate from muscles, tendons, and joints, likely from the free nerve endings in the connective tissue. Thus, signals from these receptors are conducted by the primary sensory neurons and travel to the dorsal root ganglia, or an equivalent cranial nerve ganglion, as described above.

The sensory endings are supplied by axons that differ in size and other characteristics. There is some correlation between the rate of conduction of the action potential and the fiber diameter. Different sensory endings are supplied by fibers of specific sizes. Pain and temperature information carried in the C fibers is typically carried at a slow conduction velocity, because C fibers are of a small external diameter and unmyelinated.

The type of sensation consciously perceived from the skin is referred to as a modality. These are not always easily distinguished, but traditionally they are separated into five modalities that correlate to a physical examination: fine touch, vibration, light touch, temperature, and pain. Each of these modalities is associated with a qualitative aspect. For example, pain can be aching or burning, while temperature has a quality that can vary continuously. The human skin is a patchwork of these modalities, each area responding only to one of the modalities. Another important property to note about sensory fibers is that they adapt. For a continued stimulus, there is a lessened response. The one modality that does not have adaption is pain, for safety reasons.

THE INNERVATION OF THE PERIPHERAL NERVOUS SYSTEM

The central and peripheral nervous systems are sources of clinical symptoms, particularly pain, in different ways. The spinal cord has no sensory receptors, and sensory input from the meninges is inconsistent. Thus, when direct trauma occurs to the spinal cord, the patient may or may not experience pain. Pressure-related discomfort, as with actual injection into the spinal cord, appears to be more readily sensed by patients, due to the pressure-related stimulation of afferent neurons. In the PNS, the connective tissues are highly innervated, and are believed to greatly contribute to pain with compression nerve injuries.[12] The connective tissue, nerve roots, and the autonomic nervous system have an intrinsic innervation: the "nervi nervorum" from local axonal branching. This has been considered a source of symptoms in diabetic neuropathy and inflammatory polyneuropathies. Also, free nerve endings have been observed (by electron microscopy) in the epineurium and perineurium.[6] Direct damage to the peripheral nerve results in continual ectopic spontaneous discharge of pain signals, known as neuropathic pain. Finally, there is an extrinsic vasomotor innervation from the fibers coming from the perivascular plexuses into the nerve itself. Overall, the innervation of the PNS and how it relates to particular pathological entities is an understudied area, and our understanding is thus incomplete.

NERVE INJURY

CATEGORIES OF NERVE INJURY

A less serious nerve injury is known as a moderate conduction block. Some ischemia occurs to the entire anatomically area, which is not due to any direct local mechanism. This leads to a temporary conduction block within the nerves. Recovery is usually rapid, within hours to days. No long-term structural damage is caused to the nerves.

Seddon proposed a classification of the serious nerve injuries.[24] In order to determine the extent and prognosis of the nerve injury, it must be determined whether or not the axon was preserved. In *neuropraxic injuries*, the myelin sheath is damaged, leading to dysfunction of the action potential (conduction block), but the axon, nerve trunk itself, and the endoneurial sheath are preserved. These commonly occur with stretch or compression injuries and have a better prognosis, as myelin can be regenerated. These injuries generally take 4–6 weeks to recover. The nerves with more support cells are less susceptible to injury than those larger fibers with little supporting connective tissue. If the axon is destroyed, usually either by a severe crush or traction injury, recovery is slower and usually incomplete. This occurrence is known as *axonotmesis*. The recovery is basically reliant on collateral reinnervation from surrounding nerves or axonal regrowth. After the injury, a process called *Wallerian degeneration* occurs, in which the axon degenerates after being detached from the remainder of the cells. Phagocytes remove the residual portions of axon and myelin, and they prepare the nerve to receive any axons that might regenerate into its remaining stump. The process of Wallerian degeneration affects not only the axon but its myelin sheath. Subsequent regrowth may or may not occur. The success of this regrowth mainly depends on how much of the endoneurial tubes (chains of Schwann cells) were preserved. If most of the sheath and connective tissue elements are preserved, the injury may be reversible. It takes 3–12 months to recover, as a nerve grows approximately 1 mm/day.

If there is total disruption of the axon and connective tissue elements, the growing axons have no guide to the correct peripheral target, and the injury is more severe. This injury is termed *neurotmesis*. This also results in degeneration, but no opportunity for regeneration and thus often necessitates surgery to regain some degree of partial function.

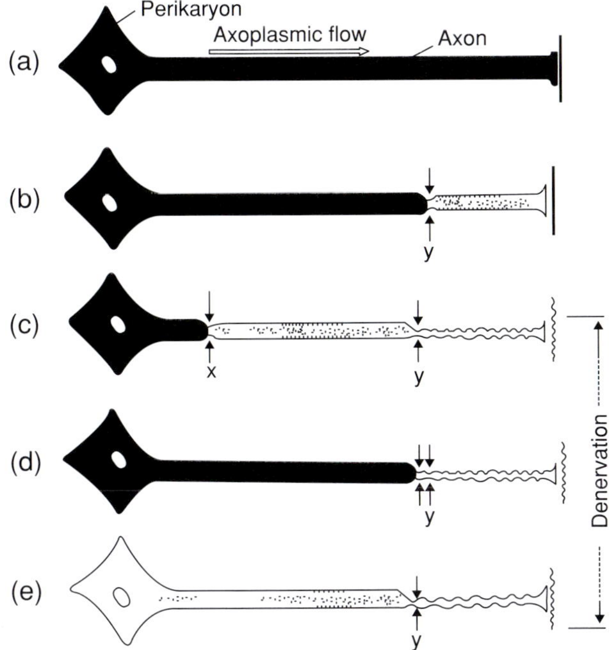

Figure 10.4 *The double crush syndrome* The different types of neural lesions leading to denervation are represented. In these sketches, the amount of axoplasmic material is indicated by the density of shading; complete loss of material causes denervation (c, d, e). X and Y are two regions of nerve compression. (a) In a healthy nerve, there is no compression. (b) Mild compression at Y is insufficient to cause denervation. (c) Mild compression at two sites causes denervation distal to Y. (d) Severe compression at one site only (Y) also causes denervation. (e) Barely sufficient trophic material is manufactured by the perikaryon of a "sick" neuron (e.g., in diabetes) and is then reduced by compression at one site, again causing denervation. Reprinted from Upton AR, McComas AJ. The double crush in nerve entrapment syndromes. *Lancet*. 1973;302: 359–362, with permission from Elsevier.

THE DOUBLE CRUSH SYNDROME

In the proposal of the double crush syndrome, Upton *et al.*[25] showed that "most patients with carpal tunnel syndromes or ulnar neuropathies not only have compressive lesions at the wrist or elbows, but they also have evidence of damage at the level of the cervical roots." The hypothesis states that if nerve function is impaired at one location with the axons being compressed at one site, the nerve is more susceptible to damage at another site. The functional integrity of an axon, as well as the sensory receptors and muscle fibers downstream, rely on chemical substances that are transported down the axon and secreted along the neuron. Any disruption to that supply, such as that which occurs at injury, can either produce symptoms or be subclinical. If the patient's injury remains subclinical, it may take a secondary injury to produce symptoms. This is the basis of the "double crush" injury hypothesis (Figure 10.4). The injury may be of a lesser degree than expected to produce symptoms, because the axon was already damaged. It has also been noted that two low-grade compressions along a nerve trunk is worse than compression at a single site, but that the damage of the dual compression far exceeds the expected additive damage caused by each isolated compression.[26]

NERVE CONDUCTION STUDIES AND LOCALIZING THE INJURY

Conduction block occurs when the nerve action potential is blocked along the path of an intact axon. It causes neurapraxia, a certain type of nerve injury in which the myelin is damaged, but not the axon. Via nerve conduction studies, conduction blocks can be identified by electrical stimulation proximal and then distal to the suspected injury. Conduction block occurs if the muscle action potential has a significant drop in amplitude across the distal, as compared to the proximal, stimulation site. This assists in definitively localizing the lesion to the site of the block and suggests neurapraxia.

BLOCKADE OF PERIPHERAL NERVE CONDUCTION

While the detection and prevention of nerve injury is extremely important, temporary blockade of peripheral nerve conduction plays an important role in surgical and perioperative management. Local anesthetics act by binding to sodium channels in their inactive state, thereby preventing subsequent channel activation and sodium channel influx. By blocking sodium channel input, the action potential cannot be propagated.[27] While this is effective in blocking afferent pain transmission, nerve fibers not associated with pain are also blocked, thereby producing motor blockade and other unwanted effects. A better understanding of genetic disorders associated with pain (erythromelalgia, paroxysmal extreme pain disorder, congenital insensitivity to pain) has led to an appreciation of mutations of specific sodium channels.[28,29] The $Na_v1.7$ appears to be a potential target of the selective blockade of nociceptors.

Another promising concept for the selective sensory blockade during peripheral nerve blocks involves the TRPV1 receptors and permanently charged local anesthetics. Normally, only local anesthetics in their nonionized form can traverse the lipophilic nerve membrane to gain access to the receptor site of the sodium channel, while the ionized form binds to the site and produces the blocking action. The TRPV1 receptor is a nonspecific, large ion channel selectively expressed on nociceptors that is activated by heat and capsaicin (the active ingredient in chili peppers). By opening these receptors using capsaicin or short-acting local anesthetics (lidocaine), a permanently charged local anesthetic (i.e. QX-314- a permanently charged form of lidocaine) can gain access to sodium channel binding sites on the internal membrane of nociceptors. The inability for a permanently charged local anesthetic to cross the membrane of other nerve types leads to a selective sensory blockade.[30,31]

CONCLUSION

The basic anatomy and function of the PNS has been a well-studied topic over the past decades, but many areas in the field, especially clinical applications, are still under development. It is imperative for the anesthesiologist to have at least a basic understanding of the PNS not only to deliver proper anesthetic care but also to follow new developments in the field. The anatomy and function of the PNS can be applied to the etiology, prevention, diagnosis, and treatment of perioperative nerve injuries, the administration of peripheral nerve blocks in all their complexity, and the administration of drugs that act directly on the PNS.

REFERENCES

1. Berthold CH. Morphology of normal peripheral axons. In: Waxman SG, ed. *Physiology and Pathobiology of Axons*. New York: Raven Press; 1978.
2. Huxley AF, Stampfli R. Evidence for saltatory conduction in peripheral myelinated nerve fibres. *J Physiol.* 1949;108:315–339.
3. Enlarger J, Gasser H. *Electrical Signs of Nervous Activity*. Philadelphia: University of Pennsylvania Press; 1937.
4. Vallee RB, Bloom GS. Mechanisms of fast and slow axonal transport. *Annu Rev Neurosci.* 1991;14:59–92.
5. Berthold CH, Fraher JP, King RHM. Microscopic anatomy of the peripheral nervous system. In: Dyke PJ, Thomas PK, eds. *Peripheral Neuropathy*, 4th ed. Philadelphia: Elsevier Saunders; 2005.
6. Thomas PK. The connective tissue of peripheral nerve: an electron microscope study. *J Anat.* 1963;97:35–44.
7. Shanthaveerappa TR, Bourne GH. The "perineural epithelium," a metabolically active, continuous, protoplasmic cell barrier surrounding peripheral nerve fasciculi. *J Anat.* 1962;96:527–537.
8. Lundborg G. *Nerve Injury and Repair*. Edinburgh: Churchill Livingston; 1988.
9. Moayeri N, Bigeleisen PE, Groen GJ. Quantitative architecture of the brachial plexus and surrounding compartments, and their possible significance for plexus blocks. *Anesthesiology.* 2008;108:299–304.
10. Millesi H. The nerve gap: theory and clinical practice. *Hand Clin.* 1986;2:651–663.
11. Wilgis EF, Murphy R. The significance of longitudinal excursion in peripheral nerves. *Hand Clin.* 1986;2:761–766.
12. Butler DS. Functional anatomy and physiology of the nervous system. In: Butler DS, ed. *Mobilisation of the Nervous System*. Philadelphia: Churchill Livingstone; 1991.
13. Neal JM. Effects of epinephrine in local anesthetics on the central and peripheral nervous systems: neurotoxicity and neural blood flow. *Reg Anesth Pain Med.* 2003;28:124–134.
14. Rechthand E, Hervonen A, Sato S, Rapoport SI. Distribution of adrenergic innervation of blood vessels in peripheral nerve. *Brain Res.* 1986;374:185–189.
15. Lundborg G. Structure and function of the intraneural microvessels as related to trauma, edema formation, and nerve function. *J Bone Joint Surg Am.* 1975;57:938–948.
16. Bell MA, Weddell AG. A descriptive study of the blood vessels of the sciatic nerve in the rat, man and other mammals. *Brain.* 1984; 107(Pt 3):871–898.
17. Lundborg G, Rydevik B. Effects of stretching the tibial nerve of the rabbit: a preliminary study of the intraneural circulation and the barrier function of the perineurium. *J Bone Joint Surg Br.* 1973; 55:390–401.
18. Dommisse GF. The blood supply of the spinal cord. In: Grieve GP, ed. *Modern Manual Therapy of the Vertebral Column*. Edinburgh: Churchill Livingston, 1986.
19. Wall EJ, Massie JB, Kwan MK, Rydevik BL, Myers RR, Garfin SR. Experimental stretch neuropathy: changes in nerve conduction under tension. *J Bone Joint Surg Br.* 1992;74:126–129.
20. Tanoue M, Yamaga M, Ide J, Takagi K. Acute stretching of peripheral nerves inhibits retrograde axonal transport. *J Hand Surg Br.* 1996;21:358–363.
21. Lundborg G, Dahlin LB. Anatomy, function, and pathophysiology of peripheral nerves and nerve compression. *Hand Clin.* 1996; 12:185–193.
22. Myers RR, Heckman HM. Effects of local anesthesia on nerve blood flow: studies using lidocaine with and without epinephrine. *Anesthesiology.* 1989;71:757–762.
23. Hodgkin AL, Huxley AF. A quantitative description of membrane current and its application to conduction and excitation in nerve. *J Physiol.* 1952;117:500–544.
24. Seddon HJ. Three types of nerve injury. *Brain.* 1942;66:237.
25. Upton AR, McComas AJ. The double crush in nerve entrapment syndromes. *Lancet.* 1973;2:359–362.
26. Osterman AL. The double crush syndrome. *Orthop Clin North Am.* 1988;19:147–155.
27. Butterworth JFt, Strichartz GR. Molecular mechanisms of local anesthesia: a review. *Anesthesiology.* 1990;72:711–734.
28. Dib-Hajj SD, Rush AM, Cummins TR, et al. Gain-of-function mutation in Nav1.7 in familial erythromelalgia induces bursting of sensory neurons. *Brain.* 2005;128:1847–1854.
29. Waxman SG. Nav1.7, its mutations, and the syndromes that they cause. *Neurology.* 2007;69:505–507.
30. Binshtok AM, Gerner P, Oh SB, et al. Coapplication of lidocaine and the permanently charged sodium channel blocker QX-314 produces a long-lasting nociceptive blockade in rodents. *Anesthesiology.* 2009;111:127–137.
31. Gerner P, Binshtok AM, Wang CF, et al. Capsaicin combined with local anesthetics preferentially prolongs sensory/nociceptive block in rat sciatic nerve. *Anesthesiology.* 2008;109:872–878.

11

THE NEUROBIOLOGY OF INCISIONAL PAIN

Timothy J. Brennan, Sinyoung Kang, and Jun Xu

Many patients experience moderate to severe pain after surgery, especially pain during physical activities. For postoperative patients, the current analgesic treatments rely largely on the generous administration of opioids.[1,2] However, these drugs have limited efficacy and produce several undesirable side effects. Furthermore, regional analgesia, as an alternative pain control approach, benefits a minority number of patients and has limitations as well as side effects. If new treatments with greater efficacy and reduced side effects become available, pain and suffering after surgery will be reduced, perioperative morbidity will decline, and health care costs could decrease.

In many cases, our understanding of pathophysiologic processes provides the rationale for particular therapies in perioperative medicine. However, this is not the case for postoperative pain management. A disease-oriented approach to postoperative pain is one model from which mechanism-based therapies should evolve. That is, surgery causes severe pain and the etiology should be better understood. Presumably, if we learn more about the sensory processes that intensify pain after surgery, new treatment methods can be developed. Thus, research to make translational links between clinical postoperative pain and basic preclinical research on pain mechanisms caused by incisions is key to translate new therapeutic targets for postoperative patients.

RAT MODEL FOR POSTOPERATIVE PAIN

We have developed and characterized a rat model for postoperative pain to understand the processes that amplify and intensify pain caused by surgery.[3] The model is produced by a simple incision that includes skin, fascia, and deep muscle tissue at the plantar aspect of the hindpaw in anesthetized rats (Figure 11.1A).

Many studies have been undertaken to examine changes in sensory processing produced by surgery. These extensive studies began by recording activity from sensory neurons with input from the plantar hindpaw and measuring their responses during and after experimental plantar hindpaw incisions.[4] Incisions into hindpaw mechanical receptive fields of lumbar dorsal horn neurons increased both ongoing and evoked sensory neuron activity. Furthermore, the effect of local anesthetic administered into the incision site before or after incision on these responses has been characterized.[5] In general, local anesthetic injection into the incision restores dorsal horn neuron activity to a level similar to the unincised preparation. Similarly, local anesthetic injection eliminates pain-related behavioral responses when administered before or after incision. Together, these studies suggest that peripheral, primary afferent nociceptors transmit the early, acute pathophysiologic signal of both increased ongoing and evoked sensory neuron activity from incisions. Additional studies at later times after incision support the concept that peripheral sensitization is a prominent feature in the sensory signature of acute postoperative pain.[6,7] Central sensitization also occurs and is easily demonstrated.[8] Nevertheless, the central sensitization is largely driven by peripheral input. Thus, nociceptor physiology and pathophysiology are of considerable importance for understanding mechanisms of acute incisional and postoperative pain.

This chapter will examine pain-related behaviors caused by incisions. Nociceptor physiology will be examined. Evidence for pathophysiologic changes in nociceptors produced by incisions that transmit abnormal pain-related behaviors will be reviewed. Potential therapeutic targets present on nociceptors for relief of postoperative pain will be discussed.

PAIN-RELATED BEHAVIORS

Pain is an unpleasant sensory and emotional experience associated with actual or potential tissue damage.[9] In disease states, increased pain sensitivity occurs, which is known as hyperalgesia. For comparison, nociception, a physiological term, describes the neural processes for transmitting and processing responses to noxious or potentially noxious stimuli. Because animals cannot describe their sensory experience, exaggerated behavioral responses are inferred to represent pain and hyperalgesia in animal models. These animal models are developed, in part, to understand pathophysiology using techniques and experiments that may not be easily

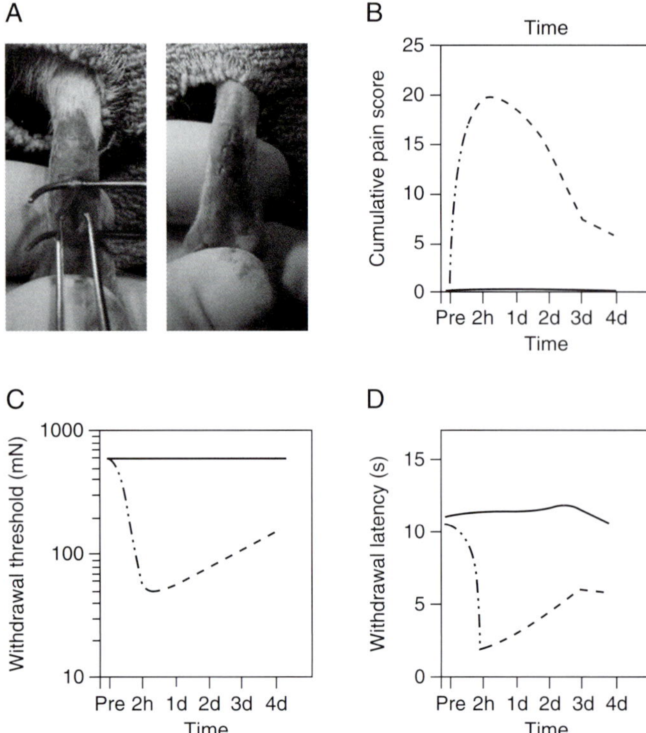

Figure 11.1 (A) Example of plantar incision of skin, fascia, and muscle. The underlying muscle is divided and retracted (left) and the skin is closed with nylon suture (right). (B) Nonevoked spontaneous guarding behavior in sham (solid line) and incised rats (broken line). (C) Paw withdrawal threshold in sham (solid line) and incised rats (broken line). (D) Heat withdrawal latency in sham (solid line) and incised rats (broken line). Pre = before incision. h = hour. d =day. S = seconds. mN = millinewtons.

undertaken in humans. The behaviors in animal models that parallel clinical postoperative pain are beginning to be understood; these responses are nociceptive behaviors that are correlates of pain and hyperalgesia in humans.

Our laboratory and others have assessed several pain-related behaviors in rats after plantar incision.[3,8] In this review we will describe three behaviors after plantar incision and propose models for their underlying neural transmission pathways from the site of injury into the central nervous system. The behavioral aspects of the model are characterized as follows: (1) nonevoked, guarding behaviors; (2) persistent, reduced withdrawal thresholds to mechanical stimuli; and (3) decreased heat withdrawal latency. All of these pain-related behaviors observed in animals are correlates of pain in postoperative patients and human subjects with incisions in terms of changes in intensity over time.

NONEVOKED GUARDING

As rats were left undisturbed in the testing environment, it was noted that they did not bear weight on the incised hindpaw for several days after plantar incision. This positioning was used to develop a cumulative pain score, to quantify guarding behavior.[3,10] Each hindpaw was scored during a 1-minute period every 5 minutes for 1 hour. A score of 0, 1, or 2 was given. Full weight-bearing of the hindpaw (score = 0) was present if the wound was blanched or distorted by the mesh floor. If the hindpaw wound was completely off the mesh, a score of 2 was recorded. If the area of the wound touched the mesh without blanching or distorting, a 1 was given. The same measurement was performed for the corresponding area in the uninjured hindpaw. The sum of the 12 scores (0–24) obtained during the 1 hr session for each hindpaw was obtained. The difference between the scores from the incised hindpaw and nonincised hindpaw was the cumulative pain score for that 1 hr period. Several pharmacologic studies indicate this behavior is different than the response to punctate mechanical stimuli.[11–13]

Example data of nonevoked guarding after incision are shown in Fig. 11.1B. Two hours after plantar incision, the median pain score increased from approximately 0 to 19. On the day after incision, the score was 16 and then was approximately 11 on the second day after incision. Pain scores continued to decrease at later times after the incision. By day 3 or 4 the guarding had largely resolved. In contrast to other pain models, no consistent flinching and licking behavior was observed except during emergence from general anesthesia and in the immediate postoperative recovery period. It is recognized that our pain score is a result of the position chosen by the rat after the incision rather than an evoked mechanical response; therefore, differences between these tests should be expected. Data indicate that this cumulative pain score may correlate to pain at rest in patients after surgery and may be driven by spontaneous activity in nociceptive pathways that occurs after incision.

MECHANICAL WITHDRAWAL THRESHOLD

Responses to punctate mechanical stimuli are determined by measuring withdrawal responses to nylon filaments with variable thickness. Application of these filaments causes them to bend and limits the force applied. Application until bending causes thin filaments to produce weak forces and thicker filaments to elicit greater forces. Nylon monofilament-induced touch may be converted to a painful stimulus after a variety of surgical procedures[14,15] as well as after experimental incisions in humans.[16,17]

Primary mechanical withdrawal threshold has been extensively characterized after hindpaw incision.[3,8] Filaments were applied from underneath the cage through openings (12 x 12 mm) in the plastic mesh floor to an area adjacent to the incision. Each filament was applied once starting with a low force like 15 millinewtons (mN) and continuing until a withdrawal response occurred or strong force like 500 mN (the cutoff value) was reached. The lowest force from the three tests producing a response was considered the withdrawal threshold. These filaments have been shown to excite large myelinated A-beta fibers and A- and C-mechanonociceptors recorded from afferents in the rat plantar hindpaw.[18,19]

Decreased response threshold to mechanical stimuli at the incision represents a nociceptive behavior similar to primary mechanical hyperalgesia noted in humans.[16,17] An example of changes in withdrawal threshold to mechanical stimuli is shown in Figure 11.1C. The median withdrawal threshold in the incised hindpaw decreased from a high force like 500 mN before incision (Pre) to approximately 50 mN at 2 hours after incision. The withdrawal thresholds were usually less than 100 mN 1, 2, and 3 days post incision (Figure 11.1C). A gradual return toward preincision values occurred over the next several days so that by 1 week the response was usually not significantly different than before incision (not shown).[3] The reduced withdrawal threshold was sustained for a greater duration than the nonevoked guarding behavior.

HEAT WITHDRAWAL LATENCY

Heat nociception is commonly studied in rodent pain models.[20] Withdrawal latencies to heat were assessed by applying a focused radiant heat source onto the incision in unrestrained rats until a withdrawal response is elicited. The heat stimulus was light from a 50 W projector lamp, with an aperture diameter of 6 mm, applied from underneath a heat-tempered glass floor (3 mm thick) on the middle of the incision in an unrestrained rat. Paw withdrawal latencies can be measured to the nearest 0.1 seconds. Three trials 5 to 10 minutes apart were used to obtain an average paw withdrawal latency; a reduced withdrawal latency indicates pain-related hyperalgesia. Decreased heat pain latency occurs in volunteers after experimental incisions[21] and in patients after surgery.[22]

After incision, the withdrawal latency to radiant heat applied directly on the incision decreased from the baseline of 10 to 12 seconds to approximately 3 seconds (Figure 11.1D). On postoperative days 1 and 2, the withdrawal latency remained decreased to less than 5 seconds. A gradual return toward preincision values occurred over 7 to 10 days (not shown). The clinical importance of heat hyperalgesia in postoperative pain patients is not yet understood. Nevertheless, heat pain testing is a common test, highly quantifiable, and used to characterize nociceptive responsiveness in animals.

NOCICEPTORS

Sensory nerve fibers are responsible for relaying information for both external and internal stimuli from visceral and somatic structures. These sensory fibers have terminals with specialized endings that respond to particular types of stimuli. If the stimulus is sufficient, such as the response to light touch of the skin, abdominal contractions, or a full urinary bladder, action potentials are generated in these sensory fibers. One group of primary afferent sensory fibers, nociceptors, is capable of responding to noxious, potentially tissue-damaging, stimuli.[23] Recording action potentials from these axons can be used to quantitate the nociceptor activity and properties. These pain-transmitting sensory fibers may not exclusively respond to noxious stimuli but may be activated by innocuous stimuli also. However, they respond to a greater degree to noxious stimulus intensities and can code the intensity of the stimulus. Nonnociceptive fibers may respond to warm, nonnoxious temperatures, cooling, and light touch, but as the strength of these stimuli increase into the noxious range, responses in these nonnociceptive fibers do not intensify correspondingly.

Nociceptors have been identified in dura, visceral structures, bone, muscle, blood vessels, and other organs. However, nociceptors have been most extensively studied in skin.[23] Thus classifications of nociceptors are largely based on detailed studies of a variety of stimuli applied to those afferent fibers innervating cutaneous and subcutaneous tissue. Nociceptors from other organs are less well characterized and in many cases are based on similar response criteria to those applied to skin nociceptors.

In the skin, nociceptors are classified as A-fiber nociceptors or C-fiber nociceptors based on conduction velocity. A-fibers are myelinated and C-fibers are unmyelinated. Typically, C-fiber nociceptors have conduction velocities less than 2 meters per second. A-fiber nociceptors conduct at velocities less than 30 meters per second and greater than 2 meters per second. Rapidly conducting A-fibers can be subdivided into Aβ (15 to 30 meters per second) and A-delta (2 to 15 meters per second) fibers. Of note, conduction velocity in nociceptors is a continuum; there is no strict cutoff for these different classes. For different species, the criteria of conduction velocity for A- and C-fibers also vary. For a detailed discussion of classifications based on conduction velocity see Djouhri and Lawson.[24]

Nociceptor responses are typically studied in two states, the normal and the postinjury state. In the normal state, nociceptors are also classified based on their responses to a variety of stimuli. Stimuli that can be used to characterize the fibers include noxious chemicals like capsaicin, mustard oil, or acid. Furthermore, noxious cold can excite nociceptors. Depending on the organ studied, other potentially noxious stimuli like stretch or distension can be evaluated. However, in general, nociceptors are classified based on their characteristic responses to mechanical and heat stimuli and conduction velocity. C-fibers responding to noxious mechanical and heat stimuli are C-fiber mechano-heat (CMH) nociceptors. Other examples are C-fiber heat (CH), A-fiber mechano-heat (AMH), mechanically insensitive afferent C-fibers (MIA), and MIA A-fibers.[23] Fibers can be further subdivided using detailed quantitative

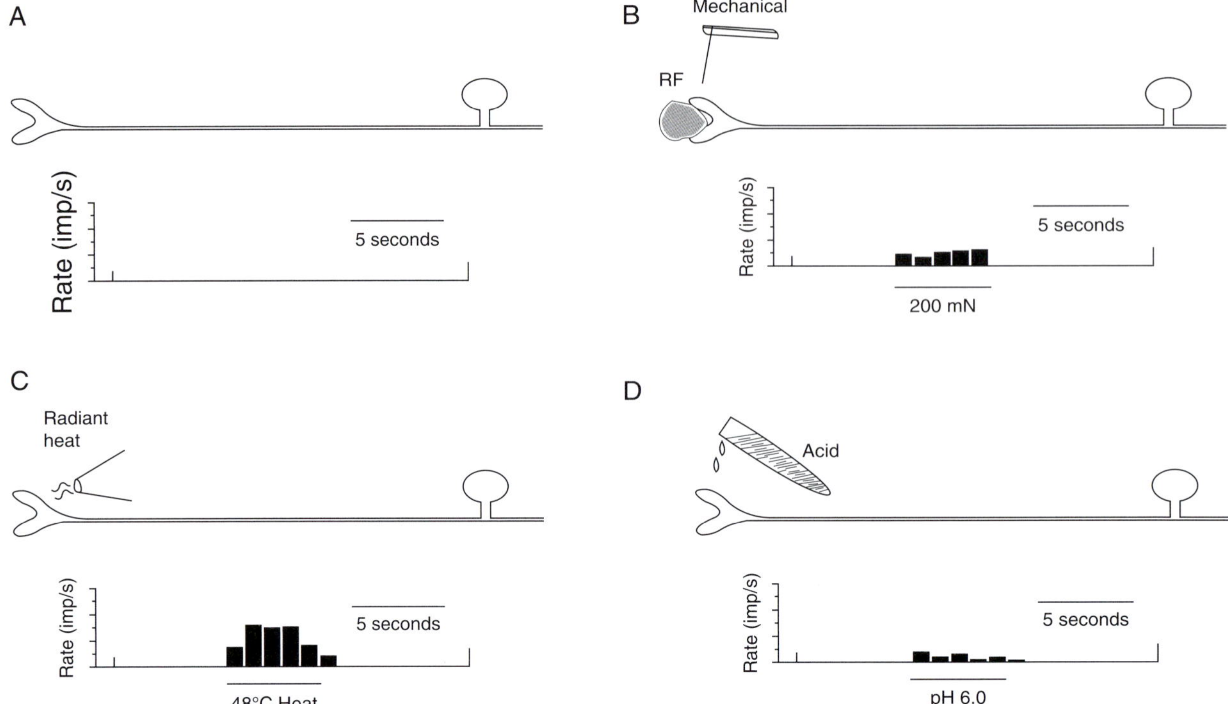

Figure 11.2 Schematic of normal nociceptor function. Nerve terminal, axon and dorsal root ganglion cell body are shown. (A) Nociceptors have minimal background activity. (B) Nociceptors typically have a mechanical receptive field mapped with a nylon monofilament that codes the intensity of noxious mechanical stimuli. (C) Heat responsive nociceptors are activated by noxious temperature usually greater than 43°C. (D) Nociceptors respond to chemical irritants like acid. Imp/s = impulses per second. RF = receptive field. mN = millinewtons.

responses to these stimuli. Immunoreactivity of the cell body in the dorsal root ganglion or nerve fiber for certain antigens like calcitonin gene-related peptide and neurofilament 200 can be used to further characterize the sensory afferents.[25]

Examples of responses of nociceptors to several types of noxious stimuli are shown in Figure 11.2. Each portion of Figure 11.2 depicts a dorsal root ganglion cell body, the afferent axon, the nerve terminal and the receptive field of the nociceptor. Nociceptors in the normative state rarely have spontaneous ongoing action potentials (Figure 11.2A). Usually they are quiescent, with minimal ongoing activity in the absence of any stimuli. Mechanical responses may occur with weak mechanical stimuli, but the magnitude of the response increases with greater mechanical stimulus strength. Vigorous responses to strong mechanical stimuli like monofilaments with 200 mN forces are typical. The response usually occurs only during the stimulation period (Figure 11.2B). There is a mechanical receptive field area, the area of mechanical responsiveness to a suprathreshold stimulus that can be mapped and quantified. For nociceptors, this area is usually well delineated (Figure 11.2B).

Noxious heat can be tested using radiant heat, a contact thermode, or a heated saline solution. Nociceptors respond to noxious heat; the threshold is usually 43 to 45°C and increasing responses are elicited with greater temperatures. In the example shown (Figure 11.2C), the 48°C heat stimulus exceeds the noxious threshold in humans and activation of the fiber occurs. Noxious chemicals, like acid, excite some nociceptors; the proportion of chemically responsive nociceptors and the degree to which they respond depends on the chemical stimulus used and the population of fibers selected for study (Figure 11.2D).

NOCICEPTOR SENSITIZATION

Nociceptors not only signal potential tissue-damaging stimuli but also become sensitized, that is, they develop increased responses to noxious and innocuous stimuli after an injury. A simple example is the response to warm stimuli. Before an injury, nonpainful warmth is perceived. After an injury the warm stimulus can produce a burning sensation. As one example of hyperalgesia, application of warm water produces a painful sensation after a sunburn. A key to translational pain research is to identify nociceptors that encode enhanced responsiveness so that targets transmitting these amplified signals on these nociceptors can be evaluated for therapeutic potential.

Hyperalgesia is the subjective response to nociceptor sensitization.[26] Hyperalgesia is divided into primary and secondary hyperalgesia. Primary hyperalgesia is an increased response at the site of injury, and secondary hyperalgesia is an enhanced response to a stimulus outside the injured area. Because nociceptors rarely sensitize to injury outside the receptive field, the generation of primary and secondary hyperalgesia have different mechanisms.[26] In general, primary hyperalgesia is a result of enhancement of nociceptor function per excitability.[23] Secondary hyperalgesia occurs as a result of sensitization of central pain-transmitting neurons both in the spinal cord and in supraspinal structures. Primary hyperalgesia may be further amplified by central sensitization. Secondary hyperalgesia is initiated by nociceptor activation but is a result of central sensitization.

This chapter will focus on primary hyperalgesia and peripheral sensitization. The changes in nociceptor physiology, sensitization, that likely transmit pain related responses after incision will be reviewed. The implications in the pathophysiology of postoperative pain in patients will be discussed.

Characteristics of nociceptor sensitization after injury include:[27,28]

- increased spontaneous activity,
- decreased threshold,
- increased response to a suprathreshold stimulus,
- after-discharge,
- expansion of the receptive field,
- an increase in the proportion of afferents responding to a stimulus.

Examples of these phenomena are shown in Figure 11.3. Again the dorsal root ganglion cell body, the afferent axon, the nerve terminal, and the receptive field of the nociceptor are shown. An incisional injury is depicted in the receptive field. Sustained background activity is present in the injured state (Figure 11.3A). Background activity in sensitized nociceptors may be regular, or activity may occur in irregular, bursting patterns (not shown). There is an increase in response to mechanical stimulation (Figure 11.3B) compared to the normative state (Figure 11.2B). The size of the mechanical receptive field is increased as well (Figure 11.3B). It is possible that MIAs are converted to mechanically sensitive fibers by the injury (not shown).

After injury, an increased response to heat is noted (Figures 11.2C and 11.3C). Usually heat threshold is decreased (not shown). In some cases the response continues after the heat stimulus is removed in a sensitized afferent. In general, the area of the heat receptive field is not measured because the size of the heat stimulus is usually large relative to the receptive field.

Response to chemical stimulation may be increased. For example, the threshold for a response to acid may be decreased, or the response to low pH increased (Figures 11.2D and 11.3D). The area of the chemoreceptive

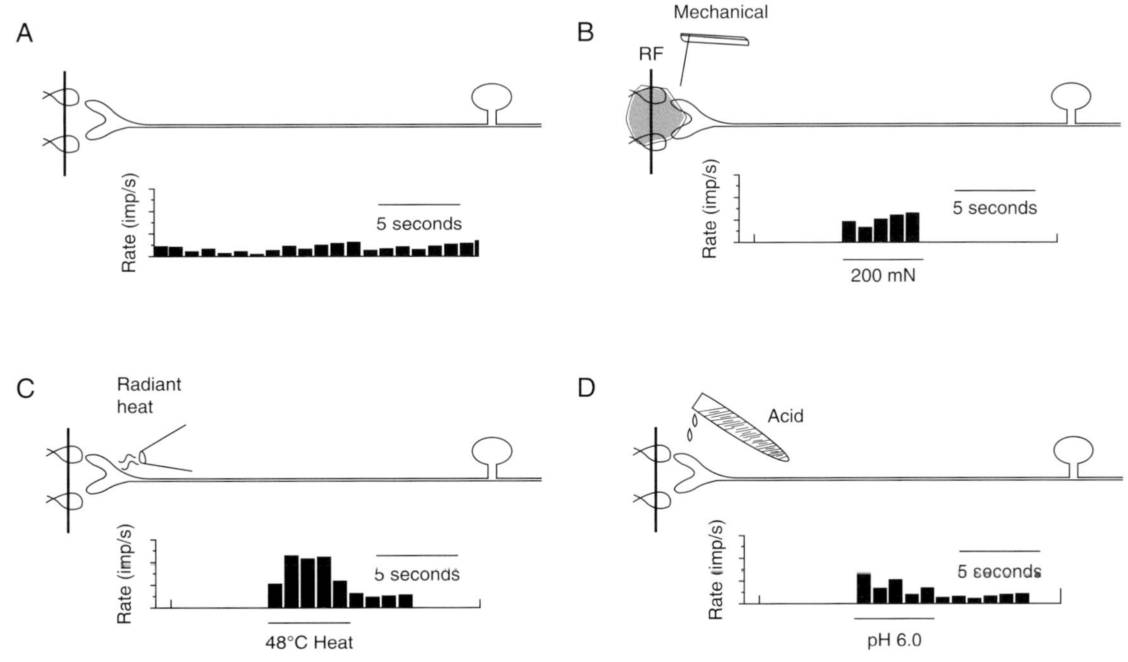

Figure 11.3 Nociceptors develop increased responses, sensitization, after injury. This is a schematic of nociceptor sensitization after incisional injury. (A) Nociceptors develop ongoing, background activity following injury. (B) Nociceptors develop decreased threshold and increased responsiveness to suprathreshold mechanical stimuli as well as expansion of the mechanical receptive fields. (C) Nociceptors develop decreased heat threshold after incisional injury. Also, increased peak responses to a heat stimulus and after discharge following the heat stimulus can occur. (D) Nociceptors may become responsive to chemical stimuli and develop enhanced responses to chemical stimuli. Imp/s = impulses per second. RF = receptive field. mN = millinewtons.

fields is generally not determined. There are few studies that have shown that the proportion of afferents responding to acid increases after injury. After-discharge, a response that continues after removal of the acid, may occur.

METHODS FOR RECORDING NOCICEPTOR ACTIVITY

Two methods are used to record electrical activity of nociceptors and evaluate the effect of incisions. These methods are briefly described. The first is in vivo primary afferent fiber recording.[29] Rats are initially anesthetized with an intraperitoneal injection of pentobarbital sodium and supplemented with additional anesthesia as needed. Rats are ventilated, mean arterial blood pressure is recorded, and body temperature is maintained at approximately 37°C. At the popliteal fossa, the tibial nerve is isolated and transected proximally. A pool for warm mineral oil is then made. Fine filaments of the tibial nerve are repeatedly teased from the cut end and placed on a platinum electrode until single-unit activity can be discriminated and recorded. Nerve activity is amplified, filtered, and displayed on a digital oscilloscope. It is then stored into a personal computer with a data acquisition system.

In the other method, recordings are made from nociceptors in vitro. A glabrous in vitro skin-nerve preparation, modeled as saphenous nerve-skin preparation,[30] has been described elsewhere.[31,32] In brief, rats are euthanized in a carbon dioxide chamber; the medial and lateral plantar nerves and their innervated territory on the glabrous hindpaw skin are dissected until the nerve and skin can be removed. The skin is placed epidermal side down in the in vitro perfusion chamber, and superfused with modified balanced salt solution, which is saturated with a gas mixture of 95% oxygen and 5% carbon dioxide. The temperature of the bath solution is maintained at 32 ± 0.5°C. The plantar nerves are drawn through a small hole into the recording chamber containing a superficial layer of mineral oil and a bottom layer of modified balanced salt solution. The nerve is desheathed on a mirror stage, and small filaments are repeatedly split with sharpened forceps to allow single fiber recording to be made using extracellular wire recording electrodes. Neural activity is amplified, filtered, and displayed using standard techniques. Amplified signals are relayed into a digital oscilloscope, an audiomonitor, and a computer via a data acquisition system.

For the in vivo preparation, the receptive fields of afferent fibers in the plantar hindpaw are identified by applying monofilaments onto the glabrous skin; for the in vitro preparation, the receptive fields are determined by probing the skin with a blunt glass rod; thus, mechanosensitive afferents are recorded. Only units with a clearly distinguished signal to noise ratio (greater than 2:1) are further studied. The conduction velocity of each unit is determined by electrical stimulation (5–20 V, 0.5–2.0 ms duration, 0.2–1.0 Hz) into the most mechanosensitive site in the receptive field. Then the distance between the receptive field and the recording electrode (conduction distance) is divided by the latency of the electrically evoked action potential. Afferent fibers are classified as C-fibers or as A-fiber nociceptors. Units are classified as mechanosensitive nociceptors on the basis of their graded response throughout the innocuous and noxious range of mechanical force stimuli.

SPONTANEOUS ACTIVITY IN NOCICEPTORS AFTER INCISION

For in vivo recording, comparisons between unincised rats and rats incised one day previously were performed. Spontaneous activity was present in both Aδ- and C-nociceptors.[18,29] Overall, the percentage of nociceptors with spontaneous activity was low, 13% (25% Aδ- and 10% C-nociceptors) in the unoperated, control group compared to 61% (60% Aδ- and 61% C-nociceptors) in the incision group, on postoperative day 1. An example is shown in Figure 11.4 (A–B). During mechanical testing, ongoing spontaneous activity is present in the fiber from the incised group. The prevalence of afferents with spontaneous activity was only 14% (0% Aδ- and 20% C-nociceptors) when pain behaviors had resolved on postoperative day 7. The mean rate of spontaneous activity was 6 ± 6 impulses per second in the sham group, the spontaneous activity also tended to be greater in the incision group (10 ± 3 impulses per second) compared with the sham group (6 ± 6) on postoperative day 1. The activity resolved by postoperative day 7 (0 ± 0 impulses per second). In a previous study, similar results were noted. One day after incision,[18] more A- and C-fibers have spontaneous activity (39% vs. 0% in the sham control group) and the activity was also greater (15 impulses per second vs. 0 impulses per second) in the incision group (postoperative day 1) compared to the sham control group.

In previous studies, however, spontaneous activity was not evident in mechanosensitive afferents acutely after plantar incision,[19] whereas significant spontaneous activity was remarkable 1 day after incision.[18] It was first suggested that nociceptors that developed spontaneous activity after incision were mechanically insensitive afferents (MIA) or chemosensitive afferents.[18] We suggested that these afferents are not easily identified using a mechanical search stimulus in normal tissue before incision,[19] but can be sensitized and distinguished 1 day after tissue injury.[18] Subsequent studies suggested that these afferents with spontaneous activity after incision likely innervate deep tissue.[29]

Several years ago, other investigators used mechanical damage or skin cuts to attempt to activate and sensitize

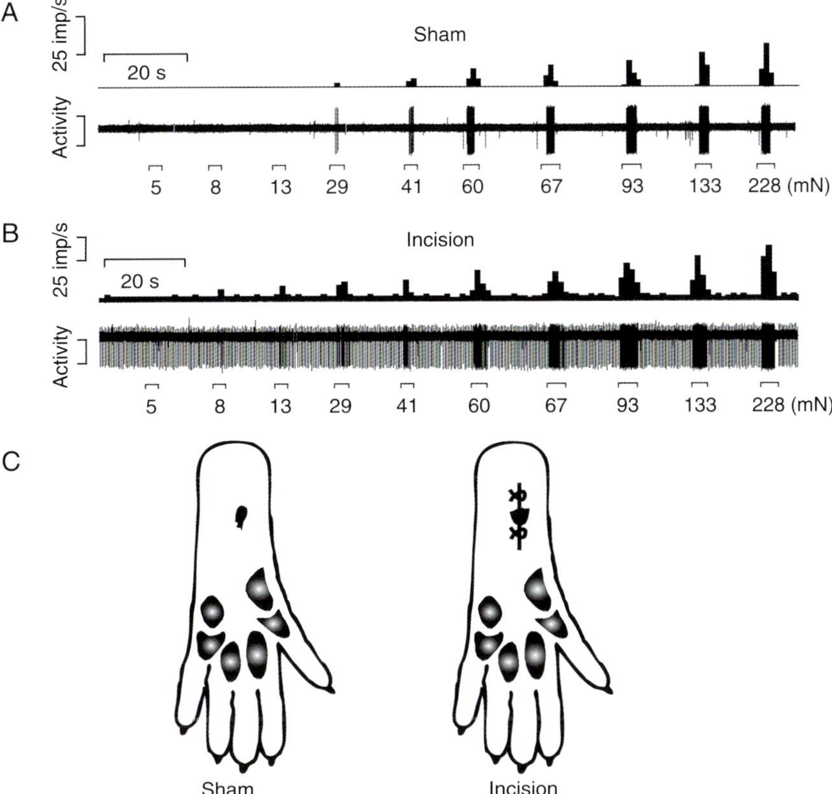

Figure 11.4 Example recordings of spontaneous activity and responses of nociceptors to mechanical stimulation. Digitized oscilloscope trace of action potentials evoked by von Frey filaments in the sham control rats (A) and in a rat that underwent incision one day earlier (B). Mechanical receptive field size of nociceptor from sham operated hindpaw (left) and incised (right) hindpaw denoted by solid black area (C). The area of the receptive fields were larger in incised rats. imp/s = impulses per second. mN = millinewtons. Reprinted with permission from Xu J, Brennan TJ. Guarding pain and spontaneous activity of nociceptors after skin versus skin plus deep tissue incision. *Anesthesiology*. 2010;112(1):153–164.

cutaneous nociceptors.[33] In these earlier studies, persistent activation of nociceptors was not reported. For example, spontaneous activity in cat cutaneous A- and C-nociceptors was not induced immediately after penetrations into the skin receptive field using a sharp (needle) point.[34,35] Even after repeated penetrations of the receptive field in skin, only a few after-discharges were occasionally produced.[35] Afferent spontaneous activity was not reported immediately after 1 mm deep cuts were made with a blade in the mechanical receptive field of cutaneous C-nociceptors of monkey in vivo.[33] And in our own in vivo studies, after determining the mechanical receptive field of cutaneous nociceptors, incision was made through the receptive field and spontaneous activity was not generated afterward[19] despite the fact that in behavioral studies, guarding pain was greatest immediately after incision.[3]

In summary, incisions do not appear to easily generate spontaneous activity of cutaneous nociceptors. Rather, deep tissue sensory afferents appear to be strongly activated by incision. With this deep tissue muscle injury, the proportion of nociceptors with spontaneous activity increases and the amount of activity is greater than the unincised control.

MECHANICAL SENSITIVITY AFTER INCISION

For in vivo recording, we attempted to induce mechanical sensitivity by making incisions within the receptive field as near as possible to the low threshold, mechanosensitive site of the nociceptor. The mechanical response threshold was determined using calibrated monofilaments applied to the low threshold, mechanosensitive site. The mapping of the area of mechanical receptive fields was also completed with von Frey filament using a bending force approximately twice the response threshold and depicted on a diagram of the plantar hindpaw. After characterization of an afferent fiber, a 5 mm–long incision of skin and fascia or sham control operation was made. The incision was closed. Forty-five minutes to 90 minutes later, mechanical responses of the fibers were tested again. Fibers that were activated only by pinch or monofilaments greater than 235 mN were considered to be MIA and were analyzed separately.[19]

Aβ-fibers did not sensitize after the incision. Only 4 of 13 mechanosensitive A-fibers exhibited at least one criterion for sensitization after the incision; response threshold decreased, response magnitude increased, or receptive field size increased. Sensitization was observed in 4 of 18 mechanosensitive C-fibers 45 minutes after the incision. In a group of MIAs, 3 of 7 A-fibers and 4 of 10 C-fibers were sensitized 45 minutes after incision. Response threshold was decreased in only 2 of 17 MIAs; receptive field size increased in 7 of 17 MIAs.

In a similar study, it was demonstrated that incision was sufficient to markedly reduce mechanical withdrawal thresholds in the hindpaw.[18,29] The same rats used for behavior underwent afferent fiber recording (see example Figure 11.4 A-B). The median mechanical threshold for A-nociceptors was 61 mN and 8 mN in both the sham control and incision groups, respectively. For C-nociceptors the thresholds were 29 mN and 13 mN in the sham and incision groups, respectively. These were not significantly different. However, the percent difference in normalized receptive field size was again increased in the incision group (Figure 11.4 C). For A-nociceptors, the receptive field size was 100 ± 18% and 202 ± 45% in the sham and skin incision group, respectively. For C-fibers, the receptive field size was 100 ± 11% and 199 ± 21% in these two groups.

From three studies in this model, the principal effect of an incision is an increase in receptive field size of the afferents, particularly those characterized as MIAs. To the extent that the mechanical hyperalgesia characterized in the same model is initiated in the periphery, spatial summation may contribute to the development of reduced withdrawal threshold. In agreement, after incision, correlation of fiber sensitization with primary mechanical hyperalgesia has been reported only rarely despite testing in a variety of peripheral injury models.[27,36–39] MIAs as a group did not develop increased responsiveness to the mechanical stimuli. Also, we could not identify any particular subpopulation of these fibers that likely by itself mediated the reduced withdrawal threshold. The major limitation of these experiments is the search strategy to find the receptive field is a mechanical stimulus that favored only certain types of afferents.

In conclusion, the search for nociceptive afferents coding for enhanced responses to mechanical stimuli after incision is not complete. The physiology likely eliciting the markedly enhanced behavioral responses to mechanical stimuli is not evident. The only consistent positive finding is that receptive field expansion of many A-delta and C-fibers could permit a far greater number of fibers to be activated by application of a single monofilament after incision. Thus, mechanical receptive field expansion could be sufficient to produce spatial summation of inputs at the dorsal horn and contribute to a withdrawal response.

HEAT SENSITIVITY AFTER INCISION

For in vivo recording, evaluation of heat sensitization has been difficult. Some heat sensitive afferents may have a very high heat threshold like 49°C;[40,41] therefore, heat testing to the threshold may damage the receptive field and damage the afferent fiber.[42] Furthermore, strong heat testing can sensitize the afferents, greatly limiting the ability to detect sensitization by another injury like incision.

Because of the limitations noted above, a series of studies using the rat glabrous skin incision and an in vitro glabrous skin nerve preparation have been undertaken as described above.[11,32] Mechanosensitive C-fiber nociceptors innervating the plantar aspect of rat hindpaw one day after incision were recorded and compared to the skin from control, unincised rats. We determined if afferent fibers were sensitized to heat stimuli one day after an incision when heat hyperalgesia was marked.

Mechanosensitive C-fibers with receptive fields in the skin were studied. The threshold temperature to excite C-fibers was less in those C-fibers innervating less than 2 mm from the incision compared to control. The responses shown in Figure 11.5 are representative of control C-fibers that generally began their response to heat stimuli at approximately 39°C, whereas the other example is representative of C-fibers innervating the incision (Figure 11.5). This afferent responded at approximately 35°C for threshold. The mean heat response threshold was significantly less (36.7°C ± 3.6) in the C-fiber innervating less than 2 mm from the incision than those from sham control skin (39.8°C ± 3.2). Those innervating well outside the incision from the incision (39.2°C ± 3.7) were not different than control. Furthermore, fibers that had receptive fields less

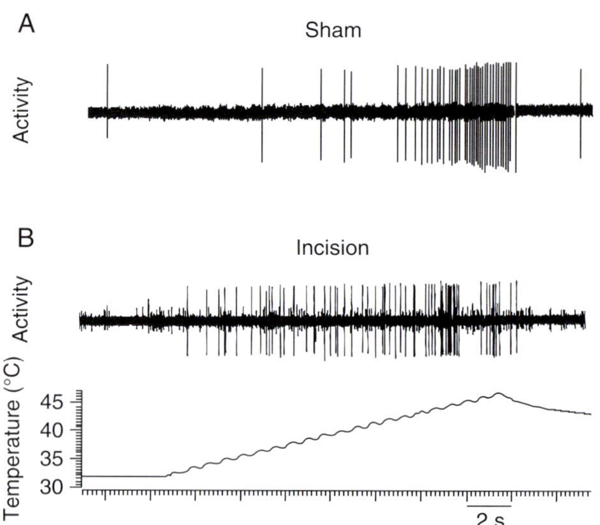

Figure 11.5 Example recordings of increased heat responses of nociceptors from incised and sham operated rat. Digitized oscilloscope trace of action potentials evoked by radiant heat in the sham control (A) and in a rat that underwent incision one day earlier (B). The heat stimulus was a 15-s heat ramp from 33 to 48°C. s = second. This figure has been reproduced with permission of the International Association for the Study of Pain (IASP). The figure may not be reproduced for any other purpose without permission. Banik RK, Brennan TJ. Spontaneous discharge and increased heat sensitivity of rat C-fiber nociceptors are present in vitro after plantar incision. *Pain.* 2004;112(1–2):204–213.

than 2 mm from the incision had significantly increased total evoked action potentials to heat (72 ± 41 impulses per second) compared to control (40 ± 22 impulses per second). Total evoked action potentials of those innervating more than 2 mm from the incision (43 ± 47 impulses per second) were not different from control.

In addition, heat responsive fibers that did not have mechanical receptive fields were also evaluated.[11,32] These heat responsive fibers that did not have mechanical receptive fields were termed "unclassified fibers" because their activity was recognized during heat stimulation. These fibers also had reduced threshold and were more prevalent in the incised skin. We did not locate mechanical receptive fields before or after the heat stimulation procedure; therefore, the conduction velocity of these units could not be measured. These may be C-fiber MIA units.

In summary, heat sensitization of C-fibers was localized to fibers less than 2 mm from the incision. Heat sensitization was evident in the form of decreased threshold, increased response to suprathreshold stimuli, and recruitment of "unclassified fibers" in the incised preparation. Thus, more fibers responsive to heat tend to be recruited by making incision. These changes in fiber activity were present at a time when animals showed behaviors indicative of heat hyperalgesia.

CHEMOSENSITIVITY AFTER INCISION

In previous studies, we have demonstrated that a decrease in tissue pH occurs immediately after incision and is sustained for several days.[43] The decreased pH is localized at the incision site, and pain related behaviors are evident during the period of low tissue pH. Pain behaviors correlate with pH. Lactate is also increased in incised tissue and this elevation also occurs at a time during which pain behaviors are present.[44]

Chemosensitivity of nociceptors in pathologic states is rarely evaluated. The rat glabrous in vitro skin-nerve preparation was used to study nociceptor chemosensitivity to determine if the acid-responsiveness of nociceptive afferents innervating the plantar aspect of the rat hindpaw 1 day after incision would be greater than the responsiveness of afferents in control sham-operated rats.[45] For testing chemosensitivity, we used lactic acid applied to the receptive field. To restrict the chemical stimuli to the isolated receptive field of the afferent fiber, a small metal ring (5 mm internal diameter), was placed on the receptive field and the modified balanced salt solution inside the ring was removed with a syringe. Then either pH 6.0 lactic acid (15 mM; 32°C) or control solution (balanced salt solution equilibrated with room air; pH 7.4; 32°C) was applied to the receptive field for 5 minutes, followed by 5-minute washout.

Similar to heat stimulation, we emphasized afferents less than 2 mm from the incision. Chemical responses to pH 6.0 lactic acid were evaluated in 17 C-fibers adjacent to the incision and 21 sham control C-fibers. A greater proportion of C-fibers adjacent to the incision was responsive (53%, 9 of 17) compared to sham control (14%, 3 of 21). The prevalence of acid responsive C-fibers innervating outside the incised area (greater than 2 mm from the incision) was not different from sham control (23%, 3 of 13). Few A-fibers responded to pH 6.0 lactic acid indicating in rat glabrous skin most chemosensitive fibers were C-fibers. Fibers from incised skin or unincised skin did not respond to pH 7.4 solution.

Responses of these units to pH 6.0 lactic acid were further quantified by counting activity during baseline, acid application, and washout period (Figure 11.6). Nociceptive afferents discharged during the acid application period in some cases after a brief delay. Total evoked potentials during acid exposure were greater in C-fibers innervating less than 2 mm from the incision compared to those of sham control. Total evoked potentials of C-fibers having

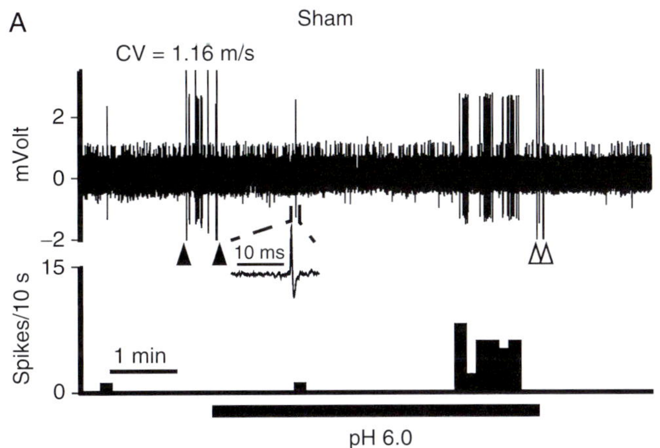

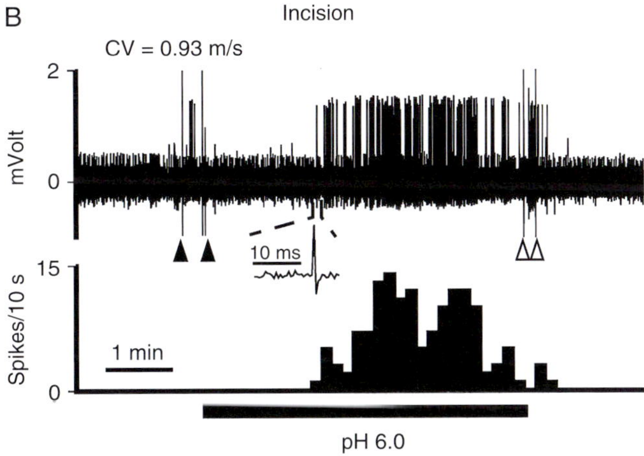

Figure 11.6 Example C-fiber responses to pH 6.0 lactic acid. Sample recordings from single C-fibers innervating sham control (A) and incised (B) skin. The solid arrows denote application and the open arrows the removal of the acid solution. S = seconds. Min = minutes. CV = conduction velocity. Reprinted with permission from Kang S, Brennan TJ. Chemosensitivity and mechanosensitivity of nociceptors from incised rat hindpaw skin. *Anesthesiology*. 2009;111(1):155–164.

receptive fields greater than 2 mm from the incision were not different from sham control. In C-fibers having receptive fields less than 2 mm from the incision, the median rate during acid application was 1.3 impulses per second, which was greater than that of sham control C-fibers, which was 0.2 impulses per second.

In summary, acid-responsive C-nociceptors showed sustained and reproducible excitation 1 day after plantar incision. Few A-fibers responded to lactic acid, with a range of pH 6.5 to 5.5 in both incisions and sham control groups; and the majority of nociceptors that responded to lactic acid in a pH-dependent manner were C-fibers. A greater proportion of C-fibers are activated by pH 6.0 lactic acid in vitro, and total evoked potentials during lactic acid exposure are greater in C-fibers less than 2 mm from the incision compared to sham control.

POTENTIAL THERAPEUTIC TARGETS ON NOCICEPTORS

Identification of receptors present on nociceptors should allow us to develop novel therapies that directly interfere with sensory transmission of pathophysiologic signals. This chapter reviews three target receptors, which are present on primary afferent nociceptors and produce analgesia by directly interfering with nociceptor function. These targets may have greater specificity for influencing sensory function rather than an effect on other processes like neovascularization or other repair processes that are occurring in wounds.

The first target is the transient receptor potential vanilloid 1 (TRPV1). The TRPV1 receptor responds to heat and acid stimuli.[46,47] Antagonism of the TRPV1 receptor interferes with heat hyperalgesia caused by incision. In support, knockout of the TRPV1 receptor gene in mice also modifies heat hyperalgesia after plantar incision.[48,49] Studies on nociceptors innervating unincised and incised skin from TRPV1 receptor knockout mice indicate that unidentified, mechanically insensitive nociceptors, may transmit heat hyperalgesia after plantar incision in mice.[48]

In addition to TRPV1, the TrkA receptor has emerged as a target for nociceptors sensitized by incision.[50] The TrkA receptor is a high affinity receptor for nerve growth factor (NGF). Several studies indicate that sequestration of NGF reduces pain-related behaviors after incision.[11,13,50] There are few nonneuronal sensory effects of NGF identified in the adult animal; thus, NGF acting at the TrkA receptor is likely one of the critical nociceptor sensitizing signals from incisions.

Other pain mediators may have receptors present on nociceptors and also receptors on nonsensory cells. Thus, these mediators may have both direct and indirect effects to sensitize nociceptors. Examples of these mediators are prostaglandins and interleukin-1 (IL-1). PGE2 receptor blockade[51] inhibits pain-related behaviors, as does locally applied sustained release ketoprofen, a nonsteroidal anti-inflammatory drug.[52] Similarly, IL-1 is increased in incisions and receptors are present on nociceptors.[53–55] Drugs blocking the IL-1 receptor affect pain behaviors. IL-1 affects immune function and could influence pain indirectly as well. The complement C5a fragment is in this category as well.[56]

Finally, there are also many factors affecting nociceptor function. These include factors affecting immune function. Other examples include substance P and calcitonin gene-related peptide.[57] Such targets may influence inflammation at incisions and indirectly affect nociceptor from transmission.

CONCLUSION

Our long-term goal is to understand how factors that activate and sensitize pain-transmitting neurons can be effectively targeted for the improved treatment of pain in patients undergoing surgery. The results are expected to have an important positive impact by targeting receptors on nociceptors whose activity is enhanced by surgery. We anticipate improved treatment of pain in patients undergoing surgery so that perhaps patients can undergo painless or nearly painless surgery.

REFERENCES

1. Kehlet H, Dahl JB. Anaesthesia, surgery, and challenges in postoperative recovery. *Lancet*. Dec 6 2003;362(9399):1921–1928.
2. Kehlet H, Werner M, Perkins F. Balanced analgesia: what is it and what are its advantages in postoperative pain? *Drugs*. Nov 1999; 58(5):793–797.
3. Brennan TJ, Vandermeulen EP, Gebhart GF. Characterization of a rat model of incisional pain. *Pain*. Mar 1996;64(3):493–501.
4. Brennan TJ, Zahn PK, Pogatzki-Zahn EM. Mechanisms of incisional pain. *Anesthesiol Clin North America*. Mar 2005;23(1):1–20.
5. Pogatzki EM, Vandermeulen EP, Brennan TJ. Effect of plantar local anesthetic injection on dorsal horn neuron activity and pain behaviors caused by incision. *Pain*. May 2002;97(1–2):151–161.
6. Xu J, Brennan TJ. Comparison of skin incision vs. skin plus deep tissue incision on ongoing pain and spontaneous activity in dorsal horn neurons. *Pain*. Jun 13 2009;144(3):329–339.
7. Xu J, Richebe P, Brennan TJ. Separate groups of dorsal horn neurons transmit spontaneous activity and mechanosensitivity one day after plantar incision. *Eur J Pain*. Dec 8 2008;13(8):820–828.
8. Zahn PK, Brennan TJ. Primary and secondary hyperalgesia in a rat model for human postoperative pain. *Anesthesiology*. Mar 1999; 90(3):863–872.
9. Loeser JD, Treede RD. The Kyoto protocol of IASP basic pain terminology. *Pain*. Jul 31 2008;137(3):473–477.
10. Zahn PK, Gysbers D, Brennan TJ. Effect of systemic and intrathecal morphine in a rat model of postoperative pain. *Anesthesiology*. May 1997;86(5):1066–1077.
11. Banik RK, Subieta AR, Wu C, Brennan TJ. Increased nerve growth factor after rat plantar incision contributes to guarding behavior and heat hyperalgesia. *Pain*. Sep 2005;117(1–2):68–76.

12. Hamalainen MM, Subieta A, Arpey C, Brennan TJ. Differential effect of capsaicin treatment on pain-related behaviors after plantar incision. *J Pain*. Jun 2009;10(6):637–645.
13. Wu C, Erickson MA, Xu J, Wild KD, Brennan TJ. Expression profile of nerve growth factor after muscle incision in the rat. *Anesthesiology*. Jan 2009;110(1):140–149.
14. Stubhaug A, Breivik H, Eide PK, Kreunen M, Foss A. Mapping of punctuate hyperalgesia around a surgical incision demonstrates that ketamine is a powerful suppressor of central sensitization to pain following surgery. *Acta Anaesthesiol Scand*. Oct 1997;41(9):1124–1132.
15. Lavand'homme PM, Roelants F, Waterloos H, De Kock MF. Postoperative analgesic effects of continuous wound infiltration with diclofenac after elective cesarean delivery. *Anesthesiology*. Jun 2007;106(6):1220–1225.
16. Kawamata M, Takahashi T, Kozuka Y, et al. Experimental incision-induced pain in human skin: effects of systemic lidocaine on flare formation and hyperalgesia. *Pain*. Nov 2002;100(1–2):77–89.
17. Kawamata M, Watanabe H, Nishikawa K, et al. Different mechanisms of development and maintenance of experimental incision-induced hyperalgesia in human skin. *Anesthesiology*. Sep 2002; 97(3):550–559.
18. Pogatzki EM, Gebhart GF, Brennan TJ. Characterization of Adelta- and C-fibers innervating the plantar rat hindpaw one day after an incision. *J Neurophysiol*. Feb 2002;87(2):721–731.
19. Hamalainen MM, Gebhart GF, Brennan TJ. Acute effect of an incision on mechanosensitive afferents in the plantar rat hindpaw. *J Neurophysiol*. Feb 2002;87(2):712–720.
20. Hargreaves K, Dubner R, Brown F, Flores C, Joris J. A new and sensitive method for measuring thermal nociception in cutaneous hyperalgesia. *Pain*. Jan 1988;32(1):77–88.
21. Pogatzki-Zahn EM, Wagner C, Meinhardt-Renner A, et al. Coding of incisional pain in the brain: a functional magnetic resonance imaging study in human volunteers. *Anesthesiology*. Feb 2010;112(2): 406–417.
22. Martinez V, Fletcher D, Bouhassira D, Sessler DI, Chauvin M. The evolution of primary hyperalgesia in orthopedic surgery: quantitative sensory testing and clinical evaluation before and after total knee arthroplasty. *Anesth Analg*. Sep 2007;105(3):815–821.
23. Meyer RA, Ringkamp M, Campbell JN, Raja SN. Peripheral mechanisms of cutaneous nociception. In: McMahon SB, Koltzenburg M, eds. *Wall and Melzack's Textbook of Pain*. 5th ed. Amsterdam: Elsevier Churchill Livingstone. 2006:3–34.
24. Djouhri L, Lawson SN. Abeta-fiber nociceptive primary afferent neurons: a review of incidence and properties in relation to other afferent A-fiber neurons in mammals. *Brain Res Rev*. Oct 2004; 46(2):131–145.
25. McMahon SB, Bennett DLH, Bevan S. Inflammatory mediators and modulators of pain. In: McMahon SB, Koltzenburg M, eds. *Wall and Melzack's Textbook of Pain*. 5th ed. Amsterdam: Elsevier Churchill Livingstone. 2006:49–72.
26. Treede RD, Meyer RA, Raja SN, Campbell JN. Peripheral and central mechanisms of cutaneous hyperalgesia. *Prog Neurobiol*. 1992; 38(4):397–421.
27. Reeh PW, Bayer J, Kocher L, Handwerker HO. Sensitization of nociceptive cutaneous nerve fibers from the rat's tail by noxious mechanical stimulation. *Exp Brain Res*. 1987;65(3):505–512.
28. Schmidt R, Schmelz M, Forster C, Ringkamp M, Torebjork E, Handwerker H. Novel classes of responsive and unresponsive C nociceptors in human skin. *J Neurosci*. Jan 1995;15(1 Pt 1):333–341.
29. Xu J, Brennan TJ. Guarding pain and spontaneous activity of nociceptors after skin versus skin plus deep tissue incision. *Anesthesiology*. 2010;24(1):153.
30. Reeh PW. Sensory receptors in mammalian skin in an in vitro preparation. *Neurosci Lett*. May 15 1986;66(2):141–146.
31. Du J, Koltzenburg M, Carlton SM. Glutamate-induced excitation and sensitization of nociceptors in rat glabrous skin. *Pain*. Jan 2001;89(2–3):187–198.
32. Banik RK, Brennan TJ. Spontaneous discharge and increased heat sensitivity of rat C-fiber nociceptors are present in vitro after plantar incision. *Pain*. Nov 2004;112(1–2):204–213.
33. Campbell JN, Khan AA, Meyer RA, Raja SN. Responses to heat of C-fiber nociceptors in monkey are altered by injury in the receptive field but not by adjacent injury. *Pain*. Mar 1988;32(3):327–332.
34. Burgess PR, Perl ER. Myelinated afferent fibres responding specifically to noxious stimulation of the skin. *J Physiol*. Jun 1967; 190(3):541–562.
35. Bessou P, Perl ER. Response of cutaneous sensory units with unmyelinated fibers to noxious stimuli. *J Neurophysiol*. Nov 1969; 32(6):1025–1043.
36. Andrew D, Greenspan JD. Mechanical and heat sensitization of cutaneous nociceptors after peripheral inflammation in the rat. *J Neurophysiol*. Nov 1999;82(5):2649–2656.
37. Handwerker HO, Kilo S, Reeh PW. Unresponsive afferent nerve fibres in the sural nerve of the rat. *J Physiol*. Apr 1991;435: 229–242.
38. Meyer RA, Davis KD, Cohen RH, Treede RD, Campbell JN. Mechanically insensitive afferents (MIAs) in cutaneous nerves of monkey. *Brain Res*. Oct 11 1991;561(2):252–261.
39. Schaible HG, Schmidt RF. Neurophysiology of chronic inflammatory pain: electrophysiological recordings from spinal cord neurons in rats with prolonged acute and chronic unilateral inflammation at the ankle. *Prog Brain Res*. 1996;110:167–176.
40. Leem JW, Willis WD, Weller SC, Chung JM. Differential activation and classification of cutaneous afferents in the rat. *J Neurophysiol*. Dec 1993;70(6):2411–2424.
41. Leem JW, Willis WD, Chung JM. Cutaneous sensory receptors in the rat foot. *J Neurophysiol*. May 1993;69(5):1684–1699.
42. Treede RD, Meyer RA, Campbell JN. Myelinated mechanically insensitive afferents from monkey hairy skin: heat-response properties. *J Neurophysiol*. Sep 1998;80(3):1082–1093.
43. Woo YC, Park SS, Subieta AR, Brennan TJ. Changes in tissue pH and temperature after incision indicate acidosis may contribute to postoperative pain. *Anesthesiology*. Aug 2004;101(2):468–475.
44. Kim TJ, Freml L, Park SS, Brennan TJ. Lactate concentrations in incisions indicate ischemic-like conditions may contribute to postoperative pain. *J Pain*. Jan 2007;8(1):59–66.
45. Kang S, Brennan TJ. Chemosensitivity and mechanosensitivity of nociceptors from incised rat hindpaw skin. *Anesthesiology*. Jul 2009; 111(1):155–164.
46. Basbaum AI, Bautista DM, Scherrer G, Julius D. Cellular and molecular mechanisms of pain. *Cell*. Oct 16 2009;139(2):267–284.
47. Julius D, Basbaum AI. Molecular mechanisms of nociception. *Nature*. Sep 13 2001;413(6852):203–210.
48. Banik RK, Brennan TJ. Trpv1 mediates spontaneous firing and heat sensitization of cutaneous primary afferents after plantar incision. *Pain*. Jan 2009;141(1–2):41–51.
49. Pogatzki-Zahn EM, Shimizu I, Caterina M, Raja SN. Heat hyperalgesia after incision requires TRPV1 and is distinct from pure inflammatory pain. *Pain*. Jun 2005;115(3):296–307.
50. Zahn PK, Subieta A, Park SS, Brennan TJ. Effect of blockade of nerve growth factor and tumor necrosis factor on pain behaviors after plantar incision. *J Pain*. Apr 2004;5(3):157–163.
51. Omote K, Kawamata T, Nakayama Y, Kawamata M, Hazama K, Namiki A. The effects of peripheral administration of a novel selective antagonist for prostaglandin E receptor subtype EP(1), ONO-8711, in a rat model of postoperative pain. *Anesth Analg*. Jan 2001; 92(1):233–238.
52. Spofford CM, Ashmawi H, Subieta A, et al. Ketoprofen produces modality-specific inhibition of pain behaviors in rats after plantar incision. *Anesth Analg*. Dec 2009;109(6):1992–1999.
53. Wolf G, Livshits D, Beilin B, Yirmiya R, Shavit Y. Interleukin-1 signaling is required for induction and maintenance of postoperative incisional pain: genetic and pharmacological studies in mice. *Brain Behav Immun*. Oct 2008;22(7):1072–1077.

54. Loram LC, Themistocleous AC, Fick LG, Kamerman PR. The time course of inflammatory cytokine secretion in a rat model of postoperative pain does not coincide with the onset of mechanical hyperalgesia. *Can J Physiol Pharmacol.* Jun 2007;85(6):613–620.
55. Honore P, Wade CL, Zhong C, et al. Interleukin-1alphabeta gene-deficient mice show reduced nociceptive sensitivity in models of inflammatory and neuropathic pain but not post-operative pain. *Behav Brain Res.* Feb 28 2006;167(2):355–364.
56. Clark JD, Qiao Y, Li X, Shi X, Angst MS, Yeomans DC. Blockade of the complement C5a receptor reduces incisional allodynia, edema, and cytokine expression. *Anesthesiology.* Jun 2006;104(6):1274–1282.
57. Sahbaie P, Shi X, Guo TZ, et al. Role of substance P signaling in enhanced nociceptive sensitization and local cytokine production after incision. *Pain.* Oct 2009;145(3):341–349.

12

SEQUELAE OF NERVE INJURY

NEUROPATHIC PAIN AND COMPLEX REGIONAL PAIN SYNDROME

Haroon Hameed, Mariam Hameed, Srinivasa Raja, and Michael Erdek

INTRODUCTION

The peripheral nervous system is a beautifully organized structure. It is essentially a skeletally unprotected extension of the central nervous system (CNS) that gives shape and meaning to its many functions by controlling the entire body both voluntarily and involuntarily, as well as transmitting sensory input centrally. Even with the most basic histology, the peripheral nervous system has many hallmarks that easily distinguish it from the CNS. One example is the proportion of myelinated axons, with myelin being produced by Schwann cells rather than oligodendrocytes. Further in contrast to the CNS, its basement membrane-lined regeneration conduits are relatively reliable when preserved and give relatively superior resilience in case of injury. Considerable advances have been made in our understanding of the plastic changes in the peripheral and central nervous systems after injury to nerves. In this chapter we will present a concise yet thorough review of the most relevant information regarding peripheral nerve injury and complex regional pain syndrome (CRPS).

NERVE INJURY

CLASSIFICATIONS AND IMPORTANT DEFINITIONS

Using a combination of the classic Seddon and Sunderland classifications is probably the ideal way to define nerve injury. Neurapraxia (Sunderland 1st degree) is related to temporary loss of function, originally defined by Seddon as lasting for weeks to months, but more correctly can be thought of as a segmental demyelination. Seddon described axonotmesis as disruption of the axon associated with Wallerian degeneration; it occurs in three types. The most optimal for regeneration is when continuity of the endoneurial basement membrane is preserved (Sunderland 2nd degree). The second type involves rupture of the endoneurial basement membrane but intact perineurium (Sunderland 3rd degree), and the third type of axonotmesis is when the perineurium is compromised and intraneural neuromas form behind an intact epineurium (Sunderland 4th degree). Seddon described neurotmesis as when the epineurium is compromised (Sunderland 5th degree), which if completely transected requires surgical correction for regeneration, if any. Most nontraumatic nerve injuries are essentially within a spectrum from segmental demyelination to axonotmesis.[1,2]

Definitions related to neuropathic pain symptoms can be found in the International Association for the Study of Pain guidelines and website—the reader is referred to them as a comprehensive learning tool. Especially important are the terms "allodynia," which is pain, due to a stimulus that does not normally provoke pain, and "hyperalgesia," which is "the increased response to a stimulus which is normally painful."[3]

MECHANISMS OF PERIPHERAL NEUROPATHIC PAIN AND THEIR TREATMENTS

In this section the origins, mechanisms, mediators, and modulators of neuropathic pain are discussed. They are outlined in Table 12.1, below.

Ectopic Impulses

Ectopic impulse generation has been directly correlated with neuroma pain in humans[4] and can be initiated by a wide variety of mechanisms causing activation of neuronal cell depolarization and impulse propagation. These impulses are defined as ectopic as they are produced at sites other than the peripheral sensory receptor, such as the neuronal soma, axonal transection endbulbs, neurite sprouts, or demyelinated areas. Ectopic impulse formation can be found in sites of neuroma formation by nerve transection, diabetic polyneuropathy, neuritis, nerve entrapment, and a variety of other conditions.[5–9] These impulses may be produced post axotomy in either the pain transmitting myelinated A- (δ and β) or the unmyelinated C-fibers. Postdemyelination ectopic impulse production has also been well described and is thought to be caused by hyperexcitability of demyelinated segments, which is possibly due to release of local tissue factors associated with remodeling of the neuronal support structures, such as the endoneurium, perineurium, and epineurium as well as other supporting cells.[10,11] Ectopy has been closely linked with the activation and upregulation of voltage-gated sodium and calcium channels.

a. Local Anesthetics and Selective Na-Channel Inhibitors

The powerful nonselective sodium channel blockade is what makes the local anesthetics such as lidocaine (and antiepileptics, see below) so effective in inhibition of ectopic impulse generation.[12] Unfortunately, research has been unable to identify definitively a single sodium channel that (when inhibited) can completely extinguish nerve injury pain. In animal studies, Nav1.3, Nav1.7, and Nav 1.8 channels have shown to be effective in relieving pain when blocked by various methods, yet knockout animals continue to sense pain.[13–20] The usefulness of newer selective sodium channel blockers in neuropathic pain and CRPS is yet to be determined in humans.

b. Tricyclic Antidepressants

Tricyclic antidepressants have a complex action in neuropathic pain states that is likely related to multiple mechanisms of action. Among those is blockade of Nav1.7 sodium channels, which occurs at therapeutic dosages and is responsible for stabilization of the membrane potential and inhibition of ectopic impulse formation.[21]

c. Calcium Channels: α_2-δ_1 Calcium Channel Subunit Inhibitors: Gabapentin and Pregabalin

Gabapentin and pregabalin bind to an α_2-δ_1 auxilliary subunit of the calcium channel and block the pore-forming action of the channel. This action thereby decreases membrane excitability and release of synaptic neurotransmitters at the central terminals of primary afferents, and transmission of nociception.[22,23] α_2-δ_1 and Cav2.2 subunits of calcium channels are upregulated in the dorsal root ganglia (DRG) post-nerve injury[22] leading to increased excitability and ectopic discharge production. Cav2.2 receptor knockout mice appear to show decreased susceptibility to neuropathic pain and an intrathecal inhibitory peptide called MVIIA that blocks Cav2.2 receptors is associated with decreased neuropathic pain in preclinical studies[22]

d. Antiepileptics

Antiepileptics also act in neuropathic pain disorders by suppression of ectopic impulse formation. Carbamazepine works both peripherally and centrally by blocking voltage-gated sodium channels and inhibition of voltage-dependent calcium channels[24] Phenytoin suppresses ectopic impulse production peripherally and centrally by inhibition of presynaptic glutamate release and blockade of sodium channels.[25] Valproic acid inhibits γ-aminobutyric acid (GABA) degradation, resulting in an increase of GABA concentrations in the brain, as well as by prolonging the repolarization phase of voltage-sensitive sodium channels.

Neurogenic Inflammation

a. Macrophages and Tumor Necrosis Factor-α

The peripheral nervous system is separated from the systemic vascular system by a blood tissue barrier. Injury to nerves can result in disruption of this barrier and accumulation of lymphocytes, immune and inflammatory cells at the injury site. Macrophages present in the peripheral nerve facilitate trafficking of T lymphocytes by expression of the major histocompatibility complex class II antigen, which presents antigens to the T-cells. This process is induced by production of tumor necrosis factor-α (TNF-α) and interleukin-1 (IL-1) and IL-6 by macrophages, T-cells, and other inflammatory cells to mediate the inflammatory response. Mast cells that are present intraneurally can cause massive endoneural edema after degranulation, which can be caused by breakdown of the blood-nerve barrier.[26–28]

The production of TNF-α and IL-1 induces leukocyte migration and leukocyte adhesion.[29] TNF-α has been shown to be directly related to hyperalgesia after nerve injury in a number of diseases and models.

b. TNF-α Antagonists and the TNF-α Fusion Protein

Current therapies such as treatment with TNF-α antagonists such as infliximab (Remicade) and adalimumab (Humira) are effective in many forms of vasculitis, such as Kawasaki's disease and rheumatoid arthritis–associated vasculitis. Recently, infliximab has had many reports of relieving sciatica after intravenous (IV) infusion, and subsequently a randomized controlled trial has shown efficacy in sciatica in those patients in whom modic changes (signal intensity changes in vertebral body marrow adjacent to the endplates of degenerative disks) were present, or those in whom disc changes were severe.[30]

Etanercept is a TNF-α receptor-binding inhibitor "fusion protein" and has also shown benefit as a long-acting analgesic in animal models of inflammatory neuropathic pain.[31] Its benefit as a perispinal agent in humans has also been shown in controlled trials both in the United States and Japan.[32] Its efficacy is multimodal and likely includes but is not limited to inhibition of inflammation (through inhibition of lymphocyte chemotaxis), direct inhibition of synaptic pain transmission, and inhibition of apoptosis through decreased mitochondrial membrane derangements.

c. Adenosine Triphosphate, Adenosine and Potential Inhibitory Targets

Adenosine triphosphate (ATP) acts in both the central and peripheral nervous system and is responsible for pain generation by way of binding to purine and pyrimidine receptors, especially the P2X3 and P2X2/3 and P2Y2 receptors.[33] Adenosine, a byproduct of ATP degradation, has also been linked to pain generation. While not classified as a neurotransmitter since it is not stored in presynaptic vesicles, it is a product of ATP degradation and can also be released from neuronal and nonneuronal tissues. Some of its receptors have been positively linked to TNF-α release, and its A2A and A2B receptors have been associated with nociception. Adenosine's anti-TNF-α releasing properties appear to be especially relevant to the lung and show promise in the treatment of asthma, while the antagonists of the A2B receptor appear to be powerful anti-inflammatory and antinociceptive agents. The A2A receptor has also a potent anti inflammatory action but its usefulness as a target seems to be limited due to immunosuppressant actions. Further, inhibitors of adenosine kinase, which phosphorylates adenosine into adenosine monophosphate, have been shown to be potent anti-inflammatory and antinociceptive agents.[34]

d. Capsaicin and Transient Receptor Potential Vanilloid-type1 (TRPV-1)

Capsaicin has long been used to desensitize tissues from nociception by transdermal application. Capsaicin's effects on the dermis include excitation and desensitization of nociceptors, with an accompanying decrease in epidermal axon terminals and decreased sensory neuropeptide expression. Nerve growth factor (NGF) can protect the sensory neurons against capsaicin toxicity. Capsaicin effects include phosphorylation of TRPV1 channels possibly via PI3K (phosphotidyl-inositide-3-kinase) and the methyl ethyl ketone/extracellular signal regulated kinase (MEK/ERK).[35–38] Capsaicin-sensitive TRPV1 activation is also thought to cause mitochondrial permeability transition by way of caspase activation, which in turn causes ATP loss and possible necrosis and or apoptosis as mentioned above. Of note, capsaicin-induced mitochondrial permeability transition change can also be inhibited by cyclosporine A.[39]

Ephaptic and Nonephaptic Interneuronal Stimulation

Ephaptic connections or abnormal connections between axons through the adjacent basement membranes of demyelinated and unmyelinated segments (secondary to trauma, virus, etc), have been long known to conduct impulses.[40] Conduction of abnormal impulses through single or multiple adjacent fibers may result in generation of pain sensation. Ephaptic impulses are known to occur soon after injury, after which there can be a short remission of pain-generating impulses.[41] Then after a few weeks there is often a resurgence of pain-generating ephaptic impulse conduction.[41] These processes have been proven posttraumatically in neuromas and postherpetically in the DRG.[41,42] Often abnormal electrical impulse transmissions through unmyelinated axon segments are few and cannot account for the degree of perceived pain.[43–45] More importantly, cross-conduction of impulses through the release of excitatory neurotransmitters and diffusion of chemical mediators to proximal axons occurs, but this requires repetitive excitation leading to a summation effect causing sufficient additive increase in local mediator concentration to effectively excite the nearby pain conducting fibers.

Tricyclic Antidepressants

Tricyclic antidepressants (TCA) may be able to inhibit ephaptic crosstalk at therapeutic dosages by their ability to block nicotinic acetylcholine receptors (nAChrs) on unmyelinated C fibers.[46] This may decrease the response of the C fibers to acetylcholine released by nearby axons with damaged myelin sheaths.

PERIPHERAL NERVE INJURY, NEUROTROPHIC FACTORS, AND CENTRAL SENSITIZATION

Pain-Related and Other Sensory-Related Factors

a. Nerve Growth Factor (NGF)

The neurotrophin class of neurotrophic factors includes nerve growth factor (NGF), brain-derived neurotrophic factor (BDNF), neurotrophin-3 (NT-3), neurotrophin 4/5 (NT-4/5) and neurotrophin-6 (NT-6) (which is not present in humans). The neurotrophins are necessary for the development and survival of certain neurons. The low-affinity p75^{NTR} receptor binds these neurotrophins, and each neurotrophin also binds to a high affinity trk receptor. NGF binds selectively to the neurotrophic tyrosine kinase receptor type A (trkA), BDNF and NT-4/5 to the neurotrophic tyrosine kinase receptor type B (trkB) and NT-3 to the neurotrophic tyrosine kinase receptor type C (trkC).[47] The trk receptor-ligand complex in turn causes activation of multiple signaling pathways that are responsible for promoting cell survival and differentiation. In fact, no neural crest–derived small sensory neurons can survive in NGF or trkA knockout animals.[48]NGF is also especially important for neurite outgrowth at axonal ends and in pain generation.[49]

NGF is especially important in sensory axonal regeneration, and NGF levels correlate directly with the amount of preferential reinnervation.[50] Further, studies have shown that the NGF-trkA complex is important in pain generation,

Table 12.1 ORIGINS, MECHANISMS, MEDIATORS, AND MODULATORS OF NEUROPATHIC PAIN

NEUROPATHIC MECHANISMS	ORIGINS	MEDIATORS	CURRENT MEDICATIONS AND POSSIBLE FUTURE TARGETS
Ectopy	Sodium channels	Nonselective	Lidocaine, and other local anesthetics
		Nav 1.3 channels	Oligosense nucleotide inhibitors*
		Nav 1.7 channels	Tricyclic antidepressants, e.g., amitriptyline Selective Nav 1.7 blockers*
		Nav 1.8 channels	Selective Nav 1.8 blockers*
	Calcium channel upregulation	Alpha2delta1 subunit of Calcium channel	Inhibitors: gabapentin, pregabalin
		Cav2.2 receptor	MVIIA*
Inflammation (Macrophages, T-cells, mast cells, B-cells and fibroblasts)	TNF-alpha	Inflammatory cascade activation (release of interleukins, TNF-alpha, inflammatory cell recruitment)	TNF-alpha antagonists: infliximab, adalimumab, etc.
			TNF-alpha binding fusion protein: etanercept
			Steroids
		Mitochondrial Permeability Transition	Inhibitor: Cyclosporine A (through TRPV1)**
		TRAIL	—
	ATP	P2X2 receptors	NMDA inhibitors: ketamine, dextromethorphan,
		P2X2/3 receptors	A-317491*,
		P2X3 receptors	TNP-ATP*, A-317491*, RO-3*
		P2Y2 receptors	—
		TRPV1	capsaicin
	Adenosine	A2A	
		A2B	
	Inflammatory cytokines	NGF production	See below
Sprouting and Sympathetic mediated pain	NGF	trkA receptor	Anti-NGF***
	BDNF	trkB receptor	Anti-BDNF*
		Phosphorylation of NR1 and NR2b subunits of NMDA receptors	
	NT-3	trk C?	NT-3 (agonist)*
Ephaptic	Acetylcholine	NAchr?	Tricyclics
Central Sensitization	Glutamate	NMDA receptor	Ketamine, dextromethorphan
	GABA		Benzodiazepines*
	Norepinephrine		SNRI, tricyclics
	Glial Modifying Agents	TLR receptor	AV411
		IL-10	AV333, Propentofylline

* denotes either more evidence or human studies are needed.
** evidence in painful bladder syndrome/interstitial cystitis only, not proven for neuropathy; may not be through mitochondrial stabilization effects.
*** NGF may be neuroprotective with GDNF.

and mice with mutations in either NGF or trkA are unresponsive to painful stimuli.[51] In trkA expressing neurons NGF increases the expression of substance P and calcitonin gene-related peptide (CGRP) mRNA and protein,[52] as well as BDNF expression in DRG neurons. Further, NGF delivery to the cut end of the sciatic nerve[53] or directly into the intrathecal space[54] can reverse axotomy-induced downregulation of CGRP and substance P as well as galanin and vasoactive intestinal polypeptide, all of which have been associated with pain generation in animal models.

NGF induces sympathetic postganglionic neurite sprouting to encase primary sensory neurons within the DRG, as well as trkA expressing nociceptor sprouting causing hyperinnervation of the epidermis.[55,56] Postaxotomy NGF enables trkA expressing sensory neurons to regrow into the CNS and restore some of the lost functions caused by the lesion. Axotomy downregulates the substance P and CGRP proteins as well as the TRPV1, Nav1.8, and Nav1.9 sodium channels.[53,54,57,58] Treatment with NGF, either delivered to the area of cut nerve or intrathecally, reverses these changes in trkA expressing neurons. Further, NGF administration by similar methods can reverse the upregulation of galanin, vasoactive intestinal polypeptide, and activating transcription factor 3, as well as protect against capsaicin toxicity in animal models.[59]

In humans it has been shown subcutaneous or intramuscular injections of NGF produces pain or hyperalgesia at the injection site immediately and persists for many hours. Small IV doses have an even more dramatic widespread effect with tenderness and deep pain lasting for days.[60] These effects are partly due to the direct action of NGF directly on trkA positive nociceptors, but indirect actions may involve mast cells, sympathetic postganglionic neurons, or chemoattraction of neutrophils to the NGF injection site.[51]

Deprivation of NGF in experimental animals by using NGF sequestering molecules or inducing autoimmune changes results in altered nociceptor properties and a net hypoalgesia to thermal and some chemical algogenic stimuli (stimuli that produce pain).[51]

NGF is produced from a variety of tissues. In the skin it is produced by basal keratinocytes and epithelial cells in hollow viscera as well as mast cells, macrophages, and Schwann cells. NGF levels are increased in inflamed tissues. Further, release of IL-1β, PDGF, TNF-α, IL-4, and TGF-β all stimulate the production of NGF.

Since NGF antagonism has shown protective effects on small-diameter nociceptive sensory neurons and since it can reverse hyperalgesia in preclinical studies, it may also be antinociceptive when applied directly to the site of injury. Yet, a study using NGF in patients with diabetic polyneuropathy (DPN) did not show any benefit. It is possible that the dosage was too low.[51] NGF was used to treat DPN to supplement the decreased NGF production at the end organ receptor site, which had been responsible for decreased trophic support to the primary sensory neurons at the dorsal horn.[51]

Conversely, anti-NGF treatments have been delivered to the injury site with the idea that there was overproduction of NGF by functioning Schwann cells, mast cells, and other local cells. Although there may have been some primary nociceptor loss, the net effect would be too much NGF available to stimulate the remaining nociceptors.[61] Interestingly, it was found that anti-NGF treatments combined with glial-derived neurotrophic factor (GDNF) had superior neuroprotective effects than NGF alone. Although NGF is currently thought to be a promising target for pain management, it will be interesting to see if negating its pain-promoting effect has a negative effect on the amount of preferential sensory reinnervation.

b. Brain-Derived Neurotrophic Factor (BDNF)

BDNF is also important in pain generation through diverse mechanisms. In inflammation-related models of neuropathic pain, an NGF dependent mechanism induces TNF-α to increase BDNF in small sensory neurons.[62] First, its receptor, trkB, is upregulated in the entire spinal cord after peripheral inflammation and also after increased neuronal activity.[63,64] BDNF given intrathecally induces the expression of c-fos, cAMP responsive element binding protein, c-jun, and other genes that have been associated with pain.[65–68] This includes activation of the mitogen-associated kinase extracellular-signal related kinase (MAK ERK) cascade, thus increasing synthesis of preprodynorphin, preproenkephalin, neuropeptide Y, and glutamic acid decarboxylase, all of which have been implicated in pain processing.[66,69,70]

Further, BDNF has been shown to potentiate postsynaptic NMDA receptors through the phosphorylation of the NR1 and NR2b subunits, which plays a significant role in central sensitization.[71,72] Evidence has also shown that BDNF is important in central sensitization and C-fiber mediated reflexes.[73,65] Interestingly, anti-BDNF antiserum has abolished the abnormally increased A-β afferent activity in animal models of inflammation important in tactile allodynia.[74]

BDNF may also be important for the sympathetic sprouting around large-diameter sensory neurons in the DRG because sympathetic sprouting is stimulated by exogenous BDNF, and both BDNF antisense oligodeoxynucleotides and BDNF antibodies partially block sprouting.[51]

Conversely, large doses of BDNF—injected intracerebroventricularly, delivered intraspinally by a viral vector, or via a BDNF-expressing cell graft applied to the spinal cord—decrease pain behavior as well as normalize some spinal neuropeptide levels.[75–79]

Central and Spinal Cord Sensitization, Disinhibition, and A-β Fiber Mediated Pain

a. Central Sensitization

Central sensitization and disinhibition at the level of the brain and spinal cord contribute significantly to the development of neuropathic pain. The continuous neuronal firing that is caused by peripheral nerve injury leads to the pre- and postsynaptic upregulation of ion channels and their properties, neurotransmitters, as well as the activity of multiple genes and kinases. Subsequent to repetitive firing after nerve injury, as can be seen in chronic pain, there can be subsequent facilitation of nociceptive input signals to the spinal cord, which is thought to be a form of long-term potentiation (LTP). LTP is a phenomenon of hyperexcitablity that is associated with plasticity of the CNS and is observed in several conditions—memory, epilepsy, and also chronic pain states.

Among other changes, upregulation of presynaptic calcium channels appears to be important. Inhibitory modulators of central calcium channels such as pregabalin and gabapentin have gained much attention because of their efficacy, which is enhanced by effects on calcium channels in the peripheral nervous system.[80,81]

b. NMDA Receptor Antagonists

Postsynaptically, the excitatory N-methyl-D-aspartate (NMDA) glutamate receptors seem to be quite important. Inhibitors such as dextromethorphan and ketamine have gained much attention as they also seem to be efficacious, but unfortunately their use appears to be limited by side effects.[81]

c. GABAergic Mediated Pain

After nerve injury there appear to be at least two mechanisms responsible for loss of GABAergic inhibitory control of pain sensations. One is related to the increased production of BDNF, which causes downregulation of a potassium chloride cotransporter isoform 2, leading to depolarization instead of hyperpolarization of pain-transmitting lamina 1 neurons after GABA release.[82,83] Another mechanism is related to inhibitory interneuron loss secondary to apoptosis after nerve injury. Modulators of $GABA_A$ receptors such as benzodiazepines have limited usefulness in neuropathic pain secondary to their side effects at analgesic doses.

d. Tricyclic Antidepressants (TCA) and Serotonin and Norepinephrine Reuptake Inhibitors (SNRIs)

Inhibition of pain sensing pathways by supratentorial structures such as the hypothalamus, amygdala, and anterior cingulate gyrus occurs by way of brainstem nuclei located in the rostroventral medulla and periaqueductal gray matter. The primary inhibitory neurotransmitters used by those tracts include 5-hydroxytryptamine, norepinephrine, and endogenous opioids.[84] Physiologically, there is a constant noradrenergic inhibitory effect present. After nerve injury this noradrenergic stimulation is suspended, and the serotonergic tone that is usually inhibitory becomes facilitatory for pain signals.[85,86] (TCA) and SNRIs increase the norepinephrine levels in these pathways. This causes a relative increase in the central norepinephrine:acetylcholine ratio, thereby enhancing descending inhibitory neuromodulation.[87]

e. Role of Glial Modifying Agents in the Management of Central Sensitization

Glial cells are abundant in the CNS, accounting for 70% of cells. Their functions include macrophage-like activity, as well as neuronal support, homeostasis, and impulse transduction.[88] Their hyperactivation is thought to play a key role in the development and maintenance of the central sensitization associated with neuropathic pain. Peripheral or central inflammatory, degenerative, or cytotoxic processes can cause activation of glial related neuropathic pain pathways via activation of substance P, NMDA- and AMPA-glutamatergic, and purinergic receptors. These receptors then utilize mitogen-activated protein kinase (MEKK) signaling pathways including the extracellular signal-related kinase (ERK), c-Jun N-terminal-kinase (JNK) and p38, which ultimately cause upregulation of pro-inflammatory mediators such as cytokines, neurotrophic factors, and nitric oxide. IL-1α, IL-1β, IL-6, TNF-α, and IL-10 appear to be especially important for central neuropathic pain processing.[89]

Currently, there is much interest in the recently elaborated toll-like receptors (TLRs) found on many cells in the body. TLR-2 and TLR-4 found on glial cells appear to play a central role in neuropathic pain, opioid tolerance, reward, and hyperalgesia.[90,91] These receptors are potential therapeutic targets. AV411 (Avigen Inc., Alameda, CA) is a potent TLR-4 antagonist and phosphodiesterase inhibitor that has been shown to decrease the production of inflammatory mediators while increasing anti-inflammatory IL-10, thereby diminishing neuropathic pain.[92] Another agent also developed by Avigen is the plasmid AV333 (Avigen Inc., Alameda, CA), which increases IL-10 and was shown to significantly reduce neuropathic pain for 90 days in animals.[93] Similar to AV411, pentoxifylline, a phosphodiesterase inhibitor, decreases inflammatory cytokines associated with neuropathic pain.[94]

Propentofylline, or SLC022 (Solace Pharmaceuticals, Canterbury, Kent, United Kingdom), a methylxanthine derivative, is a glial modifying agent that is thought to exert its effects through altering GABAergic tone.[95] Therapy targeting glial cells and their receptors hold much promise and may play a major role in the management of neuropathic pain in the future.

OTHER GENERAL ANATOMIC AND PHENOTYPIC ALTERATIONS AND SENSITIZATIONS AFTER PERIPHERAL NERVE INJURY

Skin/End Organ

Peripheral nerve injury is quickly followed by changes to the structure, quantity, and quality of the peripheral axons and nociceptors found in the skin. After nerve transection it has been shown that there is segmentation of axons within the first 24 hours, with complete axonal loss from the skin by 48 hours. Epidermal and small diameter axons are usually lost first, followed by deeper and large diameter axons. In chronic neuropathy in humans, it has been shown that distal fiber loss predominates. However, even in areas of normal fiber density the axons were abnormal and often had areas of attenuation alternating with areas of dilation that contained neurofilaments, organelles, and mitochondria. These changes are thought to be the predecessors to fiber loss and represent impaired axonal transport.[96] Postaxotomy Wallerian degeneration ensues, as the remaining Schwann cells can still be identified in the dermis for up to 50 days by their markers p75 and S100. By approximately 8 months they disappear almost completely.[96]

EVALUATION OF THE PATIENT WITH NEUROPATHIC PAIN

Evaluation of the patient with neuropathic pain should begin with a thorough history and physical exam, with special attention to a thorough neurological exam. Quantitative sensory testing with von Frey hairs, and thermal and vibratory stimuli are scientifically validated. Use of pain rating scales like the visual analog scale and numerical rating scale are useful for initial evaluation and measurement of progress but lack specificity. Special questionnaires like the McGill Pain Questionnaire and Neuropathic Pain Scale may be useful. Quality-of-life inventories may also be important for measuring disease impact and treatment efficacy.[97]

Nerve conduction studies and somatosensory-evoked potentials are useful to localize areas of damaged nerve, though they are not specific for damage to nociceptive neurons. Laser-evoked potentials and late laser evoked potentials (for A-δ fiber damage) may be the best laboratory tests to evaluate function of nociceptive pathways and may be considered if available.[97]

COMPLEX REGIONAL PAIN SYNDROME

Complex regional pain syndrome (CRPS) is a neuropathic pain syndrome characterized by burning pain that usually begins in an extremity and may progressively involve adjacent or distant regions of the body. CRPS was first described by Silas Weir Mitchell, and his colleagues Moorehouse and Keene as "causalgia" or posttraumatic nerve pain in Civil War soldiers after major limb or plexus injuries on the battlefield.[98] In 1946 Evans coined the term "reflex sympathetic dystrophy" in those patients with no evidence of nerve injury. In an effort to standardize the nomenclature and diagnosis of this disease, the International Association for the Study of Pain (IASP) consensus in 1994 changed the name to complex regional pain syndrome type I (reflex sympathetic dystrophy) and type II (causalgia) and put forth diagnostic criteria.[99,100] Classically CRPS type I has been thought of as occurring in the absence of identifiable nerve injury, and CRPS type II is thought of as occurring after a readily identifiable nerve injury, though this definition is often not clinically delineated.

PATHOPHYSIOLOGY

Somatic Sensory Nervous System

a. Trauma and Inflammation in CRPS

Axonal injury results in increased spontaneous firing of primary afferents, as well as abnormal mechanosensitivity and adrenergic sensitization peripherally and at the DRG.[101,102] Ectopic discharges leading to continuous nociceptive input may lead to central sensitization and changes in cortical sensory and motor processing.

The role of the inflammatory cascade[103] in the development of CRPS begins with tissue injury and is classically mediated by intraneural macrophages. In addition, injured nociceptive C-fibers secrete neuropeptides resulting in neurogenic inflammation peripherally[104,105] as well as the induction of microglia centrally leading to further enhanced nociception and central sensitization.[106]

b. Consequences of Sympathetic and Central Sprouting: Sympathetic Mediated Pain and Tactile Allodynia

Sympathetic-mediated pain is found in a subset of CRPS patients and is diagnosed by relief from pain after a sympathetic block. This is thought to occur through sympathetic and afferent coupling in the skin and DRG, and through increased α-adrenoreceptor mediated sensitivity of nociceptive fibers.[107] Animal studies show increased sympathetic sprouting in the DRG and increased expression of α-adrenoreceptors on DRG neurons after nerve injury.[108,109] Peripherally, aberrant migration and sprouting sympathetic fibers may develop (or be) in close proximity to sensory nerves in the upper dermis after partial nerve injury.[110,111] Human studies also show increased hyperalgesia and allodynia with norepinephrine and phenylephrine, an α1-adrenergic agonist, when administered cutaneously.[112,113,114] Clondine, an α_2-agonist, acts on presynaptic neurons blocking noradrenaline release, thus reducing activation of postsynaptic α1-receptors and consequently reducing pain.[115] Noradrenaline activation of α-adrenoreceptors can cause antidromic impulse transmission in pain carrying fibers, in addition to the release of pro-inflammatory mediators by postganglionic sympathetic neurons, thus potentially furthering nociception.[116,117]

Loss of A-δ and C-fibers often leads to sprouting of A-β fibers from lamina 3 and 4 (where they are normally present) to the nociceptive lamina 2 of the dorsal horn in the spinal cord. This mechanism is partially responsible for generation of tactile allodynia.[118,119]

c. Central Sensitization and Cortical Reorganization

In neuropathic pain states, central sensitization at the spinal cord level can occur after damage to afferent neurons starting with the dorsal horn. The NMDA glutamate receptor plays a role in central sensitization[105,120] at this level, as evidenced by the efficacy of NMDA-receptor antagonists such as ketamine and memantine in CRPS therapy. Alteration in central processing of tactile and nociceptive stimuli occurs,[121] leading to cortical reorganization and central nociceptive sensitization.[122]

Sympathetic Nervous System: Vasomotor and Sudomotor Changes

After partial nerve damage, there may be a loss of the sympathetic supply to the blood vessels leading to vasodilation and the "warm" phase in acute CRPS.[123] Later, loss of trophic support (possibly related to NGF) leads to upregulation of adrenoreceptors centrally and peripherally, causing hypersensitivity and vasoconstriction peripherally.[113,123,124] Interestingly, in normal subjects there are no sympathetic sprouts into the skin, nor is there a connection between the sympathetic nervous system and nociceptive signaling pathways.[125,126]

Motor Dysfunction

Motor dysfunction progresses over time and its prevalence may be as high as 50%.[127] Though the exact mechanism by which motor dysfunction occurs is unclear, it is thought that sympathetic activation, central sensitization, and cortical reorganization may all play a part. Evidence supporting the role of sympathetic activation in motor dysfunction is supported by amelioration of movement abnormalities after a sympathetic block.[128] Continuous nociceptive input peripherally can lead to central sensitization. At the spinal level, elevated substance P and CGRP can induce prolonged activation of motor neurons leading to spasticity and dystonia.[129] In the higher centers, cortical plasticity has also been reported in CRPS as demonstrated by bilateral disinhibition of the primary motor cortex,[130] altered integration of sensory input, reorganization in the central motor circuits,[131] and a neglect-like syndrome that can lead to disuse of the affected limb.[132]

EPIDEMIOLOGY

CRPS most commonly occurs in Caucasian females[133–135] and is most commonly precipitated by injuries,[134,136] with 10% not attributable to a precipitating cause.[127]

CLINICAL SIGNS AND SYMPTOMS

Clinical Diagnostic Criteria for *CRPS**

1. Continuing pain, which is disproportionate to any inciting event
2. Must report at least one symptom in *three of the four* following categories:
   - *Sensory*: Reports of hyperesthesia and/or allodynia
   - *Vasomotor*: Reports of temperature asymmetry and/or skin color changes and/or skin color asymmetry
   - *Sudomotor/Edema*: Reports of edema and/or sweating changes and/or sweating asymmetry
   - *Motor/Trophic*: Reports of decreased range of motion and/or motor dysfunction (weakness, tremor, dystonia) and/or trophic changes (hair, nail, skin)
3. Must display at least one sign at time of evaluation in *two or more* of the following categories:
   - *Sensory*: Evidence of hyperalgesia (to pinprick) and/or allodynia (to light touch and/or deep somatic pressure and/or joint movement)
   - *Vasomotor*: Evidence of temperature asymmetry and/or skin color changes and/or asymmetry
   - *Sudomotor/Edema*: Evidence of edema and/or sweating changes and/or sweating asymmetry
   - *Motor/Trophic*: Evidence of decreased range of motion and/or motor dysfunction (weakness, tremor, dystonia) and/or trophic changes (hair, nail, skin)
4. There is no other diagnosis that better explains the signs and symptoms

TREATMENT

Noninterventional

a. Pharmacologic

Table 12.2 outlines pharmacologic treatment options.

*Proposed clinical diagnostic criteria by Harden et al.[137]

Table 12.2 **PHARMACOLOGIC**

TARGETED PROCESS	MEDICATION	MECHANISM OF ACTION	REFERENCES	COMMENTS
Nociception	Gabapentin	$\alpha_2\delta$ ligand of calcium channels blocker	van de Vusse 2004[138]	One RCT shows significant reduction of sensory deficits, but no effect on sudomotor or motor changes.
	Local Anesthetics: i) Lidocaine	i) Sodium channel blocker	Wallace 2000,[139] Meirer 2009[140]	Lumbar sympathetic blocks have shown to be more effective in pain control than by the intravenous route.
	i) Ketamine ii)Memantine	NMDA receptor antagonists	Corell 2004,[141] Sitgerman 2009,[142] Finch 2009[143]	Subanesthetic infusions of ketamine provides significant pain relief. Also effective topically. Memantine improves autonomic, motor symptoms with pain relief.
	Antidepressants	Enhancing noradrenergic descending inhibitory pathways and by partially blocking sodium channels.	Sindrup 2005,[144] Max 1992,[145] Max 1987[146]	Have been studied extensively for neuropathic pain states, and their use has been extrapolated to CRPS. Side effects limit their use.
	Opioids	Mu receptors and inhibition of central nociceptive neurons	Watson 2003,[147] Gilron 2005,[148] Agarwal 2007,[149] Altier 2005[150]	Methadone, morphine, oxycodone, transdermal fentanyl have shown efficacy in neuropathic pain.
	Ziconotide	N-type calcium channel blocker	Wermeling 2006,[151] Kapural 2009[152]	A few case series show improved pain, edema, and mobility
Anti-inflammatory	Corticosteroids	Inhibits inflammatory mediator production	Christensen 1982[153]	RCT showed pulsed dosing effective in managing CRPS after 12 weeks of therapy.
	Inflixumab	TNF α inhibitor	Huygen 2004[154]	Though there are no RCTs, preliminary studies support its use.
	Bisphosphonates	Inhibiting osteoclastic activity	Varena 2000,[155] Manicount 2004,[156] Robinson 2004[157]	Improves pain and function.
Free Radicals	i) Dimethyl sulfoxide (DMSO) ii) *N*-acetyl-l-cysteine (NAC) iii) Vitamin C	Free radical scavengers	Perez 2003,[158] Zuurmond 1996,[159] Zollinger et al 1999[160]	DMSO more effective in managing "warm" CRPS, while NAC better for "cold" CRPS. Vitamin C has been shown to decrease incidence of CRPS in patients with wrist fractures.
Dystonia	Baclofen	$GABA_B$ agonist	Van Hilten 2000[161], Kofler 1994,[162] Becker 1995[163]	Activates GABAergic inhibition in spinal cord.
	Clonazepam	Benzodiazepine	Netherlands Association of Posttraumatic Dystrophy Patients 2006[164]	
Others	Capsaicin	TRVP1 Receptors	Winters 1995,[165] Ribbers 1990,[166] Robbins 1998[167]	Only anecdotal reports supporting its use as an adjunct to physiotherapy.
	Tadalafil	Phosphodiesterase inhibitor	Groeneweg 2008[168]	RCT showed improved pain in conjunction with physiotherapy versus placebo.

RCT=randomized controlled trial

b. Physiotherapy and Psychological Therapy

Due to the scope of this chapter, details of physiotherapy and psychological therapy will not be fully discussed. In short, the principal objective of treatment of CRPS is improving functional ability by means of physical, occupational, and recreational therapy as first-line treatment.

Psychological therapy is not recommended in the first two months of CRPS, but should symptoms persist and chronic CRPS develop, patients should have a psychological evaluation to manage any underlying anxiety, depression, or personality disorder.[169,170]

Interventional Therapies

a. Sympathetic Blocks

Sympathetic blocks can be both diagnostic and therapeutic. Diagnostic blocks divide patients into those with sympathetically maintained pain or sympathetically independent pain.[171] Stellate ganglion blocks and lumbar sympathetic blocks are often used to manage pain in the upper and lower extremity respectively. Due to poor qualitative studies, evidence based data supporting the usefulness of sympathetic ganglion blocks is somewhat lacking and it has been difficult to ascertain significant treatment responses to these blocks.[172,173] One study found no significant difference between reductions in peak pain intensity between placebo and local anesthetic injections but did find that local anesthetics provided longer duration of pain relief.[174] Further, botulinum toxin A has been shown to increase the analgesic effect of sympathetic blocks in a subset of patients.[175]

b. Spinal Cord Stimulators/Neurostimulators

Spinal cord stimulation (SCS) has been used to treat pain for over 25 years.[176] Although its mechanism of action is not completely understood, it has been theorized that SCS exerts its effects at the spinal and supraspinal levels. At the spinal level, it may exert a segmental antidromic inhibition of pain-carrying nerve fibers and/or by altering the amount of neurotransmitters or neuromodulators.[177] An experiment in nerve-lesioned rats showed SCS decreased the release of the excitatory glutamate and aspartate neurotransmitters and simultaneously increased GABA release, therefore having an inhibitory effect on dorsal horn neurons by controlling A-β fiber mediated tactile allodynia.[178,179]

Despite little evidence supporting or arguing against SCS in CRPS, evidence-based review of the literature favors SCS as treatment in patients who do not respond to standard therapies.[180] SCS has been shown to significantly decrease severe burning pain, but its efficacy, lasting about 2–3 years, diminishes with time. SCS has not been shown to improve function, but does positively affect health-related quality of life.[181,182] Peripheral nerve stimulation has also been used to manage CRPS, though there is scant literature relating to its efficacy. One prospective study showed an improvement of pain in nearly two thirds of patients with surgically placed platelike electrodes on affected nerves,[183] with some showing additional improvement in activity levels. Peripheral nerve stimulation has better outcome for CRPS limited to the involvement of one major nerve.[184]

c. Intrathecal Drug Infusions (baclofen, morphine, and clonidine)

Dystonia can be disabling and in refractory cases can be treated by intrathecal baclofen.[161] Baclofen is a GABA-type B receptor agonist, thus inhibiting sensory input to the spinal cord. In a Dutch cohort study, intrathecal baclofen was shown to improve pain, disability, quality of life, and dystonia.[161] Side effects included device-related complications (e.g., postdural headache, infection). Psychiatric adverse events[161] and, in some cases, seizures have been reported.[162] Intrathecally administered morphine and clonidine have also been independently reported to be efficacious.[163]

d. Sympathectomy

In 1950, Leriche first described the treatment of causalgia by sympathectomy, which was thought to control sympathetic mediated pain by interrupting the sympathetic system.[185] Patients who are impervious to conventional therapy and respond to sympathetic blocks by regional anesthetic procedures may be candidates for sympathectomy.[186] Sympathectomies may be done chemically, surgically, or by radiofrequency ablation. Alcohol or phenol is classically used to chemically destroy the sympathetic chain.[187] Surgical sympathectomies can be either open or percutaneous. One large case series of 73 patients showed significant to moderate improvement of pain in 75% of subjects, lasting for more than one year,[188] yet high quality evidence supporting use of sympathectomy is lacking.[189] Further, the many complications—which include a worsening of the pain or "new" CRPS, spinal cord injury, hyperhidrosis, Horner's syndrome, and wound infection—suggest that a clear and explicit discussion of adverse outcomes is necessary before proceeding with this option.[190]

REFERENCES

1. Seddon H. Three types of nerve injury. *Brain*. 1943;66:237–288.
2. Sunderland S. *Nerves and Nerve Injuries*. 2nd ed. Baltimore: Williams and Wilkins;1978.
3. www.iasp-pain.org. Last accessed September 28, 2009.
4. Nyström B, Hagbarth KE. Microelectrode recordings from transected nerves in amputees with phantom limb pain. *Neurosci Lett*. Dec 11, 1981;27(2):211–216.
5. Wall PD, Gutnick M. Ongoing activity in peripheral nerves: The physiology and pharmacology of impulses originating from a neuroma. *Exp Neurol*. 1974;43:580–593.
6. Burchiel KJ, Russell LC, Lee RP, et al. Spontaneous activity of primary afferent neurons in diabetic BB/Wistar rats. a possible mechanism of chronic diabetic neuropathic pain. *Diabetes*. 1985;34: 1210–1213.

7. Delio DA, Reuhl KR, Lowndes HE. Ectopic impulse generation in dorsal root ganglion neurons during methylmercury intoxication. an electrophysiological and morphological study. *Neurotoxicology.* 1992;13:527–540.
8. Gillespie CS, Sherman DL, Fleetwood-Walker SM, et al. Peripheral demyelination and neuropathic pain behavior in periaxin-deficient mice. *Neuron.* 2000;26:523–531.
9. McMahon SB, Koltzenburg M, eds. *Wall and Melzack's Textbook of Pain*, 5th ed. Edinburgh: Elsevier Churchill Livingstone; 2006.
10. Baker M, Bostock H. Ectopic activity in demyelinated spinal root axons of the rat. *J Physiol (Lond).* 1992;451:539–552.
11. Calvin WH, Devor M, Howe J. Can neuralgias arise from minor demyelination? Spontaneous firing, mechanosensitivity and afterdischarge from conducting axons. *Exp Neurol.* 1982;75:755–763.
12. Sheets PL, Heers C, Stoehr T, Cummins TR. Differential block of sensory neuronal voltage-gated sodium channels by lacosamide [(2R)-2-(acetylamino)-N-benzyl-3-methoxypropanamide], lidocaine, and carbamazepine. *J Pharmacol Exp Ther.* Jul 2008;326(1):89–99.
13. Hains BC, Klein JP, Saab CY, Craner MJ, Black JA, Waxman SG. Upregulation of sodium channel Nav1.3 and functional involvement in neuronal hyperexcitability associated with central neuropathic pain after spinal cord injury. *J Neurosci.* Oct 1 2003;23(26): 8881–8892.
14. Nassar MA, Baker MD, Levato A, et al. Nerve injury induces robust allodynia and ectopic discharges in Nav1.3 null mutant mice. *Mol Pain.* Oct 19 2006;2:33.
15. Nassar MA, Levato A, Stirling LC, Wood JN. Neuropathic pain develops normally in mice lacking both Na(v)1.7 and Na(v)1.8. *Mol Pain.* 2005;1:24.
16. Dong XW, Goregoaker S, Engler H, et al. Small interfering RNA-mediated selective knockdown of Na(V)1.8 tetrodotoxin-resistant sodium channel reverses mechanical allodynia in neuropathic rats. *Neuroscience.* 2007;146(2):812–821.
17. Ekberg J, Jayamanne A, Vaughan CW, et al. muO-conotoxin MrVIB selectively blocks Nav1.8 sensory neuron specific sodium channels and chronic pain behavior without motor deficits. *Proc Natl Acad Sci U S A.* 2006;103(45):17030–17035.
18. Gold MS, Weinreich D, Kim CS, et al. Redistribution of Na(V)1.8 in uninjured axons enables neuropathic pain. *J Neurosci.* 2003;23(1): 158–166.
19. Jarvis MF, Honore P, Shieh CC, et al. A-803467, a potent and selective Nav1.8 sodium channel blocker, attenuates neuropathic and inflammatory pain in the rat. *Proc Natl Acad Sci U S A.* 2007; 104(20):8520–8525.
20. Hoyt SB, London C, Ok H, et al. Benzazepinone Nav1.7 blockers: potential treatments for neuropathic pain. *Bioorg Med Chem Lett.* 2007;17(22):6172–6177.
21. Dick IE, Brochu RM, Purohit Y, et al. Sodium channel blockade may contribute to the analgesic efficacy of antidepressants. *J Pain.* 2007;8(4):315–324. Epub Dec 15, 2006.
22. McGivern JG. Targeting N-type and T-type calcium channels for the treatment of pain. *Drug Discov Today.* 2006;11(5–6):245–253.
23. Hendrich J, Van Minh AT, Heblich F, et al. Pharmacological disruption of calcium channel trafficking by the alpha2delta ligand gabapentin. *Proc Natl Acad Sci U S A.* 2008;105(9):3628–3633.
24. Ambrósio AF, Soares-Da-Silva P, Carvalho CM, Carvalho AP. Mechanisms of action of carbamazepine and its derivatives, oxcarbazepine, BIA 2–093, and BIA 2–024. *Neurochem Res.* 2002;27(1–2): 121–130.
25. Yaari Y, Devor M. Phenytoin suppresses spontaneous ectopic discharge in rat sciatic nerve neuromas. *Neurosci Lett.* 1985;58(1): 117–122.
26. Powell HC, Myers RR, Costello ML. Increased endoneurial fluid pressure following injection of histamine and compound 48/80 into rat peripheral nerves. *Lab Invest.* 1980;43(6):564–572.
27. Seitz RJ, Reiners K, Himmelmann F, Heininger K, Hartung H-P, Toyka KV. The bloodnerve barrier in Wallerian degeneration: a sequential long-term study. *Muscle Nerve.* 1989;12:627–635.
28. Harvey GK, Toyka KV, Hartung HP. Effects of mast cell degranulation on blood-nerve barrier permeability and nerve conduction in vivo. *J Neurol Sci.* 1994;125(1):102–109.
29. Ho TW, McKhann GM, Griffin JW. Human autoimmune neuropathies. *Annu Rev Neurosci.* 1998;21:187–226.
30. Korhonen T, Karppinen J, Paimela L, et al. The treatment of disc-herniation-induced sciatica with infliximab: one-year follow-up results of FIRST II, a randomized controlled trial. *Spine.* 2006; 31(24):2759–2766.
31. Zanella JM, Burright EN, Hildebrand K, et al. Effect of etanercept, a tumor necrosis factor-alpha inhibitor, on neuropathic pain in the rat chronic constriction injury model. *Spine.* 2008;33(3):227–234.
32. Cohen SP, Bogduk N, Dragovich A, et al. Randomized, double-blind, placebo-controlled, dose-response, and preclinical safety study of transforaminal epidural etanercept for the treatment of sciatica. *Anesthesiology.* 2009;110(5):1116–1126.
33. Burnstock G. Purinergic receptors and pain. *Curr Pharm Des.* 2009;15(15):1717–1735.
34. Gao ZG, Jacobson KA. Emerging adenosine receptor agonists. *Expert Opin Emerg Drugs.* 2007;12(3):479–492.
35. Chuang HH, Prescott ED, Kong H, et al. Bradykinin and nerve growth factor release the capsaicin receptor from PtdIns(4,5) P2-mediated inhibition. *Nature.* 2001;411(6840):957–962.
36. Ji RR, Samad TA, Jin SX, Schmoll R, Woolf CJ. p38 MAPK activation by NGF in primary sensory neurons after inflammation increases TRPV1 levels and maintains heat hyperalgesia. *Neuron.* 2002;36(1):57–68.
37. Khasar SG, Lin YH, Martin A, Dadgar J, McMahon T, et al. A novel nociceptor signaling pathway revealed in protein kinase C epsilon mutant mice. *Neuron.* 1999;24(1):253–260.
38. Zhuang ZY, Xu H, Clapham DE, Ji RR. Phosphatidylinositol 3-kinase activates ERK in primary sensory neurons and mediates inflammatory heat hyperalgesia through TRPV1 sensitization. *J Neurosci.* 2004;24(38):8300–8309.
39. Shin CY, Shin J, Kim BM, et al. Essential role of mitochondrial permeability transition in vanilloid receptor 1-dependent cell death of sensory neurons. *Mol Cell Neurosci.* 2003;24(1):57–68.
40. Granit R, Skoglund CR. Facilitation, inhibition and depression at the 'artificial synapse' formed by the cut end of a mammalian nerve. *J Physiol.* 1945;103(4):435–448.
41. Seltzer Z, Devor M. Ephaptic transmission in chronically damaged peripheral nerves. *Neurology.* 19791;29(7):1061–1064.
42. Fried K, Govrin-Lippmann R, Devor M. Close apposition among neighbouring axonal endings in a neuroma. *J Neurocytol.* 1993; 22(8):663–681.
43. Amir R, Devor M. Chemically-mediated cross-excitation in rat dorsal root ganglia. *J Neurosci.* 1996;16:4733–4741.
44. Matsuka Y, Neubert JK, Maidment NY, et al. Concurrent release of ATP and substance P within guinea pig trigeminal ganglia in vivo. *Brain Research.* 2001;915:248–255.
45. Oh EJ, Weinreich D: Chemical communication between vagal afferent somata in nodose ganglia of the rat and the guinea pig in vitro. *J Neurophysiol.* 2002;87:2801–2807.
46. Freysoldt A, Fleckenstein J, Lang PM, Irnich D, Grafe P, Carr RW. Low concentrations of amitriptyline inhibit nicotinic receptors in unmyelinated axons of human peripheral nerve. *Br J Pharmacol.* 2009;158(3):797–805.
47. Chao MV. Neurotrophins and their receptors: a convergence point for many signaling pathways. *Nat Rev Neurosci.* 2003;4(4):299–309.
48. Crowley C, Spencer SD, Nishimura MC, et al. Mice lacking nerve growth factor display perinatal loss of sensory and sympathetic neurons yet develop basal forebrain cholinergic neurons. *Cell.* 1994;76(6):1001–1011.
49. McMahon SB, Bennett DL, Bevan S. Inflammatory mediators and modulators. In: McMahon SB, Koltzenburg M, eds. *Textbook of Pain*. London: Elsevier; 2006:49–72.
50. Höke A, Redett R, Hameed H, Jari R, Zhou C, Li ZB, Griffin JW, Brushart TM. Schwann cells express motor and sensory

phenotypes that regulate axon regeneration. *J Neurosci.* 2006; 26(38):9646–9655.
51. Pezet S, McMahon SB. Neurotrophins: mediators and modulators of pain. *Annu Rev Neurosci.* 2006;29:507–538.
52. Pezet S, Onténiente B, Jullien J, et al. Differential regulation of NGF receptors in primary sensory neurons by adjuvant-induced arthritis in the rat. *Pain.* 2001;90(1–2):113–125.
53. Fitzgerald M, Wall PD, Goedert M, Emson PC. Nerve growth factor counteracts the neurophysiological and neurochemical effects of chronic sciatic nerve section. *Brain Res.* 1985;332(1):131–141.
54. Verge VM, Gratto KA, Karchewski LA, Richardson PM. Neurotrophins and nerve injury in the adult. *Philos Trans R Soc Lond B Biol Sci.* 1996;351(1338):423–430.
55. Ramer MS, Bisby MA. Adrenergic innervation of rat sensory ganglia following proximal or distal painful sciatic neuropathy: distinct mechanisms revealed by anti-NGF treatment. *Eur J Neurosci.* 1999;11(3):837–846.
56. Mendell LM, Albers KM, Davis BM. Neurotrophins, nociceptors, and pain. *Microsc Res Tech.* 1999;45(4–5):252–261.
57. Gould HJ 3rd, Gould TN, England JD, Paul D, Liu ZP, Levinson SR. A possible role for nerve growth factor in the augmentation of sodium channels in models of chronic pain. *Brain Res.* 2000;854(1–2):19–29.
58. Verge VM, Richardson PM, Wiesenfeld-Hallin Z, Hökfelt T. Differential influence of nerve growth factor on neuropeptide expression in vivo: a novel role in peptide suppression in adult sensory neurons. *J Neurosci.* 1995;15(3 Pt 1):2081–2096.
59. Averill S, Michael GJ, Shortland PJ, Leavesley RC, King VR, et al. NGF and GDNF ameliorate the increase in ATF3 expression which occurs in dorsal root ganglion cells in response to peripheral nerve injury. *Eur J Neurosci.* 2004;19(6):1437–1445.
60. Svensson P, Cairns BE, Wang K, Arendt-Nielsen L. Injection of nerve growth factor into human masseter muscle evokes long-lasting mechanical allodynia and hyperalgesia. *Pain.* 2003;104(1–2):241–247.
61. Fukuoka T, Noguchi K. Contribution of the spared primary afferent neurons to the pathomechanisms of neuropathic pain. *Mol Neurobiol.* 2002;26(1):57–6762.
62. Onda A, Murata Y, Rydevik B, Larsson K, Kikuchi S, Olmarker K. Infliximab attenuates immunoreactivity of brain-derived neurotrophic factor in a rat model of herniated nucleus pulposus. *Spine.* 2004;29(17):1857–1861.
63. Zhou XF, Parada LF, Soppet D, Rush RA. Distribution of trkB tyrosine kinase immunoreactivity in the rat central nervous system. *Brain Res.* 1993;622(1–2):63–70.
64. Mannion RJ, Costigan M, Decosterd I, et al. Neurotrophins: peripherally and centrally acting modulators of tactile stimulus-induced inflammatory pain hypersensitivity. *Proc Natl Acad Sci U S A.* 1999; 96(16):9385–9390.
65. Kerr BJ, Bradbury EJ, Bennett DL, et al. Brain-derived neurotrophic factor modulates nociceptive sensory inputs and NMDA-evoked responses in the rat spinal cord. *J Neurosci.* 1999;19(12): 5138–5148.
66. Kim HS, Lee SJ, Kim DS, Cho HJ. Effects of brain-derived neurotrophic factor and neurotrophin-3 on expression of mRNAs encoding c-Fos, neuropeptides and glutamic acid decarboxylase in cultured spinal neurons. *Neuroreport.* 2000;11(17):3873–3876.
67. Jongen JL, Haasdijk ED, Sabel-Goedknegt H, van der Burg J, Vecht ChJ, Holstege JC. Intrathecal injection of GDNF and BDNF induces immediate early gene expression in rat spinal dorsal horn. *Exp Neurol.* 2005;194(1):255–266.
68. Hunt SP, Pini A, Evan G. Induction of c-fos-like protein in spinal cord neurons following sensory stimulation. *Nature.* 1987;328(6131): 632–634.
69. Ji RR, Baba H, Brenner GJ, Woolf CJ. Nociceptive-specific activation of ERK in spinal neurons contributes to pain hypersensitivity. *Nat Neurosci.* 1999;2(12):1114–1119.
70. Zhuang ZY, Gerner P, Woolf CJ, Ji RR. ERK is sequentially activated in neurons, microglia, and astrocytes by spinal nerve ligation and contributes to mechanical allodynia in this neuropathic pain model. *Pain.* 2005;114(1–2):149–159. Epub Jan 26 2005.
71. Brenner GJ, Ji RR, Shaffer S, Woolf CJ. Peripheral noxious stimulation induces phosphorylation of the NMDA receptor NR1 subunit at the PKC-dependent site, serine-896, in spinal cord dorsal horn neurons. *Eur J Neurosci.* 2004;20(2):375–384.
72. Guo W, Zou S, Guan Y, et al. Tyrosine phosphorylation of the NR2B subunit of the NMDA receptor in the spinal cord during the development and maintenance of inflammatory hyperalgesia. *J Neurosci.* 2002;22(14):6208–6217.
73. Heppenstall PA, Lewin GR. BDNF but not NT-4 is required for normal flexion reflex plasticity and function. *Proc Natl Acad Sci U S A.* 2001;98(14):8107–8112.
74. Matayoshi S, Jiang N, Katafuchi T, et al. Actions of brain-derived neurotrophic factor on spinal nociceptive transmission during inflammation in the rat. *J Physiol.* Dec 1, 2005;569(Pt 2):685–695.
75. Cirulli F, Berry A, Alleva E. Intracerebroventricular administration of brain-derived neurotrophic factor in adult rats affects analgesia and spontaneous behavior but not memory retention in a Morris Water Maze task. *Neurosci Lett.* 2000;287(3):207–210.
76. Pezet S, Malcangio M, McMahon SB. BDNF: a neuromodulator in nociceptive pathways? *Brain Res Rev.* 2002;40(1–3):240–249.
77. Cejas PJ, Martinez M, Karmally S, et al. Lumbar transplant of neurons genetically modified to secrete brain-derived neurotrophic factor attenuates allodynia and hyperalgesia after sciatic nerve constriction. *Pain.* 2000;86(1–2):195–210.
78. Eaton MJ, Blits B, Ruitenberg MJ, Verhaagen J, Oudega M. Amelioration of chronic neuropathic pain after partial nerve injury by adeno-associated viral (AAV) vector-mediated over-expression of BDNF in the rat spinal cord. *Gene Ther.* 2002;9(20):1387–1395.
79. Siuciak JA, Wong V, Pearsall D, Wiegand SJ, Lindsay RM. BDNF produces analgesia in the formalin test and modifies neuropeptide levels in rat brain and spinal cord areas associated with nociception. *Eur J Neurosci.* 1995;7(4):663–670.
80. Chizh BA, Göhring M, Tröster A, Quartey GK, Schmelz M, Koppert W. Effects of oral pregabalin and aprepitant on pain and central sensitization in the electrical hyperalgesia model in human volunteers. *Br J Anaesth.* 2007;98(2):246–254.
81. Dworkin RH, O'Connor AB, Backonja M, et al. Pharmacologic management of neuropathic pain: evidence-based recommendations. *Pain.* 2007;132(3):237–251. Epub Oct 24 2007.
82. Keller AF, Coull JA, Chery N, Poisbeau P, De Koninck Y. Region-specific developmental specialization of GABA-glycine cosynapses in laminas I-II of the rat spinal dorsal horn. *J Neurosci.* 2001;21(20): 7871–7880.
83. Coull JA, Boudreau D, Bachand K, et al. Trans-synaptic shift in anion gradient in spinal lamina I neurons as a mechanism of neuropathic pain. *Nature.* 2003;424(6951):938–942.
84. Costigan M, Scholz J, Woolf CJ. Neuropathic pain: a maladaptive response of the nervous system to damage. *Annu Rev Neurosci.* 2009;32:1–32.
85. Vera-Portocarrero LP, Zhang ET, Ossipov MH, et al. Descending facilitation from the rostral ventromedial medulla maintains nerve injury-induced central sensitization. *Neuroscience.* 2006;140: 1311–1320.
86. Bee LA, Dickenson AH. Descending facilitation from the brainstem determines behavioural and neuronal hypersensitivity following nerve injury and efficacy of pregabalin. *Pain.* 2008;140(1):209–223. Epub Sep 21 2008.
87. Matsuzawa-Yanagida K, Narita M, Nakajima M, Kuzumaki N, Niikura K, et al. Usefulness of antidepressants for improving the neuropathic pain-like state and pain-induced anxiety through actions at different brain sites. *Neuropsychopharmacology.* 2008;33: 1952–1965.
88. Nakajima K, Kohsaka S. Functional roles of microglia in the brain. *Neurosci Res.* 1993;17:187–203.
89. Ji RR, Gereau RW 4th, Malcangio M, Strichartz GR. MAP kinase and pain. *Brain Res Rev.* 2009, 60:135–148.

90. Takeda K, Akira S. TLR signaling pathways. *Semin Immunol.* 2004;16:3–9.
91. Hameed H, Hameed M, Christo PJ. The effect of morphine on glial cells as a potential therapeutic target for pharmacological development of analgesic drugs. *Curr Pain Headache Rep.* 2010;14(2):96–104.
92. Ledeboer A, Hutchinson MR, Watkins LR, Johnson KW. Ibudilast (AV-411). A new class therapeutic candidate for neuropathic pain and opioid withdrawal syndromes. *Expert Opin Investig Drugs.* 2007;16:935–950.
93. Avigen, Inc. Available at www.avigen.com. Accessed November 2009.
94. Wei T, Sabsovich I, Guo TZ, et al. Pentoxifylline attenuates nociceptive sensitization and cytokine expression in a tibia fracture rat model of complex regional pain syndrome. *Eur J Pain.* 2009;13:253–262.
95. Gwak YS, Crown ED, Unabia GC, Hulsebosch CE. Propentofylline attenuates allodynia, glial activation and modulates GABAergic tone after spinal cord injury in the rat. *Pain.* 2008;138:410–422.
96. Ebenezer GJ, McArthur JC, Thomas D, Murinson B, Hauer P, Polydefkis M, Griffin JW. Denervation of skin in neuropathies: the sequence of axonal and Schwann cell changes in skin biopsies. *Brain.* 2007;130(Pt 10):2703–2714.
97. Cruccu G, Anand P, Attal N, et al. EFNS guidelines on neuropathic pain assessment. *Eur J Neurol.* 2004;11(3):153–162.
98. Mitchell, S.W. *Injuries of Nerves and Their Consequences.* Philadelphia: J. B. Lippincott & Co.; 1872.
99. Stanton Hicks M, Jänig W, Hassenbusch S, Haddox JD, Boas R, Wilson P. Reflex sympathetic dystrophy: changing concepts and taxonomy. *Pain.* 1995;63(1):127–133.
100. Merskey H, Bogduk N. *Classification of Chronic Pain: Description of Pain Syndromes and Definitions of Pain Terms.* Seattle: IASP Press; 1994.
101. Burchiel KJ. Spontaneous impulse generation in normal and denervated dorsal root ganglia: sensitivity to alpha-adrenergic stimulation and hypoxia. *Exp Neurol.* 1984;85(2):257–272.
102. Korenman EM, Devor M. Ectopic adrenergic sensitivity in damaged peripheral nerve axons in the rat. *Exp Neurol.* 1981;72(1):63–81.
103. Heijmans-Antonissen C, Wesseldijk F, Munnikes RJ, et al. Multiplex bead array assay for detection of 25 soluble cytokines in blister fluid of patients with complex regional pain syndrome type 1. *Mediators Inflamm.* 2006;2006(1):28398.
104. Birklein F. Complex regional pain syndrome. *J Neurol.* 2005;252(2):131–138.
105. de Mos M, Sturkenboom MC, Huygen FJ. Current understandings on complex regional pain syndrome. *Pain Pract.* 2009;9(2): 86–99. Epub Feb 9, 2008.
106. Del Valle L, Schwartzman RJ, Alexander G. Spinal cord histopathological alterations in a patient with longstanding complex regional pain syndrome. *Brain Behav Immun.* 2009;23(1):85–91. Epub Aug 26 2008.
107. Gibbs GF, Drummond PD, Finch PM, Phillips JK. Unravelling the pathophysiology of complex regional pain syndrome: focus on sympathetically maintained pain. *Clin Exp Pharmacol Physiol.* 2008;35(7):717–724.
108. McLachlan EM, Janig W, Devor M, Michaelis M. Peripheral nerve injury triggers noradrenergic sprouting within dorsal root ganglia. *Nature.* 1993;363:543–546.
109. Birder LA, Perl ER. Expression of alpha2-adrenergic receptors in rat primary afferent neurones after peripheral nerve injury or inflammation. *J Physiol.* 1999;515:533–542.
110. Yen LD, Bennett GJ, Ribeiro-da-Silva A. Sympathetic sprouting and changes in nociceptive sensory innervation in the glabrous skin of the rat hind paw following partial peripheral nerve injury. *J Comp Neurol.* 2006;495:679–690.
111. Grelik C, Bennett GJ, Ribeiro-da-Silva A. Autonomic fibre sprouting and changes in nociceptive sensory innervation in the rat lower lip skin following chronic constriction injury. *Eur J Neurosci.* 2005;21: 2475–2487.
112. Fuchs PN, Meyer RA, Raja SN. Heat, but not mechanical hyperalgesia, following adrenergic injections in normal human skin. *Pain.* 2001;90:15–23.
113. Ali Z, Raja SN, Wesselmann U, Fuchs PN, Meyer RA, Campbell JN. Intradermal injection of norepinephrine evokes pain in patients with sympathetically maintained pain. *Pain.* 2000;88:161–168.
114. Torebjork E, Wahren L, Wallin G, Hallin R, Koltzenburg M. Noradrenaline-evoked pain in neuralgia. *Pain.* 1995;63:11–20.
115. Davis KD, Treede RD, Raja SN, Meyer RA, Campbell JN. Topical application of clonidine relieves hyperalgesia in patients with sympathetically maintained pain. *Pain.* 1991;47:309–317.
116. Gonzales R, Sherbourne CD, Goldyne ME, Levine JD. Noradrenaline induced prostaglandin production by sympathetic postganglionic neurons is mediated by alpha 2-adrenergic receptors. *J Neurochem.* 1991;57:1145–1150.
117. Lin Q, Zou X, Fang L, Willis WD. Sympathetic modulation of acute cutaneous flare induced by intradermal injection of capsaicin in anesthetized rats. *J Neurophysiol.* 2003;89:853–861.
118. Kohama I, Ishikawa K, Kocsis JD. Synaptic reorganization in the substantia gelatinosa after peripheral nerve neuroma formation: aberrant innervation of lamina II neurons by Abeta afferents. *J Neurosci.* 2000;20(4):1538–1549.
119. Woolf CJ, Shortland P, Coggeshall RE. Peripheral nerve injury triggers central sprouting of myelinated afferents. *Nature.* 1992; 355(6355):75–78.
120. Ji RR, Kohno T, Moore KA, Woolf CJ. Central sensitization and LTP: do pain and memory share similar mechanisms? *Trends Neurosci.* 2003;26(12):696–705.
121. Pleger B, Ragert P, Schwenkreis P, et al. Patterns of cortical reorganization parallel impaired tactile discrimination and pain intensity in complex regional pain syndrome. *Neuroimage.* 2006;32(2): 503–510.
122. Maihöfner C, Neundörfer B, Birklein F, Handwerker HO. Mislocalization of tactile stimulation in patients with complex regional pain syndrome. *J Neurol.* 2006;253(6):772–779. Epub May 18, 2006.
123. Wasner G, Heckmann K, Maier C, Baron R. Vascular abnormalities in acute reflex sympathetic dystrophy (CRPS I): complete inhibition of sympathetic nerve activity with recovery. *Arch Neurol.* 1999;56(5):613–620.
124. Kurvers H, Daemen M, Slaaf D, Stassen F, van den Wildenberg F, Kitslaar P, de Mey J. Partial peripheral neuropathy and denervation induced adrenoceptor supersensitivity. *Functional studies in an experimental model Acta Orthop Belg.* 1998;64(1):64–70.
125. Elam M, Macefield VG. Does sympathetic nerve discharge affect the firing of myelinated cutaneous afferents in humans? *Auton Neurosci.* 2004;111(2):116–126.
126. Baron R, Wasner G, Borgstedt R, et al. Effect of sympathetic activity on capsaicin-evoked pain, hyperalgesia, and vasodilatation. *Neurology.* 1999;52(5):923–932.
127. Veldman PH, Reynen HM, Arntz IE, Goris RJ. Signs and symptoms of reflex sympathetic dystrophy: prospective study of 829 patients. *Lancet.* 1993;342(8878):1012–1016.
128. van de Beek WJ, Vein A, Hilgevoord AA, van Dijk JG, van Hilten BJ. Neurophysiologic aspects of patients with generalized or multifocal tonic dystonia of reflex sympathetic dystrophy. *J Clin Neurophysiol.* 2002;19(1):77–83.
129. Schwartzman RJ, Alexander GM, Grothusen J. Pathophysiology of complex regional pain syndrome. *Expert Rev Neurother.* 2006; 6(5):669–681.
130. Schwenkreis P, Janssen F, Rommel O, et al. Bilateral motor cortex disinhibition in complex regional pain syndrome (CRPS) type I of the hand. *Neurology.* 2003;61(4):515–519.
131. Geha PY, Baliki MN, Harden RN, Bauer WR, Parrish TB, Apkarian AV. The brain in chronic CRPS pain: abnormal gray-white matter interactions in emotional and autonomic regions. *Neuron.* 2008;60(4):570–581.

132. Frettlöh J, Hüppe M, Maier C. Severity and specificity of neglect-like symptoms in patients with complex regional pain syndrome (CRPS) compared to chronic limb pain of other origins. *Pain.* 2006;124(1–2):184–189.
133. Allen G, Galer BS, Schwartz L. Epidemiology of complex regional pain syndrome: a retrospective chart review of 134 patients. *Pain.* 1999;80(3):539–544.
134. Schwartzman RJ, Erwin KL, Alexander GM. The natural history of complex regional pain syndrome. *Clin J Pain.* 2009;25(4): 273–280.
135. Sharma A, Agarwal S, Broatch J, Raja SN. A web-based cross-sectional epidemiological survey of complex regional pain syndrome. *Reg Anesth Pain Med.* 2009;34(2):110–115.
136. Sandroni P, Benrud-Larson LM, McClelland RL, Low PA. Complex regional pain syndrome type I: incidence and prevalence in Olmsted county, a population-based study. *Pain.* 2003;103 (1–2):199–207.
137. Harden RN, Bruehl S, Stanton-Hicks M, Wilson PR. Proposed new diagnostic criteria for complex regional pain syndrome. *Pain Med.* 2007;8(4):326–331.
138. van de Vusse AC, Stomp-van den Berg SG, Kessels AH, Weber WE. Randomised controlled trial of gabapentin in Complex Regional Pain Syndrome type 1 [ISRCTN84121379]. *BMC Neurol.* 2004;4:13.
139. Wallace MS, Ridgeway BM, Leung AY, Gerayli A, Yaksh TL. Concentration-effect relationship of intravenous lidocaine on the allodynia of complex regional pain syndrome types I and II. *Anesthesiology.* 2000;92(1):75–83.
140. Meier PM, Zurakowski D, Berde CB, Sethna NF. Lumbar sympathetic blockade in children with complex regional pain syndromes: a double blind placebo-controlled crossover trial. *Anesthesiology.* 2009;111(2):372–380.
141. Correll GE, Maleki J, Gracely EJ, Muir JJ, Harbut RE. Subanesthetic ketamine infusion therapy: a retrospective analysis of a novel therapeutic approach to complex regional pain syndrome. *Pain Med.* 2004;5(3):263–275.
142. Sigtermans MJ, van Hilten JJ, Bauer MC, Arbous MS, Marinus J, Sarton EY, Dahan A. Ketamine produces effective and long-term pain relief in patients with Complex Regional Pain Syndrome Type 1. *Pain.* 2009;145(3):304–311.
143. Finch PM, Knudsen L, Drummond PD. Reduction of allodynia in patients with complex regional pain syndrome: a double-blind placebo-controlled trial of topical ketamine. *Pain.* 2009; 146(1-2):18–25.
144. Sindrup SH, Otto M, Finnerup NB, Jensen TS. Antidepressants in the treatment of neuropathic pain. *Basic Clin Pharmacol Toxicol.* 2005;96(6):399–409.
145. Max MB, Lynch SA, Muir J, Shoaf SE, Smoller B, Dubner R. Effects of desipramine, amitriptyline, and fluoxetine on pain in diabetic neuropathy. *N Engl J Med.* 1992;326(19):1250–1256.
146. Max MB. Endogenous monoamine analgesic systems: amitriptyline in painful diabetic neuropathy. *Anesth Prog.* 1987;34(4): 123–127.
147. Watson CP, Moulin D, Watt-Watson J, Gordon A, Eisenhoffer J. Controlled-release oxycodone relieves neuropathic pain: a randomized controlled trial in painful diabetic neuropathy. *Pain.* 2003;105(1–2):71–78.
148. Gilron I, Bailey JM, Tu D, Holden RR, Weaver DF, Houlden RL. Morphine, gabapentin, or their combination for neuropathic pain. *N Engl J Med.* 2005;352(13):1324–1334.
149. Agarwal S, Polydefkis M, Block B, Haythornthwaite J, Raja SN. Transdermal fentanyl reduces pain and improves functional activity in neuropathic pain states. *Pain Med.* 2007;8(7):554–562.
150. Altier N, Dion D, Boulanger A, Choinière M. Management of chronic neuropathic pain with methadone: a review of 13 cases. *Clin J Pain.* 2005;21(4):364–369.
151. Wermeling DP, Berger JR. Ziconotide infusion for severe chronic pain: case series of patients with neuropathic pain. *Pharmacotherapy.* 2006;26(3):395–402.
152. Kapural L, Lokey K, Leong MS, et al. Intrathecal ziconotide for complex regional pain syndrome: seven case reports. *Pain Pract.* 2009;9(4):296–303. Epub May 29, 2009.
153. Christensen K, Jensen EM, Noer I. The reflex dystrophy syndrome response to treatment with systemic corticosteroids. *Acta Chir Scand.* 1982;148(8):653–655.
154. Huygen FJ, Niehof S, Zijlstra FJ, van Hagen PM, van Daele PL. Successful treatment of CRPS 1 with anti-TNF. *J Pain Symptom Manage.* 2004;27(2):101–103.
155. Varenna M, Zucchi F, Ghiringhelli D, et al. Intravenous clodronate in the treatment of reflex sympathetic dystrophy syndrome: a randomized, double blind, placebo controlled study *J Rheumatol.* 2000;27(6):1477–1483.
156. Manicourt DH, Brasseur JP, Boutsen Y, Depreseux G, Devogelaer JP. Role of alendronate in therapy for posttraumatic complex regional pain syndrome type I of the lower extremity. *Arthritis Rheum.* 2004;50(11):3690–3697.
157. Robinson JN, Sandom J, Chapman PT. Efficacy of pamidronate in complex regional pain syndrome type I. *Pain Med.* 2004;5(3): 276–280.
158. Perez RS, Zuurmond WW, Bezemer PD, Kuik DJ, van Loenen AC, de Lange JJ, Zuidhof AJ. The treatment of complex regional pain syndrome type I with free radical scavengers: a randomized controlled study. *Pain.* 2003;102(3):297–307.
159. Zuurmond WW, Langendijk PN, Bezemer PD, Brink HE, de Lange JJ, van Loenen AC. Treatment of acute reflex sympathetic dystrophy with DMSO 50% in a fatty cream. *Acta Anaesthesiol Scand.* 1996;40(3):364–367.
160. Zollinger PE, Tuinebreijer WE, Kreis RW, Breederveld RS. Effect of vitamin C on frequency of reflex sympathetic dystrophy in wrist fractures: a randomised trial. *Lancet.* 1999;354(9195): 2025–2028.
161. van Hilten BJ, van de Beek WJ, Hoff JI, Voormolen JH, Delhaas EM. Intrathecal baclofen for the treatment of dystonia in patients with reflex sympathetic dystrophy. *N Engl J Med.* 2000; 343(9):625–630.
162. Kofler M, Kronenberg MF, Rifici C, Saltuari L, Bauer G. Epileptic seizures associated with intrathecal baclofen application. *Neurology.* 1994;44(1):25–27.
163. Becker WJ, Harris CJ, Long ML, Ablett DP, Klein GM, DeForge DA. Long-term intrathecal baclofen therapy in patients with intractable spasticity. *Can J Neurol Sci.* 1995 Aug;22(3): 208–217.
164. Netherlands Association of Posttraumatic Dystrophy Patients. EBGD guidelines CRPS type I 2006. Available at http://pdver.atvomputing.nl/english.html.
165. Winter J, Bevan S, Campbell EA. Capsaicin and pain mechanisms. *Br J Anaesth.* 1995;75(2):157–168.
166. Ribbers GM, Stam HJ. Complex regional pain syndrome type I treated with topical capsaicin: a case report. *Arch Phys Med Rehabil.* 2001;82(6):851–852.
167. Robbins WR, Staats PS, Levine J, et al. Treatment of intractable pain with topical large-dose capsaicin: preliminary report. *Anesth Analg.* 1998;86(3):579–583.
168. Groeneweg G, Huygen FJ, Niehof SP, et al. Effect of tadalafil on blood flow, pain, and function in chronic cold complex regional pain syndrome: a randomized controlled trial. *BMC Musculoskelet Disord.* 2008;9:143.
169. Stanton-Hicks M, Baron R, Boas R, et al. Complex regional pain syndromes: guidelines for therapy. *Clin J Pain.* 1998;14(2): 155–166.
170. Raja SN, Grabow TS. Complex regional pain syndrome I (reflex sympathetic dystrophy). *Anesthesiology.* 2002;96(5):1254–1260.

171. Jänig W, Baron R. Complex regional pain syndrome: mystery explained? *Lancet Neurol.* 2003;2(11):687–697.
172. Cepeda MS, Lau J, Carr DB. Defining the therapeutic role of local anesthetic sympathetic blockade in complex regional pain syndrome: a narrative and systematic review. *Clin J Pain.* 2002; 18(4):216–233.
173. Cepeda MS, Carr DB, Lau J. Local anesthetic sympathetic blockade for complex regional pain syndrome. *Cochrane Database Syst Rev.* 2005;(4):CD004598.
174. Price DD, Long S, Wilsey B, Rafii A. Analysis of peak magnitude and duration of analgesia produced by local anesthetics injected into sympathetic ganglia of complex regional pain syndrome patients. *Clin J Pain.* 1998;14(3):216–226.
175. Carroll I, Clark JD, Mackey S. Sympathetic block with botulinum toxin to treat complex regional pain syndrome. *Ann Neurol.* 2009;65(3):348–351.
176. Shealy CN, Mortimer JT, Reswick JB. Electrical inhibition of pain by stimulation of the dorsal columns: preliminary clinical report. *Anesth Analg.* 1967;46(4):489–491.
177. Krames E. Spinal cord stimulation: indications, mechanism of action, and efficacy. *Curr Rev Pain.* 1999;3(6):419–426.
178. Cui JG, O'Connor WT, Ungerstedt U, Linderoth B, Meyerson BA. Spinal cord stimulation attenuates augmented dorsal horn release of excitatory amino acids in mononeuropathy via a GABAergic mechanism. *Pain.* 1997;73(1):87–95.
179. Meyerson BA, Linderoth B. Mode of action of spinal cord stimulation in neuropathic pain. J *Pain Symptom Manage.* 2006 Apr;31 (4 Suppl):S6–12.
180. Grabow TS, Tella PK, Raja SN. Spinal cord stimulation for complex regional pain syndrome: an evidence-based medicine review of the literature. *Clin J Pain.* 2003 Nov-Dec;19(6):371–83.
181. Kemler MA, de Vet HC, Barendse GA, van den Wildenberg FA, van Kleef M. Effect of spinal cord stimulation for chronic complex regional pain syndrome Type I: five-year final follow-up of patients in a randomized controlled trial. *J Neurosurg.* 2008 Feb;108(2): 292–8.
182. Kemler MA, de Vet HC, Barendse GA, van den Wildenberg FA, van Kleef M. Spinal cord stimulation for chronic reflex sympathetic dystrophy–five-year follow-up. *N Engl J Med.* Jun 1, 2006. 354(22):2394–6.
183. Hassenbusch SJ, Stanton-Hicks M, Schoppa D, Walsh JG, Covington EC. Long-term results of peripheral nerve stimulation for reflex sympathetic dystrophy. *J Neurosurg.* 1996 Mar;84(3): 415–23.
184. Bittar RG, Teddy PJ. Peripheral neuromodulation for pain. *J Clin Neurosci.* 2009 Oct;16(10):1259–61. Epub Jun 28, 2009.
185. Leriche R. Treatment of pain by sympathectomy. *Rev Neurol (Paris).* 1950 Jul;83(1):41–2.
186. Stanton-Hicks MD, Burton AW, Bruehl SP, Carr DB, Harden RN, Hassenbusch SJ, Lubenow TR, Oakley JC, Racz GB, Raj PP, Rauck RL, Rezai AR. An updated interdisciplinary clinical pathway for CRPS: report of an expert panel. *Pain Pract.* 2002 Mar;2(1):1–16.
187. Nelson DV, Stacey BR. Interventional therapies in the management of complex regional pain syndrome. *Clin J Pain.* 2006 Jun;22(5):438–42.
188. Bandyk DF, Johnson BL, Kirkpatrick AF, Novotney ML, Back MR, Schmacht DC. Surgical sympathectomy for reflex sympathetic dystrophy syndromes. *J Vasc Surg.* 2002 Feb;35(2): 269–77.
189. Mailis A, Furlan A. Sympathectomy for neuropathic pain. *Cochrane Database Syst Rev.* 2003;(2):CD002918.
190. Sharma A, Williams K, Raja SN. Advances in treatment of complex regional pain syndrome: recent insights on a perplexing disease. *Curr Opin Anaesthesiol.* 2006 Oct;19(5):566–72.

PART V

AUTONOMIC NERVOUS SYSTEM

13

THE AUTONOMIC NERVOUS SYSTEM

David B. Glick and Gerald Glick

BACKGROUND

The autonomic nervous system (ANS) controls the body's involuntary activities (i.e., those outside of consciousness). It is, at once, the most primitive and among the most essential of the body's systems. It is primitive in that its characteristics are largely preserved across all mammalian species. It is essential in that it oversees the body's responses to immediate life-threatening challenges and the body's vital maintenance needs (including cardiovascular, gastrointestinal, and thermal homeostasis).

The ANS is divided into two subsystems, the sympathetic nervous system and the parasympathetic nervous system. A third subsystem, the enteric nervous system, has been added to the original characterization of the ANS. Activation of the sympathetic nervous system elicits what is traditionally called the fight or flight response, including redistribution of blood flow from the viscera to skeletal muscle, augmented cardiac function, sweating, and pupillary dilatation. The parasympathetic system governs activities of the body more closely associated with maintenance of function, such as digestive and genitourinary functions. The intelligent administration of anesthetic care to patients requires knowledge of ANS pharmacology to achieve optimum interactions of anesthetics with the involuntary control system and to avoid responses or interactions that produce deleterious effects. Disease states may impair ANS function to a significant extent and may thereby alter the expected responses to surgery and anesthesia. In addition, possible harmful effects produced by the human stress response have long been appreciated, and it is possible that modification or ablation of the stress response actually may improve perioperative outcomes.

FUNCTIONAL ANATOMY

Each branch of the ANS exhibits a unique anatomic motif that is recapitulated on a cellular and molecular level. The underlying theme of the sympathetic nervous system is an amplification response, whereas that of the parasympathetic nervous system is a discrete and narrowly targeted response. The enteric nervous system is arranged nontopographically, as would be appropriate for the viscera, and relies on the mechanism of chemical coding to differentiate between nerves serving different functions.

SYMPATHETIC NERVOUS SYSTEM (THORACOLUMBAR)

The sympathetic nervous system originates from the spinal cord in the thoracolumbar region, from the first thoracic through the second or third lumbar segment. The preganglionic sympathetic neurons have cell bodies within the horns of the spinal gray matter (i.e., the intermediolateral columns). Preganglionic nerve fibers from these cell bodies exit the vertebral column in the anterior nerve roots and enter the ganglion at their respective level through the white (myelinated) ramus and then extend to three types of ganglia: 1) those grouped as paired sympathetic chains, 2) various unpaired distal plexuses, and 3) terminal or collateral ganglia near the target organ.

The 22 paired ganglia lie along either side of the vertebral column. Nerve trunks formed by the preganglionic fibers connect these ganglia to one another. Gray rami communications formed by the postganglionic fibers exiting from each ganglion connect the ganglia to the spinal nerves.

Sympathetic postganglionic fibers innervate the trunk and limbs via the spinal nerves. The sympathetic distribution to the head and neck, enabling and mediating vasomotor, pupillodilator, sudomotor (sweat gland) secretory, and pilomotor functions, comes from the three ganglia of the cervical sympathetic chain. Preganglionic fibers of these cervical structures originate in the upper thoracic segments. In 80% of people, the stellate ganglion is formed by the fusion of the inferior cervical ganglion with the first thoracic ganglion.

Postganglionic fibers innervating the terminal cardiac, esophageal, and pulmonary plexuses have their origins in the upper thoracic paravertebral sympathetic ganglia.

In contrast to paravertebral ganglia, the unpaired prevertebral ganglia reside in the abdomen and pelvis anterior to the vertebral column and are the celiac, superior mesenteric, aorticorenal, and inferior mesenteric ganglia. Their postganglionic fibers innervate the viscera of the abdomen and pelvis.

Ganglia of the third type, the terminal or collateral ganglia, are small, few in number, and near their target organs (e.g., the adrenal medulla). The adrenal medulla and other chromaffin tissue are homologous to sympathetic ganglia, all being derived embryonically from neural crest cells. Unlike sympathetic postganglionic fibers, however, the adrenal medulla releases epinephrine and norepinephrine.

Sympathetic preganglionic fibers are relatively short because sympathetic ganglia are generally close to the central nervous system (CNS), but they are distant from the effector organs; therefore, postganglionic fibers run a long course before innervating effector organs. Preganglionic sympathetic fibers may pass through multiple ganglia before synapsing, and their terminal fibers may contact large numbers of postganglionic neurons. Terminal fibers of preganglionic axons may synapse with more than 20 ganglia, and, moreover, one cell may be supplied by several preganglionic fibers. Sympathetic response, therefore, is not confined to the segment from which the stimulus originates, thereby allowing an amplified, diffuse discharge.

PARASYMPATHETIC NERVOUS SYSTEM (CRANIOSACRAL)

The parasympathetic nervous system arises from cranial nerves III, VII, IX, and X, as well as from sacral segments. Unlike the sympathetic nervous system, the ganglia of the parasympathetic nervous system are in close proximity to or within the innervated organ. This location of ganglia makes the parasympathetic nervous system more targeted and less robust than the sympathetic nervous system.

Preganglionic fibers of the parasympathetic nervous system originate in three areas of the CNS: the midbrain, the medulla oblongata, and the sacral part of the spinal cord. Fibers arising in the Edinger-Westphal nucleus of the oculomotor nerve course in the midbrain to synapse in the ciliary ganglion. This pathway innervates the smooth muscle of the iris and the ciliary muscle. In the medulla oblongata lie parasympathetic components of the facial (lacrimatory nucleus), glossopharyngeal, and vagus (dorsal motor nucleus) nerves. The facial nerve gives off parasympathetic fibers to the chorda tympani, which subsequently synapses in the ganglia of the submaxillary or sublingual glands and the greater superficial petrosal nerve, which synapses in the sphenopalatine ganglion. The glossopharyngeal nerve synapses in the otic ganglion. These postganglionic fibers innervate the mucous, salivary, and lacrimal glands; they also carry vasodilator fibers.

The vagus nerve transmits fully three fourths of the traffic of the parasympathetic nervous system. It supplies the heart, tracheobronchial tree, liver, spleen, kidney, and the entire gastrointestinal tract except the distal colon. Most vagal fibers do not synapse until they arrive at small ganglia on and around the thoracic and abdominal viscera.

The second through fourth sacral segments contribute the nervi erigentes, or pelvic splanchnic nerves. They synapse in terminal ganglia associated with the rectum and genitourinary organs.

ENTERIC NERVOUS SYSTEM

Given the importance of clinical phenomena such as nausea, vomiting, and alterations in bowel function associated with anesthesia, it is surprising how little is understood about the third branch of the ANS. The enteric nervous system is the system of neurons and their supporting cells found within the walls of the gastrointestinal tract, including the neurons within the pancreas and gallbladder.[1] It is derived from neuroblasts of the neural crest that migrate to the gastrointestinal tract along the vagus nerve.

One major difference between the enteric nervous system and the sympathetic and parasympathetic branches of the ANS is its extraordinary degree of local autonomy. For example, digestion and peristalsis continue after spinal cord transection or during spinal anesthesia, although sphincter function may be impaired.

Although functionally discrete, the gut is influenced by sympathetic and parasympathetic activity. The sympathetic preganglionic fibers from T8 through L3 inhibit gut action via the celiac, superior, and inferior mesenteric ganglia. A spinal or epidural anesthetic covering the midthoracic levels removes this inhibition, yielding a contracted small intestine that may afford superior surgical conditions in combination with the profound muscle relaxation of a spinal anesthetic.[2] The sphincters are relaxed, and peristalsis is normally active.

Conversely, if the contents of the upper intestine become overly acidic or hypertonic, an adrenergically mediated enterogastric reflex may be induced that reduces the rate of gastric emptying. In the unstimulated state the adrenergic neurons of the gastrointestinal tract are usually inactive. Reflex pathways, both within and external to the alimentary tract, cause discharge of these neurons. Thus, when the viscera are handled during abdominal surgery, reflex firing of the adrenergic nerves may inhibit the motor activity of the intestine for an extended period thereby producing postoperative ileus.

Loss of parasympathetic nervous control usually decreases bowel tone and peristalsis, but over time, the increased activity of the enteric plexus compensates for the loss. Spinal cord lesions may remove sacral parasympathetic input, but cranial parasympathetics may still be carried by branches of the vagus nerve to the end-organ ganglia. As a result, colonic dilation and fecal impaction (which may precipitate hypertension in autonomic hyperreflexia) may occur. Small intestinal dysfunction is less common.

Unlike the sympathetic and parasympathetic nervous systems, in which geographic location confers selective action, in the gut an alternative pattern of chemical coding for function assumes an important organizational role. Specifically, the combination of amines and peptides and their relative concentrations within the enteric neuron are thought to code for its function.

Acetylcholine is the principal excitatory trigger of the nonsphincteric portion of the enteric nervous system, causing muscle contraction. Cholinergic neurons have several roles in the enteric nervous system, including excitation of external muscle, activation of motor neurons augmenting water and electrolyte secretion, and stimulation of gastric cells. Neural control of gastrointestinal motility is mediated through two types of motor neurons: excitatory and inhibitory. These neurons act in concert on the circular smooth muscle layer in sphincteric and nonsphincteric regions throughout the digestive tract, and they supply the muscles of the biliary tree and the muscularis mucosae. Although excitatory motor neurons supply the external longitudinal muscle, the role of inhibitory motor neurons is not well established in this muscular layer. Enteric motor neurons to the circular muscle of the small and large intestine are activated by local reflex pathways contained within the wall of the intestine. Distention evokes polarized reflexes, including contraction proximally and relaxation distally, which in synchrony constitute peristalsis. Nicotinic antagonists abolish enteric reflexes, suggesting that the sensory neurons or interneurons in the pathway are cholinergic. In cases of cholinergic overload, such as insecticide poisoning or "overreversal" of muscle relaxants (in which cholinesterase is inhibited), there is a tendency for the gut to become hyperreactive.

There are many neuroactive compounds other than norepinephrine and acetylcholine that participate in the autonomic control of intestinal function. The predominant of these nonadrenergic noncholinergic neurotransmitters appears to be nitric oxide (NO), which provides the primary intrinsic inhibitory innervation to the gastrointestinal tract. Other neuroactive chemicals and peptides identified in the gastrointestinal tract include substance P, a variety of opiate peptides, vasoactive intestinal protein (VIP), and a growing population of peptide hormones (Table 13.1). Complex interactions between these neurotransmitters underlie the local control of gastrointestinal function.

Table 13.1 **NEUROPEPTIDES AND THEIR ACTIONS IN THE GASTROINTESTINAL TRACT**

PEPTIDE	ACTION(S)
Bombesin	Multiple stimulatory effects (incl. gastrin release)
Calcitonin gene-related peptide	Gastric acid secretion, muscle constriction
CCK8	Unknown
Dynorphin	Opiate effects
Endothelin-1	Vasoconstriction
Galanin	Muscle constriction
Leu-enkephalin	Opiate effects
Met-enkephalin	Opiate effects
Neuromedin U	Muscle constriction, vasoconstriction
Neuropeptide Y	Vasoconstriction
Pituitary adenylate cyclase activating peptide	Adenylate cyclase activation
Peptide histidine methionine	Muscle relaxation, secretion
Somatostatin	Multiple inhibitory effects (incl. gastrin inhibition)
Substance P	Vasodilatation, muscle constriction
Vasoactive intestinal polypeptide	Vasodilatation, muscle relaxation, secretion

CCK8=cholecystokinin-8
Modified from Bishop A, Polak J. The gut and the autonomic nervous system. In: Mathias C, Bannister R, eds. *Autonomic Failure: A Textbook of Clinical Disorders of the Autonomic Nervous System*. 4th ed. Oxford: Oxford University Press; 1999:120.

FUNCTION

ORGANIZATION AND INTEGRATION

The sympathetic system, in response to internal or external challenges, acts to 1) increase heart rate, arterial pressure, and cardiac output; 2) dilate the bronchial tree; and 3) shunt blood away from the intestines and other viscera to voluntary muscles. Teleologically, the body is then better prepared to deal with the challenge. Parasympathetic nervous input acts primarily to conserve energy and maintain organ function and to support vegetative processes.

Most organs of the body exhibit dual innervation, with input from the sympathetic and parasympathetic systems frequently mediating opposing effects (Table 13.2).[3] Stimulation of one system may have an excitatory effect on the end organ, whereas stimulation of the other system may have an inhibitory effect. For example, sympathetic stimulation of the heart increases the rate and vigor of contraction and enhances conduction through the atrioventricular node, whereas parasympathetic stimulation decreases heart rate, atrial contractility, and conduction through the atrioventricular node. One of the two systems normally dominates the organ's function, providing its "resting tone"

Table 13.2 RESPONSES ELICITED IN EFFECTOR ORGANS BY STIMULATION OF SYMPATHETIC AND PARASYMPATHETIC NERVES

DOMINANT EFFECTOR ORGAN	ADRENERGIC RESPONSE	RECEPTOR INVOLVED	CHOLINERGIC RESPONSE	RESPONSE (A OR C)
Heart, Rate of contraction	Increase	β_1	Decrease	C
Heart, Force of contraction	Increase	β_1	Decrease	C
Blood vessels, Arteries (most)	Vasoconstriction	α_1		A
Blood vessels, Skeletal muscle	Vasodilation	β_2		A
Blood vessels, Veins	Vasoconstriction	α_2		A
Bronchial tree	Bronchodilation	β_2	Bronchoconstriction	C
Splenic capsule	Contraction	α_1		A
Uterus	Contraction	α_1	Variable	A
Vas deferens	Contraction	α_1		A
Prostatic capsule	Contraction	α_1		A
Gastrointestinal tract	Relaxation	α_2	Contraction	C
Eye, Radial muscle, iris	Contraction (mydriasis)	α_1		A
Eye, Circular muscle, iris			Contraction (miosis)	C
Eye, Ciliary muscle	Relaxation	β	Contraction	C
Kidney	Renin secretion	β_1	(accommodation)	A
Urinary bladder Detrusor	Relaxation	β	Contraction	C
Trigone and sphincter	Contraction	α_1	Relaxation	A, C
Ureter	Contraction	α_1	Relaxation	A
Insulin release from pancreas	Decrease	α_2		A
Fat cells	Lipolysis	β_1		A
Liver glycogenolysis	Increase	α_1		A
Hair follicles, smooth muscle	Contraction (piloerection)	α_1		A
Nasal secretion			Increase	C
Salivary glands	Increase secretion	α_1	Increase secretion	C
Sweat glands	Increase secretion	α_1	Increase secretion	C

A, adrenergic; C, cholinergic

Table 13.3 USUAL SYMPATHETIC OR PARASYMPATHETIC DOMINANCE AT SPECIFIC EFFECTOR SITES

SITE	PREDOMINANT TONE
Ciliary muscle	Parasympathetic
Iris	Parasympathetic
Sinoatrial node	Parasympathetic
Arterioles	Sympathetic
Veins	Sympathetic
Gastrointestinal tract	Parasympathetic
Uterus	Parasympathetic
Urinary bladder	Parasympathetic
Salivary glands	Parasympathetic
Sweat glands	Sympathetic (cholinergic)

(Table 13.3). In a few systems, the sympathetic system alone provides innervation, most notably blood vessels, the spleen, and piloerector muscles.

To predict the effects of drugs, the interaction of the sympathetic and parasympathetic systems in different organs must be understood. Blockade of sympathetic function unmasks preexisting parasympathetic activity, and the converse relation also is true. For example, basal heart rate is mainly determined by parasympathetic tone, but with administration of atropine unopposed sympathetic tone causes tachycardia.

ADRENERGIC FUNCTION

Overview of the Effects of Sympathetic Mediators

Activation of the adrenergic neurons influences many bodily functions, but the effects on circulation and respiration are among the most important. Ventilation is increased by a central effect on the ventilatory centers and by bronchodilation. Heart rate and myocardial contractility are also markedly increased. Function of the gastrointestinal and genitourinary systems is decreased as a result of the relaxation of the smooth muscle in these organs and contraction of their sphincters. Gastrointestinal secretory activity is inhibited, and adrenal medullary output is increased. Metabolism is stimulated to provide more fuel for bodily function in the form of glucose and fatty acids.

The endogenous catecholamines, norepinephrine and epinephrine, possess α- and β-receptor agonist activity. Norepinephrine has minimal β_2-receptor activity, whereas epinephrine stimulates both β_1- and β_2-receptors.

The physiologic responses mediated by α-adrenoceptors are wide ranging and important. α-Receptor-mediated activity is responsible for most of the sympathetically induced smooth muscle contraction throughout the body, namely the vascular, bronchial, and ureteral smooth muscle and the ciliary muscle of the eye.[4] The gastrointestinal and genitourinary sphincter mechanisms are stimulated by α-adrenergic receptors. α-Receptor agonism decreases pancreatic insulin secretion from the pancreatic β cells. In the peripheral vasculature, α_1- and α_2-receptors modulate vascular tone in response to humorally borne neurotransmitters and exogenously administered drugs.

β-Receptor agonism appears to be primarily responsible for sympathetic stimulation of the heart, relaxation of vascular and bronchial smooth muscle, stimulation of renin secretion by the kidney, and several metabolic consequences, including lipolysis and glycogenolysis. The β_1-receptor mechanism is thought to be primarily involved in the cardiac effects[5] and release of fatty acids and renin, whereas the β_2-receptors are primarily responsible for smooth muscle relaxation and hyperglycemia. In specialized circumstances, however, β_2-receptors may also mediate cardiac activity. Although acute changes in arterial pressure and heart rate can be caused by norepinephrine or epinephrine, chronic hypertension does not appear to be related to circulating levels of these hormones.[6] It is estimated that 85% of resting arterial pressure is controlled by the renin-angiotensin system. Psychological and physical stimuli may evoke different sympathetic compensatory responses. Public speaking activates the adrenal gland with a disproportionate rise in serum epinephrine, whereas physical exercise elicits primarily a rise in serum norepinephrine.[7] Thus, the stress response should not be conceived of as a uniform response; it can vary in mechanism, intensity, and manifestations.

Blood Glucose

Sympathetic nervous stimulation through β-receptor activation augments glycogenolysis in liver and muscle and liberates free fatty acids from adipose tissue, ultimately increasing blood glucose levels. In neonates, epinephrine plays an additional role in the exothermic breakdown of brown fat to maintain body temperature (i.e., nonshivering thermogenesis).

α_2- and β_2-Receptors also are present in the pancreas. As noted above, α_2-receptor activation suppresses insulin secretion by pancreatic islet cells. Thus, blockade of these receptors may increase insulin release and may be associated with significant lowering of blood glucose levels. β_2-Receptor stimulation increases glucagon and insulin secretion and decreases peripheral sensitivity to insulin.[8]

Potassium Shift

Plasma epinephrine also takes part in the regulation of serum potassium concentration. Transient hyperkalemia occurs as potassium shifts out of hepatic cells with the glucose efflux produced by β_2-adrenergic stimulation. This effect is followed by a more prolonged hypokalemia as the β_2-adrenergic stimulation drives potassium into muscle and red blood cells. Exogenously administered or endogenously released epinephrine stimulates the β_2-receptors of red blood cells, activating adenylate cyclase and the sodium-potassium ATPase, driving potassium into the red cells.

CHOLINERGIC FUNCTION

Overview of the Effects of Acetylcholine

Acetylcholine release is the hallmark of parasympathetic activation. The actions of acetylcholine are almost diametrically opposed to those of norepinephrine and epinephrine. In general, the muscarinic effects of acetylcholine are qualitatively the same as the effects of vagal stimulation.

The dose of exogenously administered acetylcholine determines its effect. A small intravenous dose causes generalized vasodilation (including the coronary and pulmonary circulation), whereas a larger dose demonstrates negative chronotropic and dromotropic effects. The vasodilation occurs because significant numbers of muscarinic receptors exist in vascular beds despite the absence of a cholinergic nerve supply. A second mechanism of vessel relaxation by acetylcholine is inhibition of norepinephrine release from adrenergic nerve terminals.

Acetylcholine decreases heart rate, the velocity of conduction in the sinoatrial (SA) and atrioventricular (AV) nodes, and atrial contractility. In the SA node acetylcholine causes membrane hyperpolarization, thereby delaying attainment of the threshold potential with a resultant decrease in heart rate. In the AV node, acetylcholine decreases conduction velocity and increases the effective refractory period. This decrease in AV nodal conduction accounts for the complete heart block seen when large amounts of cholinergic agonists are given. In the ventricle, acetylcholine decreases automaticity in the Purkinje system, thereby increasing the fibrillation threshold.

Parasympathetic activation has many effects outside the cardiovascular system. Cholinergic stimulation causes smooth muscle constriction, including that of the bronchial walls. In the gastrointestinal and genitourinary tracts, smooth muscle in the walls constricts, but sphincter muscles relax, leading to incontinence. Topically administered acetylcholine constricts the smooth muscle of the iris, causing miosis.

Signs and symptoms of cholinergic overload reflect all these effects as well as nausea and vomiting, intestinal cramps, belching, urination, and urgent defecation. All glands innervated by the parasympathetic nervous system are stimulated to produce secretions, including the lacrimal, tracheobronchial, salivary, digestive, and exocrine glands.

PHARMACOLOGY

ADRENERGIC PHARMACOLOGY

Synthesis of Norepinephrine

Norepinephrine is synthesized from tyrosine, which is actively transported into the varicosity of the postganglionic sympathetic nerve ending (Figure 13.1). Tyrosine is synthesized from phenylalanine. Precursors are taken up in greater amounts in shock and this increased uptake may have beneficial effects on the efforts of the sympathetic nervous system to maintain perfusion pressure.

A series of steps results in the conversion of tyrosine to norepinephrine and epinephrine (in the adrenal medulla). The first of these steps involves the cytoplasmic enzyme tyrosine hydroxylase (TH). This is the rate-limiting step in norepinephrine biosynthesis. High levels of norepinephrine inhibit TH, and low levels stimulate the enzyme. During stimulation of the sympathetic nervous system, an increased supply of tyrosine also increases synthesis of norepinephrine. TH activity is modified by phosphorylation. Whereas acute control of TH occurs by altering enzyme activity, chronic stress can elevate TH levels by stimulating synthesis of new enzyme. Under the influence of TH, tyrosine is converted to dihydroxyphenylalanine (DOPA), which is decarboxylated to dopamine by an aromatic amino acid decarboxylase (DOPA decarboxylase).

Dopamine can and does act as a neurotransmitter in some cells, but most of the produced dopamine is β-hydroxylated within the vesicles to norepinephrine by the enzyme dopamine β-hydroxylase (DBH). In the adrenal medulla, and to a limited extent in discrete regions of the brain, another enzyme, phenylethanolamine N-methyl transferase (PNMT), methylates about 85% of the norepinephrine to epinephrine. Glucocorticoids from the adrenal cortex pass through the adrenal medulla and can activate the system, and stress-induced steroid release can increase epinephrine production. This local circulation amplifies the effects of glucocorticoid release.[9]

Storage of Norepinephrine

Norepinephrine is stored within large, dense-core vesicles. These vesicles also contain calcium and a variety of peptides and adenosine 5′-triphosphate (ATP). Although norepinephrine is the predominant neurotransmitter at sympathetic nerve endings, depending on the nature and frequency of physiologic stimuli, the ATP can be released selectively for an immediate postsynaptic effect through purinoreceptors.

The vesicles containing norepinephrine are heterogeneous and exist within functionally defined compartments. An actively recycling population of synaptic vesicles has been defined, together with a reserve population of vesicles that is mobilized only on extensive stimulation. Newly

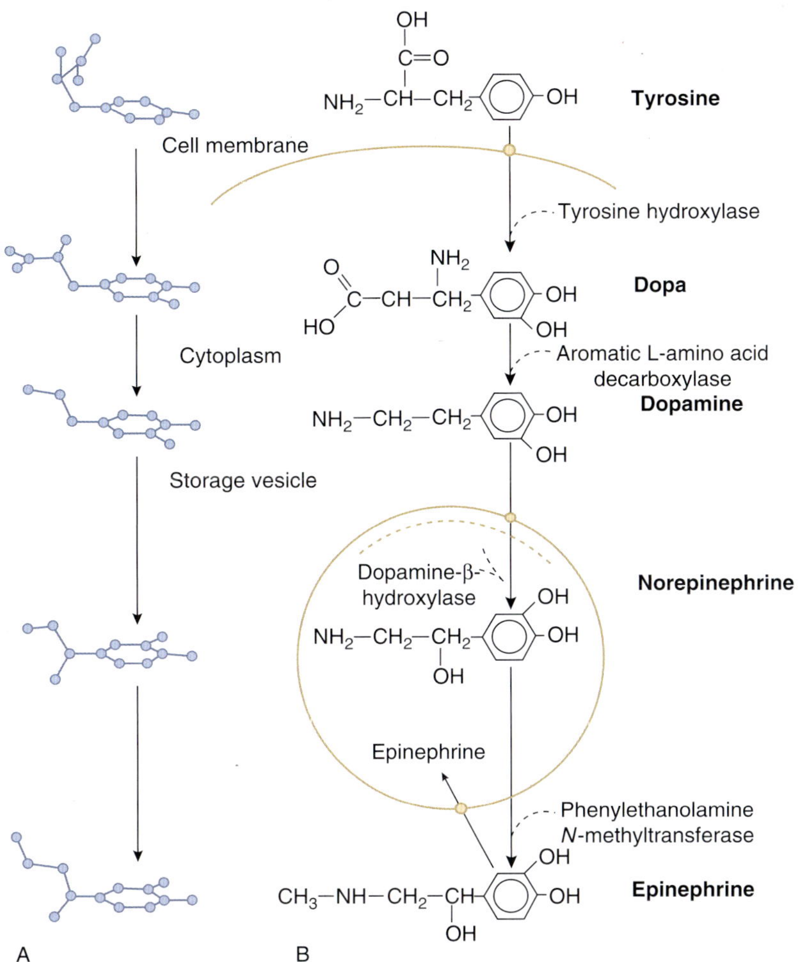

Figure 13.1 Biosynthesis of norepinephrine and epinephrine in sympathetic nerve terminal (and adrenal medulla). A, Perspective view of molecules. B, Enzymatic processes. From Tollenaeré JP. *Atlas of the Three-Dimensional Structure of Drugs*. Amsterdam: Elsevier North-Holland; 1979, as modified by Vanhoutte PM. Adrenergic neuroeffector interaction in the blood vessel wall. *Fed Proc*. 1978;37:181.

synthesized or taken up transmitters are incorporated preferentially into the actively recycling vesicles and are the first ones released on stimulation. These readily releasable vesicles make up approximately 10% of the total norepinephrine containing vesicular population of the neuron. In general, 1% of stored norepinephrine is released with each depolarization, implying a significant functional reserve.

The vesicles have two fundamentally different functions: They take up and store neurotransmitters, and they fuse with and bud from the presynaptic plasma terminal membrane. The proteins of vesicles can be divided into two functionally discrete classes. The first class, transport proteins, provides the channels and pumps for the uptake and storage of neurotransmitters. The second class of proteins directs movement and docking reactions of the vesicle membrane.

Release of Norepinephrine

There are several different processes by which the contents of the vesicle enter the synaptic cleft. The dominant physiologic mechanism of release is exocytosis, during which the vesicle responds to the entry of calcium by initiating the sequence of vesicular docking, fusion, release of vesicular contents, and ultimately endocytosis (the process by which vesicular membrane and proteins are recaptured).

Various specific soluble and membrane-bound proteins have been identified that participate in docking, fusion, and endocytosis. Synaptotagmin serves as the intermediary between calcium entry and docking.[10] Although the mechanisms of docking and fusion are still incompletely understood, it appears to be a highly differentiated process in which a pair of soluble binding proteins—soluble N-ethyl maleimide sensitive factor (NSF) attachment proteins (SNAPs) and soluble NSF receptors (SNAREs)—interact.[11,12]

SNARE proteins are present on both the vesicular and neuronal membranes. A core complex of SNARE proteins is formed when three or four of these proteins (two reactive sites each from the vesicle and the cell membranes) are brought into close proximity. The apposition of the two membranes allows them to fuse and the vesicular contents

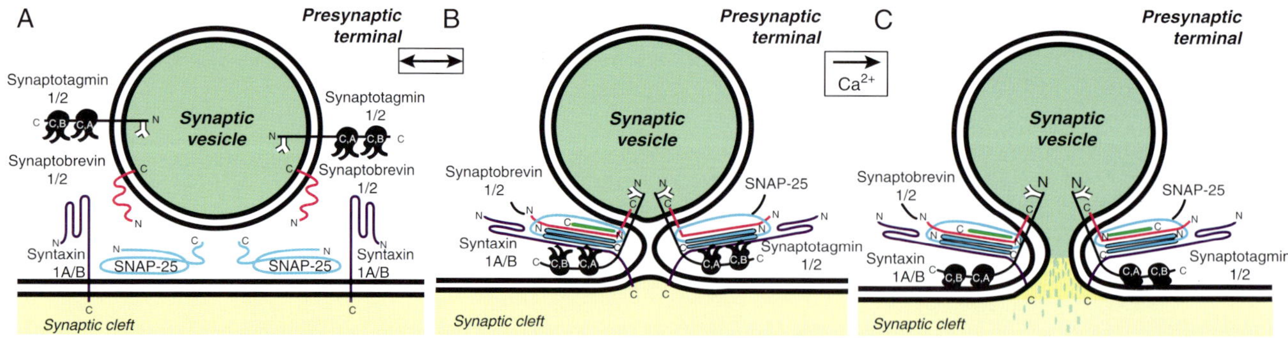

Figure 13.2 Model for the functions of SNARE proteins. A. Vesicle is docked, SNAREs, synaptotagmins are not engaged. B. SNARE complexes are formed, and the vesicle and plasma membranes are brought into close proximity. C. Ca^{2+} triggers the opening of the fusion pore and the release of the vesicular contents. Reprinted with permission from Sudhof T. The synaptic vesicle cycle. *Annu Rev Neurosci*. 2004; 27:509–547.

to be released into the synaptic cleft. Three SNARE proteins involved in synaptic exocytosis have been identified: synaptobrevin (on the vesicular membrane) and syntaxin-1 and SNAP-25 (on the neuronal membrane). Other proteins, including synaptophysins, have been identified that can bind to synaptobrevin and inhibit SNARE complex formation and exocytosis (Figure 13.2).[13]

Evidence for the biologic relevance of these proteins is derived from observations that tetanus toxin and botulinum toxin block vesicular release by binding to the docking and fusion proteins,[14] whereas microinjection of SNAP into neurons enhances exocytosis.[10, 15] In vesicular docking and release, a subpopulation of vesicles is tethered to the active zone of the prejunctional neuron. These are the readily releasable vesicles noted previously (Figure 13.3).[13,16,17] The short latency between excitation and vesicle release[18] has functional implications, particularly in facilitating rapid transmission in the sympathetic nervous system.

Although chromaffin cells in the adrenal medulla synthesize epinephrine and norepinephrine, the two compounds are stored in and secreted from distinct chromaffin cell subtypes. Data suggest that there may be a preferential release from one or another form of chromaffin cell depending on the stimulus.[19] Nicotinic agonists or depolarizing agents cause the preferential release of norepinephrine, whereas histamine elicits predominantly epinephrine release.[20–22]

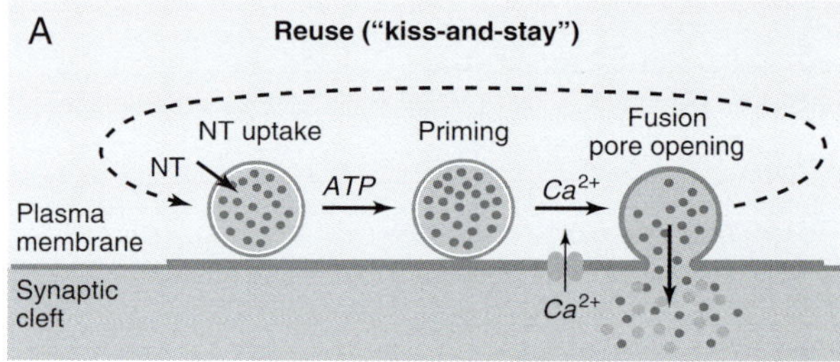

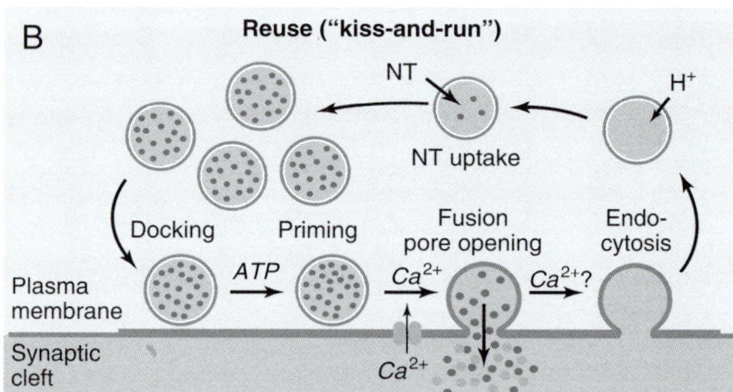

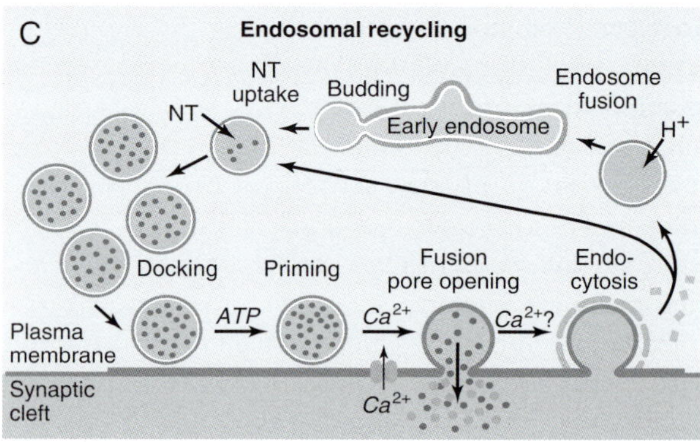

Figure 13.3 Synaptic vesicle recycling pathways. A. Vesicles refill with neurotransmitters while still docked to the active zone along the postganglionic sympathetic neural membrane. B. Vesicles are returned to the cytoplasm, where they are quickly refilled with neurotransmitters (i.e., "kiss-and-run"). C. Vesicles return to the cytoplasm via endocytosis and are incorporated into endosomes before reforming vesicles and filling with neurotransmitters. Reprinted with permission from Sudhof T. The synaptic vesicle cycle. *Annu Rev Neurosci*. 2004;27:509–547.

Inactivation

Most of the norepinephrine released is rapidly removed from the synaptic cleft via active reuptake mechanisms in the neuron. If a transmitter is to exert fine control over an effector system its half-life in the biophase (i.e., the extracellular space close to the receptor) must be short. The active reuptake mechanism ensures that norepinephrine's time in the synaptic cleft is appropriately short. Most released norepinephrine is transported into the storage vesicle for reuse. This neurotransmitter uptake into synaptic vesicles is driven by an electrochemical proton gradient across the synaptic vesicle membrane. After reuptake, the small amounts of norepinephrine not taken up into the vesicle are deaminated by cytoplasmic monoamine oxidase (MAO).

Uptake of norepinephrine into the nerve varicosity and its return to the storage vesicle, albeit efficient, is not specific for the neurotransmitter. Some compounds structurally similar to norepinephrine may enter the nerve by the same mechanism and may result in depletion of the neurotransmitter. These false transmitters can be of great clinical importance. Moreover, some drugs that block reuptake into the vesicle or into the nerve ending itself may enhance response to catecholamines; that is, more norepinephrine remains available to receptors. These drugs include cocaine and tricyclic antidepressants.

Activity of the reuptake system varies greatly among different tissues. Peripheral blood vessels have almost no reuptake of norepinephrine, consequently, norepinephrine must be metabolized within the synaptic cleft to be inactivated. As a result, rapid rates of norepinephrine synthesis within the vesicle are necessary to modulate vascular tone. On the other hand, the highest rate of reuptake is found in the heart.

Metabolism

During storage and reuptake, the norepinephrine that escapes uptake into the nerve ending enters the circulation where it is metabolized by MAO or catechol-O-methyl transferase (COMT) in the blood, liver, and kidney.[23]

Epinephrine is inactivated by the same enzymes. The final metabolic product of inactivation is vanillylmandelic acid (VMA). The two catabolic enzymes (MAO and COMT) and the vigorous uptake system account for the efficient clearance of catecholamines. Because of this rapid clearance, the half-life of norepinephrine (and most biogenic amines) in plasma is short, less than 1 minute. Consequently, a more ideal measure of catecholamine production may be metabolic products, rather than catecholamine levels in the blood or urine.

Inhibition of MAO would be expected to have a great impact on the sympathetic function of a patient. MAO inhibitors (MAOIs) are generally well tolerated, but the stability of the patient belies the fact that amine handling is fundamentally changed.

Other compounds can produce sympathomimetic effects by acting as false transmitters. Although it is not used therapeutically, tyramine is the prototypic drug studied. It is present in many foods, particularly aged cheese and wines. Tyramine enters the sympathetic nerve terminal through the reuptake mechanism, displacing norepinephrine from the vesicles into the cytoplasm. Released norepinephrine leaks out from the cytoplasm and is responsible for the hypertensive effect of tyramine. However, a secondary effect can occur. In the vesicle, tyramine is converted by DBH into octopamine, which is eventually released as a false transmitter in place of norepinephrine, but without the hypertensive effect, because it has only 10% of the potency of norepinephrine.[24]

ADRENERGIC RECEPTORS

Ahlquist originally identified α- and β-adrenergic receptors by their different responses to pharmacologic antagonists.[25] Adrenergic receptors have been subclassified as α_1, α_2, β_1, β_2, or β_3 based on responses to specific drugs.

α-Adrenergic Receptors

Within α_1–adrenergic receptors, $\alpha_{1A/D}$, α_{1B}, and α_{1C} receptors have been characterized.[26] Several α_2-isoreceptors (α_{2A}, α_{2B}, and α_{2C}) have been described.[27] The α_2-receptors are usually expressed presynaptically or even in nonneuronal tissue. The α_2-receptors are found in the peripheral nervous system, in the CNS, and in a variety of organs, including platelets, liver, pancreas, kidney, and eyes, where specific physiologic functions have been identified.[28] The predominant α_2-receptor of the human spinal cord has been identified as the α_{2A}-subtype.[29,30] It appears that mammalian genomes contain two sets of at least three unique genes encoding the α-adrenoceptors. The genes encoding α_2-receptors have been localized in chromosomes 2, 4, and 10.

There is more than theoretical relevance in subclassification of receptors.[31] For example, the α-adrenergic receptors in the prostate gland are predominantly α_{1A}. Therapy with selective α_{1A}-antagonists for benign prostatic hypertrophy may avoid some of the postural hypotension and other deleterious effects that occur with less specific α-antagonists. Amino acid sequence comparisons indicate that α-receptors are members of the seven transmembrane segment gene superfamily using G protein for signal transduction. A core of 175 amino acids constitutes the seven transmembrane regions that are highly conserved among different family members.[32]

Receptors can be presynaptic as well as postsynaptic. Presynaptic receptors may act as heteroreceptors or autoreceptors. An autoreceptor is a presynaptic receptor that reacts with the neurotransmitter released from its own nerve terminal, providing feedback regulation. A heteroreceptor is a presynaptic receptor that responds to substances other than the neurotransmitter released from that specific nerve terminal. This regulatory scheme is present throughout the nervous system but is particularly important in the sympathetic nervous system.[33]

Although several presynaptic receptors have been identified, the α_2-receptor may be of the greatest clinical import. Presynaptic α_2-receptors regulate the release of norepinephrine and ATP through a negative-feedback mechanism.[34] Activation of presynaptic α_2-receptors by norepinephrine inhibits subsequent norepinephrine release in response to nerve stimulation.

β-Adrenergic Receptors

The structure of the β-adrenergic receptor was among the first to be ascertained and is well characterized. Like the α-receptor, the β-receptor is one of the superfamily of proteins that have seven helices woven through the cellular membrane. These transmembrane domains are labeled M_1 through M_7; antagonists have specific binding sites, whereas agonists are more diffusely attached to hydrophobic membrane-spanning domains (Figure 13.4). The extracellular portion of the receptor ends in an amino group. A carboxyl group occupies the intracellular terminus, where phosphorylation occurs. At the cytoplasmic domains, there is interaction with G proteins and kinases, including β-adrenergic receptor kinase. The β-receptor has mechanistic and structural similarities with muscarinic, but not nicotinic, receptors, primarily in the transmembrane sections. Muscarinic receptors and β-receptors are coupled to adenylate cyclase through G proteins, and both can initiate the opening of ion channels.

β-receptors have been further divided into β_1-, β_2-, and β_3-subtypes, all of which increase cyclic adenosine monophosphate (cAMP) through adenylate cyclase and the mediation of G proteins.[35,36] Traditionally, the β_1-receptors were thought to be isolated to cardiac tissue, and β_2-receptors were believed to be restricted to vascular and bronchial smooth muscle. Although this model of distribution is still useful because it reflects the primary clinical effects of pharmacologic manipulation of the β_1- and β_2-receptor subtypes, β_2-receptors are more important in cardiac function than indicated by this model. The β_2-receptor population in human cardiac tissue is substantial, accounting for 15% of the β-receptors in the ventricles and 30% to 40% in the atria.[37] β_2-receptors may help to compensate for disease by maintaining response to catecholamine stimulation when β_1-receptors are downregulated during chronic catecholamine stimulation and in congestive heart failure (CHF).[38] The β_2-population is almost unaffected in end-stage congestive cardiomyopathy.[39] In addition to positive inotropic effects, β_2-receptors in the human atria participate in the regulation of heart rate. Localization of β_3-receptors to fat cells suggests a new therapeutic target for obesity.

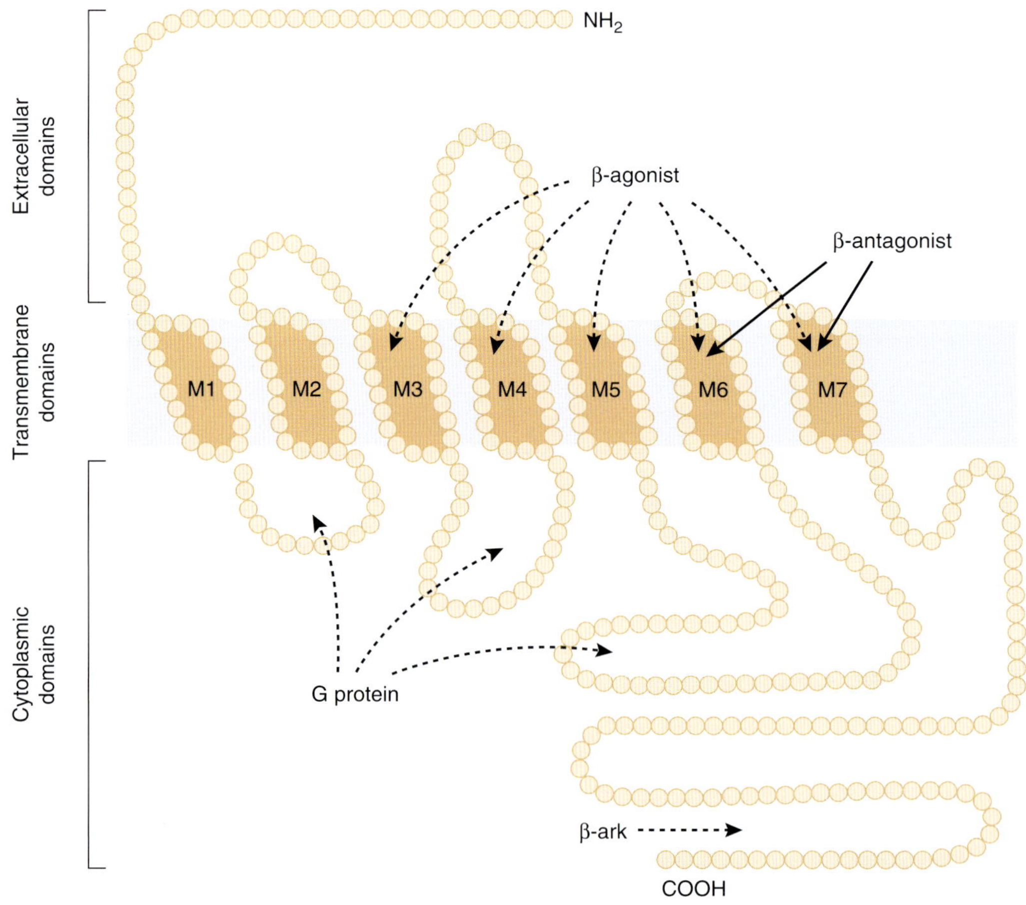

Figure 13.4 Molecular structure of the β-adrenergic receptor. Notice the three domains. The transmembrane domains act as a ligand-binding pocket. Cytoplasmic domains can interact with G proteins and kinases, such as β-adrenergic receptor kinase (β-ARK). The latter can phosphorylate and desensitize the receptor. Reprinted with permission from Opie LH. *The Heart: Physiology and Metabolism*. New York: Raven Press; 1991;154.

Polymorphism of the β_3-receptor subtype is associated with obesity and the potential for the development of diabetes.[40–42] Point mutations in genes encoding β_2-receptors are correlated with enhanced downregulation of β-receptors and nocturnal asthma.[43,44]

Dopamine Receptors

Dopamine exists as an intermediate in norepinephrine biosynthesis and exogenously administered dopamine exerts predominantly α- or β-adrenergic effects depending on the dose administered. Furthermore, Goldberg and Rajfer[45] demonstrated physiologically distinct dopamine type 1 (DA_1) and dopamine type 2 (DA_2) receptors, and these remain the most important of the five dopamine receptors that have been cloned. DA_1 receptors are postsynaptic and act on renal, mesenteric, splenic, and coronary vascular smooth muscle to mediate vasodilation through stimulation of adenylate cyclase and consequent increased cAMP production. The vasodilatory effect tends to be strongest in the renal arteries. Additional renal DA_1 receptors located in the tubules modulate natriuresis through the sodium potassium ATPase pump and the sodium-hydrogen exchanger.[45–48] The DA_2 receptors are presynaptic; they may inhibit norepinephrine and perhaps acetylcholine release. There are also central DA_2 receptors that may mediate nausea and vomiting.

GTP-BINDING REGULATORY PROTEINS (G PROTEINS)

Each class of adrenergic receptor couples to a different major subfamily of G proteins, which are linked to different secondary messengers. α_1-Receptors are linked to phospholipase C activation.

β-Receptor stimulation activates G_s proteins, enhancing adenylate cyclase activity and cAMP formation. The briefest encounter of plasma membrane β-adrenergic receptors with epinephrine or norepinephrine results in profound increases in the intracellular levels of cAMP (up to 400-fold higher than the basal level). Increased cAMP synthesis activates protein kinases, which phosphorylate target proteins thereby eliciting various cellular responses that complete the path between β–receptor and effect. In contrast, stimulation of α_2-receptors results in G_i inhibition of adenylate cyclase.

There is a relative abundance of G proteins, resulting in amplification of receptor agonism at the signal transduction step. The number of G protein molecules greatly exceeds the number of β-adrenergic receptors and adenylate cyclase molecules. It is the receptor concentration and ultimately adenylate cyclase activity, rather than G protein availability, that limit the response to catecholamines.

Upregulation and Downregulation

β-Adrenergic receptors are not fixed; they change significantly in dynamic response to the amount of norepinephrine present in the synaptic cleft or in plasma. For β-adrenergic receptors, this response is fast; within 30 minutes of denervation or adrenergic blockade, the number of receptors increases. This upregulation may explain why sudden discontinuation of β-adrenergic receptor blocking drugs sometimes cause rebound tachycardia and may increase the incidence of ischemia and myocardial infarction. Many chronic conditions, such as varicose veins[49] or aging, can decrease adrenergic receptor number (downregulation) or responsiveness.

Clinically, and at the cellular level, responses to many hormones and neurotransmitters wane rapidly despite continuous exposure to adrenergic agonists.[50] This phenomenon, called desensitization, has been particularly well studied for the stimulation of cAMP levels by plasma membrane β-adrenergic receptors.[32] Mechanisms postulated for desensitization include uncoupling (e.g., phosphorylation), internalization, and downregulation. The molecular mechanisms underlying rapid β-adrenergic receptor desensitization do not appear to require internalization of the receptors, but rather an alteration in the functioning of β-receptors themselves that uncouples the receptors from the stimulatory G_s protein.

Agonist-induced desensitization involves phosphorylation of G protein–coupled receptors by two classes of serine-threonine kinases. One of these initiates receptor-specific or homologous desensitization. The other works through second messenger–dependent kinases, mediating a general cellular hyporesponsiveness, called heterologous desensitization. Ultimately, an inhibitory arrestin protein binds to the phosphorylated receptor, causing desensitization by blocking signal transduction. Because enzymatic phosphorylation occurs only in the activated state, transient β-blockade has been used in states of receptor desensitization such as CHF or cardiopulmonary bypass to achieve a "receptor holiday."[51] Regeneration of a functional β-adrenergic receptor is contingent on internalization of the receptor, with dephosphorylation and consequent recycling. Receptor populations can thus change rapidly through internalization and subsequent recycling.

In contrast, downregulation occurs after prolonged exposure to an agonist (as in chronic stress or CHF). New receptors must be synthesized before a return to a baseline state is possible.

CHOLINERGIC PHARMACOLOGY

Acetylcholine Synthesis

Acetylcholine is synthesized intraneuronally from acetyl coenzyme A and choline through the action of the enzyme choline acetyl transferase in the synaptosomal mitochondria.[52] Sources of choline include dietary phospholipids, hepatic synthesis of phosphatidylcholine from dietary precursors such as ethanolamines, and choline released by hydrolysis of acetylcholine. Choline is transported as the phospholipid and is taken up by a high-affinity transport system. This system appears to be largely responsible for determining acetylcholine levels, although there is some evidence that precursor availability may limit cholinergic activity. The level of circulating choline can affect the release of acetylcholine when rapid firing takes place.

Storage and Release

On the nerve or presynaptic side, the nerve ending contains many vesicles that contain acetylcholine. When a nerve impulse arrives at the presynaptic nerve terminal, it causes an influx of calcium ions across the membrane. This induces 100 to 300 synaptic vesicles to fuse with the presynaptic membrane at specific release sites at the active zone, resulting in the liberation of acetylcholine from vesicles into the synaptic cleft.

Inactivation

Acetylcholine is an ester that hydrolyzes spontaneously in alkaline solutions into acetate and choline, neither of which has significant pharmacologic activity. In vivo, the rate of hydrolysis is increased enormously by enzymatic catalysis. The two most important hydrolytic enzymes are acetylcholinesterase and butyrylcholinesterase.

Acetylcholinesterase, sometimes called tissue esterase or true esterase, is a membrane-bound enzyme that is present in all cholinergic synapses, where it functions to destroy the neurotransmitter released from the nerve endings. Acetylcholinesterase is one of the most efficient of enzymes, terminating transmission within milliseconds after acetylcholine release. The substrate turnover is 2500 molecules per second, and one catalytic event lasts 40 μsec. The enzyme also is present in tissues that are not innervated, such as erythrocytes. Its function in these tissues is unknown.

Inhibition of acetylcholinesterase prevents the destruction of acetylcholine in cholinergic synapses and can activate all cholinergic systems simultaneously. In addition to their therapeutic use, cholinesterase inhibitors are the active ingredients in insecticides and many nerve gases.

Butyrylcholinesterase, sometimes called plasma esterase or pseudocholinesterase, is a soluble enzyme that is made primarily in the liver and circulates in the blood. Its function in normal situations is not known. Individuals who are genetically incapable of making the enzyme are normal in all other respects. It is important for the destruction of some cholinergic drugs, such as succinylcholine, which are not metabolized by acetylcholinesterase.

Cholinergic Receptors

Traditionally, cholinergic receptors have been organized into two major subdivisions, muscarinic and nicotinic. Muscarinic receptors are present mostly in peripheral visceral organs; nicotinic receptors are found on parasympathetic and sympathetic ganglia and on the neuromuscular junctions of skeletal muscle.

Although these two structurally and functionally distinct classes of receptors have significantly different responses to acetylcholine, the chemical itself exhibits no specificity. However, specific antagonists can exploit the difference between the muscarinic and nicotinic receptors. All cholinergic agonists appear to need a quaternary ammonium group as well as an atom capable of forming a hydrogen bond through an unshared pair of electrons. The distance between the two sites may determine whether the agonism is muscarinic or nicotinic. With muscarinic agonists, the distance appears to be about 4.4 Å, whereas for nicotinic agonists, the distance is 5.9 Å.

The nicotinic receptors are pentameric membrane proteins, which form nonselective cation channels. There are two α-units (each 40 kd) and one each of the β-, ε-, and δ-units. The α-subunits represent the binding sites for acetylcholine or nicotinic antagonists. These five subunits surround each ion channel through which sodium or calcium may enter the cell or potassium may exit. For the channel to open, acetylcholine must occupy a receptor site on each of the two α-subunits. If only one site is occupied and the other is empty, the channel remains closed and there is no flow of ions or change in electrical potential. If one site is occupied by acetylcholine and the other site is occupied by an antagonist such as D-tubocurarine, or if both sites are occupied by D-tubocurarine, the channel also remains closed. The ion channel response to acetylcholine is instantaneous and usually lasts only a few milliseconds because acetylcholine is rapidly destroyed by acetylcholinesterase in the synapse.

Compared with adrenergic receptors, cholinergic receptors turn over slowly. When a nerve to a muscle is transected, it takes 1 to 3 days to increase the number of cholinergic receptors. These new receptors are no longer confined to the motor end plate, and that change has important clinical ramifications. For example, overwhelming hyperkalemia can result from the stimulation of these abundant ectopic cholinergic receptors by succinylcholine.

In contrast to the ion-gated nicotinic receptors, muscarinic receptors belong to the superfamily of G protein–coupled receptors. Muscarinic receptors, therefore, have a greater homology to α- and β-adrenergic receptors than to nicotinic receptors. Like the other members of the family of receptors with seven helices, muscarinic receptors use G proteins for signal transduction. Five muscarinic receptors (i.e., M_1 through M_5) exist with the primary structural variability residing in a cytoplasmic loop between the fifth and sixth membrane-spanning domains.

The muscarinic receptors have diverse signal transduction mechanisms. The odd-numbered receptors (i.e., M_1, M_3, and M_5) work predominantly through the hydrolysis of polyphosphoinositide, whereas the even-numbered receptors work primarily to regulate adenylate cyclase.[53]

Muscarinic receptors are found on central and peripheral neurons; a single neuron may have muscarinic receptors with excitatory as well as inhibitory effects. Presynaptic muscarinic receptors may inhibit the release of acetylcholine from postganglionic parasympathetic neurons; presynaptic nicotinic receptors may increase its release.

Because of the complex coupling, the response of the muscarinic system is sluggish. No response is seen for seconds to minutes after the application of acetylcholine. The effect, however, long outlives the presence of the agonist. Even though the transmitter is destroyed rapidly, the train of events it initiates causes the cellular response to continue for many minutes. Muscarinic receptors are desensitized through agonist-dependent phosphorylation in a mechanism similar to that described earlier for β-adrenergic receptors.

NONADRENERGIC, NONCHOLINERGIC NEUROTRANSMISSION IN THE AUTONOMIC NERVOUS SYSTEM

Classically, norepinephrine has been considered the moderator of vascular tone. Beginning in the early 1960s, however, various other compounds, including monoamines, purines, amino acids, and polypeptides, were identified that fulfilled the criteria of functional neurotransmitters.[54,55] Other transmitter candidates demonstrated in perivascular nerves using histochemical and immunohistochemical techniques include ATP, adenosine, VIP, substance P, 5-hydroxytryptamine, neuropeptide Y (NPY), and calcitonin gene–related peptide (CGRP). Immunocytochemical studies show that more than one transmitter or putative transmitter may be colocalized in the same nerve. The most common combinations of transmitters in perivascular nerves are norepinephrine, ATP, and NPY in sympathetic nerves (Figure 13.5); acetylcholine and VIP in parasympathetic nerves; and substance P, CGRP, and ATP in sensory-motor nerves. Many of these putative transmitters act through cotransmission, which is the synthesis, storage, and release of more than one transmitter by a nerve.[56] Autonomic nerves exhibit chemical coding—individual neurons serving a specific physiologic function contain distinct combinations of transmitter substances.[57]

The concepts of cotransmission and neuromodulation have become accepted mechanisms in autonomic nervous control. To establish that transmitters coexisting in the same nerves act as cotransmitters, it is necessary to demonstrate that, on release, each substance acts postjunctionally on its own specific receptor to produce a response.

For many perivascular sympathetic nerves, there is evidence that norepinephrine and ATP act as cotransmitters and are released from the same nerves but act on α_1-adrenoceptors and P_2-purinoceptors, respectively, to produce vasoconstriction[58,59] (Figure 13.5). ATP, once thought to act only as an electrical buffer for the charged norepinephrine, is believed to mediate contraction through P_2-receptors by voltage-dependent calcium channels.[60] The fast component of contraction appears to be mediated by these purinoceptors, whereas norepinephrine sustains contraction of muscle by acting on the α_1-adrenoreceptor through receptor-operated calcium channels. ATP is stored in vesicles along nerve varicosities. It is released into the synaptic cleft via exocytosis and then binds to postsynaptic purinergic receptors. ATP is then broken down to adenosine by membrane-bound ATPases and 5'-nucleotidases. Adenosine is then taken up into the presynaptic neuron, where ATP is resynthesized and incorporated into vesicles for subsequent release.[61]

NPY is also colocalized with norepinephrine and ATP. However, in some vessels, NPY has little or no direct action.

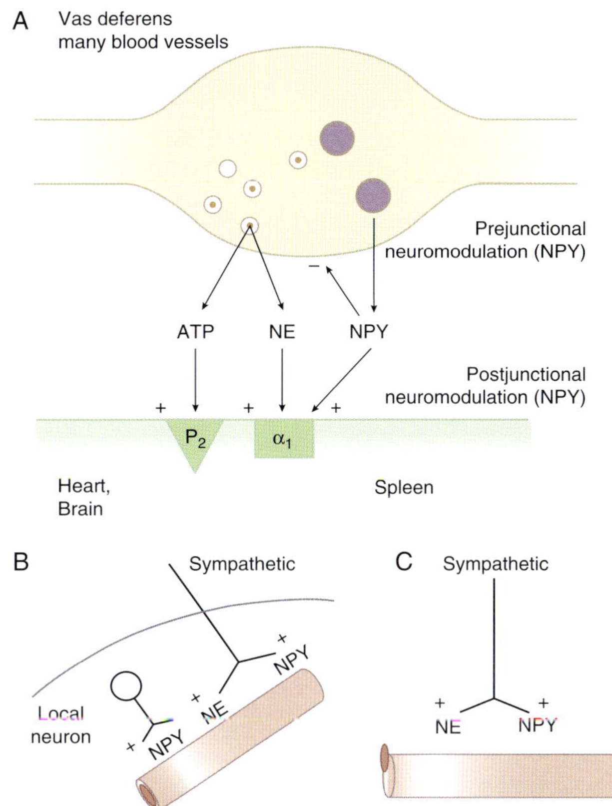

Figure 13.5 Schematic representation of different interactions that occur between neuropeptide Y (NPY) and adenosine triphosphate (ATP), and norepinephrine (NE) released from single sympathetic nerve varicosities. A, Diagram shows what occurs in the vas deferens and many blood vessels, where NE and ATP, probably released from small granular vesicles, act synergistically to contract (+) the smooth muscle through α_1-adrenoceptors and P_2-purinoceptors, respectively. B and C, Sympathetic neurotransmission in the heart and brain (B) and spleen (C). Reprinted with permission from Lincoln J, Burnstock G. Neural-endothelial interactions in control of local blood flow. In: Warren J, ed. *The Endothelium: An Introduction to Current Research*. New York: Wiley-Liss; 1990:21.

Instead, NPY acts as a neuromodulator prejunctionally to inhibit the release of norepinephrine from the nerve or postjunctionally to enhance the action of norepinephrine (Figure 13.5A).[62,63] In other vessels, notably those of the spleen, skeletal muscle, and cerebral and coronary vasculature, NPY has direct vasoconstrictor actions. In the heart and brain, local intrinsic (nonsympathetic) neurons use NPY as the principal transmitter (see Figure 13.5B). In the spleen, NPY appears to act as a genuine cotransmitter with norepinephrine in perivascular sympathetic nerves (see Figure 13.5C).[64] The frequency of stimulation determines which vesicles are mobilized to release their transmitters.

A classic transmitter such as acetylcholine coexists with VIP in the parasympathetic nerves of many organs, but in this instance, the two transmitters are stored in separate vesicles. They can be released differentially at different stimulation frequencies, depending on where they are located.[65,66] For example, in the salivary gland, they can act independently on acinar cells and glandular blood vessels.[67] Cooperation is achieved by the selective release of acetylcholine at low frequencies and of VIP at high frequencies of stimulation. Elements of prejunctional and postjunctional modulation have also been described. It is becoming increasingly apparent that in many biologic states, including pregnancy,[68] hypertension, and aging, the relationships among cotransmitters may be an important determinant of a compensatory response, allowing finer control of important physiologic function. Additionally, the large number of different receptors may provide targets for potential pharmacologic interventions.

GENETIC CONTRIBUTORS TO AUTONOMIC FUNCTION

In the past 5 years an explosion in the knowledge of non-Mendelian genetic contributors to human physiologic and pathophysiologic function has occurred. Genetic variations as small as a single nucleotide polymorphism and to a lesser extent larger deletion and insertion sequences have been identified in the genes that code for nearly every adrenergic and dopaminergic receptor subtype. The genetic coding for the muscarinic receptor subtypes, on the other hand, is remarkably well conserved.[69] In addition to variants in the coding for the autonomic receptors, genetic mutations in the codes for the proteins responsible for catecholamine synthesis, reuptake, and breakdown have also been identified as have variants for the receptor coupled G proteins.[70] Though many potential genetic contributors to autonomic-related disease states (e.g., essential hypertension, lipid and glucose metabolism, and postural tachycardia syndrome[71]) have been identified, no single genetic mutation has completely explained any of the examined autonomic dysfunctions. Therefore, abnormalities in autonomic function are likely polygenic in origin with significant environmental inputs. Once the collection of genetic variants responsible for the majority of the autonomic findings of a given disease are identified, the impact of the combined genetic contribution on responsiveness to a given drug or class of drugs will need to be assessed through directed clinical trials.

REFERENCES

1. Furness JB, Costa M. *The Enteric Nervous System*. New York: Churchill Livingstone; 1987.
2. Bridenbaugh PO, Greene NM. Spinal (subarachnoid) neural blockade. In: Cousins M, Bridenbaugh P, eds. *Neural Blockade in Clinical Anesthesia and Pain Management*. 2nd ed. Philadelphia: JB Lippincott; 1988:213.
3. Bylund DB. Introduction to the autonomic nervous system. In: Minneman KP, Wecker L, Larner J, et al, eds. *Brody's Human Pharmacology: Molecular to Clinical*. Philadelphia: Elsevier-Mosby; 2005: 99.
4. Lefkowitz R, Hoffman B, Taylor P. Drugs acting at synaptic and neuroeffector junctional sites. In Gilman A, Rall T, Nies A, et al, eds. *Goodman and Gilman's The Pharmacological Basis of Therapeutics*. 8th ed. New York: Pergamon Press; 1990:84.
5. Hoffman B, Lefkowitz R. Adrenergic receptors in the heart. *Annu Rev Physiol.* 1982;44:475.
6. Goldstein DS, Ziegler MG, Lake CR. Plasma norepinephrine in essential hypertension. In: Ziegler M, Lake C, eds. *Frontiers of Clinical Neuroscience*, vol. 2. Baltimore: Williams & Wilkins; 1984:389.
7. Dimsdale J, Moss J. Plasma catecholamines in stress and exercise. *JAMA.* 1980;243:340.
8. Philipson LH. beta-agonists and metabolism. *J Allergy Clin Immunol.* 2001;110:S313.
9. Nussdorfer GG. Pancrine control of adrenal cortical function by medullary chromaffin cells. *Pharmacol Rev.* 1996;48:495.
10. DeBello WM, O'Connor V, Dresbach T, et al. SNAP-mediated protein-protein interactions essential for neurotransmitter release. *Nature.* 1995;373:626.
11. Jahn R, Sudhof TC. Membrane fusion and exocytosis. *Annu Rev Biochem.* 1999;68:863.
12. Sudhof TC. The synaptic vesicle cycle revisited. *Neuron.* 2000;28:317.
13. Sudhof TC. The synaptic vesicle cycle. *Annu Rev Neurosci.* 2004;27:509.
14. Schiavo G, Rossetto O, Montecucco C. Clostridial neurotoxins as tools to investigate the molecular events of neurotransmitter release. *Semin Cell Biol.* 1994;5:221.
15. Morgan A, Burgoyne RD. A role for soluble NSF attachment proteins (SNAPs) in regulated exocytosis in adrenal chromaffin cells. *EMBO J.* 1995;14:232.
16. Bennett MK, Scheller RH. A molecular description of synaptic vesicle membrane trafficking. *Annu Rev Biochem.* 1994;63:63.
17. Rothman JE. Mechanisms of intracellular protein transport. *Nature.* 1994;372:55.
18. Katz B, Miledi R. The effect of temperature on the synaptic delay at the neuromuscular junction. *J Physiol.* 1965;181:656.
19. Moro MA, Lopez MG, Gandia L, et al. Separation and culture of living adrenaline and noradrenaline-containing cells from bovine adrenal medulla. *Anal Biochem.* 1990;185:243.
20. Livett BG, Marley PD. Effects of opioid peptides and morphine on histamine-induced catecholamine secretion from cultured, bovine adrenal chromaffin cells. *Br J Pharmacol.* 1986;89:327.
21. Marley PD, Livett BG. Differences between the mechanism of adrenaline and noradrenaline secretion from isolated, bovine, adrenal chromaffin cells. *Neurosci Lett.* 1987;77:81.
22. Owen PJ, Plevin R, Boarder MR. Characterization of bradykinin-stimulated release of noradrenaline from cultured bovine adrenal chromaffin cells. *J Pharmacol Exp Ther.* 1989;248:1231.

23. Lake CR, Chernow B, Feuerstein G, et al. The sympathetic nervous system in man, its evaluation and the measurement of plasma norepinephrine. In: Ziegler M, Lake C, eds. *Frontiers of Clinical Neuroscience*, vol. 2. Baltimore: Williams & Wilkins; 1984:1.
24. Kopin IJ. False neurochemical transmitters and the mechanism of sympathetic blockade by monoamine oxidase inhibitors. *J Pharmacol Exp Ther.* 1965;147:186.
25. Ahlquist RP. A study of the adrenotropic receptors. *Am J Physiol.* 1998;153:586–600.
26. Docherty JR. Subtypes of functional α1-adrenoceptor. *Cell Mol Life Sci.* 2010;67:405–417.
27. Gyires K, Zádosi ZS, Török T, et al. α2-adrenoceptor subtypes-mediated physiological, pharmacological actions. *Neurochem Int.* 2009;55:447–453.
28. Szabo B, Hedler L, Starke K. Peripheral presynaptic and central effects of clonidine, yohimbine and rauwolscine on the sympathetic nervous system in rabbits. *Naunyn Schmiedebergs Arch Pharmacol.* 1989;340:648.
29. Lawhead R, Blaxall H, Bylund D. α2A is the predominant α2-adrenergic receptor subtype in human spinal cord. *Anesthesiology.* 1992;77:983.
30. Ongioco RR, Richardson CD, Rudner XL, et al. Alpha2-adrenergic receptors in human dorsal root ganglia: predominance of alpha2b and alpha2c subtype mRNAs. *Anesthesiology.* 2000;92:968.
31. Michelotti GA, Price DT, Schwinn DA. α1-adrenergic receptor regulation: basic science and clinical implications. *Pharmacol Ther.* 2000;88:281.
32. Hausdorff WP, Caron MG, Lefkowitz RJ. Turning off the signal: desensitization of β-adrenergic receptor function. *FASEB J.* 1990; 4:2881.
33. Boehm S, Kubista H. Fine tuning of sympathetic transmitter release via ionotropic and metabotropic presynaptic receptors. *Pharmacol Rev.* 2002;54:43.
34. Szabo B, Schramm A, Starke K. Effect of yohimbine on renal sympathetic nerve activity and renal norepinephrine spillover in anesthetized rabbits. *J Pharmacol Exp Ther.* 1992;260:780.
35. Opie L. Receptors and signal transduction. In: Opie LH, ed. *The Heart: Physiology and Metabolism*. New York: Raven Press; 1991;152.
36. Raymond J, Hnatowich M, Lefkowitz R, et al. Adrenergic receptors: models for regulation of signal transduction processes. *Hypertension.* 1990;15:119.
37. Vanhees L, Aubert A, Fagard R, et al. Influence of β1- versus β2-adrenoceptor blockade on left ventricular function in humans. *J Cardiovasc Pharmacol.* 1986;8:1086.
38. Opie L. Ventricular overload and heart failure. In: Opie LH, ed. *The Heart: Physiology and Metabolism*. 2nd ed. New York, Raven Press, 1991:386.
39. Brodde O. The functional importance of β1 and β2 adrenoceptors in the human heart. *Am J Cardiol.* 1988;62:24C.
40. Walston J, Silver K, Bogardus C, et al. Time of onset of non–insulin dependent diabetes mellitus and genetic variation in the β3-adrenergic-receptor gene. *N Engl J Med.* 1995;333:343.
41. Widen E, Lehto M, Kanninen T, et al. Association of a polymorphism in the β3-adrenergic receptor gene with features of the insulin resistance syndrome in Finns. *N Engl J Med.* 1995;333:348.
42. Clement K, Vaisse C, Manning BSF, et al. Genetic variation in the β3-adrenergic receptor and an increased capacity to gain weight in patients with morbid obesity. *N Engl J Med.* 1995;333:352.
43. Hall IP, Wheatley A, Wilding P, et al. Association of Glu27 β2-adrenoceptor polymorphism with lower airway reactivity in asthmatic subjects. *Lancet.* 1995;345:1213.
44. Turki J, Pak J, Green SA, et al. Genetic polymorphisms of the β2-adrenergic receptor in nocturnal and non-nocturnal asthma: evidence that Gly 16 correlates with the nocturnal phenotype. *J Clin Invest.* 1995;95:1635.
45. Goldberg LI, Rajfer SI. Dopamine receptors: applications in clinical cardiology. *Circulation.* 1985;72:245.
46. Bertorello A, Aperia A. Both DA1 and DA2 receptor agonists are necessary to inhibit Na+/K+ ATPase activity in proximal tubules from the rat kidney. *Acta Physiol Scand.* 1988;132:441.
47. Bertorello A, Aperia A. Regulation of Na+/K+ ATPase activity in kidney proximal tubules: involvement of GTP binding proteins. *Am J Physiol.* 1989;256:F57.
48. Gesek FA, Schoolwerth AC. Hormonal interactions with the proximal Na+/H+ exchanger. *Am J Physiol.* 1990;258:F514.
49. Blochl-Daum B, Schuller-Petrovic S, Wolzt M, et al. Primary defect in α-adrenergic responsiveness in patients with varicose veins. *Clin Pharmacol Ther.* 1991;49:49.
50. Insel PA. Adrenergic receptors: evolving concepts and clinical implications. *N Engl J Med.* 1996;334:580.
51. Bristow MR, Ginsburg R, Minobe W, et al. Decreased catecholamine sensitivity and β-adrenergic receptor density in failing human hearts. *N Engl J Med.* 1982;307:205.
52. Ehlert FJ. Drugs affecting the parasympathetic nervous system and autonomic ganglia. In: Minneman KP, Wecker L, Larner J, et al, eds. *Brody's Human Pharmacology: Molecular to Clinical*. Philadelphia: Elsevier-Mosby; 2005:104.
53. Hosey MM. Diversity of structure, signaling and regulation within the family of muscarinic cholinergic receptors. *FASEB J.* 1992;12:845.
54. Burnstock G. The first von Euler lecture in physiology: the changing face of autonomic neurotransmission. *Acta Physiol Scand.* 1986;126:67.
55. Burnstock G. Autonomic neuromuscular junctions: Current developments and future directions. *J Anat.* 1986;146:1.
56. Burnstock G. Do some nerve cells release more than one transmitter? *Neuroscience.* 1976;1:239.
57. Bartfai T, Iverfeldt K, Fisone G, et al. Regulation of the release of coexisting neurotransmitters. *Annu Rev Pharmacol Toxicol.* 1988; 28:285.
58. Von Kügelgen I, Starke K. Noradrenaline-ATP co-transmission in the sympathetic nervous system. *Trends Pharmacol Sci.* 1991;12:319.
59. Burnstock G. Local mechanisms of blood flow control by perivascular nerves and endothelium. *J Hypertens Suppl.* 1990;8:S95.
60. Ralevic V, Burnstock G. Receptors for purines and pyrimidines. *Pharmacol Rev.* 1998;50:413.
61. Jacobson KA, Trivedi BK, Churchill PC, et al. Novel therapeutics acting via purine receptors. *Biochem Pharmacol.* 1991;41:1399.
62. Walker P, Grouzmann E, Burnie M, et al. The role of neuropeptide Y in cardiovascular regulation. *Trends Pharmacol Sci.* 1991;12:111.
63. Lincoln J, Burnstock G. Neural-endothelial interactions in control of local blood flow. In: Warren J, ed. *The Endothelium: An Introduction to Current Research*. New York: Wiley-Liss; 1990:21.
64. Lundberg JM, Rudehill A, Sollevi A, et al. Frequency- and reserpine-dependent chemical coding of sympathetic transmission: differential release of noradrenaline and neuropeptide Y from pig spleen. *Neurosci Lett.* 1986;63:96.
65. Bloom S, Edwards A. Vasoactive intestinal polypeptide in relation to atropine resistant vasodilatation in the submaxillary gland of the cat. *J Physiol.* 1980;300:41.
66. Lundberg JM. Evidence for coexistence of vasoactive intestinal polypeptide (VIP) and acetylcholine in neurons of cat exocrine glands: morphological, biochemical and functional studies. *Acta Physiol Scand Suppl.* 1981;112:1.
67. Burnstock G. Local mechanisms of blood flow control by perivascular nerves and endothelium. *J Hypertens Suppl.* 1990;8:S95.
68. Mione M, Cavanagh J, Lincoln J, et al. Pregnancy reduces noradrenaline but not neuropeptide levels in the uterine artery of the guinea-pig. *Cell Tissue Res.* 1990;259:503.
69. Kirstein Sl, Insel PA. autonomic nervous system pharmacogenomics: a progress report. *Pharmacol Rev.* 2004;56(1):31–52.
70. H Zhu, J Poole, Y Lu, GA Harshfield, et al. Sympathetic nervous system, genes and human essential hypertension. *Curr Neurovasc Res.* 2005;2:303–317.
71. G Jacob, EM Garland, F Costa, et al. β2-Adrenoceptor genotype and function affect hemodynamic profile heterogeneity in postural tachycardia syndrome. *Hypertension.* 2006;47:421–427.

14

ANESTHETIC PHARMACOLOGY OF THE AUTONOMIC NERVOUS SYSTEM

Timothy Angelottiv

INTRODUCTION

Vital organs communicate with the central nervous system (CNS) via highly specialized peripheral nerves within the autonomic nervous system (ANS). More than one hundred years ago, Langley distinguished two separate parts to the ANS, a sympathetic nervous system (SNS) and a parasympathetic nervous system (PaNS), located at the thoracolumbar and craniosacral regions respectively.[1] In fact, the identification and development of specific toxins and drugs to modulate these two arms of the ANS led in many ways to the modern research specialties of physiology and pharmacology. Using such toxins, drugs, and electrical stimulation, early researchers were able to identify spinal segments responsible for regulating various organs and determine that the two parts of the ANS often regulate the same organ; however, stimulation of organ function was often opposed. Around the same time as Langley, the preeminent physiologist Walter B. Cannon described the concept of physiological homeostasis and suggested that the ANS was the peripheral system responsible for its regulation.[2]

The ANS operates as an integrative structure, connecting afferent and efferent signaling of multiple vital organs with the CNS. Though the ANS is primarily an efferent system, transmitting electrical impulses from the CNS to various organs, such as the heart, lung, vasculature, and gastrointestinal tract, it is also highly important for afferent trafficking of information concerning the state of our vital organs back to the CNS. Research has advanced our understanding of the efferent arm of the ANS and we are beginning to understand the importance of ANS afferent signaling.[3]

Modulation of the ANS can arise from various mechanisms, including drugs and acute or chronic pathophysiological conditions. Primary neurodegenerative disorders that involve the ANS include pure autonomic failure, multiple system atrophy (Shy-Drager syndrome), and Parkinson's disease. Such dysfunction, termed dysautonomia, can be manifested as orthostatic hypotension, bradycardia, and other abnormal functions of various organ systems.[4–5] Secondary dysfunction of the ANS can also occur, as seen in autonomic dysreflexia following spinal cord injury, diabetic dysautonomia, and certain cancers.[6–8] Equally important to our specialty is the finding that compensatory alterations in SNS function (i.e., increased neurotransmitter release) can be seen in various disease states, such as congestive heart failure. In this case, this abnormal elevation of SNS function eventually leads to worsening of the disease, if left untreated.[9] Acute disease states can also lead to dysfunction of the ANS. The decrease in heart rate variability seen in critically ill patients may relate to dysregulation of normal autonomic heart reflexes, and may be a predictor of 28-day mortality.[10–12]

Given the various mechanisms listed above where dysregulation of the ANS can appear as or arise in response to a disease state, a thorough understanding of the ANS and how it can be modulated is of utmost importance to many different specialists. In the perioperative setting, management of sympathetic dysfunction can be the major challenge facing an anesthesiologist. Alterations in blood pressure and heart rate are common occurrences, and when they occur in the setting of a patient with cardiovascular comorbidities, effective management can be difficult. Though general and local anesthetics can modulate these functions, direct and indirect acting pharmacological agents active on end organ systems often are better choices for management (e.g., beta blockers).

The aim of this chapter is to utilize the ANS as a model system for anesthesiology-based research. However, unlike several excellent textbooks of anesthetic pharmacology, it will not merely list various ANS drugs and describe their pharmacokinetic and pharmacodynamic parameters. Instead of a drug-based approach to understand ANS pharmacology, this chapter will be organized by receptors and systems biology with specific emphasis on G-protein coupled receptors (GPCR), which are often the target for various ANS neurotransmitters and drugs. Basic science and clinical research from anesthesiology and critical care regarding GPCRs and the ANS will be used to illustrate not only pharmacological principles, but also the important contributions of anesthesiology based physician-scientists in this field. Lastly, the role of pharmacogenomics in physiology and pathophysiology of the

ANS will be described, as well as future directions for ANS research.

NEUROPHARMACOLOGY OF THE ANS

The previous chapter presented a complete neuroanatomical description of the various neurons in the SNS and PaNS, as well as the basic neurotransmitters utilized by these two systems (Please see Chapter 13, "The Autonomic Nervous System"). Briefly, the SNS and PaNS are somewhat similar in structure, they both utilize preganglionic neurons that synapse on postganglionic neurons, and the postganglionic neurons ultimately reach their target effector organs, where they modulate physiological functions. The two systems differ in the anatomical site of the ganglion, with the SNS localized to thoracolumbar prevertebral ganglia, whereas the PaNS tends to be localized to distal ganglion localized near or in the target organ.

In both the SNS and PaNS, acetylcholine (ACh) acts as the neurotransmitter within ganglia. Acetylcholine released from the preganglionic neuron travels across the synapse to activate nicotinic receptors on the postganglionic neuron. In the postganglionic neuron of the PaNS, ACh also acts as the neurotransmitter, activating muscarinic receptors in the effector organ. In most postganglionic neurons of the SNS, norepinephrine (NE) is released, which in turn activates various adrenergic receptor subtypes located within the effector target organ. A specialized form of SNS postganglionic neuron can be found in the adrenal medulla[13] Here, the postganglionic neurons have specialized to become an endocrine organ and they do not travel to an effector target organ. Instead, epinephrine (Epi) released from these specialized "neurons" is transported via the blood stream to reach its targets. This relatively straightforward model for PaNS and SNS neurotransmission has been challenged as of late, and new concepts such as neuromodulation and co-transmission have been developed.[14] New co-neurotransmitters or neuromodulators that have been suggested include dopamine, adenosine triphosphate (ATP), angiotensin II, neuropeptide Y, enkephalin, somatostatin, and vasoactive intestinal peptide.[15]

The respective neurotransmitters NE/Epi and ACh are synthesized within the nerve terminals by the action of specific enzymes. Once synthesized, these neurotransmitters are packaged into secretory vesicles, where they remain until activation of the postganglionic neuron causes their release (please see Chapter 13 and Figures 14.1 and 14.2 for further details). Though the synthetic enzymes are highly regulated and are vital for the production of catecholaminergic and cholinergic neurotransmission, they have not proven to be efficacious targets for recent ANS drug development and they will not be discussed further.

Following an action potential–induced release, both types of neurotransmitters travel across the synapse to their effector site of action, where they undergo two possible processes. In the case of NE, the predominant mode of terminating neurotransmission occurs when released NE is transported back into the presynaptic neuron via the action of specific norepinephrine transporter proteins.[16–17] In addition, two enzymes found either in the effector cell or liver can metabolize both NE and Epi to products that can be excreted. In the case of ACh, the enzyme acetylcholinesterase is localized to the synaptic site, causing breakdown of ACh to choline and acetate, which are recycled and transported back into the neuron and utilized for resynthesis of ACh.

THE NEUROEFFECTOR MODEL

The relationship between sympathetic neurons and cardiac myocytes is a well described example of SNS-neuroeffector interaction (Figure 14.1).[18] NE released from the sympathetic postganglionic neuron activates various ß adrenergic receptors (AR) on the cardiac myocyte, leading to changes in cardiac performance, such as increases in heart rate or contractility. In addition, released NE can activate extra- and presynaptic α_2A&C ARs to decrease further release of NE from nerve terminals (i.e., autoreceptors). As feedback regulators of neurotransmitter release, α_2A&C ARs act as "brakes" on the SNS, thus playing key roles in the modulation of sympathetic neurotransmission. Similar autoreceptors serve as negative feedback loops to regulate SNS and PaNS activation at most neuroeffector sites. Though the neuroeffector model is similar to a synapse, it has not been considered a true synapse. This concept is beginning to change, as recent work has shown that sympathetic innervation of cardiac myocytes can lead to the development of specialized zones for membrane signaling, akin to synapses.[19] Similar neuroeffector sites can be found in the PaNS, where various muscarinic receptor subtypes function on effector organ sites to mediate the response to acetylcholine; other muscarinic receptor subtypes function as presynaptic autoreceptors.

The pharmacology of the neuroeffector site, including receptor subtypes, receptor dynamics, and even receptor pharmacogenomics, is complex and still evolving. However, it is this receptor model system that has allowed for the development of newer specific drugs, as well as a more complete understanding of ANS function. The remainder of this chapter will explore the basics of receptor nomenclature, signal transduction, and pharmacogenomics in order to understand clinically relevant concepts of ANS pharmacology. In addition, effects of various anesthetic agents on the complete ANS system will be detailed.

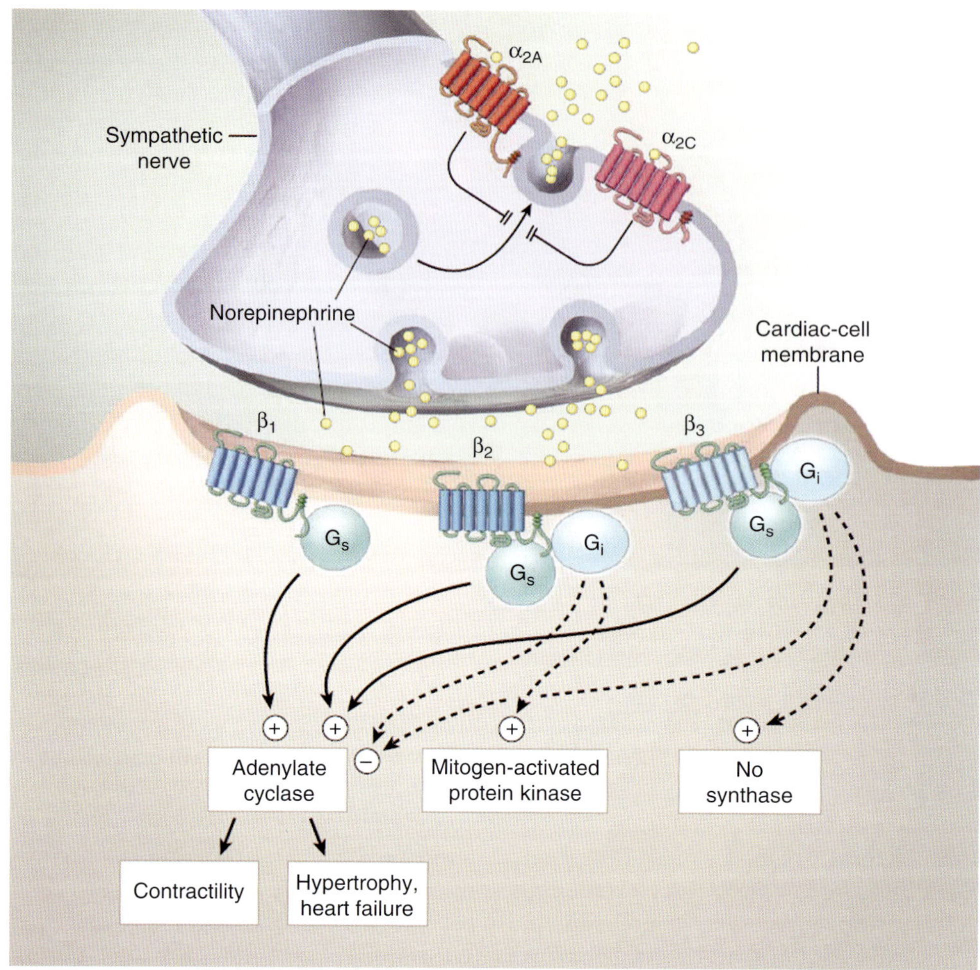

Figure 14.1 Schematic of ARs as a model sympathetic neuroeffector site. α2A&C ARs are shown localized to an axon terminal, where they function as autoreceptors to regulate norepinephrine release. β ARs are shown on the neuroeffector cell plasma membrane (e.g., cardiac myocyte). Reprinted with permission from Hajjar RJ and MacRae CA. Adrenergic-receptor polymorphisms and heart failure. *N Engl J Med.* 2002;347(15):1196–1199.

G-PROTEIN COUPLED RECEPTORS

Most receptors found at neuroeffector sites in the ANS belong to the superfamily of G-protein coupled receptors (GPCRs) or seven transmembrane receptors. In vertebrates, there are between 1000 and 2000 GPCRs, which account for about 1 to 2% of the genome.[20] All GPCRs are integral proteins that possess seven helical transmembrane domains with the amino terminus being extracellular and the carboxyl terminus being intracellular (Figure 14.2). Upon activation, these receptors activate heterotrimeric G-proteins that then can activate and/or inhibit various cytosolic signal transduction pathways and/or modulate membrane ion channels. The superfamily of GPCRs has been divided primarily into five subfamilies based on their sequence/structural characteristics (see reviews[20–22]). The class A GPCRs are the largest subfamily of receptors, whose members are activated by small ligands (i.e., catecholamines, acetylcholine, or serotonin) binding to a pocket formed by specific transmembrane domains. Our knowledge of GPCRs has exploded in the last three decades, and a complete review of the topic is beyond the scope of this chapter. However, there are several good Web sites that offer a more complete description of GPCRs.[23]

From the 1940s to the 1980s, current GPCR classification evolved from a systems-based approach dependent on physiological responses to various pharmacological agents, to a classification scheme based on pharmacological binding profiles with relatively selective ligands. During the last 25 years, the advent of molecular biology and cloning of genes allowed for a more definitive characterization of GPCR receptors based on structure and function (see review[24]).

In 1949, Ahlquist proposed that application of synthetic adrenaline elicited two behaviors due to effects at an activating receptor (α AR) and an inhibiting receptor (β AR). When it was discovered that the β-adrenergic

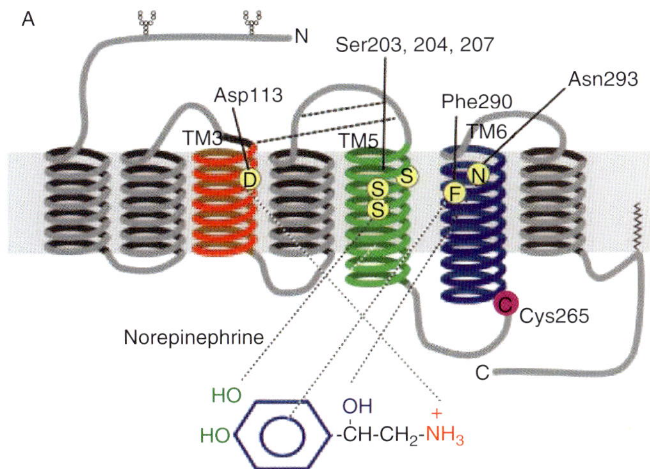

Figure 14.2 Schematic of the β_2 AR, a prototypical seven transmembrane G-protein coupled receptor. The seven alpha helices that traverse the cell membrane are shown as coils. Specific amino acid residues involved with norepinephrine binding are shown. Note the extracellular (top) and intracellular (bottom) portions of the receptor. Reprinted with permission from Swaminath G, Deupi X, Lee TW, et al. Probing the β_2 adrenoceptor binding site with catechol reveals differences in binding and activation by agonists and partial agonists. *J Biol Chem*. 2005;280:22165–22171. © 2005 The American Society for Biochemistry and Molecular Biology.

agonist, isoproterenol, had both activating (increased heart rate and contractility) and inhibitor effects (bronchial relaxation), this classification scheme was adapted and expanded to include β_1 and β_2 ARs respectively. Similarly, α ARs were later shown to have both activating and inhibitor effects, and the classification of ARs was expanded again. The next generation of classification schemes was based on the nature of the drug effect (activation vs. inhibition) and the site (presynaptic vs. postsynaptic). Over the next several decades, the development of more specific agonists and antagonists, as well as radioactive ligands, led to further refinement of the receptor concept, and not only for ARs. However, the application of molecular biology and genetic cloning paved the way to a more complete understanding of receptor function, biology, and structure.[24]

To date, nine different adrenergic receptors have been cloned from humans, though previous pharmacological data suggested that roughly only four different subtypes existed. With respect to the activating α AR, the family of $\alpha_{1A/D}$, α_{1B}, and α_{1C} ARs was described. In general, members of the α_1 AR family are found on various smooth muscle cells (such as arteries), where agonist activation leads to contraction.[24] Molecular cloning revealed a bigger surprise when the inhibiting α_2 ARs were discovered; there were three different isoforms, α_{2A}, α_{2B}, and α_{2C}.[25] In general, family members of a receptor subtype are delineated by their relative amino acid and nucleotide homology, but differing pharmacology, when compared to other subtypes. One could question the importance of any given subtype (e.g., is the receptor subtype a species variant?), however all α_2 AR subtypes have been conserved throughout evolution. Most interesting was the finding that the transmembrane domains are the most conserved within a family, but the extracellular and intracellular portions are the most divergent. Such a finding suggests that ligand binding most likely resides in the transmembrane regions, whereas the divergent extracellular and intracellular domains must lend some specificity to receptor function. Lastly, the β AR family was found to have three members, named β_1, β_2, and β_3.[24] Similar to α_2 AR family members, the β AR family is also conserved throughout evolution and can be delineated by tissue specificity, signal transduction mechanisms, cellular localization, and ligand specificity.

Prior to cloning GPCRs, Rodbell and associates noted that agonist activation of the glucagon receptor led to stimulation of adenylate cyclase, producing the second messenger cAMP.[26] It was subsequently determined that a protein, termed the G_s protein, was responsible for transducing receptor binding to second messenger generation, via turnover of GTP (Figure 14.3A). Further work by others demonstrated that multiple subtypes of G-proteins existed, including inhibitors of adenylate cyclase (e.g., $G_{i/o}$), activators of phospholipase Cβ (e.g., G_q), and also direct activators of G-protein coupled inwardly rectifying potassium (GIRK) channels (e.g., $G_{i/o}$).[27–29]

At the level of the cell, GPCR function is a highly complex intersection of multiple pathways and cascades. To more fully understand GPCR function, one must also take into account the localization of GPCRs within a system, such as the ANS. Once GPCR proteins are synthesized by the endoplasmic reticulum, they must travel within the cell to their final destination, the plasma membrane. This process is termed receptor trafficking. However, many cells of the ANS are specialized to subserve different functions, and GPCRs have evolved to assist in this process. Specifically in some neurons, some GPCRs may be found only at a presynaptic site, or possibly at an extrasynaptic site. Alternatively, they may be localized within specialized membrane regions linking ligand binding to physiological effects, such as cardiac muscle contraction. In general, structural determinants within GPCRs are responsible for fine-tuning membrane expression. Trafficking and localization of GPCRs are important attributes that further define their physiological roles. In fact, some diseases arise from mutations that alter GPCR folding, processing, and/or trafficking.[30–31]

RECEPTOR BIOLOGY

In both the SNS and PaNS, the preganglionic neurotransmitter acetylcholine activates nicotinic acetylcholine receptors (e.g., nAchRs) on the postganglionic neuron. Activation of these ligand-gated ion channels by acetylcholine leads to depolarization of the postganglionic neuron and bursts

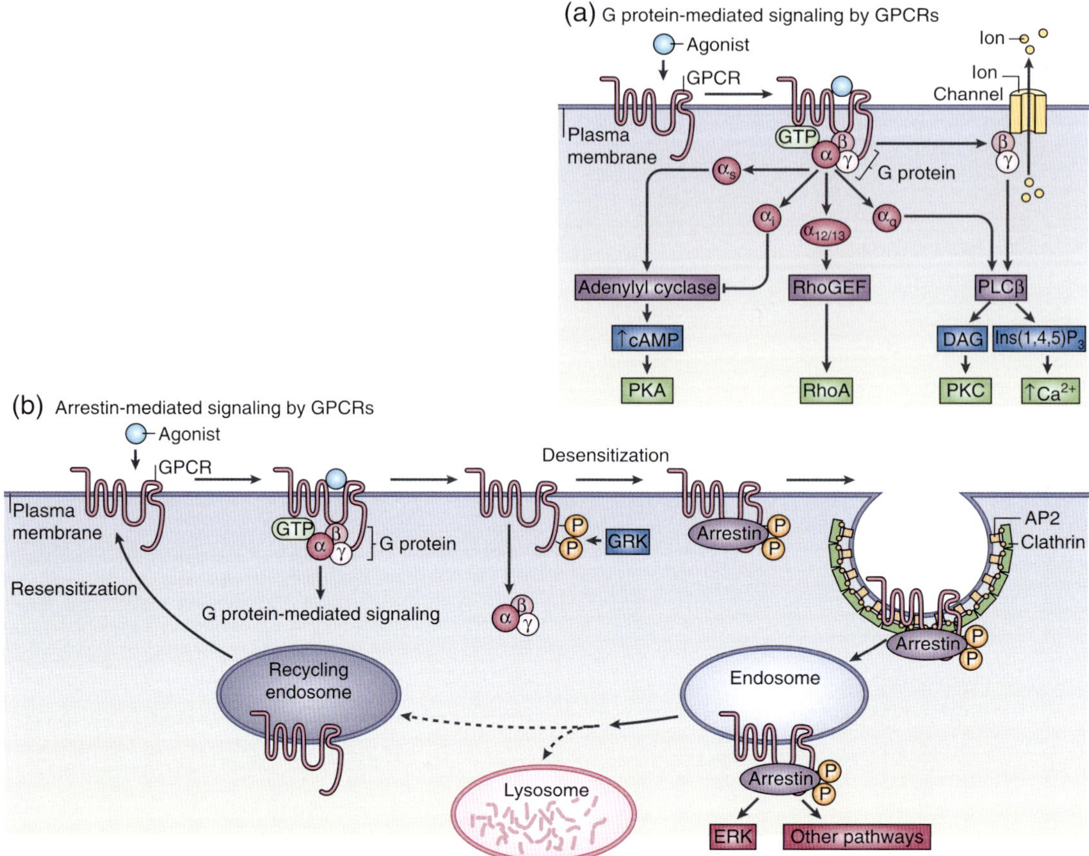

Figure 14.3 GPCR signaling mechanisms are shown. **Top:** Classic GPCR signaling occurs when receptor activation leads to binding of a G-protein, triggering a cascade of signal transduction that can include activation of adenylate cyclase or ion channels. Alternative second messenger systems are shown (e.g., PLCβ, RhoGEF). **Bottom:** Arrestin-mediated GPCR signaling occurs following phosphorylation of the receptor by GRK, leading to arrestin binding. This event is followed by either activation of another kinase cascade starting with ERK or degradation/recycling of the receptor. Reprinted by permission from Macmillan Publishers Ltd: Ritter SL, Hall RA. Fine-tuning of GPCR activity by receptor-interacting proteins. *Nat Rev Mol Cell Biol.* 2009;10:819–830.

of action potentials that ultimately lead to release of neurotransmitter from the postganglionic neuron to the neuroeffector site. nAchRs are made up of pentameric combinations of α and β subunits in either a homomeric or heteromeric format. To date, eight α and three β subunits have been cloned from humans, leading to a multitude of possible combinations, with α_3, α_4, α_5, α_7, β_2, and β_4 subunits predominating in the ANS.[32–33] It appears that homomeric α_7 and heteromeric $\alpha_3\beta_4$ combinations are the predominant combinations found on autonomic ganglia. Recently, it has been shown that hyperglycemia-induced reactive oxygen species may be responsible for diabetic dysautonomia, by altering α_3 nAchR gating.[34]

In humans, five different subtypes of muscarinic receptors (mAchRs) have been cloned, m1–m5. These GPCRs can be subclassified based on second messenger signaling. For example, m1, m3, and m5 subtypes preferentially couple to G_q, leading to activation of phospholipase C, culminating in protein kinase C activation and inositol phosphate (IP3) production. The mAchR subtypes m2 and m4 couple to $G_{i/o}$, leading to inhibition of adenylate cyclase, and activation of inwardly rectifying K+ channels. In addition, these two subtypes also are localized to presynaptic terminals, where they function as autoreceptors. There is some controversy regarding the possible roles of nitric oxide and cGMP as second messengers following mAchR activation.[35]

Within the ANS, certain mAchR subtypes predominate, specifically m2 and m3. In heart atria and ventricles, where activation leads to differential negative chronotropic and inotropic effects, m2 mAchRs are the predominant subtype found.[36] In the sinoatrial and atrioventricular nodes, m2 density is much higher, consistent with the dense parasympathetic innervation to these regions. In addition, m2 mAchRs are also found in smooth muscles, such as stomach, urinary bladder, and trachea. However, m3 mAchRs are the major subtype found throughout the remaining PaNS; they are abundant in smooth muscle of the entire gastrointestinal tract, urinary system, exocrine glands, trachea and bronchi, and the eye.[36–37]

To date, there are three subtypes of α_1 ARs: α_1a, α_1b, and α_1d. The nomenclature was confusing due to higher than expected DNA sequence variability between species.[38] Overall, all three α_1 AR subtypes have very similar pharmacological properties. First, all three subtypes couple to the G_q pathway, thus leading to phospholipase C activation and inositol phosphate turnover. Second, they all appear to mediate smooth muscle contraction, however they have different tissue expression profiles. Though subtype-specific agonists and antagonists exist, there are really no clinically useful subtype specific drugs.

Following the cloning of various adrenergic receptors, the α_2 AR family has been subdivided into four pharmacologically distinct subtypes: α_2A, α_2B, α_2C, and α_2D.[24] However, most mammalian species possess only three genes encoding α_2B, α_2C, and either α_2A or α_2D ARs, and thus the third gene has now been renamed α_2A/D (termed α_2A for this chapter). Both α_2A&C ARs couple to pertussis toxin-sensitive G_i/G_o signaling pathways to inhibit cAMP production as well as to regulate Ca^{2+} and K^+ channel signaling.[25] The α_2B AR subtype is found mostly in certain types of smooth muscle where activation by agonists leads to contraction, in a similar manner as α_1 AR subtypes. It appears to have little role in regulating sympathetic neurotransmission.[39] Molecular cloning of murine α_2A&C AR genes revealed structural features required for differential agonist and antagonist binding and led to the development of gene knockout (KO) models for in vivo and in vitro physiological research.[40–42]

Both α_2A&C ARs have important, but overlapping roles in regulating neurotransmitter release (for a more complete review please see reference[43]). Modulation of norepinephrine release by α_2A&C ARs is distinguishable by their responsiveness to neuronal action potential frequencies (Figure 14.4). ARs of the α_2A subtype inhibit release more quickly and at higher stimulation frequencies, whereas α_2C ARs appear to operate at lower frequencies,[44] suggesting that α_2A and α_2C ARs may serve as coarse vs. fine regulators of norepinephrine release, respectively. The dissimilarity observed may reflect differences in receptor trafficking and/or localization. Traditionally, α_2A&C ARs are thought of as presynaptic autoreceptors, however, recent work with cultured sympathetic ganglion neurons has suggested that only α_2C ARs truly colocalize to presynaptic sites, whereas α_2A ARs do not colocalize to these sites. Therefore, α_2A ARs may actually be classified as extrasynaptic receptors, where they regulate membrane hyperpolarization and thus NE release.[45] Given their differential effects on regulating NE release and localization in sympathetic neurons, subtype specific drugs may be beneficial for treating various forms of acute and chronic dysautonomia. However, no such specific α_2A&C AR agonists or antagonists are clinically available.

Functions within the SNS that are regulated by β ARs include heart rate, contractility, smooth muscle relaxation, and even metabolism. Originally, it was believed that all three β ARs coupled to the G_s protein to activate cAMP

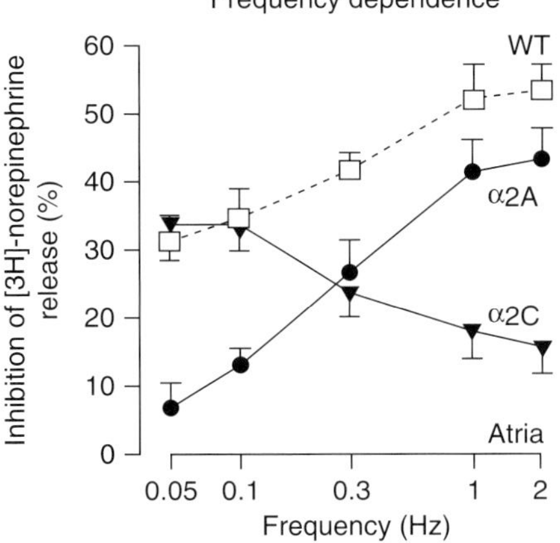

Figure 14.4 α_2A&C AR modulation of norepinephrine release from intact tissue. Field stimulation of isolated atrial slices from WT and either α_2A or α_2C AR KO mice revealed frequency dependence of norepinephrine release. α_2A ARs inhibit at higher stimulation frequencies that α_2C ARs. Reprinted with permission from Philipp M, Brede M, Hein L. Physiological significance of α_2-adrenergic receptor subtype diversity: one receptor is not enough. *Am J Physiol Regul Integr Comp Physiol.* 2002;283:R287–295.

production and thus PKA, however, recent work has shown that β_2 ARs can also couple to G_i, thus inhibiting cAMP production and accounting for some of the differences in agonist effects at β_1 and β_2 ARs.[46–47] In general, β_1 ARs are the predominant β AR in heart, where stimulation by epinephrine, norepinephrine, or synthetic sympathomimetics leads to enhanced inotropic, chronotropic, and lusitropic responses.

The role of β_2 ARs in the heart has been investigated, and a simple interpretation was that they existed in cardiac tissues as a redundant receptor to β_1 ARs. However, recent knowledge that they can couple to auxiliary G proteins besides G_s, suggested that they may have other roles as well. As mentioned above for α_2 ARs, differential localization of β ARs in cardiac tissue may account for some of their differences. Analysis of sympathetic neuron-cardiac myocyte co-cultures has revealed membrane compartment specializations for both β_1 and β_2 ARs.[19] Specifically, at sites of neuron-myocyte contact, submembrane accumulation of scaffolding proteins appears to retain β_1 ARs at these sites so that they can respond quickly to NE release. Of interest, once NE is released and β ARs are activated, β_2 ARs appear to move away from these sites, either by endocytosis or desensitization. A similar differential localization has been found on cultured ventricular myocytes, where it was determined that β_1 ARs are spread out across the entire cell surface membrane, whereas β_2 ARs are localized to deep transverse tubules, hence leading to compartmentalization of second messenger production and hence physiological effects.[48]

An interesting aspect of β AR signaling has been the recent discovery that stimulation of β_1 ARs by agonists can lead to enhanced myocyte death or apoptosis, whereas stimulation of β_2 ARs was cytoprotective or anti-apoptotic.[49] Thus, clinical use of subtype specific agonists or antagonists may impact cardiac remodeling following myocardial infarctions or in uncompensated congestive heart failure.

KNOCKOUT MICE AND ANS FUNCTION

The creation of genetic knockout (KO) mice has proven to be a powerful technology for analysis of receptor function within a physiological system, such as the ANS. However, the results of physiological studies on these mice must be interpreted cautiously, since KO mice can develop changes, such as genetic alterations of other receptor systems, to compensate for the loss of a specific gene.[50–51] Alternatively, the creation of the genetic KO can affect neighboring genes, and this alteration, rather than the gene KO itself, may actually account for the phenotype observed.[52] Despite these limitations, useful information has been obtained from KO mice concerning the role of different ion channels and GPCRs within the ANS.

The development of specific nAchR KO mice has demonstrated the importance of the α_3 subunit in autonomic control. It was observed that α_3 KO mice have altered cardiac activity and bladder function, among other defects, and die within two weeks of birth. Single β_2 or β_4 subunit KO mice have no real neurological or autonomic defects and can survive into adulthood; however, double β_2/β_4 KO mice have similar autonomic dysfunction as α_3 KO mice, along with poor intestinal peristalsis, and die within several days of birth. Lastly, α_7 KO mice show defects in afferent signaling, specifically impaired baroreflexes.[33] The differential effects of nAchR KO mice on organ function further demonstrate that autonomic function of various organs is a balance between the PaNS and SNS and that the KO phenotype is usually created by loss of the dominant autonomic system in that organ.

The creation of various mAchR KO mice has confirmed the physiological roles of these subtypes within the PaNS. Specifically, spontaneously beating mouse atria obtained from m2 KO mice do not demonstrate muscarinic agonist-induced bradycardia. In addition, m2 KO mice still demonstrated smooth muscle contraction in response to a muscarinic agonist, suggesting a more dominant role for m3 mAchRs in that tissue.[37] However, these studies were somewhat complicated by the fact that the m2 subtype also functions as a presynaptic autoreceptor. With respect to the m3 mAchR KO mice, it has been shown that loss of this subtype drastically reduces smooth muscle contraction from stomach, trachea, and particularly urinary bladder, demonstrating that the predominant mAchR subtype in the PaNS is m3.

The development of α_1 AR KO mouse models has helped reveal the relative contribution of each subtype to blood pressure control. In vas deferens, renal artery, lower urinary tract, and prostate, α_1a ARs are important regulators of contraction, but do not appear to be the major subtype responsible for blood pressure regulation in response to α_1 AR-mediated vasopressors, such as phenylephrine or norepinephrine. Instead, α_1d ARs appear to be the major contributor to vasopressor responses, since they are expressed in the larger arteries (e.g., carotid, mesenteric, and pulmonary) and aorta. KO of this AR subtype leads to an antihypertensive effect.[38,53] The physiological role for the α_1b AR is less clear, with little difference in blood pressure found in KO mice of this subtype.

Analysis of KO mice aided the delineation of the different roles that α_2A&C ARs play in central and peripheral SNS function mediated by endogenous catecholamines and other drugs.[39] For example, agonist stimulation of centrally located α_2A ARs led to decreased SNS activation and thus decreased blood pressure. However α_2C ARs are more prevalent in peripheral sympathetic adrenergic neurons and adrenal chromaffin cells.[54–56] Both α_2A&C ARs are physiologically important regulators of norepinephrine release from sympathetic neurons, since mice lacking both α_2A&C ARs exhibit sympathetic hyperactivity and develop heart failure at 4 months of age.[44] However, single α_2A or α_2C AR KO mice do not develop symptoms of heart failure, suggesting a functional overlap.[41–42]

Single, double, and even triple β AR KO mice have been created, but with respect to the ANS, most relevant information has been obtained from β_1 and β_2. AR KO mice. Genetic deletion of β_1 ARs led to complete loss of chronotropic and inotropic responses to epinephrine and other adrenergic drugs, thus demonstrating that β_2 ARs do not functionally overlap with β_1 ARs. In addition, in some strains of mice, β_1 AR KO led to prenatal death, demonstrating that functional genetic compensation must occur.[57] Targeted disruption of the β_2 AR did not lead to lethality and in fact did not alter chronotropic or inotropic responses to catecholamines. In fact, resting heart rates and blood pressure did not differ between these mice and wild type controls. These mice did demonstrate a loss of vasodilation in response to exercise or other stress, consistent with the role of β_2 ARs on vascular smooth muscle.[58] Double β_1 and β_2 KO mice also had similar resting heart rates and blood pressure as wild type mice, suggesting that the PaNS is more relevant than the SNS in setting basal physiological homeostatic set points in the heart.[59]

ANS PHARMACOGENOMICS

Molecular cloning of various ARs added a new level of sophistication to the investigation of ANS pharmacology. However, it was the discovery of naturally occurring variant forms of these different genes in humans that led in part to the development of the field of pharmacogenetics, now termed pharmacogenomics. In short, pharmacogenomics can be defined as the inherited basis for interindividual differences in drug effects. Such naturally occurring variant forms are termed human polymorphisms and they have been found in almost every α_1, α_2, and β AR subtype.[14,60] These polymorphisms can impact AR pharmacology in several manners including:

1. Amino acid–coding polymorphisms, which can change an encoded amino acid and alter ligand binding, signal transduction, or other cellular processes.
2. Noncoding polymorphisms, which alter transcription, translation, or mRNA stability, and thus receptor expression.
3. Both amino acid–coding and noncoding polymorphisms can occur in the same gene at the same time and such a complex polymorphism is termed a haplotype.

Usually, these changes occur by single nucleotide polymorphisms (SNPs), either in the coding or noncoding regions. Alternatively, small nucleotide deletions or insertions can also occur to alter the encoded protein. When such SNPs are prevalent within a population or ethnicity, then it is possible that the variant form may be responsible for a pathophysiological condition.

Though many studies have been published linking various SNPs with physiological and pathophysiological conditions, truly strong associations across various populations have not been commonly seen. For example, human polymorphisms of α_3, α_7, β_2, and β_4 nAchR subunits have been identified, however, none have been linked to any clinically relevant autonomic defect, despite causing some alterations in receptor desensitization and activation when studied in vitro.[14] In addition, few SNPs have been found for any of the mAchRs.[14] It would seem plausible that polymorphic forms of m2 and m3 mAchRs could play a role in heart rhythm abnormalities or gastrointestinal/bronchial diseases, however, no such linkages have been found to date. With respect to adrenergic receptors, only a few SNPs have actually been tightly linked to ANS dysfunction. α_2 AR SNPs have been identified and, more importantly, linked to various pathophysiological states.[14,61,62] Two α_2A&C AR variants occur within the third intracellular loop of the receptor, α_2ALys251 (single amino acid exchange) and α_2cDel322–325 (a three amino acid deletion). The α_2ALys251 polymorphism exhibits a low prevalence in Caucasians (0.4%), but occurs at a much higher level in African Americans (4.0%). The prevalence rate of α_2cDel322–325 is roughly 10-fold higher in each population (4.0% and 40% respectively).[63] To date, no disease linkage has been found for the α_2ALys251 polymorphism, however, recent genetic linkage studies have suggested that α_2cDel322–325 may be an important risk factor for cardiovascular disease, specifically congestive heart failure.[64–65] In addition to heart failure, this α_2c AR polymorphism may have genetic linkage with chronic pain and NE release, since human α_2cDel322–325 homozygotes have increased sympathoneural drive.[66]

Few SNPs for α_1 ARs and β ARs have been described that have been linked to any ANS dysfunction such as arrhythmias, congestive heart failure, or hypertension.[14] A β_1 AR SNP (Arg389Gly) has been described that has enhanced cell signaling, a gain of function variant, though it has not been linked to any disease unless coupled with the α_2cDel322–325 variant.[65]

GPCR SIGNAL TRANSDUCTION

The vast array of GPCR gene products and the importance of these receptors to physiological and pathophysiological functions illustrates the utility of developing drugs that target GPCRs. Given the variety of different GPCR families, recent research into their signal transduction mechanisms has revealed several common themes as well as some specializations.[67] Agonist-stimulated GPCR signal transduction can be fine-tuned by several mechanisms, including desensitization and downregulation. Desensitization is a process by which an activated GPCR response is quickly dampened. This dampening can occur by several mechanisms; however, it generally involves termination of signal transduction by phosphorylation of the receptor via a variety of kinase enzymes. For some GPCRs, phosphorylation of the receptor by protein kinase A (PKA), following its activation by cAMP, is involved. Alternatively, distinct G-protein coupled receptor kinases (GRKs) can phosphorylate the receptor to induce desensitization, or uncouple the signal transduction cascade. The GRK family consists of seven separate gene products, with specificity toward different classes of GPCRs. Once a GPCR is phosphorylated by a GRK, a regulatory protein termed arrestin is recruited.[68] As with GRKs and GPCRs, there are several arrestin family members.

Following recruitment of an arrestin molecule to a GRK-phosphorylated GPCR, a cascade of protein-protein interactions occurs that can lead to further specialization of the signal. First, binding of arrestin leads to interactions with adapter proteins (e.g., clathrin and AP2), causing GPCR internalization to endosomes and possible destruction by the lysosome or recycling back to the cell surface, a process termed resensitization (Figure 14.3B). The process of lysosomal destruction of GPCRs, which ultimately terminates its signal, is termed downregulation. Downregulation is an extreme form of desensitization, since it effects receptor expression at the cell surface. Additionally, recruitment of arrestin by a phosphorylated GPCR can initiate a secondary, yet distinct, arrestin-mediated signaling pathway. This cascade ultimately culminates in activation of another protein kinase system, the mitogen-activated/extracellular signal-regulated kinase (ERK) pathway.[67] Activation of this system can lead to changes in cellular function due to alterations of gene transcription and/or translation.

In essence, agonist binding to a GPCR can lead to activation of two separate signaling cascades (e.g., PKA, ERK), as well as modification of receptor expression (e.g., downregulation, desensitization). Obviously, with over 1000 GPCR family members, multiple second messenger systems, GRKs, and arrestins, the intricacies of cell signaling by GPCRs are immense. The level of detail that is now known about various receptor systems, the cells in which they are expressed, and the network of proteins involved is beyond the scope of this chapter. It is quite clear that the concepts of receptor/G-protein activation are much more complex than originally envisioned, and there are more targets for drugs than just GPCRs. Obviously, gene polymorphisms anywhere along the pathway can have great impact on receptor function.

The concepts of GPCR downregulation and desensitization have been known in anesthesiology for decades. It is well known and accepted that patients on chronic narcotics require more opiates intraoperatively than their naive counterparts, because of alterations in opiate receptor signaling. However, with respect to the SNS, these concepts have also been demonstrated intraoperatively. Studying a canine model of cardiopulmonary bypass (CPB), Schwinn and associates demonstrated that myocardial β AR desensitization occurs in healthy nonischemic myocardium and that it is reversed 30 minutes after discontinuation of CPB.[69] In addition, they demonstrated that β AR downregulation continues after stoppage of CPB. A similar study performed with human atrial samples from patients undergoing CPB, revealed that desensitization also occurs, specifically by altering adenylate cyclase function, even if β AR antagonists are administered.[70] Thus, the critical period of weaning from CPB may be influenced by GPCR dynamics.

CONCEPTS OF GPCR AGONISM

Original drug-receptor theory suggested that drugs worked by acting like a "key" to a receptor "lock." Therefore, turning the "key" activated the receptor leading to intracellular signaling. This theory evolved over several decades to delineate the fundamental concepts of basic pharmacology, specifically agonists, antagonists, and partial agonists. Simply defined, agonists are drugs or neurotransmitters that bind to a GPCR and activate intracellular signaling. Partial agonists are drugs that bind in a similar fashion as agonists, but cannot elicit the same full biological response as an agonist, even at saturating conditions (Figure 14.5). Lastly, antagonists are drugs that competitively block access for agonist binding and thus inhibit intracellular signaling.[71] However, with time, these concepts have been modified and expanded. Today, the full spectrum of pharmacology ranges from inverse agonists, neutral antagonists, and even biased agonists.

Originally, GPCRs were viewed as static proteins floating in a membrane, in one of two states (ligand bound or unbound). Once bound by agonists or ligands, they underwent a sudden change in conformation, allowing for coupling to G-proteins, thus initiating the intracellular signal transduction cascade. However, more recent work has suggested that GPCRs, like all ion channels and proteins, are constantly transitioning between different conformational states in the absence of ligand. These states can exist in several forms, including a nonliganded active state, an inactive state, or even a desensitized state.[72] Such a model suggests two important new caveats to GPCR signaling. First, it is possible for a GPCR to transition between active and inactive states in the absence of ligand, though at a very low frequency. Second, various ligands can help to stabilize these different states, thus leading to the development of new terms to describe ligand effects.

The realization of such receptor dynamics led to further clarification of GPCR pharmacology. For example, it was noted that some GPCRs can initiate measurable signaling in the absence of ligand (e.g., basal or constitutive activity), and that binding by an antagonist can lead to a decrease in basal activity (Figure 14.5). Such ligands were subsequently reclassified from antagonists to *inverse agonists*, since they had the ability to bind GPCRs and prevent the nonliganded active state from stabilizing. In the process, a newer term was added, *neutral antagonist*, which now describes a drug that, once bound to receptor, neither stimulates nor inhibits signaling, hence it truly only blocks agonist binding. Lastly, the concept of *biased agonism* was recently introduced to describe a ligand that preferentially activates one GPCR signaling cascade over another, for instance activation of the arrestin pathway over the adenylate cyclase pathway.[73]

The recent derivation of the crystal structure of the β_2 AR has allowed the foregoing descriptions to move from concept to proven theory, and the structural mechanisms involved have been revealed.[74–76] Previously, it was determined that ligand binding to β_2 ARs involved amino acid residues found within transmembrane domains TMIII, TMV, and TMVI.[77] It was determined that agonist binding did not simply cause the transition from an inactive to an active receptor, a two-state model, but instead agonist binding caused a shift in equilibrium between several different receptor conformations, ultimately leading to G-protein signaling. In other words, the key (i.e., drug) was flexible, as was the lock (i.e., GPCR), and together they altered each other until an energy minimum was reached and signaling occurred.

Agonists (full, partial, or inverse) and antagonists bind to the orthosteric site within the GPCR. The orthosteric site is defined as the ligand binding site for the natural neurotransmitter. It had been previously believed that all

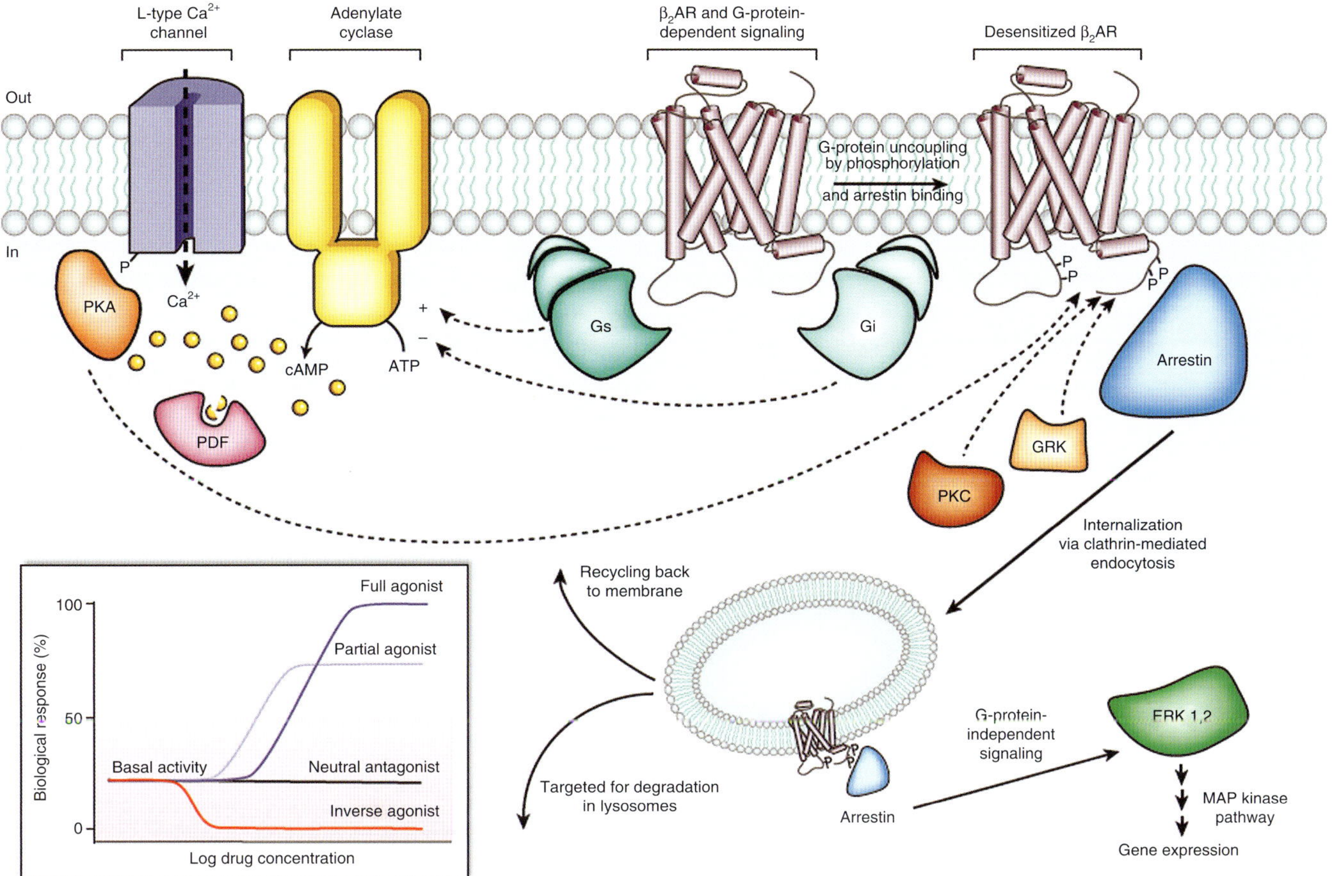

Figure 14.5 Classification of GPCR ligands by pharmacological efficacy. Some GPCRs exhibit basal activity in the absence of ligand, inverse agonists inhibit this activity and neutral antagonists have no effect. Full agonists and partial agonists differ in the extent to which they can elicit a full biological response upon binding. Reprinted by permission of Macmillan Publishers Ltd: *Nature*. Rosenbaum DM, Rasmussen SG, Kobilka BK. The structure and function of G-protein-coupled receptors. *Nature*. 2009;459:356–363.

GPCR-based drugs act only within this site, however, recent analysis of drug candidates and GPCR targets by high throughput screening has revealed that some newer agents can modify GPCR function and signal transduction in the absence of binding to the orthosteric site. These newer sites of GPCR modulation have been termed allosteric sites, and drugs that bind to these sites have been termed *allosteric modulators*.[78–79] Allosteric modulation of GPCR function has added another level of complexity, since allosteric modulators only work in the presence of the orthosteric drug. Allosteric modulators may modify the affinity of the drug at the orthosteric site and/or modify G-protein affinity for the GPCR, thus altering signal transduction.

Though the newer pharmacological concepts of inverse agonism, biased agonism, and neutral antagonist may appear esoteric, the proper application of these terms to describe GPCR ligands has led to a better understanding of several ANS drugs. Various β AR ligands are commonly used intraoperatively for management of blood pressure, including the relatively weak drug dopamine and the more potent drug epinephrine. Various studies using purified receptor preparations have revealed the structural basis for agonist efficacy, specifically that different agonists activate different molecular switches within GPCRs, stabilizing different conformations and thus activating them to varying degrees.[77,80,81] For example, dopamine is a partial agonist at β_2 ARs, when compared to the full agonist epinephrine, because of differential changes in receptor conformation. Though similar studies have not been performed with α_1 ARs, such molecular mechanisms may in part explain why dopamine is a weaker vasopressor than epinephrine or phenylephrine.

Carvedilol is a relatively new, nonspecific β and α_1 AR antagonist that is commonly utilized to treat patients with congestive heart failure. However, why this drug showed survival benefit over other β AR antagonists was not known. Recent work has suggested that carvedilol has weak inverse agonism compared to other β AR antagonists. In addition, it may act as a biased agonist for β arrestin signaling, not only as an antagonist for G_s signaling.[82–83]

Allosteric modulation of GPCRs has been seen clinically within the specialty of anesthesiology. It recently has been demonstrated that a previously unknown combination of mAchR antagonism and allosteric modulation by the nondepolarizing neuromuscular blocker rapacuronium may have led to fatal bronchospasm in susceptible people. Specifically, m2 mAchR antagonism by rapacuronium can lead to elevated release of acetylcholine at PaNS postganglionic neurons, which would then activate m3 mAchRs on bronchial smooth muscle. However, the effect of the released acetylcholine was enhanced by the concomitant allosteric modulation of m3 mAchR by rapacuronium, leading to severe bronchospasm.[84–86] Though new pharmacological terminology may appear to be the realm of laboratory science, newer drugs that take advantage or disadvantage of these differences are being discovered.

ANS CLINICAL PHARMACOLOGY

In the specialties of anesthesiology and critical care medicine, vasopressors are a commonly used class of medications. However, there are few solid randomized clinical trials dictating which vasopressor should be utilized for different clinical scenarios.[87–89] In the disease state of shock (e.g., septic, neurogenic, or cardiogenic), several vasopressors are commonly used to activate α_1 ARs (e.g., dopamine, epinephrine, and phenylephrine), and often they are combined with inotropes to activate β ARs (e.g., dobutamine and epinephrine). A major concern with many of the studies was that surrogate markers for patients, such as blood pressure and cardiac output, were utilized instead of patient outcomes, such as mortality. In the SOAP II study, mortality was utilized, and no difference was seen between patients treated with NE vs. dopamine, however, more adverse events (e.g., arrhythmias) were noted with the latter drug. Given that dopamine is a partial agonist compared to NE, and also activates multiple GPCRs (i.e., dopamine, α_1 and β_1 ARs) to cause unwanted effects, NE has become the recommended vasopressor for septic shock.[89]

The role for perioperative β AR antagonists ("beta blockers") in noncardiac surgery patients has also been challenged. The original study by Mangano and colleagues provided evidence supporting the use of these drugs to limit adverse cardiovascular events,[90] however, more recent studies examining other types of mortality including perioperative stroke has suggested that generalized use of these drugs in all patients may not be appropriate.[91] As mentioned above, β AR antagonists can now be classified with respect to subtype specificity and the presence or absence of inverse agonism or neutral antagonism. The combination of these various parameters can make for differences in β AR antagonists, possibly impacting future decisions about perioperative beta blockade.

Agonists for α_2 ARs have been utilized clinically for hemodynamic control as well as sedation, and they have proven to be potent analgesics that can potentiate the effects of opioids. Investigation of α_2 AR KO mice has revealed that various anesthetic agents possess sedative and hypnotic effects due to activation of various α_2 AR subtypes. For instance, α_2A ARs are necessary for the antinociception effects of various α_2 AR agonists, such as clonidine and dexmedetomidine.[92] Dexmedetomidine is commonly used in intensive care units as a potent sedative, and with increasing frequency in operating rooms. Dexmedetomidine is approximately 1600x more potent at α_2 ARs than at α_1 ARs (compared to 200x for clonidine); however, it is not subtype selective. Analysis of various α_2 AR KO mice revealed that the α_2A AR subtype is necessary and sufficient for mediating the central sedative effects of this drug.[93]

ANS PHYSIOLOGY

The two divisions of the ANS, the SNS and PaNS, both contain afferent and efferent pathways for nerve traffic to and from the CNS in order to regulate and monitor vital organs. Over the last several decades, neurophysiological methods have been developed to allow for direct recording and study of both of these pathways in the SNS (for a more complete description please see reference[3]). For investigations of efferent signaling, microneurography has been developed to record muscle sympathetic activity (MSA).[94] Though there are limitations to these methods in terms of recording duration, stability, and intraindividual variability, it has become possible to measure MSA amplitude and action potential frequency in response to drugs or pathophysiological conditions.[95] In addition, NE plasma concentrations can be measured for the total body ("spillover"); renal and cardiac NE spillover levels can also be determined.[96] Combining these methods, it has been determined that NE spillover levels correlate with MSA, blood pressure does not correlate with MSA, and the concept of whole-body activation of the SNS in response to stimuli has been disproven. The SNS can selectively activate its subdivisions to control individual organ systems.[3]

Afferent signaling with the SNS can also be measured; however, unlike MSA measurements, the methods are more indirect. Specifically, a major afferent pathway of the SNS is the arterial baroreceptor reflex. In this reflex arc, stretch/pressure changes sensed in the aortic arch can trigger efferent neural traffic to counteract the change seen. For example, a sudden increase in blood pressure will signal a decrease in SNS activity.[97] By administering pharmacological vasoconstrictors or vasodilators and plotting MSA burst activity as a function of the preceding diastolic pressure, the slope of the line has been shown to correlate to baroreflex sensitivity (BRS). Such experimental methods have allowed for analysis of SNS afferent signaling without contamination by PaNS effects.[98] It is now possible to study the systemic effects of drugs and anesthetic agents on both efferent and afferent SNS signaling.

INTRAVENOUS ANESTHETIC EFFECTS ON SNS FUNCTION

Ketamine is the only commonly used intravenous anesthetic agent that can increase both heart rate (HR) and arterial blood pressure (ABP). It has been postulated that ketamine administration activates the SNS and thus maintains HR and ABP. However, studies of racemic and S(+) ketamine have demonstrated an isomeric effect. Specifically, racemic ketamine reduced MSA due to baroreflex inhibition, whereas S(+) ketamine increased MSA and NE spillover. Ketamine appears to show differential effects on SNS activation and does not increase SNS outflow in a generalized manner. MSA responses to arterial hypotension appeared to be maintained, hence accounting for ketamine-induced cardiovascular stability.[99–100]

Though opioids are not considered to be classic intravenous anesthetic agents, they are commonly utilized to provide a balanced anesthetic. A variety of studies have been done to investigate the effects of opioids on SNS function, but such studies were limited by opioid-induced sedation and respiratory depression that also impact SNS activity. Despite these limitations it has been determined that acute administration of opioids alone has little impact on SNS function and that chronic opioid administration may lead to SNS depression.[101–102]

The differential effects of various sedatives and induction agents on SNS function can in part explain the observed differences in cardiovascular function when these agents are administered. Injection of barbiturates such as methohexital has been shown to lead to a variety of cardiovascular effects due to a complex interplay with the SNS and PaNS. For example, induction of anesthesia with methohexital commonly leads to tachycardia. This tachycardia is not due to SNS activation, but instead appears to be due to inhibition of vagal outflow.[103] In addition to a direct negative inotropic effect of methohexital, the decrease in HR and ABP observed upon induction is due in part to the rapid suppression of MSA and BRS.[104]

Traditionally, benzodiazepines are thought to have minimal effects on cardiovascular parameters compared to other intravenous induction agents. However, analysis of SNS function has revealed that diazepam does lead to lower NE plasma levels and attenuated BRS.[105] In addition, when coadministered with opioids, a more profound reduction in MSA and BRS occurs, suggesting a synergistic effect of these two classes of drugs on SNS function.[106]

Hypotension induced by injection of propofol has been attributed to a variety of mechanisms, including direct myocardial depression, a reduction in vascular resistance, and/or reduced cardiac preload.[107] Analysis of efferent and afferent SNS function has revealed that propofol, at both sedative and anesthetic doses, can decrease MSA by up to 92% and also greatly reduces BRS, thus altering the body's ability to counteract hypotensive episodes.[108–110] The loss of BRS appears to be responsible for the large decrease in ABP seen upon administration of propofol, over a variety of doses.

Etomidate is the induction agent most commonly associated with hemodynamic stability, and therefore has been recommended for patients with cardiovascular disease or hypovolemia (e.g., trauma patients). It has been commonly taught that etomidate has less direct myocardial and vascular depressant effects than either propofol or barbiturates and that the lack of this direct effect is responsible for its hemodynamic stability. Recordings of MSA and analysis of BRS have demonstrated that the SNS may be the actual site of these effects of etomidate. Administration of etomidate does not appear to impair either efferent SNS signaling or BRS.[110]

INHALATIONAL ANESTHETIC EFFECTS ON SNS FUNCTION

Different inhalational agents have varying effects on cardiovascular function. Examination of SNS effects by inhalational agents in humans and animals can explain in part some of the observed effects. Halothane, enflurane, sevoflurane, and isoflurane have all been shown to decrease SNS activity and to diminish baroreflex activation in animals.[109, 111–114] The effect on baroreflex activity appears to involve all components of the reflex arc from efferent and afferent nerves, the CNS, ganglia, and muscle. Some agents do exhibit differences that may explain some of the clinical thinking about these agents. For example, desflurane and isoflurane both induce vasodilation and have similar cardiac depressant effects. However, at equal anesthetic doses, desflurane maintained a higher resting MSA than isoflurane.[115] In fact, rapidly increasing the inhaled concentration of desflurane caused a surge in MSA, resulting in an increase in HR and ABP.[116] This finding is consistent with the belief that desflurane is not a good sole anesthetic agent for induction of patients with coronary artery disease. On the other hand, administration of low concentrations of isoflurane (but not desflurane) preserved BRS, which may explain the tachycardia seen with low isoflurane anesthetic concentration.[115] Lastly, sevoflurane has neither effect described above, thus increasing inspired concentrations does not lead to MSA activation, nor does low sevoflurane concentration preserve BRS.[117]

Unlike the potent inhalational anesthetic agents, nitrous oxide actually stimulates SNS efferent activity. Administration of nitrous oxide has been shown to increase MSA, while slightly decreasing BRS.[118] Interestingly, nitrous oxide has a slightly different effect on the pediatric population, where it is does not appear to activate the SNS to the same extent, if at all.[119] Sellgren and colleagues observed an interesting clinical finding when nitrous oxide was coadministered with isoflurane. Namely, withdrawal of nitrous oxide from an isoflurane anesthetic led to a decrease in MSA, a slight increase in HR, and an unchanged BP.[109] Therefore, nitrous oxide may counteract the SNS depression seen with other more potent inhalational agents, and thus argue for the continued use of nitrous oxide with inhalational agents in order to limit cardiovascular depression seen with the more potent agents alone.[120]

Various studies of intravenous and inhalational anesthetics on human physiology have uncovered various nuances of these different agents. In general, it would appear that different agents within the same class (e.g., inhalational agents), should have similar mechanisms of action and thus similar cardiovascular effects. However, clinical experience and research has demonstrated that these agents do have some unique characteristics. By examining the SNS in addition to vital signs and CNS effects, it has become apparent that part of the unique hemodynamic signatures of the individual agents may be due in part to differential activation or inhibition of the SNS.

CONCLUSIONS AND FUTURE DIRECTIONS

As described above, regulation of the ANS by drugs and inhalational anesthetics is an important part of the daily practice of anesthesiology and critical care medicine. However, most drugs utilized daily in the operating room were not developed to take advantage of the broad array of receptors and signaling mechanisms. For example, what effect would an α_2A or α_2C AR specific agonist have on SNS control of heart or arterial smooth muscle function? Development of such subtype specific drugs could allow for fine-tune control of sympathetic activity without resorting to drugs that affect the end organ (e.g., heart) only. Alternatively, it should follow that since various inhalational agents have different effects on the SNS and PaNS, the choice of agent should depend on the intended effects and not which vaporizer is available on a given anesthetic machine.

Research in the area of autonomic pharmacology also could be taken into the direction of pharmacogenomics. The fact that the administration of some drugs to certain patients does not lead to the expected dose-response effect may be due to genetic variability. Genetic screening of patients for all polymorphisms may be impractical, but molecular medicine is advancing and such knowledge may become available in the future. Lastly, real-time monitoring of SNS function in the operating room or ICU may also become a relevant method for assessing anesthetic drug effect or possibly be predictive of a patient's responsiveness to drugs or even mortality.[121]

Compared to other specialties, anesthesiology can be seen as limited in its research appeal, for the specialty does not "own" an organ system, nor has many specific disease entities to investigate, aside from malignant hyperthermia. However, the opposite statement is probably closer to the truth. Every organ system is affected by anesthetic agents and thus can be a research interest. As well, pathophysiological states are a disease entity, as described above, and thus fall within our domain. As anesthesiologists, our clinical expertise intersects with all organ systems and all diseases, hence making our specialty broadly relevant for medical research. It could be argued that the CNS and ANS are two major organ systems that can be rightfully claimed by anesthesiology.

REFERENCES

1. Langley J. Das sympatische und verwandt nervoise System der Wirbeltiere (autonomes nervoeses system). *Ergebn Physiol.* 1903; 27(II):818–872.
2. Cannon W. Organization for physiological homeostasis. *Physiol Rev.* 1929;9:399–431.
3. Neukirchen M, Kienbaum P. Sympathetic nervous system: evaluation and importance for clinical general anesthesia. *Anesthesiology.* 2008;109(6):1113–1131.
4. Mathias CJ, Polinsky RJ. Separating the primary autonomic failure syndromes, multiple system atrophy, and pure autonomic failure from Parkinson's disease. *Adv Neurol.* 1999;80:353–361.
5. Chaudhuri KR. Autonomic dysfunction in movement disorders. *Curr Opin Neurol.* 2001;14(4):505–511.
6. Mathias CJ. Disorders of the autonomic nervous system. In: Bradley W, et al. eds. *Neurology in Clinical Practice.* Boston: Butterworth-Heinemann; 2000:2131–2165.
7. Karlsson AK. Autonomic dysreflexia. *Spinal Cord.* 1999;37(6): 383–391.
8. Greene DA, Stevens MJ, Feldman EL. Diabetic neuropathy: scope of the syndrome. *Am J Med.* 1999;107(2B):2S–8S.
9. Cohn JN. The management of chronic heart failure. *N Engl J Med.* 1996;335(7):490–498.
10. Schmidt HB, Werdan K, Muller-Werdan U. Autonomic dysfunction in the ICU patient. *Curr Opin Crit Care.* 2001;7(5):314–322.
11. Gang Y, Malik M. Heart rate variability in critical care medicine. *Curr Opin Crit Care.* 2002;8(5):371–375.
12. Schmidt H, et al. Autonomic dysfunction predicts both 1- and 2-month mortality in middle-aged patients with multiple organ dysfunction syndrome. *Crit Care Med.* 2008;36(3):967–970.
13. Francis NJ, Landis SC. Cellular and molecular determinants of sympathetic neuron development. *Annu Rev Neurosci.* 1999;22: 541–566.
14. Kirstein SL, Insel PA. Autonomic nervous system pharmacogenomics: a progress report. *Pharmacol Rev.* 2004;56(1):31–52.
15. Lundberg JM. Pharmacology of cotransmission in the autonomic nervous system: integrative aspects on amines, neuropeptides, adenosine triphosphate, amino acids and nitric oxide. *Pharmacol Rev.* 1996;48(1):113–178.
16. Robertson SD, Matthies HJ, Galli A. A closer look at amphetamine-induced reverse transport and trafficking of the dopamine and norepinephrine transporters. *Mol Neurobiol.* 2009;39(2):73–80.
17. Goldstein DS, Eisenhofer G, Kopin IJ. Clinical catecholamine neurochemistry: a legacy of Julius Axelrod. *Cell Mol Neurobiol.* 2006; 26(4–6):695–702.
18. Hajjar RJ, MacRae CA. Adrenergic-receptor polymorphisms and heart failure. *N Engl J Med.* 2002;347(15):1196–1199.
19. Shcherbakova OG, et al. Organization of beta-adrenoceptor signaling compartments by sympathetic innervation of cardiac myocytes. *J Cell Biol.* 2007;176(4):521–533.
20. Bockaert J, Pin JP. Molecular tinkering of G protein-coupled receptors: an evolutionary success. *Embo J.* 1999;18(7):1723–1729.

21. Kristiansen K. Molecular mechanisms of ligand binding, signaling, and regulation within the superfamily of G-protein-coupled receptors: molecular modeling and mutagenesis approaches to receptor structure and function. *Pharmacol Ther.* 2004;103(1):21–80.
22. Horn F, et al. GPCRDB information system for G protein-coupled receptors. *Nucleic Acids Res.* 2003;31(1):294–297.
23. Rana BK, Insel PA. G-protein-coupled receptor websites. *Trends Pharmacol Sci.* 2002;23(11):535–536.
24. Bylund DB, et al. International Union of Pharmacology nomenclature of adrenoceptors. *Pharmacol Rev*, 1994;46(2):121–136.
25. MacDonald E, Kobilka BK, Scheinin M. Gene targeting—homing in on alpha 2-adrenoceptor-subtype function. *Trends Pharmacol Sci.* 1997;18(6):211–219.
26. Rodbell M, et al. The glucagon-sensitive adenyl cyclase system in plasma membranes of rat liver, V: an obligatory role of guanylnucleotides in glucagon action. *J Biol Chem.* 1971;246(6):1877–1882.
27. Ritter SL, Hall RA. Fine-tuning of GPCR activity by receptor-interacting proteins. *Nat Rev Mol Cell Biol.* 2009;10(12):819–830.
28. Gilman AG. G proteins: transducers of receptor-generated signals. *Annu Rev Biochem.* 1987;56:615–649.
29. Oldham WM, Hamm HE. Heterotrimeric G protein activation by G-protein-coupled receptors. *Nat Rev Mol Cell Biol.* 2008;9(1): 60–71.
30. Tan C, et al. Membrane trafficking of G protein-coupled receptors. *Annu Rev Pharmacol Toxicol.* 2004;44:559–609.
31. Edwards SW, Tan CM, Limbird LE. Localization of G-protein-coupled receptors in health and disease. *Trends in Pharmacol Sci.* 2000;21(8):304–308.
32. De Biasi M. Nicotinic mechanisms in the autonomic control of organ systems. *J Neurobiol.* 2002;53(4):568–579.
33. De Biasi M. Nicotinic receptor mutant mice in the study of autonomic function. *Curr Drug Targets CNS Neurol Disord.* 2002;1(4): 331–336.
34. Campanucci V, Krishnaswamy A, Cooper E. Diabetes depresses synaptic transmission in sympathetic ganglia by inactivating nAChRs through a conserved intracellular cysteine residue. *Neuron.* 2010; 66(6):827–834.
35. Lanzafame AA, Christopoulos A, Mitchelson F. Cellular signaling mechanisms for muscarinic acetylcholine receptors. *Receptors Channels.* 2003;9(4):241–260.
36. Brodde OE, Michel MC. Adrenergic and muscarinic receptors in the human heart. *Pharmacol Rev.* 1999;51(4):651–690.
37. Bymaster FP, et al. Use of M1-M5 muscarinic receptor knockout mice as novel tools to delineate the physiological roles of the muscarinic cholinergic system. *Neurochem Res.* 2003;28(3–4):437–442.
38. Docherty JR. Subtypes of functional alpha1-adrenoceptor. *Cell Mol Life Sci.* 2010;67(3):405–417.
39. Philipp M, Brede M, Hein L. Physiological significance of alpha(2)-adrenergic receptor subtype diversity: one receptor is not enough. *Am J Physiol Regul Integr Comp Physiol.* 2002;283(2):R287–295.
40. Link R, et al. Cloning of two mouse genes encoding alpha 2-adrenergic receptor subtypes and identification of a single amino acid in the mouse alpha 2-C10 homolog responsible for an interspecies variation in antagonist binding. *Mol Pharmacol.* 1992;42(1):16–27.
41. Link RE, et al. Targeted inactivation of the gene encoding the mouse alpha 2c-adrenoceptor homolog. *Mol Pharmacol.* 1995;48(1):48–55.
42. Altman JD, et al. Abnormal regulation of the sympathetic nervous system in alpha2A- adrenergic receptor knockout mice. *Mol Pharmacol.* 1999;56(1):154–161.
43. Hurt CM, Angelotti T. Molecular insights into alpha2 adrenergic receptor function: clinical implications. *Seminars in Anesthesia, Perioperative Medicine and Pain.* 2007;26:28–34.
44. Hein L, Altman JD, Kobilka BK. Two functionally distinct alpha2-adrenergic receptors regulate sympathetic neurotransmission. *Nature.* 1999;402(6758):181–184.
45. Brum PC, et al. Differential targeting and function of alpha(2A) and alpha(2C) adrenergic receptor subtypes in cultured sympathetic neurons. *Neuropharmacology.* 2006;51(3):397–413.
46. Kilts JD, et al. Beta(2)-adrenergic and several other G protein-coupled receptors in human atrial membranes activate both G(s) and G(i). *Circ Res.* 2000;87(8):705–709.
47. Xiang Y, Kobilka BK. Myocyte adrenoceptor signaling pathways. *Science.* 2003;300(5625):1530–1532.
48. Nikolaev VO, et al. Beta2-adrenergic receptor redistribution in heart failure changes cAMP compartmentation. *Science.* 2010;327(5973): 1653–1657.
49. Patterson AJ, et al. Protecting the myocardium: a role for the beta2 adrenergic receptor in the heart. *Critical Care Medicine.* 2004;32(4): 1041–1048.
50. Gingrich JA, Hen R. The broken mouse: the role of development, plasticity and environment in the interpretation of phenotypic changes in knockout mice. *Curr Opin Neurobiol.* 2000;10(1): 146–152.
51. Godecke A, Schrader J. Adaptive mechanisms of the cardiovascular system in transgenic mice—lessons from eNOS and myoglobin knockout mice. *Basic Res Cardiol.* 2000;95(6):492–498.
52. Eisener-Dorman AF, Lawrence DA, Bolivar VJ. Cautionary insights on knockout mouse studies: the gene or not the gene? *Brain Behav Immun.* 2009;23(3):318–324.
53. Koshimizu TA, Tanoue A, Tsujimoto G. Clinical implications from studies of alpha1 adrenergic receptor knockout mice. *Biochem Pharmacol.* 2007;73(8):1107–1112.
54. Trendelenburg AU, et al. Occurrence, pharmacology and function of presynaptic alpha2-autoreceptors in alpha2A/D-adrenoceptor-deficient mice. *Naunyn Schmiedebergs Arch Pharmacol.* 1999;360(5): 540–551.
55. Trendelenburg AU, et al. A study of presynaptic alpha2-autoreceptors in alpha2A/D-, alpha2B- and alpha2C-adrenoceptor-deficient mice. *Naunyn Schmiedebergs Arch Pharmacol.* 2001;364(2):117–130.
56. Brede M, et al. Differential control of adrenal and sympathetic catecholamine release by alpha 2-adrenoceptor subtypes. *Mol Endocrinol.* 2003;17(8):1640–1646.
57. Rohrer DK, et al. Targeted disruption of the mouse beta1-adrenergic receptor gene: developmental and cardiovascular effects. *Proc Natl Acad Sci U S A.* 1996;93(14):7375–7380.
58. Chruscinski A, et al. Targeted disruption of the beta2 adrenergic receptor gene. *J Biological Chem.* 1999;274(24):16701–16708.
59. Rohrer DK, et al. Cardiovascular and metabolic alterations in mice lacking both beta1- and beta2-adrenergic receptors. *J Biol Chem.* 1999;274(24):16701–16708.
60. Rosskopf D, Michel MC. Pharmacogenomics of G protein-coupled receptor ligands in cardiovascular medicine. *Pharmacol Rev.* 2008;60(4):513–535.
61. Garland EM, Biaggioni I. Genetic polymorphisms of adrenergic receptors. *Clin Auton Res.* 2001;11(2):67–78.
62. Zaugg M, Schaub MC. Genetic modulation of adrenergic activity in the heart and vasculature: implications for perioperative medicine. *Anesthesiology.* 2005;102(2):429–446.
63. Small KM, Liggett SB. Identification and functional characterization of alpha(2)-adrenoceptor polymorphisms. *Trends Pharmacol Sci.* 2001;22(9):471–477.
64. Small KM, et al. Polymorphisms of cardiac presynaptic alpha2C adrenergic receptors: diverse intragenic variability with haplotype-specific functional effects. *Proc Natl Acad Sci U S A.* 2004;101(35): 13020–13025.
65. Small KM, et al. Synergistic polymorphisms of beta1- and alpha2C-adrenergic receptors and the risk of congestive heart failure. *N Engl J Med.* 2002;347(15):1135–1142.
66. Neumeister A, et al. Sympathoneural and adrenomedullary functional effects of alpha2C-adrenoreceptor gene polymorphism in healthy humans. *Pharmacogenetics.* 2005;15(3):143–150.
67. Pierce KL, Premont RT, Lefkowitz RJ. Seven-transmembrane receptors. *Nat Rev Mol Cell Biol.* 2002;3(9):639–650.
68. Krupnick JG, Benovic JL. The role of receptor kinases and arrestins in G protein-coupled receptor regulation. *Annu Rev Pharmacol Toxicol.* 1998;38:289–319.

69. Schwinn DA, et al. Desensitization of myocardial beta-adrenergic receptors during cardiopulmonary bypass: evidence for early uncoupling and late downregulation. *Circulation.* 1991;84(6): 2559–2567.
70. Booth JV, et al. Acute depression of myocardial beta-adrenergic receptor signaling during cardiopulmonary bypass: impairment of the adenylyl cyclase moiety; Duke Heart Center Perioperative Desensitization Group. *Anesthesiology.* 1998;89(3):602–611.
71. Rosenbaum DM, Rasmussen SG, Kobilka BK. The structure and function of G-protein-coupled receptors. *Nature.* 2009;459(7245): 356–363.
72. Kenakin T. Efficacy at G-protein-coupled receptors. *Nat Rev Drug Discov.* 2002;1(2):103–110.
73. Kenakin T. Functional selectivity through protean and biased agonism: who steers the ship? *Mol Pharmacol.* 2007;72(6):1393–1401.
74. Cherezov V, et al. High-resolution crystal structure of an engineered human beta2-adrenergic G protein-coupled receptor. *Science.* 2007; 318(5854):1258–1265.
75. Rasmussen SG, et al. Crystal structure of the human beta2 adrenergic G-protein-coupled receptor. *Nature.* 2007;450(7168):383–387.
76. Rosenbaum DM, et al. GPCR engineering yields high-resolution structural insights into beta2-adrenergic receptor function. *Science.* 2007;318(5854):1266–1273.
77. Swaminath G, et al. Probing the beta2 adrenoceptor binding site with catechol reveals differences in binding and activation by agonists and partial agonists. *J Biol Chem.* 2005;280(23):22165–22171.
78. Leach K, Sexton PM, Christopoulos A. Allosteric GPCR modulators: taking advantage of permissive receptor pharmacology. *Trends Pharmacol Sci.* 2007;28(8):382–389.
79. May LT, et al. Allosteric modulation of G protein-coupled receptors. *Annu Rev Pharmacol Toxicol.* 2007;47:1–51.
80. Swaminath G, et al. Sequential binding of agonists to the {beta}2 adrenoceptor: kinetic evidence for intermediate conformational states. *J Biol Chem.* 2004;279(1):686–691.
81. Yao X, et al. Coupling ligand structure to specific conformational switches in the beta2-adrenoceptor. *Nat Chem Biol.* 2006;2(8): 417–422.
82. Wisler JW, et al. A unique mechanism of beta-blocker action: carvedilol stimulates beta-arrestin signaling. *Proc Natl Acad Sci U S A.* 2007;104(42):16657–16662.
83. Violin JD, Lefkowitz RJ. Beta-arrestin-biased ligands at seven-transmembrane receptors. *Trends Pharmacol Sci.* 2007;28(8):416–422.
84. Jooste E, et al. A mechanism for rapacuronium-induced bronchospasm: M2 muscarinic receptor antagonism. *Anesthesiology.* 2003; 98(4):906–911.
85. Jooste EH, et al. Rapacuronium augments acetylcholine-induced bronchoconstriction via positive allosteric interactions at the M3 muscarinic receptor. *Anesthesiology.* 2005;103(6):1195–1203.
86. Jakubik J, et al. Divergence of allosteric effects of rapacuronium on binding and function of muscarinic receptors. *BMC Pharmacol.* 2009;9:15.
87. Mullner M, et al. Vasopressors for shock. *Cochrane Database Syst Rev.* 2004;(3):CD003709.
88. Sakr Y, et al. Does dopamine administration in shock influence outcome? results of the sepsis occurrence in acutely ill patients (SOAP) study. *Crit Care Med.* 2006;34(3):589–597.
89. De Backer D, et al. Comparison of dopamine and norepinephrine in the treatment of shock. *N Engl J Med.* 2010;362(9):779–789.
90. Mangano DT, et al. Effect of atenolol on mortality and cardiovascular morbidity after noncardiac surgery: multicenter study of perioperative ischemia research group. *N Engl J Med.* 1996;335(23): 1713–1720.
91. Effects of extended-release metoprolol succinate in patients undergoing non-cardiac surgery (POISE trial): a randomised controlled trial. *The Lancet.* 2008;371(9627):1839–1847.
92. Stone LS, et al. The alpha2a adrenergic receptor subtype mediates spinal analgesia evoked by alpha2 agonists and is necessary for spinal adrenergic-opioid synergy. *J Neurosci.* 1997;17(18): 7157–7165.
93. Lakhlani PP, et al. Substitution of a mutant alpha2a-adrenergic receptor via "hit and run" gene targeting reveals the role of this subtype in sedative, analgesic, and anesthetic-sparing responses in vivo. *Proc Natl Acad Sci U S A.* 1997;94(18):9950–9955.
94. Wallin BG, Charkoudian N. Sympathetic neural control of integrated cardiovascular function: insights from measurement of human sympathetic nerve activity. *Muscle Nerve.* 2007;36(5): 595–614.
95. Wallin BG. Interindividual differences in muscle sympathetic nerve activity: a key to new insight into cardiovascular regulation? *Acta Physiol (Oxf).* 2007;190(4):265–275.
96. Wallin BG, et al. Simultaneous measurements of cardiac noradrenaline spillover and sympathetic outflow to skeletal muscle in humans. *J Physiol.* 1992;453:45–58.
97. Sellgren J, et al. Sympathetic muscle nerve activity, peripheral blood flows, and baroreceptor reflexes in humans during propofol anesthesia and surgery. *Anesthesiology.* 1994. 80(3):534–544.
98. Sundlof G, Wallin BG. Human muscle nerve sympathetic activity at rest: relationship to blood pressure and age. *J Physiol.* 1978; 274:621–637.
99. Kienbaum P, et al. Racemic ketamine decreases muscle sympathetic activity but maintains the neural response to hypotensive challenges in humans. *Anesthesiology.* 2000;92(1):94–101.
100. Kienbaum P, et al. S(+)-ketamine increases muscle sympathetic activity and maintains the neural response to hypotensive challenges in humans. *Anesthesiology.* 2001;94(2):252–258.
101. Taneyama C, et al. Effects of fentanyl, diazepam, and the combination of both on arterial baroreflex and sympathetic nerve activity in intact and baro-denervated dogs. *Anesth Analg.* 1993;77(1): 44–48.
102. Kienbaum P, et al. Chronic mu-opioid receptor stimulation alters cardiovascular regulation in humans: differential effects on muscle sympathetic and heart rate responses to arterial hypotension. *J Cardiovasc Pharmacol.* 2002;40(3):363–369.
103. Inoue K, Arndt JO. Efferent vagal discharge and heart rate in response to methohexitone, althesin, ketamine and etomidate in cats. *Br J Anaesth.* 1982;54(10):1105–1116.
104. Sellgren J, Ponten J, Wallin BG. Characteristics of muscle nerve sympathetic activity during general anaesthesia in humans. *Acta Anaesthesiol Scand.* 1992;36(4):336–345.
105. Marty J, et al. Effects of diazepam and midazolam on baroreflex control of heart rate and on sympathetic activity in humans. *Anesth Analg.* 1986;65(2):113–119.
106. Kotrly KJ, et al. Effects of fentanyl-diazepam-nitrous oxide anaesthesia on arterial baroreflex control of heart rate in man. *Br J Anaesth.* 1986;58(4):406–414.
107. Lepage JY, et al. Left ventricular performance during propofol or methohexital anesthesia: isotopic and invasive cardiac monitoring. *Anesth Analg.* 1991;73(1):3–9.
108. Ebert TJ. Sympathetic and hemodynamic effects of moderate and deep sedation with propofol in humans. *Anesthesiology.* 2005; 103(1):20–24.
109. Sellgren J, Ponten J, Wallin BG. Percutaneous recording of muscle nerve sympathetic activity during propofol, nitrous oxide, and isoflurane anesthesia in humans. *Anesthesiology.* 1990;73(1):20–27.
110. Ebert TJ, et al. Sympathetic responses to induction of anesthesia in humans with propofol or etomidate. *Anesthesiology.* 1992;76(5): 725–733.
111. Muzi M, Ebert TJ. Randomized, prospective comparison of halothane, isoflurane, and enflurane on baroreflex control of heart rate in humans. *Adv Pharmacol.* 1994;31:379–387.
112. Takeshima R, Dohi S. Comparison of arterial baroreflex function in humans anesthetized with enflurane or isoflurane. *Anesth Analg.* 1989;69(3):284–290.
113. Kotrly KJ, et al. Baroreceptor reflex control of heart rate during isoflurane anesthesia in humans. *Anesthesiology.* 1984;60(3): 173–179.
114. Ebert TJ. Cardiovascular and autonomic effects of sevoflurane. *Acta Anaesthesiol Belg.* 1996;47(1):15–21.

115. Ebert TJ, Muzi M. Sympathetic hyperactivity during desflurane anesthesia in healthy volunteers: a comparison with isoflurane. *Anesthesiology.* 1993;79(3):444–453.
116. Muzi M, Lopatka CW, Ebert TJ. Desflurane-mediated neurocirculatory activation in humans. effects of concentration and rate of change on responses. *Anesthesiology*. 1996;84(5):1035–1042.
117. Ebert TJ, Muzi M, Lopatka CW. Neurocirculatory responses to sevoflurane in humans: a comparison to desflurane. *Anesthesiology.* 1995;83(1):88–95.
118. Ebert TJ, Kampine JP. Nitrous oxide augments sympathetic outflow: direct evidence from human peroneal nerve recordings. *Anesth Analg.* 1989;69(4):444–449.
119. Constant I, et al. Non-invasive assessment of cardiovascular autonomic activity induced by brief exposure to 50% nitrous oxide in children. *Br J Anaesth.* 2002;88(5):637–643.
120. Bahlman SH, et al. The cardiovascular effects of nitrous oxide-halothane anesthesia in man. *Anesthesiology.* 1971;35(3):274–285.
121. Storm H. Changes in skin conductance as a tool to monitor nociceptive stimulation and pain. *Curr Opin Anaesthesiol.* 2008;21(6): 796–804.

PART VI

NEUROMUSCULAR JUNCTION

15

REVIEW OF NEUROMUSCULAR JUNCTION ANATOMY AND FUNCTION

Sorin J. Brull and Mohamed Naguib

NEUROMUSCULAR JUNCTION ARCHITECTURE

The neuromuscular junction (NMJ) is a synapse that develops between a motor neuron and a muscle fiber, and is made up of several components: the presynaptic nerve terminal, the postsynaptic muscle membrane, and the intervening cleft (or gap). The vertebrate NMJ is the focal point of contact where motor neurons transmit impulses to skeletal muscle fibers in a 1:1 ratio. Thus, its function is merely that of an impedance adapter between the (high input impedance) motor neuron and the (low input impedance) muscle fiber. The integrity of neuromuscular transmission is dependent on a highly orchestrated mechanism involving: 1) synthesis, storage, and release of acetylcholine (ACh) from motor nerve endings (presynaptic region) at the neuromuscular junction, and ACh reuptake from the cleft into the nerve terminal; 2) binding of ACh to nicotinic receptors on the muscle membrane (postsynaptic region) and generation of action potentials; and 3) rapid hydrolysis of ACh by the enzyme acetylcholinesterase, which is present in the synaptic cleft.[1]

The motor unit, first named by Liddell and Sherrington,[2] is defined as the motor neuron and all of the muscle fibers it innervates. Within the motor unit, the number of muscle fibers that are innervated by a single motor neuron defines the innervation ratio. For muscle groups that require fine control (such as the hand muscles, and ocular and facial muscles), the innervation ratio is low (a ratio close to 1:5).[3] For muscles requiring only gross movement, such as the back or leg antigravity muscles, the innervation ratio is high (1:2000).[4]

DEVELOPMENT OF NEUROMUSCULAR JUNCTION

During embryonic development, the formation of the NMJ requires three components: 1) the committed myogenic cells originating from the somite in the neural crest, 2) motor axons that are derived from somata in the neural tube, and 3) Schwann cell precursor cells from the neural crest. All three cells migrate to meet at the NMJ. Myogenic cells differentiate into myoblasts. The myoblasts fuse to form multinucleated myotubes expressing many contractile and synaptic proteins required for the development and maturation of the NMJ.[5] Motor axons contact myotubes and are followed closely by Schwann cells. Despite comigration of axons and Schwann cells, the latter are not required for the initial formation of the NMJ. In mutant mice lacking Schwann cells, axons still navigate to their targets and form initial synaptic contacts.[6] At these newly formed synapses, Schwann cells continue to depend on motor neurons to survive. At the area of contact between the axon and myotube, the axon differentiates into a motor nerve terminal (presynaptic area) packed with synaptic vesicles containing ACh, while the muscle forms a postsynaptic apparatus. Schwann cells cap the entire synaptic structure except at the interface of the presynaptic and postsynaptic membranes.

At birth, the NMJ in the vertebrate is fully functional and multiply innervated. Nicotinic acetylcholine receptors (nAChRs) (Figure 15.1) are present at a moderate level throughout the myotube surface. Such nAChRs, termed "fetal" due to their expression early in development, are assembled from five subunits: there are two α subunits, as well as one β, one γ, and one δ subunit (denoted as $\alpha_2\beta\gamma\delta$), each encoded by a different gene (Figure 15.2).[7] During the first two postnatal weeks, each postsynaptic motor site is innervated by multiple presynaptic nerve terminals. Beyond this time, a transition occurs and most of the nerve terminals are destroyed, such that each postsynaptic site receives neuronal input from a single motor axon.[8] With maturation, adult nAChRs are restricted in high concentrations (10,000/μm^2) in the postsynaptic membrane, but are virtually absent extrasynaptically.

Synapses are restricted to the endplate region in the middle of the muscle cell. Synapse maturation involves the formation of a motor nerve terminal. At the mature NMJ, pre- and postsynaptic membranes are separated by a synaptic cleft containing extracellular proteins that form the basal lamina. Acetylcholinesterase, the enzyme that hydrolyzes ACh, is present in the basal lamina. Synaptic basal lamina plays an integral role in maintaining the NMJ structure and

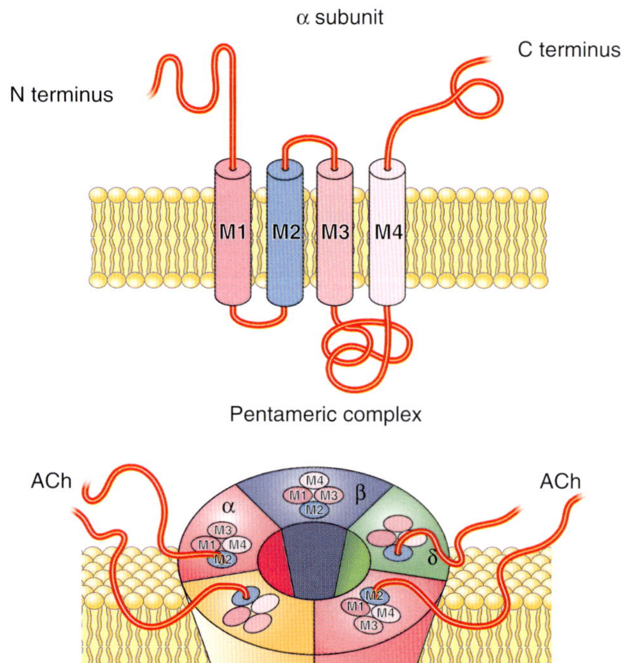

Figure 15.1 Subunit composition of the nicotinic acetylcholine receptor (nAChR) at the endplate surface of adult mammalian muscle. The adult nAChR is an intrinsic membrane protein with five distinct subunits ($\alpha_2\beta\delta\varepsilon$). Each subunit contains four helical domains labeled M1 to M4. The M2 domain forms the channel pore. The upper panel shows a single α subunit with its N and C termini on the extracellular surface of the membrane lipid bilayer. Between the N and C termini, the α subunit forms four helices (M1, M2, M3, and M4), which span the membrane bilayer. The lower panel shows the pentameric structure of the nAChR of adult mammalian muscle. The N termini of two subunits cooperate to form two distinct binding pockets for acetylcholine. These pockets occur at the ε-α and the δ-α subunit interface. The M2 membrane spanning domain of each subunit lines the ion channel. The doubly liganded ion channel has equal permeability to Na^+ and K^+; Ca^{2+} contributes approximately 2.5% to the total permeability. Reprinted with permission from Naguib M, Flood P, McArdle JJ, Brenner HR. Advances in neurobiology of the neuromuscular junction: implications for the anesthesiologist. *Anesthesiology*. 2002;96(1):202–231.

reorganization of the postsynaptic apparatus after denervation.[9] The postsynaptic region is further characterized by the presence of cytoskeletal and membrane proteins thought to be involved in its structural maintenance, and in the anchoring of nAChRs and of voltage-activated Na^+ channels; this region is also involved in the accumulation of several myonuclei, which selectively begin to express a new nAChR subunit (ε) at the synapse.[10,11] This ε subunit gives rise to a new, functionally distinct nAChR subtype (termed "adult"), with the subunit composition of 2α, β, δ, and ε in the synaptic muscle membrane (denoted as $\alpha_2\beta\delta\varepsilon$) (Figure 15.3).[7] This mature nAChR has shorter burst duration and a higher conductance to Na^+, K^+, and Ca^{2+} than the fetal nAChR.[12] As discussed below, fetal nAChRs gradually disappear both from synaptic and nonsynaptic muscle membranes as the muscle matures.

The development of the NMJ, like any other synapse, is controlled by complex dynamic interactions between the presynaptic and postsynaptic terminals. The postsynaptic apparatus is organized and maintained by signals from the presynaptic nerve terminal. The key processes in the differentiation, formation, and maintenance of postsynaptic structures at the NMJ include the release of agrin from the nerve terminal. Agrin is a proteoglycan that is involved in the aggregation of ACh receptors during synaptogenesis.[13] Typically, more than 90% of the nAChRs in a skeletal muscle fiber are found at the synapse, an area that only accounts for less than 0.1% of the total muscle membrane surface area.[14] The release of agrin activates muscle-specific tyrosine kinase (MuSK) located in the postsynaptic membrane. MuSK mediates agrin-induced aggregation and localization of nAChRs through their association with the cytoplasmic anchoring protein rapsyn.[1,15] An important role is played by rapsyn, a 43kD peripheral cytoplasmic membrane protein that is associated in a 1:1 ratio with the β-subunit of synaptic nAChRs.[14] Agrin is considered the key organizer of the postsynaptic apparatus at the NMJ. However, additional key components contribute to this pathway.[16,17] Although muscle fibers also express agrin, neural agrin is 1,000 times more active than muscle agrin in inducing nAChR clustering.[18]

THE NICOTINIC ACETYLCHOLINE RECEPTOR AT THE NEUROMUSCULAR JUNCTION

In the adult mammalian skeletal muscle the nAChR is a pentameric complex of two α subunits in association with a single β, δ, and ε subunit (Figure 15.3). These subunits are organized to form a transmembrane pore (a channel) as well as extracellular binding pockets for ACh and other agonists or antagonists.[1] Each of the two α-subunits has an acetylcholine-binding site (the α recognition site). These recognition sites are proteins located in pockets approximately 3.0 nm above the surface membrane at the interfaces of the α_H-ε and α_L-δ subunits.[19] The α_H and α_L indicate, respectively, the high- and low-affinity binding sites for *d*-tubocurarine (dTc), and probably are the result of the contribution from the different neighboring subunits.[20,21] For instance, the binding affinity of dTc for the α_H-ε site is ≈100- to 500-fold higher than that for the α_L-δ site.[19,21,22] As described above, the fetal nAChR contains a γ subunit instead of the adult ε subunit. This change explains, in part, why the mature nAChR exhibits shorter burst duration and a higher conductance to Na^+, K^+, and Ca^{2+} ions than the fetal nAChR.[1,12]

The fetal nAChR is a low conductance channel, in contrast to the high conductance channel of the adult nAChR. Thus, ACh release causes brief activation and

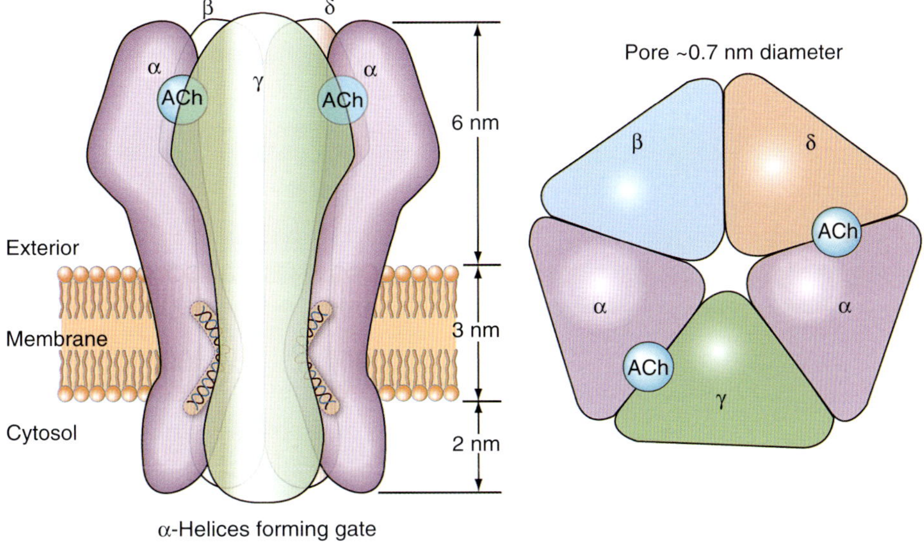

Figure 15.2 Nicotinic acetylcholine receptors (nAChRs) termed "fetal" (due to their expression early in development) consist of five subunits: two α subunits, as well as one β, one γ, and one δ subunit (denoted as $\alpha_2\beta\gamma\delta$). During the first two postnatal weeks, each postsynaptic motor site is innervated by multiple presynaptic nerve terminals. The α subunits contain the recognition site for ACh and all neuromuscular blocking agents.

reduced probability of channel opening.[1] Upregulation of nicotinic nAChRs, which occurs in states of functional or surgical denervation, is characterized by the spreading of predominantly fetal type nAChRs. These receptors are resistant to nondepolarizing neuromuscular blockers, but more sensitive to succinylcholine.[23] When depolarized, the immature receptor isoform has a prolonged open-channel time that exaggerates the K^+ efflux,[24] and results in high concentrations of plasma K^+ (hyperkalemia reported with the use of succinylcholine, for instance).

NEUROMUSCULAR TRANSMISSION AND EXCITATION-CONTRACTION COUPLING

When the motor neuron reaches the threshold current, it discharges an action potential that is propagated to the nerve terminal. This action potential usually activates all of the muscle fibers in the motor unit. This "all-or-none" property allows the nervous system to control the muscular force of contraction; thus, a variable but precise number of motor

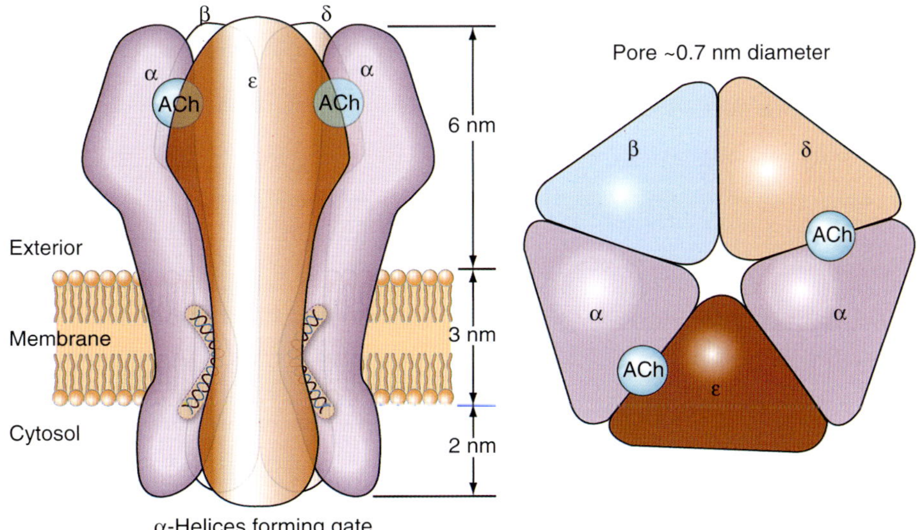

Figure 15.3 Nicotinic acetylcholine receptors (nAChRs) termed "adult" (due to their expression later in development) consist of five subunits: two α subunits, as well as one β, one δ, and one ε subunit (denoted as $\alpha_2\beta\delta\varepsilon$). Each postsynaptic adult motor site receives neuronal input from a single motor axon,[8] and the adult nAChRs are restricted in high concentrations (10,000/μm^2) in the postsynaptic membrane, but are virtually absent extrasynaptically. As with fetal nAChRs, the α subunit contains the recognition site for ACh and all neuromuscular blocking agents.

units in a particular muscle can be recruited (activated) and the intensity of muscle fiber activity is modulated by the rate and pattern of the action potentials. For instance, when the force of muscle contraction must be increased gradually, the number of individual motor units recruited increases, and the frequency of action potentials increases.[25] There are differences in the morphology of motor units, such as different innervation ratios, different muscle cross-sectional areas, different spatial alignment of muscle fibers within muscle, etc. These differences explain why the force of contraction within a particular motor neuron pool can vary by more than 50 times.[25] In contrast, the force of a single motor unit can only vary by a maximum of 15 times as the neuronal discharge rate is increased maximally.

The following is a summary of the processes that occur sequentially and result in muscle contraction:

(1) Motor nerve:

a. Depolarization of the motor nerve will open the voltage-gated Ca^{2+} channels that trigger both mobilization of synaptic vesicles and the fusion machinery in the nerve terminal to release ACh.

b. Several forms of K^+ channel present in the nerve terminal serve to limit the extent of Ca^{2+} entry and transmitter release (i.e., initiate repolarization of nerve terminal).[26]

(2) Muscle:

a. The released ACh binds to the α-subunits of the nAChRs. These ligand-gated cation channels open almost instantaneously when two ACh molecules bind cooperatively to sites on the extracellular surface of the protein, causing a conformational shift in the subunits. When the channel opens as a result of this conformational shift, Na^+ ions flow down their electrochemical gradient and into the muscle cell, depolarizing the muscle cell membrane at the neuromuscular junction; simultaneously, K^+ exits the cytosol of the fiber.[26,27]

b. The depolarization activates voltage-gated Na^+ channels that are present in the muscle membrane. These channels mediate the initiation and propagation of action potentials across the surface of the muscle membrane and into the transverse tubules (T-tubules), resulting in the upstroke of the action potential.[26–28]

c. There are two types of Ca^{2+} channels, dihydropyridine (DHP) receptor in the T-tubules, and the ryanodine receptor (RyR1) in the sarcoplasmic reticulum (SR) (Figure 15.4). The DHP receptors (DHPRs) act as "voltage sensors"[29,30] and are activated by membrane depolarization, which in turn activates RyR1 receptors.

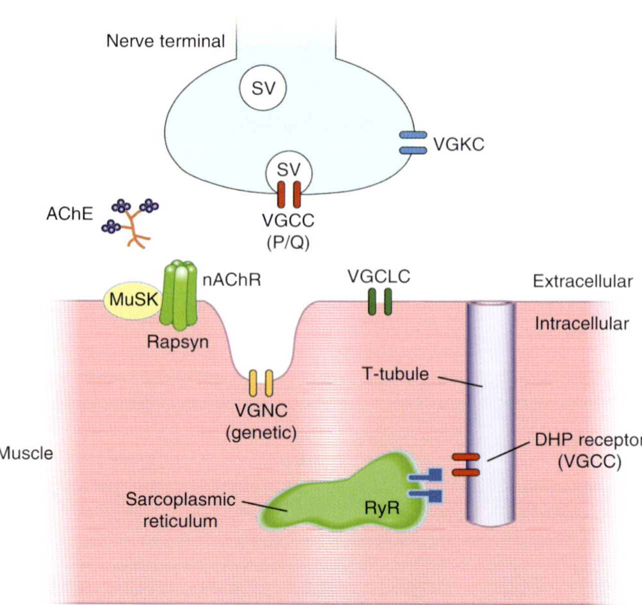

Figure 15.4 The two types of Ca^{2+} channels: the dihydropyridine (DHP) receptor in the T-tubules (the voltage-gated calcium channel), and the ryanodine receptor (RyR) in the sarcoplasmic reticulum. The DHP receptors (DHPRs) act as "voltage sensors"[29,30] and are activated by membrane depolarization, which in turn activates the RyR receptors. VG=voltage-gated, for each of the following channels: KC=potassium, CC=calcium, NC=sodium, CLC=chloride.

d. DHPR-RyR1 interaction[31] releases large amounts of Ca^{2+} from the sarcoplasmic reticulum, resulting in a transient increase in myoplasmic free Ca^{2+}, which binds to troponin C (Figure 15.5). This initiates the interaction between tropomyosin and troponin to form cross-bridges to the thin filament (actin), eventually resulting in development of tension (force of contraction). This process is known as excitation-contraction coupling.[32]

e. Repolarization of the muscle membrane is initiated by the closing of the Na^+ channels and by the opening of K^+ ion channels that conduct an outward K^+ current.[33]

f. The return of the muscle membrane potential to its resting level (approximately −70 to −90 mV) is achieved by allowing Cl^- to enter the cell through voltage-sensitive chloride channels.[26]

MOTOR UNIT RECRUITMENT AND DISCHARGE RATE

During low-force, isometric contraction, an increase in discharge rate (stimulation frequency) will result in a concurrent

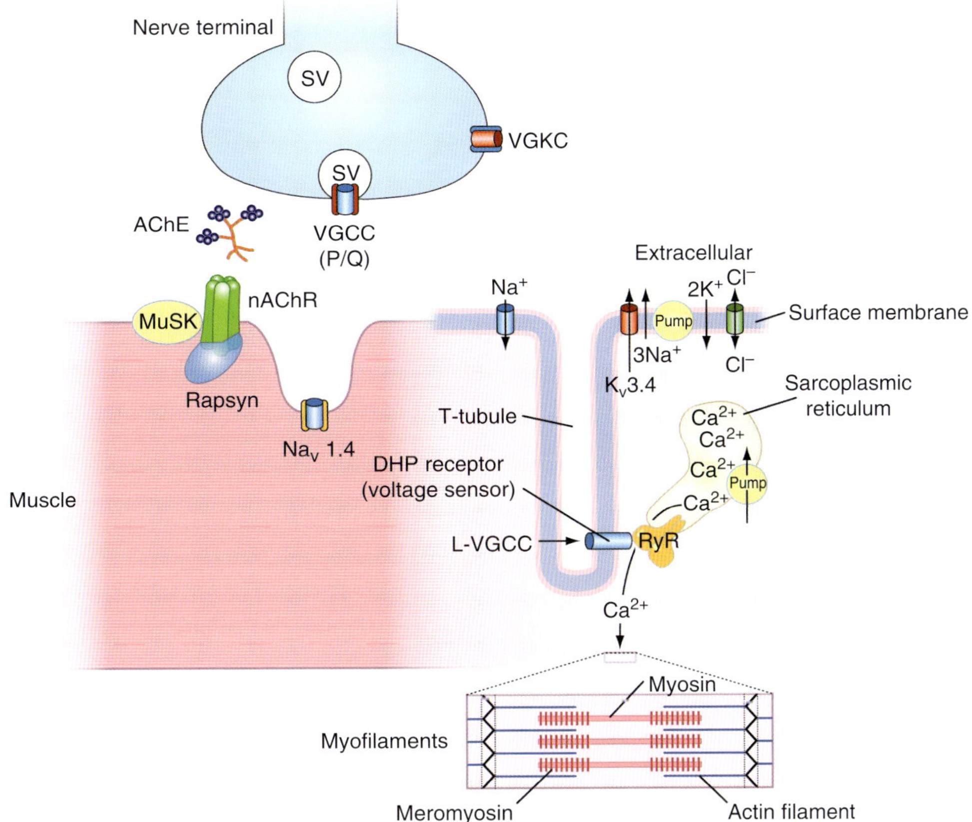

Figure 15.5 The interaction between the dihydropyridine (DHP) receptor and the ryanodine receptor (RyR)[31] releases large amounts of Ca^{2+} from the sarcoplasmic reticulum, resulting in a transient increase in myoplasmic free Ca^{2+}, which binds to troponin C. This binding initiates the interaction between tropomyosin and troponin to form cross-bridges to the thin filament (actin), eventually resulting in development of tension (force of contraction). This process is known as excitation-contraction coupling.[32]

increase in recruitment of motor units and a gradual increase in the force of muscle contraction.[34] For most muscles, maximal recruitment of motor units is reached at approximately 80% of the maximum contraction force, and the remaining 20% to maximal contraction is achieved by variation of discharge rate.[35]

GRADUAL RECRUITMENT OF MOTOR UNITS (FORCE GRADATION)

For seven decades, we have known that a particular voluntary movement appears always to begin with discharge of the same motor unit.[36] Force of contraction is increased by the recruitment of additional motor units. This addition, however, occurs in an orderly sequence that is always maintained. Thus, the initial force of contraction will activate smaller muscle fibers, and as the need for more force progresses, larger and more powerful motor units are recruited. This graded response has been termed the size principle, and states that motor units are recruited according to their increasing size.[37]

REFERENCES

1. Naguib M, Flood P, McArdle JJ, Brenner HR. Advances in neurobiology of the neuromuscular junction: implications for the anesthesiologist. *Anesthesiology.* 2002;96:202–231.
2. Liddell EGT, Sherrington CS. Recruitment and some other factors of reflex inhibition. *Proc R Soc Lond.* 1925;B97:488–518f.
3. Torre M. Number and dimensions of the motor units of the extrinsic eye muscles and, in general, of skeletal muscles connected with the sensory organs. *Schweiz Arch Neurol Psychiatr.* 1953;72:362–376.
4. Feinstein B, Lindegard B, Nyman E, Wohlfart G. Morphologic studies of motor units in normal human muscles. *Acta Anat.* 1955;23:127–142.
5. Riethmacher D, Sonnenberg-Riethmacher E, Brinkmann V, Yamaai T, Lewin GR, Birchmeier C. Severe neuropathies in mice with targeted mutations in the ErbB3 receptor. *Nature.* 1997;389:725–730.
6. Lin W, Sanchez HB, Deerinck T, Morris JK, Ellisman M, Lee K-F. Aberrant development of motor axons and neuromuscular synapses in erbB2-deficient mice. *Proc Natl Acad Sci U S A.* 2000;97:1299–1304.
7. Mishina M, Takai T, Imoto K, a;. Molecular distinction between fetal and adult forms of muscle acetylcholine receptor. *Nature.* 1986;321:406–411.
8. Redfern PA. Neuromuscular transmission in new-born rats. *J Physiol (Lond).* 1970;209:701–709.

9. Bezakova G, Ruegg MA. New insights into the roles of agrin. *Nat Rev Mol Cell Biol.* 2003;4:295–309.
10. Brenner HR, Witzemann V, Sakmann B. Imprinting of acetylcholine receptor messenger RNA accumulation in mammalian neuromuscular synapses. *Nature.* 1990;344:544–547.
11. Sanes JR, Johnson YR, Kotzbauer PT, et al. Selective expression of an acetylcholine receptor-lacZ transgene in synaptic nuclei of adult muscle fibers. *Development.* 1991;113:1181–1191.
12. Villarroel A, Sakmann B. Calcium permeability increase of endplate channels in rat muscle during postnatal development. *J Physiol (Lond).* 1996;496:331–338.
13. Magill C, Reist NE, Fallon JR, Nitkin RM, Wallace BG, McMahan UJ. Agrin. *Prog Brain Res.* 1987;71:391–396.
14. Froehner SC. The submembrane machinery for nicotinic acetylcholine receptor clustering. *J Cell Biol.* 1991;114:1–7.
15. Sanes JR, Lichtman JW. Induction, assembly, maturation and maintenance of a postsynaptic apparatus. *Nat Rev Neurosci.* 2001;2: 791–805.
16. Lin W, Burgess RW, Dominguez B, Pfaff SL, Sanes JR, Lee K-F. Distinct roles of nerve and muscle in postsynaptic differentiation of the neuromuscular synapse. *Nature.* 2001;410:1057–1064.
17. Okada K, Inoue A, Okada M, et al. The muscle protein Dok-7 is essential for neuromuscular synaptogenesis. *Science.* 2006;312: 1802–1805.
18. Ferns M, Hoch W, Campanelli JT, Rupp F, Hall ZW, Scheller RH. RNA splicing regulates agrin-mediated acetylcholine receptor clustering activity on cultured myotubes. *Neuron.* 1992;8:1079–1086.
19. Machold J, Weise C, Utkin Y, Tsetlin V, Hucho F. The handedness of the subunit arrangement of the nicotinic acetylcholine receptor from Torpedo californica. *Eur J Biochem.* 1995;234:427–430.
20. Yu XM, Hall ZW. Extracellular domains mediating epsilon subunit interactions of muscle acetylcholine receptor. *Nature.* 1991;352: 64–67.
21. Willcockson IU, Hong A, Whisenant RP, et al. Orientation of d-tubocurarine in the muscle nicotinic acetylcholine receptor-binding site. *J Biol Chem.* 2002;277:42249–42258.
22. Neubig RR, Cohen JB. Equilibrium binding of [3H]tubocurarine and [3H]acetylcholine by Torpedo postsynaptic membranes: stoichiometry and ligand interactions. *Biochemistry.* 1979;18: 5464–5475.
23. Martyn JA. Basic and clinical pharmacology of the acetylcholine receptor: implications for the use of neuromuscular relaxants. *Keio J Med.* 1995;44:1–8.
24. Kallen RG, Sheng ZH, Yang J, Chen LQ, Rogart RB, Barchi RL. Primary structure and expression of a sodium channel characteristic of denervated and immature rat skeletal muscle. *Neuron.* 1990;4: 233–242.
25. Enoka RM. Morphological features and activation patterns of motor units. *J Clin Neurophysiol.* 1995;12:538–559.
26. Cooper EC, Jan LY. Ion channel genes and human neurological disease: recent progress, prospects, and challenges. *Proc Natl Acad Sci U S A.* 1999;96:4759–4766.
27. Jurkat-Rott K, Lerche H, Lehmann-Horn F. Skeletal muscle channelopathies. *J Neurol.* 2002;249:1493–1502.
28. Lehmann-Horn F, Jurkat-Rott K. Voltage-gated ion channels and hereditary disease. *Physiol Rev.* 1999;79:1317–1372.
29. Rios E, Pizarro G. Voltage sensor of excitation-contraction coupling in skeletal muscle. *Physiol Rev.* 1991;71:849–908.
30. Fill M, Copello JA. Ryanodine receptor calcium release channels. *Physiol Rev.* 2002;82:893–922.
31. MacKrill JJ. Protein-protein interactions in intracellular $Ca2^+$-release channel function. *Biochem J.* 1999;337(Pt 3):345–361.
32. Hoffman EP. Voltage-gated ion channelopathies: inherited disorders caused by abnormal sodium, chloride, and calcium regulation in skeletal muscle. *Annu Rev Med.* 1995;46:431–441.
33. Lehmann-Horn F, Jurkat-Rott K, Rudel R. Periodic paralysis: understanding channelopathies. *Curr Neurol Neurosci Rep.* 2002;2: 61–69.
34. Person RS, Kudina LP. Discharge frequency and discharge pattern of human motor units during voluntary contraction of muscle. *Electroencephalogr Clin Neurophysiol.* 1972;32:471–483.
35. Kukulka CG, Clamann HP. Comparison of the recruitment and discharge properties of motor units in human brachial biceps and adductor pollicis during isometric contractions. *Brain Res.* 1981; 219:45–55.
36. Denny-Brown D, Pennybacker JB. Fibrillation and fasciculation in voluntary muscle. *Brain.* 1938;61:311–334.
37. Hanneman E. Functional organization of motoneuron pools: the size-principle. In: Asanuma H, Wilson VJ, eds. Integration in the Nervous System. Tokyo: Igaku-Shoin; 1977:13–25.

16

PHARMACOLOGY OF NEUROMUSCULAR BLOCKERS

Mohamed Naguib and Sorin J. Brull

INTRODUCTION

Investigation of the use of neuromuscular blockers in medicine was spurred in part by important findings at the beginning of the 20th century. In the 19th century and early years of the 20th century, the true nature of neurotransmission was disputed—it was debated whether transmission across synapses was chemical or electrical. Originally, there was broad support for the concept that impulses in the nerves acted directly on muscle, resulting in muscular contraction—the "electrical theory." The electrical theory was eventually refuted with the discovery of the role of acetylcholine in neuromuscular transmission,[1,2] and in 1936, the Nobel Prize in Physiology or Medicine was awarded to Sir Henry Hallett Dale (1875–1968) and Otto Loewi (1873–1961) "for their discoveries relating to chemical transmission of nerve impulses." This was followed by the discovery that a muscle membrane–bound allosteric protein, the nicotinic acetylcholine receptor, was involved in the pharmacological response to acetylcholine.[3]

The first successful administration of a neuromuscular blocker (curare) to produce surgical relaxation in an anesthetized patient occurred in 1912, when Arthur Läwen, a German surgeon from Leipzig, used a partially purified preparation of the substance.[4] Läwen's findings were subsequently ignored for nearly three decades until January 23, 1942, when Enid Johnson, following Harold Griffith's instructions, administered 5 mL of curare intravenously to a 20-year-old man who had been anesthetized with cyclopropane via a facemask for an appendectomy.[5] The use of neuromuscular blockers in clinical anesthesia has increased exponentially since that time.

Neuromuscular blockers that are currently available for clinical use are classified as: 1) nondepolarizing neuromuscular blockers; or 2) depolarizing neuromuscular blockers. Nondepolarizing neuromuscular blockers compete with acetylcholine for the active binding sites at the postsynaptic nicotinic acetylcholine receptor and are also called competitive antagonists. Depolarizing neuromuscular blockers act as agonists (i.e., they are similar in structure to acetylcholine) at postsynaptic nicotinic acetylcholine receptors and cause prolonged membrane depolarization. Prolonged depolarization results in neuromuscular blockade, as described in detail in the section "Characteristics of Nondepolarizing and Depolarizing Neuromuscular Block" later in this chapter. Succinylcholine is the only depolarizing neuromuscular blocker currently in clinical use.

PRINCIPLES OF ACTION OF NEUROMUSCULAR BLOCKERS AT THE NEUROMUSCULAR JUNCTION

Functionally, in the resting state, the ion channel of the acetylcholine receptor is closed. Simultaneous binding of two acetylcholine molecules to the α-subunits[6] initiates conformational changes that open the channel (see Chapter 15 for details).[7–9] On the other hand, binding of a single molecule of a nondepolarizing neuromuscular blocker (a competitive antagonist) to one α-subunit is sufficient to produce neuromuscular block.[10]

Depolarizing neuromuscular blockers, such as succinylcholine, produce prolonged depolarization of the endplate region that results in 1) desensitization of nicotinic acetylcholine receptors; 2) inactivation of voltage-gated sodium channels at the neuromuscular junction; and 3) increases in potassium permeability in the surrounding membrane. The end result is failure of action potential generation due to membrane hyperpolarization, and block ensues. It should be noted that although acetylcholine also produces depolarization, under physiological conditions it results in muscle contraction but not paralysis because it has a very short (1 ms) duration of action. However, administration of large doses of acetylcholine in experimental animals produces neuromuscular block.[10]

With respect to neuromuscular pharmacology, two enzymes of importance are known to hydrolyze choline esters: acetylcholinesterase and butyrylcholinesterase. Acetylcholinesterase (similar to red cell cholinesterase and also known as "true" cholinesterase) is present at the neuromuscular junction[11] and is responsible for the rapid hydrolysis of released acetylcholine to acetic acid and choline. Acetylcholinesterase has one of the highest catalytic efficiencies known. It can catalyze acetylcholine hydrolysis at near diffusion-limited rates (4,000 molecules of acetylcholine hydrolyzed per active site per second).[12] Butyrylcholinesterase (also known as plasma cholinesterase or pseudocholinesterase) is synthesized in the liver. Butyrylcholinesterase is present in only very small amounts at the neuromuscular junction and catalyzes the hydrolysis of butyrylcholine. Butyrylcholinesterase also catalyzes the hydrolysis of succinylcholine.

Succinylcholine is not metabolized by acetylcholinesterase, so succinylcholine administration results in a prolonged activation of the postsynaptic nicotinic acetylcholine receptors. Metabolism of succinylcholine by butyrylcholinesterase occurs mainly in the plasma.

STRUCTURE OF NEUROMUSCULAR BLOCKING DRUGS

All neuromuscular blockers, being quaternary ammonium compounds, are structurally related to acetylcholine. The majority of neuromuscular blocking drugs currently available for clinical use are synthetic alkaloids. An exception is tubocurarine, which is extracted from plants. Although tubocurarine can be synthesized, it is less expensive to isolate this drug from the Amazonian vine *Chondrodendron tomentosum*. In terms of chemical structures, some neuromuscular blocking drugs contain two quaternary ammonium cations (e.g., succinylcholine, pancuronium, and atracurium). Other neuromuscular blocking drugs contain one quaternary and one tertiary nitrogen atom (e.g., tubocurarine, vecuronium, and rocuronium). Bisquaternary amines are more potent than monoquaternary amines.

CHARACTERISTICS OF NONDEPOLARIZING AND DEPOLARIZING NEUROMUSCULAR BLOCK

During complete neuromuscular block, no response can be elicited by any pattern of nerve stimulation—single twitch, train-of-four stimulation (four stimuli delivered every 0.5 seconds), or a tetanic stimulus. However, during partial neuromuscular block, the pattern of muscle response varies with the type of neuromuscular blocker administered and the degree of block.

NONDEPOLARIZING NEUROMUSCULAR BLOCK

Nondepolarizing neuromuscular block is characterized by: 1) decrease in twitch tension; 2) fade during repetitive stimulation (train-of-four or tetanic); and 3) posttetanic potentiation (Figure 16.1).

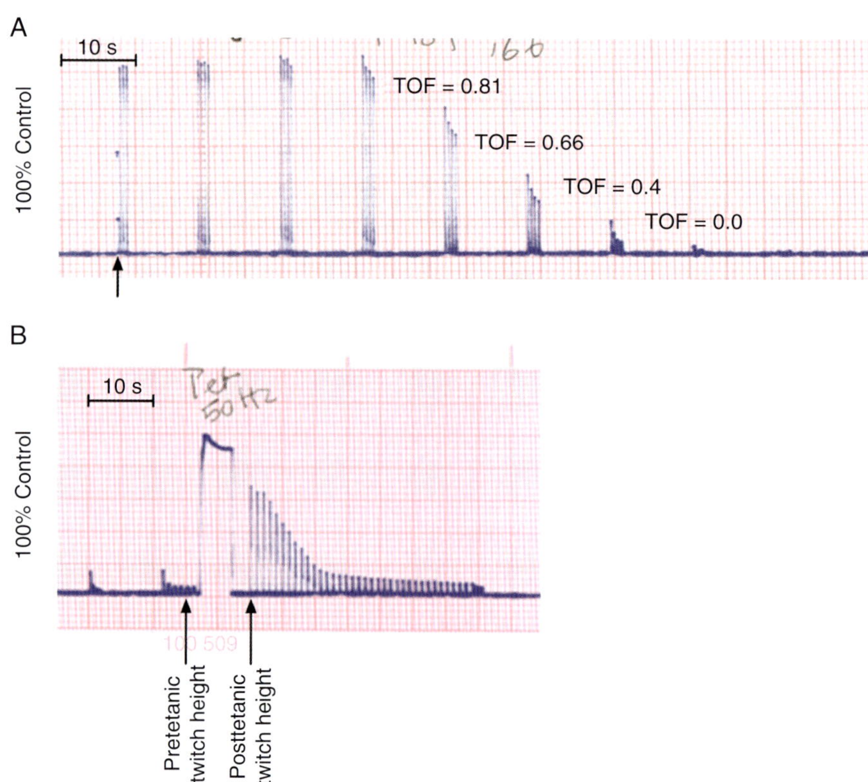

Figure 16.1 Mechanomyographic recording during the course of neuromuscular blockade induced by a nondepolarizing agent. A) Train-of-four (TOF) fade is noted during the onset of block. B) During partial recovery, tetanic fade and posttetanic potentiation are present after application of a 5-second, 50-Hz tetanic stimulation (Tet 50 Hz).

It is generally believed that twitch depression and tetanic or train-of-four fade are independent phenomena. Studies with nondepolarizing blockers have demonstrated that when twitch height has returned to baseline, significant degrees of fade in the train-of-four response may still be present.[13] It is generally believed that twitch depression results from block of postsynaptic nicotinic acetylcholine receptors, whereas tetanic or train-of-four fade results from block of presynaptic nicotinic acetylcholine receptors.[14,15] Blockade of the presynaptic nicotinic acetylcholine receptors by neuromuscular blockers prevents acetylcholine from being made available (released from presynaptic nerve terminal) to sustain muscle contraction during high-frequency (tetanic or train-of-four) stimulation. Because the released acetylcholine does not match the demand, muscle fade is observed in response to stimulation.[16]

However, there is also strong contrary evidence indicating that fade could be simply a postjunctional (postsynaptic) phenomenon. This latter argument is supported by the fact that the snake α-bungarotoxin—which binds irreversibly to muscle (postjunctional) nicotinic acetylcholine receptors but does not bind to neuronal (prejunctional) nicotinic acetylcholine receptors—does produce fade.[17,18]

DEPOLARIZING NEUROMUSCULAR BLOCK

In the case of administration of a depolarizing neuromuscular blocking agent, such as succinylcholine, the muscle response that has been "classically" described is quite different. Depolarizing block (also called phase I block) is often preceded by muscle fasciculation. During partial neuromuscular block, depolarizing block is characterized by: 1) decrease in twitch tension; 2) no fade during repetitive stimulation (tetanic or train-of-four); and 3) no posttetanic potentiation (Figure 16.2).

However, with prolonged exposure of the neuromuscular junction to succinylcholine or with administration of a single dose in patients with an abnormal genetic variant of butyrylcholinesterase, the characteristics of the neuromuscular block can be changed from those of the classic depolarizing (phase I) block to those of phase II block (characterized by fade during train-of-four and tetanic stimulation and posttetanic potentiation—similar to that induced by nondepolarizing neuromuscular blockers). A recent study, however, showed that posttetanic potentiation and fade in response to train-of-four and tetanic stimuli are characteristics of neuromuscular block even after a single bolus administration of different doses of succinylcholine.[19] It seems that some characteristics of a phase II block are evident from an initial dose (i.e., as small as 0.3 mg/kg) of succinylcholine.[19]

PHARMACOLOGY OF SUCCINYLCHOLINE

STRUCTURE-ACTIVITY RELATIONSHIPS FOR SUCCINYLCHOLINE

The depolarizing neuromuscular blocker succinylcholine is a long, thin, flexible molecule comprised of two molecules of acetylcholine linked back-to-back through the acetate methyl groups (Figure 16.3). Like acetylcholine, succinylcholine stimulates cholinergic receptors at the neuromuscular junction and at nicotinic (ganglionic) and muscarinic autonomic sites, opening the ionic channel in the acetylcholine receptor.

PHARMACOKINETICS, PHARMACODYNAMICS, AND PHARMACOGENOMICS OF SUCCINYLCHOLINE

Succinylcholine, introduced by Thesleff[20] in 1951 and Foldes et al in 1952,[21] is the only available neuromuscular blocker with a rapid onset of action and an ultrashort

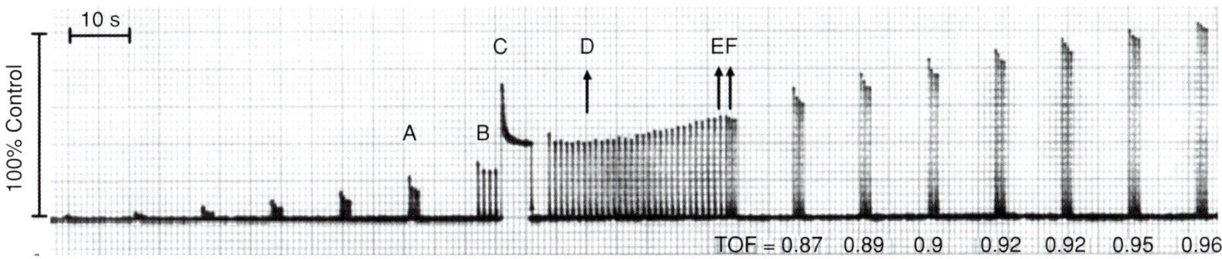

Figure 16.2 Mechanomyographic recording during recovery from 1.0 mg/kg succinylcholine. Note the fade in the train-of-four (TOF) response (A) during recovery. At 12% recovery of T1 (the first twitch in the train-of-four), the TOF ratio was 0.58 (A). Thereafter, the mode of stimulation was changed to 1-Hz single-twitch stimulation (B) followed by a tetanic stimulus (50 Hz) for 5 s (C). Three seconds later, the 1-Hz single twitch was again applied for 33 s, followed by TOF stimulation. The pretetanic twitch height (B) was 25% of control. Tetanic fade (C) was also present. The tetanic fade ratio (C) was 0.55 (measured as the amplitude of the contraction at the end of the 5-s tetanic stimulation divided by the amplitude of the contraction at the beginning of the tetanic stimulation). The minimum (D) and maximum (E) posttetanic twitch heights were 40% and 56% of control, respectively. This represents an increase of 160% and 224%, respectively, compared with the pretetanic value. Thereafter, posttetanic TOF ratio (F) recovery proceeded at a higher value (TOF = 0.95) than that noted before tetanic stimulation.

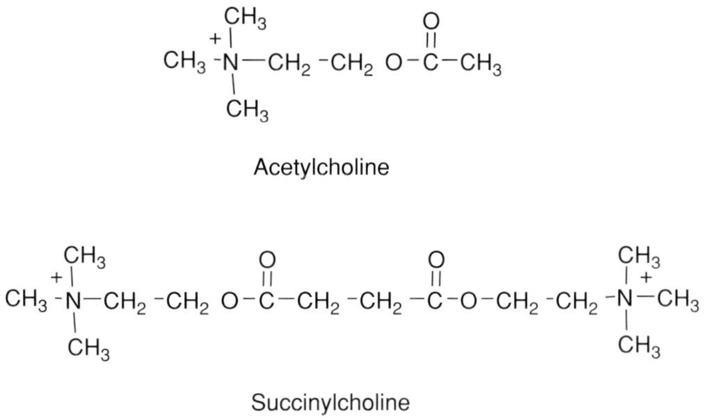

Acetylcholine

Succinylcholine

Figure 16.3 Structural relationship of succinylcholine, a depolarizing neuromuscular blocking agent, to acetylcholine. Succinylcholine consists of two acetylcholine molecules linked through the acetate methyl groups. Like acetylcholine, succinylcholine stimulates nicotinic receptors at the neuromuscular junction.

duration of action. It has an elimination half-life of 47 s (95% confidence interval of 24 to 70 s).[22] The elimination of succinylcholine appears to follow first-order kinetics.[22,23] The $t_{1/2}K_{e0}$ and Hill coefficient (after fitting two doses of 1 mg/kg succinylcholine) were 244 s (standard deviation 157) and 7.9 (standard deviation 3.3), respectively.[22] The dose of succinylcholine causing on average 95% suppression of twitch height (the ED_{95}) is approximately 0.3 mg/kg.[24,25]

The usual dose of succinylcholine required for tracheal intubation in adults is 1.0 mg/kg. Administration of 1.0 mg/kg succinylcholine results in complete suppression of response to neuromuscular stimulation in approximately 60 seconds.[26–28] In patients with genotypically normal butyrylcholinesterase activity, time to recovery to 90% muscle strength following administration of 1 mg/kg succinylcholine ranges from 9 to 13 minutes.[29,30] In one study, administration of 0.6 mg/kg of succinylcholine resulted in acceptable intubating conditions at 60 s in 95% of patients.[31] The reported proportions of patients with acceptable intubating conditions after administration of 1.0 mg/kg succinylcholine varies from 91.8% to 97%.[32–34] It also appears that there are no advantages to using succinylcholine doses larger than 1.5 mg/kg in a rapid sequence induction of anesthesia. Paradoxically, succinylcholine doses as large as 2.0 mg/kg guaranteed excellent intubating conditions at 60 s in only 86.7% of patients.[35] It should be noted that the adequacy of intubating conditions is related not only to the use of a neuromuscular blocker but also to the depth of anesthesia, airway anatomy, and the experience of the laryngoscopist.

The short duration of action of succinylcholine is due to its rapid hydrolysis by butyrylcholinesterase to succinylmonocholine and choline, such that only 10% of the administered drug reaches the neuromuscular junction.[36] Succinylmonocholine is a much weaker neuromuscular blocking agent than succinylcholine[37] and is metabolized much more slowly to succinic acid and choline.

Because there is little or no butyrylcholinesterase at the neuromuscular junction itself, butyrylcholinesterase influences the onset and duration of action of succinylcholine by controlling the rate at which the drug is hydrolyzed in the plasma before it reaches, and after it leaves, the neuromuscular junction. Recovery from succinylcholine-induced blockade occurs as succinylcholine diffuses away from the neuromuscular junction, down a concentration gradient as the plasma concentration decreases.

FACTORS AFFECTING BUTYRYLCHOLINESTERASE ACTIVITY

Butyrylcholinesterase is synthesized by the liver and found in the plasma. The enzyme consists of four identical subunits (574 amino acids each) and nine carbohydrate chains, with a total molecular weight of approximately 342,000 daltons. It contains two active sites, one anionic and the other catalytic.[38,39] Butyrylcholinesterase is responsible for metabolism of succinylcholine, mivacurium, procaine, chloroprocaine, tetracaine, cocaine, and heroin. Neuromuscular block induced by succinylcholine or mivacurium is prolonged when there is a significant reduction in the concentration or activity of butyrylcholinesterase. The activity of the enzyme refers to the number of substrate molecules (µmol) hydrolyzed per unit of time, often expressed in international units.

Factors that have been described as lowering butyrylcholinesterase activity are liver disease,[40] advanced age,[41] malnutrition, pregnancy, burns, oral contraceptives, monoamine oxidase inhibitors, echothiophate, cytotoxic drugs, neoplastic disease, anticholinesterase drugs,[42,43] metoclopramide,[44] and bambuterol.[45,46] The beta-blocker esmolol inhibits butyrylcholinesterase but causes only a minor prolongation of succinylcholine block.[47,48]

Large reductions in butyrylcholinesterase activity result in only moderate increases in the duration of action of succinylcholine. For instance, in severe liver disease when butyrylcholinesterase activity is reduced to 20% of normal, the duration of apnea following succinylcholine administration increases from a normal duration of 3 minutes to only 9 minutes.

GENETIC VARIANTS OF BUTYRYLCHOLINESTERASE

Neuromuscular block induced by succinylcholine or mivacurium can be significantly prolonged if the patient has an abnormal genetic variant of butyrylcholinesterase. The *butyrylcholinesterase* gene is located at the E_1 locus on the long arm of chromosome 3 (3q26.1–q26.2). Over 20 genetic variants of butyrylcholinesterase have been described.[49] Analysis of butyrylcholinesterase involves the determination of both enzyme activity and biochemical phenotypes. Phenotype is determined by the use of specific enzyme inhibitors (such as dibucaine or fluoride) that produce phenotype-specific patterns of dibucaine or fluoride numbers. Molecular genetic analyses can determine the true genotypes. For reviews, see Pantuck[50] and Goodall.[51]

Among the variants of butyrylcholinesterase is a dibucaine-resistant variant, a result of a point mutation in exon 2 (nt 209A→G), which is manifested by an amino acid change Asp70→Gly. Dibucaine inhibits normal butyrylcholinesterase to a far greater extent than the abnormal enzyme. The dibucaine number indicates the percentage inhibition of butyrylcholinesterase in the presence of dibucaine. In the case of the usual butyrylcholinesterase genotype ($E_1^uE_1^u$), the dibucaine number is 70 or higher, while in individuals homozygous for the atypical gene ($E_1^aE_1^a$) (frequency in general population of 1 in 3,500), the dibucaine number is less than 30. In individuals with the heterozygous atypical variant ($E_1^uE_1^a$) (frequency in general population of 1 in 480), the dibucaine number is in the range of 40 to 60.[52,53] In individuals with the homozygous atypical genotype ($E_1^aE_1^a$), the neuromuscular block induced by succinylcholine or mivacurium is prolonged to 4 to 8 hours, and in individuals with the heterozygous atypical genotype ($E_1^uE_1^a$), the period of neuromuscular block induced by succinylcholine or mivacurium is about 1.5 to 2 times that seen in individuals with the usual genotype ($E_1^uE_1^u$).[54] The longest period of apnea after the administration of succinylcholine was found in patients homozygous for the silent gene ($E_1^sE_1^s$).[54] In those patients, train-of-four stimulation will help in detecting the development of phase II block. The decision whether to attempt antagonism of a phase II block has always been controversial. However, if the train-of-four ratio is less than 0.4, administration of edrophonium or neostigmine should result in prompt antagonism.[55] The alternative is to keep the patient adequately sedated and maintain artificial ventilation until the train-of-four ratio has recovered to 0.9 or more.

Fluoride-resistant butyrylcholinesterase variants have also been described. In the case of the fluoride-resistant gene, two amino acid substitutions are possible, namely, methionine for threonine at position 243 and valine for glycine at position 390. The fluoride number indicates the percentage inhibition of butyrylcholinesterase in the presence of fluoride. In case of the usual butyrylcholinesterase genotype ($E_1^uE_1^u$), the fluoride number is 60, while in individuals with the homozygous atypical genotype ($E_1^fE_1^f$), the fluoride number is 36. The fluoride-resistant gene was found in 2.7% of patients with prolonged apnea after administration of succinylcholine.[54] Individuals with homozygous fluoride-resistant genotype exhibit mild to moderate prolongation of succinylcholine-induced paralysis. The heterozygous fluoride-resistant genotype usually produces clinically insignificant prolongation of succinylcholine block, unless accompanied by a second abnormal allele or by a coexisting acquired cause of butyrylcholinesterase deficiency.

Although the dibucaine or fluoride number indicates the genetic makeup of an individual with respect to butyrylcholinesterase, it does not measure the concentration of the enzyme in the plasma, nor does it indicate the efficiency of the enzyme in hydrolyzing a substrate such as succinylcholine or mivacurium. Both of these latter factors are determined by measuring butyrylcholinesterase activity—which may be influenced by genotype.

There are also some so-called quantitative cholinesterase variants of butyrylcholinesterase (K, H, and J type). The K-variant is the most common one, with an allele frequency of 13%, and it results in a 30% decrease in activity due to the reduction of circulating active enzyme molecules. A G→A base change at position 1615 causes an amino acid alteration Ala539→Thr.[56] The SC variant refers to an enzyme that is identified as normal by usual phenotyping methods although it displays impaired activity in hydrolyzing succinylcholine.[57]

Although most genetic variants of serum butyrylcholinesterase are associated with decreased activity, some rare variants are associated with increased enzyme activity (2 to 3 times normal).[58] These variants have normal dibucaine and fluoride numbers, and the enhanced activity has been attributed to either an increased number of enzyme molecules[58] or increased activity per active site.[59] Resistance to succinylcholine[60] and mivacurium[61] as a result of increased butyrylcholinesterase activity has been described.

SIDE EFFECTS OF SUCCINYLCHOLINE

Cardiovascular Effects

Succinylcholine—because of its inherent activities on all cholinergic autonomic sites—can induce a wide range of cardiac dysrhythmias,[62] ranging from sinus bradycardia to junctional rhythms to ventricular dysrhythmias. Succinylcholine may show a paradoxical effect. In low doses, succinylcholine has negative inotropic and chronotropic effects. In large doses, these effects may become positive,[63] causing tachycardia.

Sinus bradycardia (resulting from stimulation of cardiac muscarinic receptors) is frequently seen in children[64] and in adults after a repeated dose of succinylcholine.[65] Atropine is effective in treating or preventing bradycardia. Ventricular dysrhythmias after succinylcholine administration have been attributed to increases in circulating catecholamines and potassium concentrations[66–68] and to other autonomic stimuli associated with laryngoscopy and tracheal intubation.[69]

Hyperkalemia

The administration of succinylcholine is associated with a modest increase in the plasma potassium concentration—approximately 0.5 mEq/dL in healthy individuals. This slight increase in potassium concentration is well tolerated and generally does not cause dysrhythmias. Patients with renal failure are no more susceptible to an exaggerated hyperkalemic response to succinylcholine than are patients with normal renal function.[70,71]

Succinylcholine has been associated with severe hyperkalemia in patients with burn, severe abdominal infections,[72] severe metabolic acidosis,[73] closed head injury,[74] or conditions associated with upregulation of extrajunctional acetylcholine receptors (e.g., hemiplegia or paraplegia, muscular dystrophies, Guillain-Barré syndrome, and burn). For reviews, see Naguib et al[11] and Martyn and Richtsfeld.[75] Because of the risk of massive rhabdomyolysis, hyperkalemia, and death in children with undiagnosed muscle disease, succinylcholine is not recommended for use in children except for emergency tracheal intubation.[76–78]

Increased Intraocular Pressure

Succinylcholine usually causes an increase in intraocular pressure. The intraocular pressure peaks at 2 to 4 minutes after administration and returns to normal by 6 minutes.[79] This increase has been attributed to contraction of tonic myofibrils and/or transient dilatation of choroidal blood vessels. The use of succinylcholine is not widely accepted in open eye injury (when the anterior chamber is open) even though succinylcholine was shown to cause no adverse events in a series of 73 patients with penetrating eye injuries.[80] The efficacy of precurarization in attenuating increases in intraocular pressure following succinylcholine administration is controversial.[81–83]

Increased Intragastric Pressure

Administration of succinylcholine is associated with a variable increase in intragastric pressure and a corresponding increase in lower esophageal sphincter pressure. The increase in intragastric pressure appears to be related to: 1) the intensity of fasciculations of the abdominal skeletal muscles,[84] which could be prevented by prior administration of a nondepolarizing neuromuscular blocker; and 2) a direct increase in vagal tone. Administration of succinylcholine does not predispose to regurgitation in patients with an intact lower esophageal sphincter because the increase in intragastric pressure does not exceed the "barrier pressure."[85]

Increased Intracranial Pressure

Succinylcholine has the potential to increase intracranial pressure.[86] This increase can be attenuated or prevented by pretreatment with a nondepolarizing neuromuscular blocker.[87]

Myalgias

The incidence of muscle pain following administration of succinylcholine varies from 0.2% to 89%.[88] Muscle pain occurs more frequently in patients undergoing ambulatory surgery, especially in women, than in bedridden patients.[89] The pain characteristically affects the neck, shoulders, and chest. The mechanism of succinylcholine-induced myalgia appears to be complex and is not fully understood. One hypothesis proposes that myalgia is secondary to muscle damage by succinylcholine-induced fasciculations.[89] This hypothesis is supported by findings of myoglobinemia and increases in serum creatine kinase level following succinylcholine administration.[90–92] However, although prior administration of a small dose of a nondepolarizing neuromuscular blocker prevents fasciculations due to succinylcholine, this approach is not always effective in preventing succinylcholine-induced myalgia.[88,93] Another hypothesis suggests a possible role for prostaglandins and cyclooxygenases in succinylcholine-induced myalgias.[94,95] Pretreatment with a prostaglandin inhibitor (lysine acetyl salicylate or diclofenac) has been shown to be effective in decreasing the incidence of muscle pain after succinylcholine administration.[94,96] Other investigators, however, have found that myalgias following outpatient surgery occur even in the absence of succinylcholine.[97,98]

Masseter Spasm

Succinylcholine is a known trigger agent for malignant hyperthermia. While an increase in tone of the masseter muscle may be an early indicator of malignant hyperthermia,[99] it is not consistently associated with malignant hyperthermia.[100–102] It has been suggested that the high incidence of masseter spasm in children given succinylcholine may be due to inadequate succinylcholine dosage.[103]

PHARMACOLOGY OF NONDEPOLARIZING NEUROMUSCULAR BLOCKERS

Available nondepolarizing neuromuscular blockers can be classified according to chemical class (the steroidal, benzylisoquinolinium, and other blockers) or according to rapidity of onset or duration of action (long-acting, intermediate-acting, or short-acting) of equipotent doses (Table 16.1). The pharmacodynamic and pharmacokinetic behaviors of currently used and new nondepolarizing neuromuscular blockers are shown in Tables 16.2 and 16.3, respectively.

STRUCTURE-ACTIVITY RELATIONSHIPS

The currently used nondepolarizing neuromuscular blocking agents have either a benzylisoquinoline or aminosteroidal structure. Nondepolarizing neuromuscular blocking drugs were originally classified by Bovet[104] as pachycurares, or bulky molecules having the amine functions incorporated into rigid ring structures. Detailed structure-activity relationships have been described elsewhere.[105–108]

Table 16.1 CLASSIFICATION OF COMMONLY USED AND NEW NONDEPOLARIZING NEUROMUSCULAR BLOCKERS ACCORDING TO DURATION OF ACTION (TIME TO T1 = 25% OF CONTROL) AFTER ADMINISTRATION OF 2 × ED_{95}[a]

	DURATION OF ACTION			
	LONG (> 50 min)	INTERMEDIATE (20–50 min)	SHORT (10–20 min)	ULTRASHORT (< 10 min)
Steroidal compounds	**Pancuronium**	**Vecuronium Rocuronium**	—	—
Benzylisoquinolinium compounds	**Tubocurarine**	**Atracurium Cisatracurium**	**Mivacurium**	—
Olefinic isoquinolinium diester compounds	—	**CW002 (AV002)**	—	**Gantacurium**

ED_{95} is the dose that results in 95% depression of twitch height.
[a] The majority of nondepolarizing neuromuscular blockers are bisquaternary ammonium compounds. Tubocurarine, vecuronium, and rocuronium are monoquaternary compounds.

Table 16.2 DOSE-RESPONSE RELATIONSHIPS AND PHARMACODYNAMIC PARAMETERS FOR NONDEPOLARIZING NEUROMUSCULAR BLOCKING DRUGS IN HUMAN SUBJECTS[a]

	ED_{50} (mg/kg)	ED_{95} (mg/kg)	CE_{50} (ng/ml)	K_{E0} (min^{-1})	INTUBATING DOSE (mg/kg)	MAXIMUM BLOCK (%)	TIME TO MAXIMUM BLOCK (min)	CLINICAL DURATION OF RESPONSE[b] (min)
				Long-acting				
***d*-Tubocurarine**	0.23	0.48	370	0.13	0.6	97	5.7	81
Pancuronium	0.036	0.067	88	—	0.08	100	2.9	86
				Intermediate-acting				
Rocuronium	0.147	0.305	3510	0.405	0.6	100	1.7	36
Vecuronium	0.027	0.043	92	0.17	0.1	100	2.4	44
Atracurium	0.12	0.21	449	0.13	0.5	100	3.2	46
Cisatracurium	0.026	0.04	126–158	0.07–0.09	0.1	100	5.2	45
				Short-acting				
Mivacurium	0.039	0.067	79.9	0.18	0.15	100	3.3	16.8
				Ultrashort-acting				
Gantacurium	0.09	0.19			0.4	100	1.5	8.9

ED_{50} and ED_{95} are the doses of each drug that produce, respectively, 50% and 95% decrease in the force of contraction or amplitude of the electromyogram of the adductor pollicis muscle following ulnar nerve stimulation.
CE_{50} is the neuromuscular junction concentration of each drug that produces a 50% decrease in the force of contraction or amplitude of the electromyogram of the adductor pollicis muscle following ulnar nerve stimulation.
k_{e0} is the rate constant for equilibration of drug between the plasma and the neuromuscular junction.
[a] Derived using simultaneous pharmacokinetic/pharmacodynamic modeling.
[b] Time from injection of the intubating dose to recovery of twitch to 25% of control.

Table 16.3 **PHARMACOKINETIC PARAMETERS FOR NEUROMUSCULAR BLOCKING DRUGS**

	PLASMA CLEARANCE (mL/kg/min)	VOLUME OF DISTRIBUTION (mL/kg)	ELIMINATION HALF-LIFE (min)	REFERENCE
		Short-acting		
Mivacurium isomers				219
Cis-trans	106	278	2.0	
Trans-trans	57	211	2.3	
Cis-cis	3.8	227	68	
		Intermediate-acting		
Atracurium	6.1	182	21	121
	10.9	280	17.3	220
Cisatracurium	5.2	31	—	129
Vecuronium	3.0	194	78	147
	5.3	199	53	221
Rocuronium	2.9	207	71	155
		Long-acting		
***d*-Tubocurarine**	2.4	250	84	222
Pancuronium	1.7	261	132	223

BENZYLISOQUINOLINIUM COMPOUNDS

The South American Indians' arrow poisons, known as curare, served as the basis for the development of the benzylisoquinoline-type relaxants. Tubocurarine, the most important curare alkaloid, was introduced as a neuromuscular blocking drug for use during surgical anesthesia.[4,5]

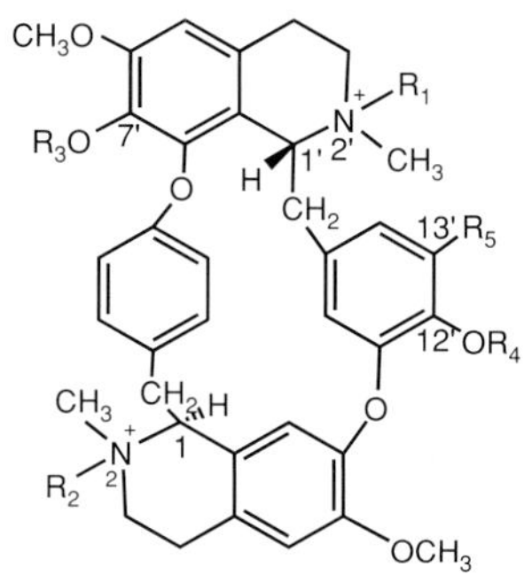

Cyclic benzylisoquinoline

Cyclic benzylisoquinoline derivatives

Name	R_1	R_2	R_3	R_4	R_5	1	1'
Tubocurarine	CH_3	H	H	H	H	*S*	*R*
Chondrocurine	CH_3	CH_3	H	H	H	*S*	*R*

R and *S* represent the stereochemical configuration about the designated carbon

Figure 16.4 Chemical structures of tubocurarine and chondrocurine.

Tubocurarine

Tubocurarine is a monoquarternary, long-acting neuromuscular blocker in which the amines are present in the form of two benzyl-substituted tetrahydroisoquinoline structures (Figure 16.4). Tubocurarine contains only three *N*-methyl groups.[109] One amine is quaternary (permanently charged with four nitrogen substituents), and the other is tertiary (pH-dependent charge with three nitrogen substituents). At physiological pH, the tertiary nitrogen is protonated to render it positively charged. Both the ganglion-blocking and the histamine-releasing properties of tubocurarine are probably due to the presence of the tertiary amine function. Bisquaternary compounds are more potent than their monoquaternary analogs.[110]

There is no active metabolism of tubocurarine. It is excreted unchanged in the urine, and the liver is probably a secondary route of elimination. Therefore, and because more suitable agents are available, tubocurarine is not indicated for use in patients with either renal[111] or hepatic failure. The onset of action of tubocurarine is slow, its duration of action is long, and its recovery is slow (Table 16.2).

The usual intubating dose is 0.5 to 0.6 mg/kg; maintenance doses are 0.1 to 0.2 mg/kg.

Atracurium

Atracurium consists of a racemic mixture of 10 stereoisomers.[112,113] These isomers have been separated into three geometrical isomer groups that are designated *cis-cis*, *cis-trans*, and *trans-trans* based on their configuration about the tetrahydroisoquinoline ring system.[112,113] The ratio of the *cis-cis*, *cis-trans*, and *trans-trans* isomers is approximately 10:6:1, corresponding to about 50% to 55% *cis-cis*, 35% to 38% *cis-trans*, and 6% to 7% *trans-trans* isomers.[114]

Atracurium has been designed to undergo spontaneous degradation (Figure 16.5) at physiological temperature and pH by a mechanism called Hofmann elimination, yielding laudanosine (a tertiary amine) and a monoquaternary acrylate as metabolites.[112,115] Furthermore, atracurium can undergo ester hydrolysis. Hofmann elimination is a purely chemical process that results in loss of the positive charges by molecular fragmentation to laudanosine and a monoquaternary acrylate.[116,117] Laudanosine easily crosses the blood-brain barrier, and it has central nervous system stimulating properties. Although the seizure threshold is not known in humans, the seizure threshold in animals ranges from 5.0 µg/ml in rabbits[118] to 17 µg/ml in dogs.[119] In patients in the intensive care unit, blood levels of laudanosine can be as high as 5.0 to 6.0 µg/ml.[120] There is no evidence to suggest that prolonged administration of atracurium in the operating room or in the intensive care unit in patients with normal or impaired renal function is likely to result in concentrations of laudanosine capable of producing convulsions. The plasma elimination half-life of laudanosine is similar in patients with normal and impaired renal function—197±38 and 234±81 min, respectively.[121,122] Interestingly, laudanosine activates $\alpha_4\beta_2$ nicotinic acetylcholine receptors and δ- and κ-opioid receptors. It has been suggested that this activation has neuroprotective effects.[123–126]

Cisatracurium

Cisatracurium is the 1R *cis*–1′R *cis* isomer of atracurium and represents about 15% of the marketed atracurium mixture by weight but more than 50% of the mixture in terms of potency or neuromuscular blocking activity (Figure 16.5). Like atracurium, cisatracurium is metabolized by Hofmann elimination to laudanosine and a monoquaternary alcohol metabolite.[127–129] There is no ester hydrolysis of the parent molecule.[127] Hofmann elimination accounts for 77% of the total clearance of 5 to 6 ml/kg/min.[130] Twenty-three percent of the drug is cleared through organ-dependent means, with renal elimination accounting for 16% of this.[129] Because cisatracurium is about four to five times as potent as atracurium, about five times less laudanosine is produced, and accumulation of this metabolite is not thought to be of any consequence in clinical practice. Unlike atracurium, cisatracurium in the clinical dose range does not cause histamine release.[131,132] This indicates that the phenomenon of histamine release may be stereospecific.[131,133]

Mivacurium

Mivacurium is the only currently available short-acting neuromuscular blocker in the European Union, but its use in the United States has been discontinued by the manufacturer (Table 16.2). Mivacurium differs from atracurium by the presence of an additional methylated phenolic group (Figure 16.5). Mivacurium has a longer interonium chain (16 atoms) than

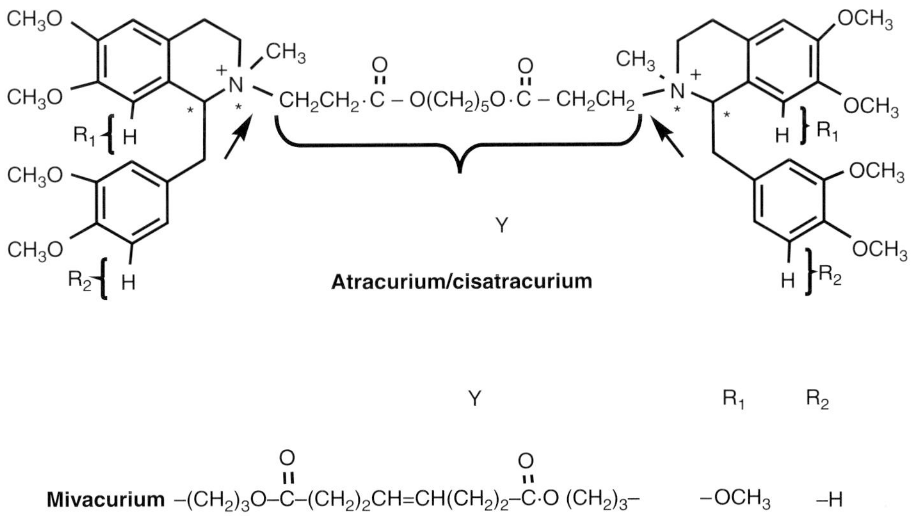

Figure 16.5 Chemical structures of atracurium, cisatracurium, and mivacurium.* Indicates the chiral centers; arrows show cleavage sites for Hofmann elimination.

other isoquinolinium neuromuscular blockers.[106] Mivacurium consists of a mixture of three stereoisomers.[134] The two most active are the *trans-trans* and *cis-trans* isomers (57% and 37% w/w respectively), which are equipotent; the *cis-cis* isomer (6% w/w) has only one-tenth of the activity of the other isomers in cats and monkeys.[134] Mivacurium is metabolized by butyrylcholinesterase at about 70% to 88% the rate of succinylcholine to a monoester, a dicarboxylic acid.[135,136] Mivacurium may produce histamine release, especially if administered rapidly.[137]

STEROIDAL COMPOUNDS

The steroid skeleton possesses onium centers at different positions. In the steroidal compounds, it is probably essential that one of two nitrogen atoms in the molecule be quaternized.[138] The presence of acetyl ester (acetylcholine-like moiety) is thought to facilitate interaction of steroidal compounds with nicotinic acetylcholine receptors at the postsynaptic muscle membrane.[10,139]

Pancuronium

Pancuronium is a potent long-acting neuromuscular blocking drug with both vagolytic and butyrylcholinesterase-inhibiting properties (Figure 16.6).[140] Incorporation of an acetylcholine-like structural unit into the D-ring at positions 16 and 17 enhanced the neuromuscular blocking activity of pancuronium. About 40% to 60% of pancuronium is cleared by the kidney[141] and 11% is excreted in the bile. A small amount (15% to 20%) is metabolized, mainly by deacetylation in the liver. The metabolites (3-OH, 17-OH, and 3,7-di-OH) are considerably less potent as neuromuscular blockers and are excreted in the urine.[142] Accumulation of the 3-OH metabolite is responsible for prolongation of the duration of block induced by pancuronium.

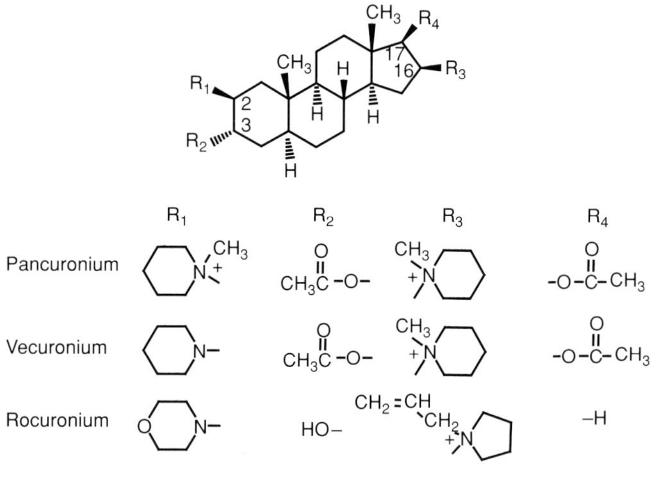

Figure 16.6 Chemical structures of the steroidal neuromuscular blockers pancuronium, vecuronium, and rocuronium.

Vecuronium

Vecuronium is a monoquarternary neuromuscular blocker with an intermediate duration of action. Vecuronium is simply pancuronium without the quaternizing methyl group in the 2-piperidino substitution (Figure 16.6).[10,143] At physiological pH, the tertiary amine is largely protonated, similar to tubocurarine. The minor molecular difference between vecuronium and pancuronium means that vecuronium is characterized by: 1) a slight decrease in potency; 2) virtual loss of the vagolytic properties of pancuronium; 3) molecular instability in solution (this explains in part the shorter duration of action of vecuronium compared with pancuronium); and 4) increased lipid solubility, which results in a greater biliary elimination of vecuronium than pancuronium.[10,106]

The liver is the principal organ of elimination for vecuronium, and renal excretion accounts for excretion of approximately 30% of the administered dose. Approximately 30% to 40% of vecuronium is cleared in the bile as parent compound.[144] The combined hepatic and renal elimination gives vecuronium a clearance rate of 3 to 6 mL/kg/min.[145,146] The duration of the vecuronium-induced neuromuscular block is therefore dependent primarily on hepatic function and, to a lesser extent, on renal function.[147,148] Vecuronium is metabolized in the liver by deacetylation into three possible metabolites: 3-OH, 17-OH, and 3,17-di-OH vecuronium. The 3-OH metabolite has 80% the neuromuscular blocking potency of vecuronium. Therefore, during prolonged administration of vecuronium, this metabolite may contribute to prolonged neuromuscular blockade.[149]

Vecuronium is prepared as a lyophilized powder because it is less stable in solution. The lower stability in solution is due to the group effect of the adjacent basic piperidine at the 2 position, which facilitates hydrolysis of the acetate at the 3 position. Vecuronium cannot be prepared as a ready-to-use solution with a sufficient shelf life, even as a buffered solution.[150] In pancuronium, the 2-piperidine is quaternized and no longer basic (charged). Thus, it does not participate in catalysis of the 3-acetate hydrolysis.[150]

Rocuronium

Rocuronium (Figure 16.6) is an intermediately acting monoquarternary neuromuscular blocker with a faster onset of action than either pancuronium or vecuronium. Rocuronium lacks the acetyl ester that is found in the steroid nucleus of pancuronium and vecuronium in the A ring (Figure 16.6). The introduction of cyclic substituents other than piperidine at the 2- and 16- positions resulted in a fast-onset-of-action compound.[151] The methyl group attached to the quaternary nitrogen of vecuronium and pancuronium is replaced by an allyl group in rocuronium. As a result, rocuronium is about six times less potent than vecuronium.[151,152]

Rocuronium is primarily eliminated by the liver and excreted in bile. It is taken up into the liver by a carrier-mediated active transport system.[153] The putative metabolite, 17-desacetylrocuronium, has not been detected in significant quantities. Approximately 30% of rocuronium is excreted unchanged in the urine.[154,155]

The replacement of the acetyl ester attached to the A ring by a hydroxy group makes it possible to prepare rocuronium as a stable solution. At room temperature, rocuronium is stable for 60 days, while pancuronium is stable for 6 months. The reason for this difference in shelf-life is related to the fact that rocuronium is terminally sterilized in manufacturing and pancuronium is not—terminal sterilization causes some degree of degradation.[150]

SZ1677

SZ1677 is a nonsteroidal nondepolarizing neuromuscular blocking agent (pyrrolidinium bromide compound) that is structurally related to rocuronium.[156] It was first synthesized by Gedeon Richter in Hungary. Its main degradation product is the 17-OH derivative (SZ1823), which is 27.5 times less potent than the parent compound. The other form, 3-acetoxy derivative (SZ1676), is considered an impurity. SZ1677 has been shown to have less presynaptic inhibitory effect than rocuronium[157], so it may induce less fade because of less interference with presynaptic acetylcholine release and reuptake. In laboratory animals, doses up to 8× ED_{95} had minimal effects on blood pressure and heart rate. At similar doses, SZ1677 has no vagal blocking effects. The potency (ED_{95}) of SZ1677 in laboratory animals is 25 μg/kg, and when measured at the airway musculature, onset time at this dose is about 1 min (0.5–2 min range). Spontaneous recovery (recovery 25%–75%) takes an average of 192 s (range of 80–390 s). It is reported to have significant variability in onset and duration at different muscle groups, such as peripheral skeletal vs. central airway muscles. The further development of this compound for clinical use is uncertain at this time.

OLEFINIC (DOUBLE-BONDED) ISOQUINOLINIUM DIESTER COMPOUNDS

Gantacurium

The investigational drug gantacurium (AV430A or GW 280430A) has a pharmacodynamic profile similar to succinylcholine's and was developed to replace succinylcholine (Figure 16.7).[158] Gantacurium is an asymmetrical isoquinolinium diester of chlorofumaric acid in which the central olefinic (double-bonded) carbons are activated by a halogen (chlorine) substitution designed to facilitate the adduction reaction.[159] The absence of halogen in such compounds (as in CW002 and CW011) results in less activation of the olefinic carbons and prolongation of the duration of neuromuscular block. Gantacurium appears to be degraded by two chemical mechanisms, neither of which is enzymatic: (1) rapid formation of an apparently inactive cysteine adduction product; and (2) slower hydrolysis of the ester bond adjacent to the chlorine substitution to presumably inactive hydrolysis products.[159] Gantacurium does not undergo Hofmann degradation. Exogenous administration of cysteine or glutathione can accelerate the antagonism of gantacurium-induced neuromuscular blockade.

A study in anesthetized human volunteers using an earlier formulation of gantacurium estimated the ED_{95} to be 0.19 mg/kg.[160] The time to onset of 90% blockade was 2.1 ± 0.6 minutes (mean ± standard deviation) at 0.18 mg/kg of gantacurium (approximately 1× ED_{95}) in four volunteers. Doubling the dose to 0.36 mg/kg shortened the time to onset of 90% blockade to 1.3 ± 0.2 minutes (again, in four volunteers).[160] Clinical durations of action ranged from 4.7 to 10.1 minutes and increased with increasing dose. Spontaneous recovery to train-of-four of 0.9 developed at the thumb within 12 to 15 minutes after administration of doses as large as 0.54 mg/kg (3× ED_{95}). The recovery was further accelerated by administration of edrophonium. Transient cardiovascular adverse effects were observed at doses beginning at 3× ED_{95} and were suggestive of histamine release.[160] Bronchospasm has not been reported in humans at doses up to 4× ED_{95}.

A multicenter, phase 2, randomized, controlled, observer-blinded, dose-response study of gantacurium involving 230 subjects with an American Society of Anesthesiologists physical status classification of 1 or 2 was recently conducted in Europe (http://clinicaltrials.gov/show/NCT00235976). The study was designed to evaluate the efficacy and safety of gantacurium chloride for injection into healthy adult patients undergoing endotracheal intubation before surgery under general anesthesia. The results of this study have not yet been published.

CW002

CW002 (AV002), a benzylisoquinolinium fumarate ester-based compound, is an investigational neuromuscular blocking drug of intermediate duration of action (Figure 16.8).[161] CW002 was designed to undergo cysteine adduction and possibly chemical hydrolysis more slowly than gantacurium. In dogs, administration of 0.08 mg/kg (10× ED_{95}) of CW002 resulted in a duration of action of 71 ± 4 minutes.[162] No signs of histamine release were observed in cats in doses up to 0.8 mg/kg (40× ED_{95}).

Animal data also showed that residual neuromuscular effects of CW002 could be antagonized with neostigmine. CW002, like gantacurium, is degraded in the bloodstream by endogenous cysteine to an inactive addition product in a chemical (nonenzymatic) reaction. In animals, intravenous administration of exogenous cysteine resulted in rapid antagonism from profound neuromuscular blockade. Cysteine reversal of 10× ED_{95} for CW002 in dogs is rapid and is maximal at cysteine doses of 20 mg/kg.[162] Cysteine degrades the parent compound into products that are 60 times less

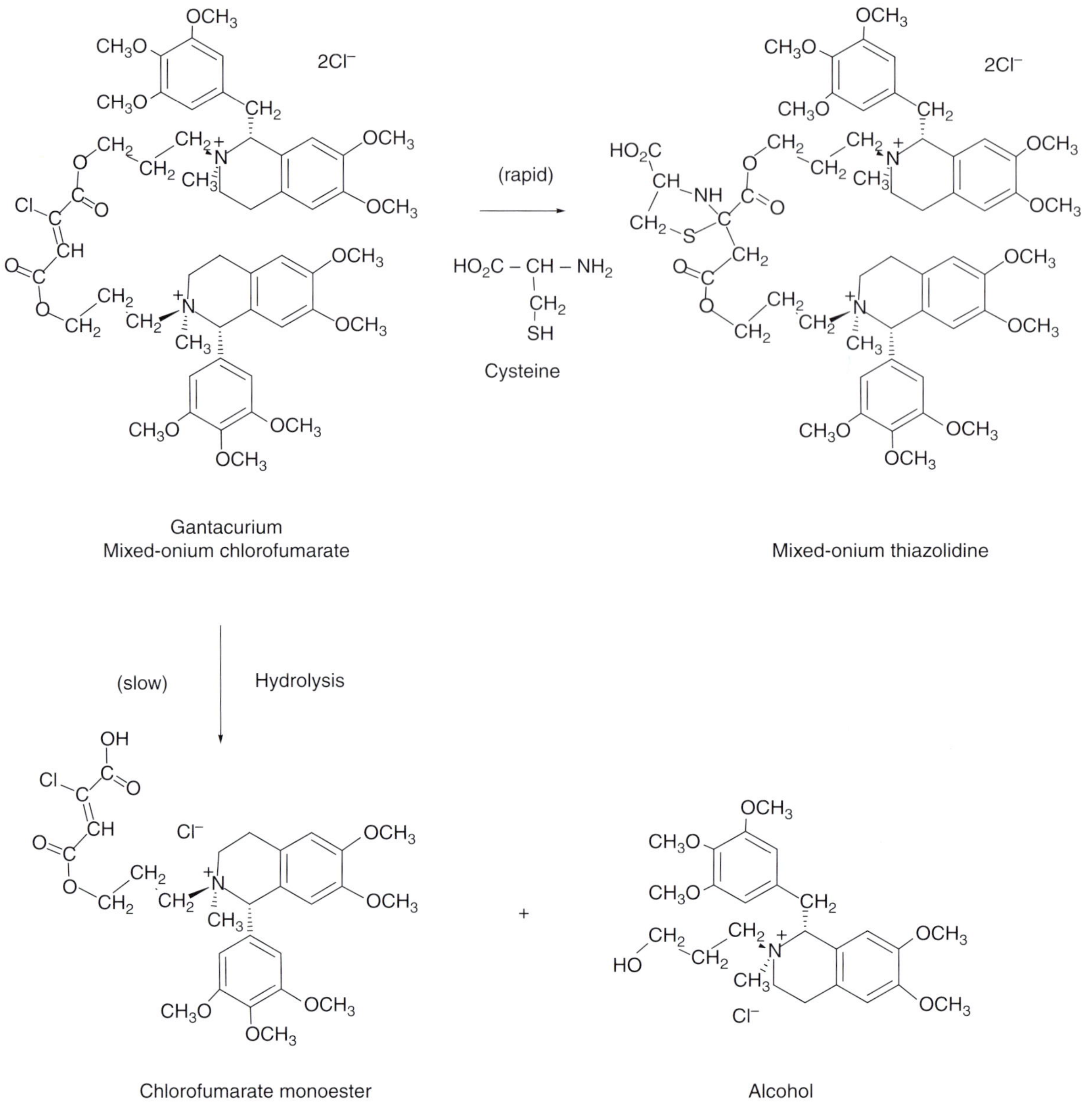

Figure 16.7 Chemical structure of gantacurium (a mixed-onium chlorofumarate). In whole human blood, two pathways of deactivation occur, neither of which is enzymatic: (1) rapid formation of an apparently inactive cysteine adduction product, with cysteine replacing chlorine; and (2) slower hydrolysis of the ester bond adjacent to the chlorine substitution, to chlorofumarate monoester and alcohol. Reprinted with permission from Boros EE, Samano V, Ray JA, et al. Neuromuscular blocking activity and therapeutic potential of mixed-tetrahydroisoquinolinium halofumarates and halosuccinates in rhesus monkeys. *J Med Chem*. 2003;46:2502–2515. Copyright 2003 American Chemical Society.

potent than CW002. Cysteine then further degrades these metabolites into 2 other molecules that are 500 times less potent than the parent compound—essentially eliminating the risk of drug accumulation (personal communication, Dr. John Savarese).

POTENCY OF NONDEPOLARIZING NEUROMUSCULAR BLOCKERS

Drug potency is commonly expressed in terms of the dose-response relationship. The potency of neuromuscular blockers can be expressed as the dose of drug required to produce an effect—e.g., 50% or 95% depression of twitch height, commonly expressed as ED_{50} and ED_{95}, respectively.[163] The neuromuscular blocking drugs have different potencies, as illustrated in Table 16.2. The dose-response curve for nondepolarizing neuromuscular blockers is sigmoidal, and different ED values have been derived in a variety of ways. The most commonly used technique is linear regression analysis after log-dose and probit- or logit-data transformation.

Recently, Kopman et al[164] reported that the ED_{50} value is a very robust parameter and should be employed rather than

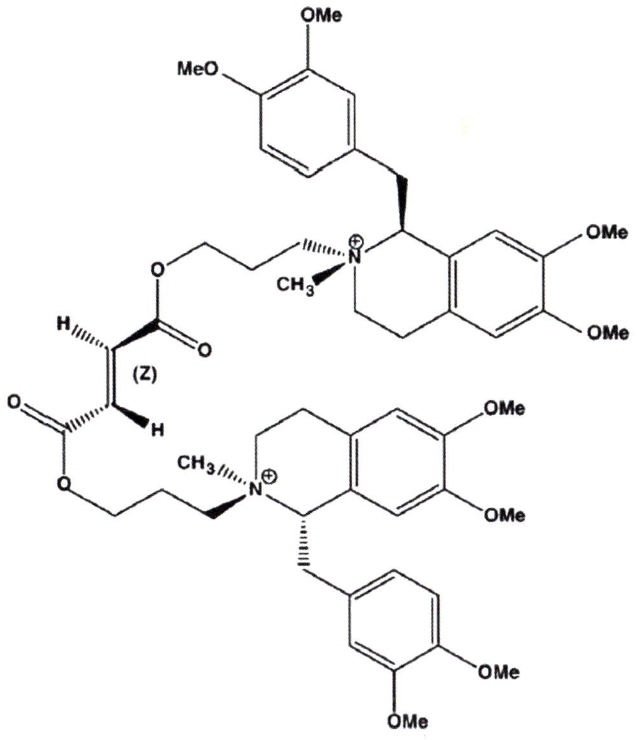

Figure 16.8 Chemical structure of CW002 (AV002).

the ED_{95} value when comparing the potency of neuromuscular blockers. They noted that the ED_{50} values calculated by different methods (nonlinear regression analysis, linear regression analysis, or Hill's equation) were interchangeable, and that the ED_{95} value was not a precise parameter because the confidence intervals of the ED_{95} were so wide.[164]

FACTORS THAT INCREASE THE POTENCY OF NONDEPOLARIZING NEUROMUSCULAR BLOCKERS

Inhalational anesthetics potentiate the neuromuscular blocking effect of nondepolarizing neuromuscular blockers. This potentiation results mainly in a decrease in the required dosage of neuromuscular blocker and prolongation of both the duration of action of the relaxant and recovery from neuromuscular block.[165] The magnitude of this potentiation depends on several factors, including the duration of inhalational anesthesia,[166–168] the specific inhalational anesthetic used,[169] and the concentration of inhalational agent used.[170] The rank order of potentiation is desflurane > sevoflurane > isoflurane > halothane > nitrous oxide–barbiturate–opioid or propofol anesthesia.[171–173] The mechanisms proposed for this potentiation include: 1) a central effect on α motoneurons and interneuronal synapses;[174] 2) inhibition of postsynaptic nicotinic acetylcholine receptors;[175] and 3) augmentation of the antagonist's affinity at the receptor site.[176]

Several antibiotics can also potentiate neuromuscular blockade. The aminoglycoside antibiotics, the polymyxins, lincomycin and clindamycin primarily inhibit the prejunctional release of acetylcholine and also depress postjunctional nicotinic acetylcholine receptor sensitivity to acetylcholine.[177] The tetracyclines, on the other hand, exhibit postjunctional activity only.[177]

Hypothermia or magnesium sulfate potentiates the neuromuscular blockade induced by nondepolarizing neuromuscular blockers.[178–181] The mechanism(s) underlying this potentiation may be pharmacodynamic, pharmacokinetic, or both.[180] High magnesium concentrations inhibit calcium channels at the presynaptic nerve terminals that trigger the release of acetylcholine.[11]

In large intravenous doses, most local anesthetics potentiate neuromuscular block; in smaller doses, no clinically significant potentiation occurs.[182] Antidysrhythmic drugs, such as quinidine, also potentiate neuromuscular block.[183]

FACTORS THAT DECREASE THE POTENCY OF NONDEPOLARIZING NEUROMUSCULAR BLOCKERS

Resistance to nondepolarizing muscle blockers has been demonstrated in patients receiving chronic anticonvulsant therapy, as evidenced by accelerated recovery from neuromuscular blockade and the need for increased doses to achieve complete neuromuscular blockade. This resistance has been attributed to increased clearance,[184] increased binding of the neuromuscular blockers to α1-acid glycoproteins, and/or upregulation of neuromuscular acetylcholine receptors.[185]

In hyperparathyroidism, hypercalcemia is associated with decreased sensitivity to atracurium and thus a shortened duration of neuromuscular blockade.[186] Increasing calcium concentrations also decreased the sensitivity to tubocurarine and pancuronium in a muscle-nerve model.[187]

EFFECT OF DRUG POTENCY ON SPEED OF ONSET

The speed of onset of action is inversely proportional to the potency of nondepolarizing neuromuscular blockers.[188,189] Low potency is predictive of rapid onset, and high potency is predictive of slow onset. Except for atracurium,[190] molar potency (the ED_{50} or ED_{95} expressed in µM/kg) is highly predictive of a drug's time to onset of effect (at the adductor pollicis muscle).[189] Rocuronium has a molar potency (ED_{95} ≈ 0.54 µM/kg) which is about 13% that of vecuronium and only 9% that of cisatracurium. Thus, rapid onset of rocuronium is to be expected. It should be noted that a drug's measured molar potency is the end result of many contributing factors: the drug's intrinsic potency (the CE_{50}, the biophase concentration resulting in 50% twitch depression), the rate of equilibration between plasma and biophase (k_{e0}), the initial rate of plasma clearance, and probably other factors as well.[191]

The onset of action of a neuromuscular blocker depends on binding to a certain population of nicotinic acetylcholine receptors at the neuromuscular junction[192] and this is the end result of the interplay between the number of available molecules of a neuromuscular blocker and the total number of receptors. The influence of potency on speed of onset could be simply explained by the fact that, for an equipotent dose (e.g., a dose that results in 50% receptor occupancy), a low-potency drug (such as rocuronium) will have a higher number of molecules than a high-potency drug (such as tubocurarine). The higher number of drug molecules will result in a greater diffusion gradient of the low-potency drug from capillary to the neuromuscular junction (faster rate of drug transfer from plasma to biophase) and a greater biophase concentration of low-potency drug resulting in a fast onset. Therefore, the high rate of drug delivery to the neuromuscular junction resulting from the higher concentration becomes the dominant element controlling onset time when all other factors are equal.

The concept of "buffered diffusion" must be invoked to explain the slow recovery of long-acting neuromuscular blockers and to understand biophase kinetics.[193] Buffered diffusion is the process in which diffusion of a drug (e.g., diffusion of a neuromuscular blocker from the neuromuscular junction) is impeded because it binds to extremely high-density receptors within a restricted space (neuromuscular junction). This process is seen with high-potency but not low-potency drugs. Buffered diffusion causes repetitive binding to and unbinding from receptors, keeping potent drugs such as tubocurarine in the neighborhood of effector sites and potentially lengthening the duration of effect.[194]

Bevan[195] also proposed that rapid plasma clearance is associated with a rapid onset of action. The fast onset of succinylcholine is related to its rapid metabolism and plasma clearance.

ADVERSE EFFECTS OF NEUROMUSCULAR BLOCKERS

Neuromuscular blocking agents seem to play a prominent role in adverse reactions that occur during anesthesia. The Committee on Safety of Medicines in the United Kingdom reported that 10.8% (218 of 2,014) of adverse drug reactions and 7.3% of deaths (21 of 286) were attributable to neuromuscular blocking drugs.[196]

AUTONOMIC EFFECTS

Neuromuscular blocking agents interact with nicotinic and muscarinic cholinergic receptors within the sympathetic and parasympathetic nervous systems and at the nicotinic receptors of the neuromuscular junction. Administration of tubocurarine is associated with marked ganglion blockade resulting in hypotension; in susceptible patients, manifestations of histamine release such as flushing, hypotension, reflex tachycardia, and bronchospasm can be seen. Pancuronium has a direct vagolytic effect. Pancuronium can block muscarinic receptors on sympathetic postganglionic nerve terminals,[197] resulting in inhibition of a negative-feedback mechanism whereby excessive catecholamine release is modulated or prevented.[198] Pancuronium may also stimulate catecholamine release from adrenergic nerve terminals.[199] Since succinylcholine consists of two linked acetylcholine molecules, it is also associated with autonomic perturbations (such as bradycardia).

HISTAMINE RELEASE

Histamine release by benzylisoquinolinium compounds such as mivacurium, atracurium, and tubocurarine can cause skin flushing, decreases in blood pressure and systemic vascular resistance, and increases in pulse rate.[137,200–203] In contrast, steroidal neuromuscular blocking drugs are not associated with histamine release in typical clinical doses.[204–206] The clinical effects of histamine are seen when plasma concentrations increase to 200% to 300% of baseline values, especially if such concentrations are achieved quickly by rapid drug administration. The effect is usually of short duration (1 to 5 minutes), is dose related, and is clinically insignificant in healthy patients. Histamine has positive inotropic and chronotropic effects on the myocardial H_2 receptors, and there is some evidence that its chronotropic effect may result in part from the liberation of catecholamines.[207] While ganglionic block secondary to the administration of tubocurarine has been demonstrated to occur in various species,[208] the peripheral venous and arteriolar dilatation via stimulation of vascular H_1 and H_2 receptors can result in a significant degree of hypotension as well as carotid-sinus-mediated reflex response to histamine-induced peripheral vasodilatation.[202] Other substances liberated by mast-cell degranulation, such as tryptase or prostaglandins, may also play a role.[209] The serosal mast cell, located in the skin and connective tissue and near blood vessels and nerves, is principally involved in the degranulation process.[209]

For patients who may be compromised hemodynamically, selecting a drug with less or no histamine release (cisatracurium, vecuronium, or rocuronium) may be appropriate. Another strategy for maintaining cardiovascular stability involves slow administration of benzylisoquinolinium neuromuscular blocking drugs (over 60 s), or the prophylactic use of the combined histamine H_1- and H_2-receptor antagonists.

RESPIRATORY EFFECTS

Three muscarinic acetylcholine receptors (M_1, M_2, and M_3) exist in the airways and play an important role in regulating airway function.[210,211] M_1 receptors are under sympathetic control, and they mediate bronchodilation.[212] M_2 receptors are located presynaptically at the postganglionic parasympathetic nerve endings, and they function in a negative feedback mechanism to limit the release of acetylcholine. M_3 receptors, which are located postsynaptically, mediate bronchoconstriction.[212] Nondepolarizing neuromuscular blockers have different antagonistic activities at both M_2 and M_3 receptors.[213]

The administration of benzylisoquinolinium neuromuscular blocking drugs (with the exception of cisatracurium) is associated with histamine release, which may result in increased airway resistance and bronchospasm in patients with hyperactive airway disease.

ALLERGIC REACTIONS

Life-threatening anaphylactic (immune-mediated) or anaphylactoid reactions during anesthesia have been estimated to occur in 1 in 1,000 to 1 in 25,000 administrations and are associated with a mortality rate of about 5%.[214,215] In France, the most common causes of anaphylaxis in patients who experienced allergic reactions were reported to be neuromuscular blocking drugs (58.2%), latex (16.7%), and antibiotics (15.1%).[216] Anaphylactic reactions are mediated through immune responses involving immunoglobulin E antibodies fixed to mast cells. Anaphylactoid reactions are not immune mediated and represent exaggerated pharmacologic responses in very sensitive individuals who represent a very small proportion of the population.

Neuromuscular blocking drugs contain two quaternary ammonium ions, which are the epitopes commonly recognized by specific immunoglobulin E.[217] Cross-reactivity has been reported between neuromuscular blocking drugs and food, cosmetics, disinfectants, and industrial materials.[217] Cross-reactivity is seen in 70% of patients with a history of anaphylaxis to a neuromuscular blocking drug.[216]

Steroidal compounds (e.g., rocuronium, vecuronium, or pancuronium) result in no significant histamine release.[137] For example, four times the ED_{95} of rocuronium (1.2 mg/kg) causes no significant histamine release.[206] Nevertheless, in the aforementioned series from France, 43.1% were due to rocuronium and 22.6% to succinylcholine among cases of anaphylaxis due to neuromuscular blocking drugs.[216] There are currently no standards regarding which diagnostic tests (skin prick test, interdermal test, or immunoglobulin E testing) should be performed to identify patients at risk.[218]

REFERENCES

1. Loewi O. Über humorale Übertragbarkeit der Herznervenwirkung. *Pflügers Arch ges Physiol.* 1921;189:239–242.
2. Dale HH, Feldberg W, Vogt M. Release of acetylcholine at voluntary motor nerve endings. *J Physiol.* 1936;86:353–380.
3. Changeux JP. The acetylcholine receptor: an "allosteric" membrane protein. *Harvey Lect.* 1981;75:85–254.
4. Läwen A. Über die Verbindung der Lokalanästhesie mit der Narkose, über hohe Extraduralanästhesie und epidurale Injektionen anästhesierender Lösungen bei tabischen Magenkrisen. *Beitr Klin Chir.* 1912;80:168–180.
5. Bodman RI, Gillies D, Griffith, H. *The Evolution of Modern Anaesthesia.* 1st ed. Toronto: Hannah Institute & Dundurn Press; 1992.
6. Sine SM, Claudio T, Sigworth FJ. Activation of Torpedo acetylcholine receptors expressed in mouse fibroblasts: single channel current kinetics reveal distinct agonist binding affinities. *J Gen Physiol.* 1990;96:395–437.
7. Devillers-Thiery A, Galzi JL, Eisele JL, Bertrand S, Bertrand D, Changeux JP. Functional architecture of the nicotinic acetylcholine receptor: a prototype of ligand-gated ion channels. *J Membr Biol.* 1993;136:97–112.
8. Grosman C, Zhou M, Auerbach A. Mapping the conformational wave of acetylcholine receptor channel gating. *Nature.* 2000;403:773–776.
9. Grosman C, Salamone FN, Sine SM, Auerbach A. The extracellular linker of muscle acetylcholine receptor channels is a gating control element. *J Gen Physiol.* 2000;116:327–340.
10. Bowman WC. *Pharmacology of Neuromuscular Function.* 2nd ed. London: Wright; 1990.
11. Naguib M, Flood P, McArdle JJ, Brenner HR. Advances in neurobiology of the neuromuscular junction: implications for the anesthesiologist. *Anesthesiology.* 2002;96:202–231.
12. Rosenberry TL. Acetylcholinesterase. *Adv Enzymol Relat Areas Mol Biol.* 1975;43:103–218.
13. Kopman AF, Klewicka MM, Neuman GG. The relationship between acceleromyographic train-of-four fade and single twitch depression. *Anesthesiology.* 2002;96:583–587.
14. Bowman WC. Prejunctional and postjunctional cholinoceptors at the neuromuscular junction. *Anesth Analg.* 1980;59:935–943.
15. Prior C, Tian L, Dempster J, Marshall IG. Prejunctional actions of muscle relaxants: synaptic vesicles and transmitter mobilization as sites of action. *Gen Pharmacol.* 1995;26:659–666.
16. Faria M, Oliveira L, Timoteo MA, Lobo MG, Correia-De-Sa P. Blockade of neuronal facilitatory nicotinic receptors containing alpha3beta2 subunits contribute to tetanic fade in the rat isolated diaphragm. *Synapse.* 2003;49:77–88.
17. Chang CC, Hong SJ. Dissociation of the end-plate potential run-down and the tetanic fade from the postsynaptic inhibition of acetylcholine receptor by alpha-neurotoxins. *Exp Neurol.* 1987;98:509–517.
18. Nagashima M, Yasuhara S, Frick CG, Martyn JA. Alpha-Bungarotoxin but not botulinum toxin causes fade during repetitive stimulation. *ASA Meeting*; 2008:A1399.
19. Naguib M, Lien CA, Aker J, Eliazo R. Posttetanic potentiation and fade in the response to tetanic and train-of-four stimulation during succinylcholine-induced block. *Anesth Analg.* 2004;98:1686–1691.
20. Thesleff S. Farmakologisks och kliniska forsok med L.T. I. (O,O-succinylcholine jodid). *Nord Med.* 1951;46:1045.
21. Foldes FF, McNall PG, Borrego-Hinojosa JM. Succinylcholine, a new approach to muscular relaxation in anaesthesiology. *N Engl J Med.* 1952;247:596–600.
22. Torda TA, Graham GG, Warwick NR, Donohue P. Pharmacokinetics and pharmacodynamics of suxamethonium. *Anaesth Intensive Care.* 1997;25:272–278.
23. Cook DR, Wingard LB, Taylor FH. Pharmacokinetics of succinylcholine in infants, children, and adults. *Clin Pharmacol Ther.* 1976;20:493–498.
24. Smith CE, Donati F, Bevan DR. Dose-response curves for succinylcholine: single versus cumulative techniques. *Anesthesiology.* 1988;69:338–342.
25. Kopman AF, Klewicka MM, Neuman GG. An alternate method for estimating the dose-response relationships of neuromuscular blocking drugs. *Anesth Analg.* 2000;90:1191–1197.
26. Ferguson A, Bevan DR. Mixed neuromuscular block: the effect of precurarization. *Anaesthesia.* 1981;36:661–666.
27. Curran MJ, Donati F, Bevan DR. Onset and recovery of atracurium and suxamethonium-induced neuromuscular blockade with simultaneous

train-of-four and single twitch stimulation. *Br J Anaesth.* 1987;59: 989–994.
28. Mehta MP, Sokoll MD, Gergis SD. Accelerated onset of non-depolarizing neuromuscular blocking drugs: pancuronium, atracurium and vecuronium. A comparison with succinylcholine. *Eur J Anaesthesiol.* 1988;5:15–21.
29. Viby-Mogensen J. Correlation of succinylcholine duration of action with plasma cholinesterase activity in subjects with the genotypically normal enzyme. *Anesthesiology.* 1980;53:517–520.
30. Katz RL, Ryan JF. The neuromuscular effects of suxamethonium in man. *Br J Anaesth.* 1969;41:381–390.
31. Naguib M, Samarkandi A, Riad W, Alharby SW. Optimal dose of succinylcholine revisited. *Anesthesiology.* 2003;99:1045–1049.
32. Blobner M, Mirakhur RK, Wierda JM, et al. Rapacuronium 2.0 or 2.5 mg kg-1 for rapid-sequence induction: comparison with succinylcholine 1.0 mg kg-1. *Br J Anaesth.* 2000;85:724–731.
33. Andrews JI, Kumar N, van den Brom RH, Olkkola KT, Roest GJ, Wright PM. A large simple randomized trial of rocuronium versus succinylcholine in rapid-sequence induction of anaesthesia along with propofol. *Acta Anaesthesiol Scand.* 1999;43:4–8.
34. Sparr HJ, Mellinghoff H, Blobner M, Noldge-Schomburg G. Comparison of intubating conditions after rapacuronium (Org 9487) and succinylcholine following rapid sequence induction in adult patients. *Br J Anaesth.* 1999;82:537–541.
35. Naguib M, Samarkandi AH, El-Din ME, Abdullah K, Khaled M, Alharby SW. The dose of succinylcholine required for excellent endotracheal intubating conditions. *Anesth Analg.* 2006; 102:151–155.
36. Gissen AJ, Katz RL, Karis JH, Papper EM. Neuromuscular block in man during prolonged arterial infusion with succinylcholine. *Anesthesiology.* 1966;27:242–29.
37. Foldes FF, McNall PG, Birch JH. The neuromuscular activity of succinylmonocholine iodide in man. *Br Med J.* 1954;1:967.
38. Lockridge O, Bartels CF, Vaughan TA, Wong CK, Norton SE, Johnson LL. Complete amino acid sequence of human serum cholinesterase. *J Biol Chem.* 1987;262:549–557.
39. Jensen FS, Schwartz M, Viby-Mogensen J. Identification of human plasma cholinesterase variants using molecular biological techniques. *Acta Anaesthesiol Scand.* 1995;39:142–149.
40. Foldes FF, Rendell-Baker L, Birch JH. Causes and prevention of prolonged apnea with succinylcholine. *Anesth Analg.* 1956;35:609.
41. Lepage L, Schiele F, Gueguen R, Siest G. Total cholinesterase in plasma: biological variations and reference limits. *Clin Chem.* 1985;31:546–550.
42. Kopman AF, Strachovsky G, Lichtenstein L. Prolonged response to succinylcholine following physostigmine. *Anesthesiology.* 1978;49: 142–143.
43. Sunew KY, Hicks RG. Effects of neostigmine and pyridostigmine on duration of succinylcholine action and pseudocholinesterase activity. *Anesthesiology.* 1978;49:188–191.
44. Kao YJ, Tellez J, Turner DR. Dose-dependent effect of metoclopramide on cholinesterases and suxamethonium metabolism. *Br J Anaesth.* 1990;65:220–224.
45. Fisher DM, Caldwell JE, Sharma M, Wiren JE. The influence of bambuterol (carbamylated terbutaline) on the duration of action of succinylcholine-induced paralysis in humans. *Anesthesiology.* 1988; 69:757–759.
46. Bang U, Viby-Mogensen J, Wiren JE, Skovgaard LT. The effect of bambuterol (carbamylated terbutaline) on plasma cholinesterase activity and suxamethonium-induced neuromuscular blockade in genotypically normal patients. *Acta Anaesthesiol Scand.* 1990;34:596–599.
47. Barabas E, Zsigmond EK, Kirkpatrick AF. The inhibitory effect of esmolol on human plasmacholinesterase. *Can Anaesth Soc J.* 1986;33:332–335.
48. Murthy VS, Patel KD, Elangovan RG, et al. Cardiovascular and neuromuscular effects of esmolol during induction of anesthesia. *J Clin Pharmacol.* 1986;26:351–357.
49. La Du BN, Bartels CF, Nogueira CP, et al. Phenotypic and molecular biological analysis of human butyrylcholinesterase variants. *Clin Biochem.* 1990;23:423–431.
50. Pantuck EJ. Plasma cholinesterase: gene and variations. *Anesth Analg.* 1993;77:380–386.
51. Goodall R. Cholinesterase: phenotyping and genotyping. *Ann Clin Biochem.* 2004;41:98–110.
52. Kalow W, Staron N. On distribution and inheritance of atypical forms of human serum cholinesterase, as indicated by dibucaine numbers. *Can J Biochem Physiol.* 1957;35:1305–1320.
53. Kalow W, Genest K. A method for the detection of atypical forms of human serum cholinesterase: determination of dibucaine numbers. *Can J Biochem.* 1957;35:339.
54. Viby-Mogensen J, Hanel HK. Prolonged apnoea after suxamethonium: an analysis of the first 225 cases reported to the Danish Cholinesterase Research Unit. *Acta Anaesthesiol Scand.* 1978;22:371–380.
55. Ramsey FM, Lebowitz PW, Savarese JJ, Ali HH. Clinical characteristics of long-term succinylcholine neuromuscular blockade during balanced anesthesia. *Anesth Analg.* 1980;59:110–116.
56. Bartels CF, Jensen FS, Lockridge O, et al. DNA mutation associated with the human butyrylcholinesterase K-variant and its linkage to the atypical variant mutation and other polymorphic sites. *Am J Hum Genet.* 1992;50:1086–1103.
57. Greenberg CP, Primo-Parmo SL, Pantuck EJ, la Du BN. Prolonged response to succinylcholine: a new variant of plasma cholinesterase that is identified as normal by traditional phenotyping methods. *Anesth Analg.* 1995;81:419–421.
58. Yoshida A, Motulsky AG. A pseudocholinesterase variant (E Cynthiana) associated with elevated plasma enzyme activity. *Am J Hum Genet.* 1969;21:486–498.
59. Krause A, Lane AB, Jenkins T. A new high activity plasma cholinesterase variant. *J Med Genet.* 1988;25:677–681.
60. Warran P, Theeman M, Bold AM, Jones S. Hypercholinesterasaemia and suxamethonium resistance. *Anaesthesia.* 1987;42:855–857.
61. Naguib M, Gomaa M, Samarkandi AH, et al. Increased plasma cholinesterase activity and mivacurium resistance: report of a family. *Anesth Analg.* 1999;89:1579–1582.
62. Galindo AHF, Davis TB. Succinylcholine and cardiac excitability. *Anesthesiology.* 1962;23:32.
63. Goat VA, Feldman SA. The dual action of suxamethonium on the isolated rabbit heart. *Anaesthesia.* 1972;27:149–153.
64. Craythorne NW, Turndorf H, Dripps RD. Changes in pulse rate and rhythm associated with the use of succinylcholine in anesthetized patients. *Anesthesiology.* 1960;21:465.
65. Stoelting RK, Peterson C. Heart-rate slowing and junctional rhythm following intravenous succinylcholine with and without intramuscular atropine preanesthetic medication. *Anesth Analg.* 1975;54:705–709.
66. Leiman BC, Katz J, Butler BD. Mechanisms of succinylcholine-induced arrhythmias in hypoxic or hypoxic:hypercarbic dogs. *Anesth Analg.* 1987;66:1292–1297.
67. Nigrovic V, McCullough LS, Wajskol A, Levin JA, Martin JT. Succinylcholine-induced increases in plasma catecholamine levels in humans. *Anesth Analg.* 1983;62:627–632.
68. Derbyshire DR. Succinylcholine-induced increases in plasma catecholamine levels in humans. *Anesth Analg.* 1984;63:465–467.
69. Derbyshire DR, Chmielewski A, Fell D, Vater M, Achola K, Smith G. Plasma catecholamine responses to tracheal intubation. *Br J Anaesth.* 1983;55:855–860.
70. Walton JD, Farman JV. Suxamethonium hyperkalaemia in uraemic neuropathy. *Anaesthesia.* 1973;28:666–668.
71. Powell JN, Golby M. The pattern of potassium liberation following a single dose of suxamethonium in normal and uraemic rats. *Br J Anaesth.* 1971;43:662–668.
72. Kohlschutter B, Baur H, Roth F. Suxamethonium-induced hyperkalaemia in patients with severe intra-abdominal infections. *Br J Anaesth.* 1976;48:557–562.

73. Schwartz DE, Kelly B, Caldwell JE, Carlisle AS, Cohen NH. Succinylcholine-induced hyperkalemic arrest in a patient with severe metabolic acidosis and exsanguinating hemorrhage. *Anesth Analg.* 1992;75:291–293.
74. Stevenson PH, Birch AA. Succinylcholine-induced hyperkalemia in a patient with a closed head injury. *Anesthesiology.* 1979;51:89–90.
75. Martyn JA, Richtsfeld M. Succinylcholine-induced hyperkalemia in acquired pathologic states: etiologic factors and molecular mechanisms. *Anesthesiology.* 2006;104:158–169.
76. Rosenberg H, Gronert GA. Intractable cardiac arrest in children given succinylcholine. *Anesthesiology.* 1992;77:1054.
77. Morell RC, Berman JM, Royster RI, Petrozza PH, Kelly JS, Colonna DM. Revised label regarding use of succinylcholine in children and adolescents. *Anesthesiology.* 1994;80:242–245.
78. Badgwell JM, Hall SC, Lockhart C. Revised label regarding use of succinylcholine in children and adolescents. *Anesthesiology.* 1994;80:243–245.
79. Pandey K, Badola RP, Kumar S. Time course of intraocular hypertension produced by suxamethonium. *Br J Anaesth.* 1972;44:191–196.
80. Libonati MM, Leahy JJ, Ellison N. The use of succinylcholine in open eye surgery. *Anesthesiology.* 1985;62:637–640.
81. Meyers EF, Krupin T, Johnson M, Zink H. Failure of nondepolarizing neuromuscular blockers to inhibit succinylcholine-induced increased intraocular pressure, a controlled study. *Anesthesiology.* 1978;48:149–151.
82. Konchigeri HN, Lee YE, Venugopal K. Effect of pancuronium on intraocular pressure changes induced by succinylcholine. *Can Anaesth Soc J.* 1979;26:479–481.
83. Miller RD, Way WL, Hickey RF. Inhibition of succinylcholine-induced increased intraocular pressure by non-depolarizing muscle relaxants. *Anesthesiology.* 1968;29:123–126.
84. Miller RD, Way WL. Inhibition of succinylcholine-induced increased intragastric pressure by nondepolarizing muscle relaxants and lidocaine. *Anesthesiology.* 1971;34:185–188.
85. Smith G, Dalling R, Williams TI. Gastro-oesophageal pressure gradient changes produced by induction of anaesthesia and suxamethonium. *Br J Anaesth.* 1978;50:1137–1143.
86. Minton MD, Grosslight K, Stirt JA, Bedford RF. Increases in intracranial pressure from succinylcholine: prevention by prior nondepolarizing blockade. *Anesthesiology.* 1986;65:165–169.
87. Stirt JA, Grosslight KR, Bedford RF, Vollmer D. "Defasciculation" with metocurine prevents succinylcholine-induced increases in intracranial pressure. *Anesthesiology.* 1987;67:50–53.
88. Brodsky JB, Brock-Utne JG, Samuels SI. Pancuronium pretreatment and post-succinylcholine myalgias. *Anesthesiology.* 1979;51:259–261.
89. Waters DJ, Mapleson WW. Suxamethonium pains: hypothesis and observation. *Anaesthesia.* 1971;26:127–141.
90. Ryan JF, Kagen LJ, Hyman AI. Myoglobinemia after a single dose of succinylcholine. *N Engl J Med.* 1971;285:824–827.
91. Maddineni VR, Mirakhur RK, Cooper AR. Myalgia and biochemical changes following suxamethonium after induction of anaesthesia with thiopentone or propofol. *Anaesthesia.* 1993;48:626–628.
92. McLoughlin C, Elliott P, McCarthy G, Mirakhur RK. Muscle pains and biochemical changes following suxamethonium administration after six pretreatment regimens. *Anaesthesia.* 1992;47:202–206.
93. Demers-Pelletier J, Drolet P, Girard M, Donati F. Comparison of rocuronium and d-tubocurarine for prevention of succinylcholine-induced fasciculations and myalgia. *Can J Anaesth.* 1997;44:1144–1147.
94. Naguib M, Farag H, Magbagbeola JA. Effect of pre-treatment with lysine acetyl salicylate on suxamethonium-induced myalgia. *Br J Anaesth.* 1987;59:606–610.
95. Jackson MJ, Wagenmakers AJ, Edwards RH. Effect of inhibitors of arachidonic acid metabolism on efflux of intracellular enzymes from skeletal muscle following experimental damage. *Biochem J.* 1987;241:403–407.
96. Kahraman S, Ercan S, Aypar U, Erdem K. Effect of preoperative i.m. administration of diclofenac on suxamethonium-induced myalgia. *Br J Anaesth.* 1993;71:238–241.
97. Zahl K, Apfelbaum JL. Muscle pain occurs after outpatient laparoscopy despite the substitution of vecuronium for succinylcholine. *Anesthesiology.* 1989;70:408–411.
98. Smith I, Ding Y, White PF. Muscle pain after outpatient laparoscopy—influence of propofol versus thiopental and enflurane. *Anesth Analg.* 1993;76:1181–1184.
99. Donlon JV, Newfield P, Sreter F, Ryan JF. Implications of masseter spasm after succinylcholine. *Anesthesiology.* 1978;49:298–301.
100. Van der Spek AF, Fang WB, Ashton-Miller JA, Stohler CS, Carlson DS, Schork MA. The effects of succinylcholine on mouth opening. *Anesthesiology.* 1987;67:459–465.
101. Leary NP, Ellis FR. Masseteric muscle spasm as a normal response to suxamethonium. *Br J Anaesth.* 1990;64:488–492.
102. Habre W, Sims C. Masseter spasm and elevated creatine kinase after intravenous induction in a child. *Anaesth Intensive Care.* 1996;24:496–499.
103. Meakin G, Walker RW, Dearlove OR. Myotonic and neuromuscular blocking effects of increased doses of suxamethonium in infants and children. *Br J Anaesth.* 1990;65:816–818.
104. Bovet D. Some aspects of the relationship between chemical constitution and curare-like activity. *Ann N Y Acad Sci.* 1951;54:407–437.
105. Waser PG. Chemistry and pharmacology of natural curare compounds, neuromuscular blocking and stimulating agents. In: Cheymol J, ed. *International Encyclopedia of Pharmacology and Therapeutics*. Oxford: Pergamon Press; 1972:205–239.
106. Hill SA, Scott RPF, Savarese JJ. Structure-activity relationships: from tubocurarine to the present day. *Bailliere's Clin Anesthesiol.* 1994;8:317–348.
107. Lee C. Structure, conformation, and action of neuromuscular blocking drugs. *Br J Anaesth.* 2001;87:755–769.
108. Tuba Z, Maho S, Vizi ES. Synthesis and structure-activity relationships of neuromuscular blocking agents. *Curr Med Chem.* 2002;9:1507–1536.
109. Everett AJ, Lowe LA, Wilkinson S. Revision of the structures of (+)-tubocurarine chloride and (+)-chondocurine. *J Chem Soc.* 1970;D:1020–1021.
110. Gandiha A, Marshall IG, Paul D, Singh H. Neuromuscular and other blocking actions of a new series of mono and bisquaternary aza steroids. *J Pharm Pharmacol.* 1974;26:871–877.
111. Miller RD, Matteo RS, Benet LZ, Sohn YJ. The pharmacokinetics of d-tubocurarine in man with and without renal failure. *J Pharmacol Exp Ther.* 1977;202:1–7.
112. Stenlake JB, Waigh RD, Dewar GH, et al. Biodegradable neuromuscular blocking agents, 6: stereochemical studies on atracurium and related polyalkylene di-esters. *Eur J Med Chem.* 1984;19:441–450.
113. Tsui D, Graham GG, Torda TA. The pharmacokinetics of atracurium isomers in vitro and in humans. *Anesthesiology.* 1987;67:722–728.
114. Nehmer U. Simultaneous determination of atracurium besylate and its major decomposition products and related impurities by reversed-phase high-performance liquid chromatography. *J Chromatogr.* 1988;435:425–433.
115. Stenlake JB, Waigh RD, Urwin J, Dewar GH, Coker GG. Atracurium: conception and inception. *Br J Anaesth.* 1983;55(Suppl 1):3S–10S.
116. Neill EA, Chapple DJ, Thompson CW. Metabolism and kinetics of atracurium: an overview. *Br J Anaesth.* 1983;55(Suppl 1):23S–25S.
117. Chapple DJ, Clark JS. Pharmacological action of breakdown products of atracurium and related substances. *Br J Anaesth.* 1983;55(Suppl 1):11S–15S.

118. Shi WZ, Fahey MR, Fisher DM, Miller RD. Modification of central nervous system effects of laudanosine by inhalation anaesthetics. *Br J Anaesth.* 1989;63:598–600.
119. Chapple DJ, Miller AA, Ward JB, Wheatley PL. Cardiovascular and neurological effects of laudanosine: studies in mice and rats, and in conscious and anaesthetized dogs. *Br J Anaesth.* 1987;59: 218–225.
120. Yate PM, Flynn PJ, Arnold RW, Weatherly BC, Simmonds RJ, Dopson T. Clinical experience and plasma laudanosine concentrations during the infusion of atracurium in the intensive therapy unit. *Br J Anaesth.* 1987;59:211–217.
121. Fahey MR, Rupp SM, Fisher DM, et al. The pharmacokinetics and pharmacodynamics of atracurium in patients with and without renal failure. *Anesthesiology.* 1984;61:699–702.
122. Ward S, Boheimer N, Weatherley BC, Simmonds RJ, Dopson TA. Pharmacokinetics of atracurium and its metabolites in patients with normal renal function, and in patients in renal failure. *Br J Anaesth.* 1987;59:697–706.
123. Zhang J, Haddad GG, Xia Y. delta-, but not mu- and kappa-, opioid receptor activation protects neocortical neurons from glutamate-induced excitotoxic injury. *Brain Res.* 2000;885:143–153.
124. Belluardo N, Mudo G, Blum M, Fuxe K. Central nicotinic receptors, neurotrophic factors and neuroprotection. *Behav Brain Res.* 2000;113:21–34.
125. Tassonyi E, Fathi M, Hughes GJ, et al. Cerebrospinal fluid concentrations of atracurium, laudanosine and vecuronium following clinical subarachnoid hemorrhage. *Acta Anaesthesiol Scand.* 2002; 46:1236–1241.
126. Fodale V, Pratico C, Signer MR, Santamaria LB. Perinatal neuroprotection by muscle relaxants against hypoxic-ischemic lesions: is it a possible hypothesis? *J Matern Fetal Neonatal Med.* 2005;18: 133–136.
127. Welch RM, Brown A, Ravitch J, Dahl R. The in vitro degradation of cisatracurium, the R, cis-R'-isomer of atracurium, in human and rat plasma. *Clin Pharmacol Ther.* 1995;58:132–142.
128. Lien CA, Schmith VD, Belmont MR, Abalos A, Kisor DF, Savarese JJ. Pharmacokinetics of cisatracurium in patients receiving nitrous oxide/opioid/barbiturate anesthesia. *Anesthesiology.* 1996; 84:300–308.
129. Kisor DF, Schmith VD, Wargin WA, Lien CA, Ornstein E, Cook DR. Importance of the organ-independent elimination of cisatracurium. *Anesth Analg.* 1996;83:1065–1071.
130. Ornstein E, Lien CA, Matteo RS, Ostapkovich ND, Diaz J, Wolf KB. Pharmacodynamics and pharmacokinetics of cisatracurium in geriatric surgical patients. *Anesthesiology.* 1996;84:520–525.
131. Wastila WB, Maehr RB, Turner GL, Hill DA, Savarese JJ. Comparative pharmacology of cisatracurium (51W89), atracurium, and five isomers in cats. *Anesthesiology.* 1996;85:169–177.
132. Lien CA, Belmont MR, Abalos A, et al. The cardiovascular effects and histamine-releasing properties of 51W89 in patients receiving nitrous oxide/opioid/barbiturate anesthesia. *Anesthesiology.* 1995; 82:1131–1138.
133. Savarese JJ, Wastila WB. The future of the benzylisoquinolinium relaxants. *Acta Anaesthesiol Scand Suppl.* 1995;106:91–93.
134. Lien CA, Schmith VD, Embree PB, Belmont MR, Wargin WA, Savarese JJ. The pharmacokinetics and pharmacodynamics of the stereoisomers of mivacurium in patients receiving nitrous oxide/ opioid/barbiturate anesthesia. *Anesthesiology.* 1994;80:1296–1302.
135. Savarese JJ, Ali HH, Basta SJ, et al. The clinical neuromuscular pharmacology of mivacurium chloride (BW B1090U). A short-acting nondepolarizing ester neuromuscular blocking drug. *Anesthesiology.* 1988;68:723–732.
136. Head-Rapson AG, Devlin JC, Parker CJ, Hunter JM. Pharmacokinetics of the three isomers of mivacurium and pharmacodynamics of the chiral mixture in hepatic cirrhosis. *Br J Anaesth.* 1994;73:613–618.
137. Naguib M, Samarkandi AH, Bakhamees HS, Magboul MA, el-Bakry AK. Histamine-release haemodynamic changes produced by rocuronium, vecuronium, mivacurium, atracurium and tubocurarine. *Br J Anaesth.* 1995;75:588–592.
138. Buckett WR, Hewett CL, Savage DS. Pancuronium bromide and other steroidal neuromuscular blocking agents containing acetylcholine fragments. *J Med Chem.* 1973;16:1116–1124.
139. Durant NN, Marshall IG, Savage DS, Nelson DJ, Sleigh T, Carlyle IC. The neuromuscular and autonomic blocking activities of pancuronium, Org NC 45, and other pancuronium analogues, in the cat. *J Pharm Pharmacol.* 1979;31:831–836.
140. Stovner J, Oftedal N, Holmboe J. The inhibition of cholinesterases by pancuronium. *Br J Anaesth.* 1975;47:949–954.
141. Agoston S, Vermeer GA, Kertsten UW, Meijer DK. The fate of pancuronium bromide in man. *Acta Anaesthesiol Scand.* 1973;17: 267–275.
142. Miller RD, Agoston S, Booij LH, Kersten UW, Crul JF, Ham J. The comparative potency and pharmacokinetics of pancuronium and its metabolites in anesthetized man. *J Pharmacol Exp Ther.* 1978;207:539–543.
143. Savage DS, Sleigh T, Carlyle I. The emergence of ORG NC 45, 1- [2 beta,3 alpha,5 alpha,16 beta,17 beta)-3, 17-bis(acetyloxy)-2-(1-piperidinyl)-androstan-16-yl]-1-methylpiperidinium bromide, from the pancuronium series. *Br J Anaesth.* 1980;52(Suppl 1): 3S–9S.
144. Lebrault C, Berger JL, D'Hollander AA, Gomeni R, Henzel D, Duvaldestin P. Pharmacokinetics and pharmacodynamics of vecuronium (ORG NC 45) in patients with cirrhosis. *Anesthesiology.* 1985;62:601–605.
145. Caldwell JE, Szenohradszky J, Segredo V, et al. The pharmacodynamics and pharmacokinetics of the metabolite 3-desacetylvecuronium (ORG 7268) and its parent compound, vecuronium, in human volunteers. *J Pharmacol Exp Ther.* 1994;270:1216–1222.
146. Arden JR, Lynam DP, Castagnoli KP, Canfell PC, Cannon JC, Miller RD. Vecuronium in alcoholic liver disease: a pharmacokinetic and pharmacodynamic analysis. *Anesthesiology.* 1988;68:771–776.
147. Fahey MR, Morris RB, Miller RD, Nguyen TL, Upton RA. Pharmacokinetics of Org NC45 (norcuron) in patients with and without renal failure. *Br J Anaesth.* 1981;53:1049–1053.
148. Bencini AF, Scaf AH, Sohn YJ, Meistelman C, Lienhart A, Kersten UW, et al. Disposition and urinary excretion of vecuronium bromide in anesthetized patients with normal renal function or renal failure. *Anesth Analg.* 1986;65:245–251.
149. Wright PM, Hart P, Lau M, Sharma ML, Gruenke L, Fisher DM. Cumulative characteristics of atracurium and vecuronium: a simultaneous clinical and pharmacokinetic study. *Anesthesiology.* 1994; 81:59–68.
150. Data on file. Organon Inc.
151. Wierda JM, Proost JH. Structure-pharmacodynamic-pharmacokinetic relationships of steroidal neuromuscular blocking agents. *Eur J Anaesthesiol Suppl.* 1995;11:45–54.
152. Naguib M, Samarkandi AH, Bakhamees HS, Magboul MA, el-Bakry AK. Comparative potency of steroidal neuromuscular blocking drugs and isobolographic analysis of the interaction between rocuronium and other aminosteroids. *Br J Anaesth.* 1995;75:37–42.
153. Smit JW, Duin E, Steen H, Oosting R, Roggeveld J, Meijer DK. Interactions between P-glycoprotein substrates and other cationic drugs at the hepatic excretory level. *Br J Pharmacol.* 1998;123: 361–370.
154. Khuenl-Brady K, Castagnoli KP, Canfell PC, Caldwell JE, Agoston S, Miller RD. The neuromuscular blocking effects and pharmacokinetics of ORG 9426 and ORG 9616 in the cat. *Anesthesiology.* 1990;72:669–674.
155. Szenohradszky J, Fisher DM, Segredo V, et al. Pharmacokinetics of rocuronium bromide (ORG 9426) in patients with normal renal function or patients undergoing cadaver renal transplantation. *Anesthesiology.* 1992;77:899–904.
156. Vizi ES, Tuba Z, Mahó S, et al. A new short-acting non-depolarizing muscle relaxant (SZ1677) without cardiovascular side-effects. *Acta Anaesthesiol Scand.* 2003;47:291–300.

157. Takagi S, Adachi YU, Saubermann AJ, Vizi ES. Presynaptic inhibitory effects of rocuronium and SZ1677 on [3H]acetylcholine release from the mouse hemidiaphragm preparation. *Neurochem Intl.* 2002;40:655–659.
158. Savarese JJ, Belmont MR, Hashim MA, et al. Preclinical pharmacology of GW280430A (AV430A) in the rhesus monkey and in the cat: a comparison with mivacurium. *Anesthesiology.* 2004;100: 835–845.
159. Boros EE, Samano V, Ray JA, et al. Neuromuscular blocking activity and therapeutic potential of mixed-tetrahydroisoquinolinium halofumarates and halosuccinates in rhesus monkeys. *J Med Chem.* 2003;46:2502–2515.
160. Belmont MR, Lien CA, Tjan J, et al. Clinical pharmacology of GW280430A in humans. *Anesthesiology.* 2004;100:768–773.
161. Savarese JJ, Belmont MR, Kraus K, Cross WM, Tg LA, Vasquez A. AV002: a promising cysteine-reversible intermediate duration neuromuscular blocker in rhesus monkeys. *ASA Meeting.* San Francisco, CA; 2007:A986.
162. Sunaga H, Malhotora JK, Savarese JJ, Heerdt PM. Dose response relationship for cysteine reversal of the novel muscle relaxant AV002 in dogs. *ASA Annual Meeting.* Orlando, FL; 2008:A364.
163. Donlon JV Jr., Ali HH, Savarese JJ. A new approach to the study of four nondepolarizing relaxants in man. *Anesth Analg.* 1974; 53:934–939.
164. Kopman AF, Lien CA, Naguib M. Determining the potency of neuromuscular blockers: are traditional methods flawed? *Br J Anaesth.* 2010;104(6):705–710.
165. Saitoh Y, Toyooka H, Amaha K. Recoveries of post-tetanic twitch and train-of-four responses after administration of vecuronium with different inhalation anaesthetics and neuroleptanaesthesia. *Br J Anaesth.* 1993;70:402–404.
166. Miller RD, Way WL, Dolan WM, Stevens WC, Eger EI 2nd. The dependence of pancuronium- and d-tubocurarine-induced neuromuscular blockades on alveolar concentrations of halothane and forane. *Anesthesiology.* 1972;37:573–581.
167. Miller RD, Crique M, Eger EI 2nd. Duration of halothane anesthesia and neuromuscular blockade with d-tubocurarine. *Anesthesiology.* 1976;44:206–210.
168. Kelly RE, Lien CA, Savarese JJ, et al. Depression of neuromuscular function in a patient during desflurane anesthesia. *Anesth Analg.* 1993;76:868–871.
169. Rupp SM, Miller RD, Gencarelli PJ. Vecuronium-induced neuromuscular blockade during enflurane, isoflurane, and halothane anesthesia in humans. *Anesthesiology.* 1984;60:102–105.
170. Gencarelli PJ, Miller RD, Eger EI 2nd, Newfield P. Decreasing enflurane concentrations and d-tubocurarine neuromuscular blockade. *Anesthesiology.* 1982;56:192–194.
171. Miller RD, Way WL, Dolan WM, Stevens WC, Eger EI 2nd. Comparative neuromuscular effects of pancuronium, gallamine, and succinylcholine during forane and halothane anesthesia in man. *Anesthesiology.* 1971;35:509–514.
172. Wulf H, Ledowski T, Linstedt U, Proppe D, Sitzlack D. Neuromuscular blocking effects of rocuronium during desflurane, isoflurane, and sevoflurane anaesthesia. *Can J Anaesth.* 1998;45: 526–532.
173. Bock M, Klippel K, Nitsche B, Bach A, Martin E, Motsch J. Rocuronium potency and recovery characteristics during steady-state desflurane, sevoflurane, isoflurane or propofol anaesthesia. *Br J Anaesth.* 2000;84:43–47.
174. Pereon Y, Bernard JM, Nguyen The Tich S, Genet R, Petitfaux F, Guiheneuc P. The effects of desflurane on the nervous system: from spinal cord to muscles. *Anesth Analg.* 1999;89:490–495.
175. Franks NP, Lieb WR. Molecular and cellular mechanisms of general anaesthesia. *Nature.* 1994;367:607–614.
176. Paul M, Fokt RM, Kindler CH, Dipp NC, Yost CS. Characterization of the interactions between volatile anesthetics and neuromuscular blockers at the muscle nicotinic acetylcholine receptor. *Anesth Analg.* 2002;95:362–367.
177. Singh YN, Harvey AL, Marshall IG. Antibiotic-induced paralysis of the mouse phrenic nerve-hemidiaphragm preparation, and reversibility by calcium and by neostigmine. *Anesthesiology.* 1978;48:418–424.
178. Heier T, Caldwell JE, Sessler DI, Miller RD. Mild intraoperative hypothermia increases duration of action and spontaneous recovery of vecuronium blockade during nitrous oxide-isoflurane anesthesia in humans. *Anesthesiology.* 1991;74:815–819.
179. Leslie K, Sessler DI, Bjorksten AR, Moayeri A. Mild hypothermia alters propofol pharmacokinetics and increases the duration of action of atracurium. *Anesth Analg.* 1995;80:1007–1014.
180. Caldwell JE, Heier T, Wright PM, et al. Temperature-dependent pharmacokinetics and pharmacodynamics of vecuronium. *Anesthesiology.* 2000;92:84–93.
181. Sinatra RS, Philip BK, Naulty JS, Ostheimer GW. Prolonged neuromuscular blockade with vecuronium in a patient treated with magnesium sulfate. *Anesth Analg.* 1985;64:1220–1222.
182. Usubiaga JE, Wikinski JA, Morales RL, Usubiaga LE. Interaction of intravenously administered procaine, lidocaine and succinylcholine in anesthetized subjects. *Anesth Analg.* 1967;46:39–45.
183. Miller RD, Way WL, Katzung BG. The potentiation of neuromuscular blocking agents by quinidine. *Anesthesiology.* 1967;28: 1036–1041.
184. Alloul K, Whalley DG, Shutway F, Ebrahim Z, Varin F. Pharmacokinetic origin of carbamazepine-induced resistance to vecuronium neuromuscular blockade in anesthetized patients. *Anesthesiology.* 1996;84:330–339.
185. Kim CS, Arnold FJ, Itani MS, Martyn JA. Decreased sensitivity to metocurine during long-term phenytoin therapy may be attributable to protein binding and acetylcholine receptor changes. *Anesthesiology.* 1992;77:500–506.
186. Al-Mohaya S, Naguib M, Abdelatif M, Farag H. Abnormal responses to muscle relaxants in a patient with primary hyperparathyroidism. *Anesthesiology.* 1986;65:554–556.
187. Waud BE, Waud DR. Interaction of calcium and potassium with neuromuscular blocking agents. *Br J Anaesth.* 1980;52:863–866.
188. Bowman WC, Rodger IW, Houston J, Marshall RJ, McIndewar I. Structure:action relationships among some desacetoxy analogues of pancuronium and vecuronium in the anesthetized cat. *Anesthesiology.* 1988;69:57–62.
189. Kopman AF, Klewicka MM, Kopman DJ, Neuman GG. Molar potency is predictive of the speed of onset of neuromuscular block for agents of intermediate, short, and ultrashort duration. *Anesthesiology.* 1999;90:425–431.
190. Kopman AF, Klewicka MM, Neuman GG. Molar potency is not predictive of the speed of onset of atracurium. *Anesth Analg.* 1999;89:1046–1049.
191. Naguib M, Kopman AF. Low dose rocuronium for tracheal intubation. *Middle East J Anesthesiol.* 2003;17:193–204.
192. Paton WD, Waud DR. The margin of safety of neuromuscular transmission. *J Physiol.* 1967;191:59–90.
193. Adams PR. Drug interactions at the motor endplate. *Pflugers Arch.* 1975;360:155–164.
194. Donati F, Meistelman C. A kinetic-dynamic model to explain the relationship between high potency and slow onset time for neuromuscular blocking drugs. *J Pharmacokinet Biopharm.* 1991;19:537–552.
195. Bevan DR. The new relaxants: are they worth it? *Can J Anaesth.* 1999;46: R88–100.
196. Anaesthetists and the reporting of adverse drug reactions. *Br Med J (Clin Res Ed).* 1986;292:949.
197. Vercruysse P, Bossuyt P, Hanegreefs G, Verbeuren TJ, Vanhoutte PM. Gallamine and pancuronium inhibit pre- and postjunctional muscarine receptors in canine saphenous veins. *J Pharmacol Exp Ther.* 1979;209:225–230.
198. Savarese JJ, Lowenstein E. The name of the game: no anesthesia by cookbook. *Anesthesiology.* 1985;62:703–705.
199. Domenech JS, Garcia RC, Sastain JM, Loyola AQ, Oroz JS. Pancuronium bromide: an indirect sympathomimetic agent. *Br J Anaesth.* 1976;48:1143–1148.

200. Savarese JJ, Ali HH, Basta SJ, et al. The cardiovascular effects of mivacurium chloride (BW B1090U) in patients receiving nitrous oxide-opiate-barbiturate anesthesia. *Anesthesiology.* 1989; 70:386–394.
201. Scott RP, Savarese JJ, Basta SJ, et al. Atracurium: clinical strategies for preventing histamine release and attenuating the haemodynamic response. *Br J Anaesth.* 1985;57:550–553.
202. Moss J, Rosow CE, Savarese JJ, Philbin DM, Kniffen KJ. Role of histamine in the hypotensive action of d-tubocurarine in humans. *Anesthesiology.* 1981;55:19–25.
203. Basta SJ, Savarese JJ, Ali HH, Moss J, Gionfriddo M. Histamine-releasing potencies of atracurium, dimethyl tubocurarine and tubocurarine. *Br J Anaesth.* 1983;55(Suppl 1):105S–106S.
204. Naguib M, Abdulatif M, Absood A. Comparative effects of pipecuronium and tubocurarine on plasma concentrations of histamine in humans. *Br J Anaesth.* 1991;67:320–322.
205. Cannon JE, Fahey MR, Moss J, Miller RD. Large doses of vecuronium and plasma histamine concentrations. *Can J Anaesth.* 1988;35:350–353.
206. Levy JH, Davis GK, Duggan J, Szlam F. Determination of the hemodynamics and histamine release of rocuronium (Org 9426) when administered in increased doses under N2O/O2-sufentanil anesthesia. *Anesth Analg.* 1994;78:318–321.
207. Moss J, Rosow CE. Histamine release by narcotics and muscle relaxants in humans. *Anesthesiology.* 1983;59:330–339.
208. Flacke W, Gillis RA. Impulse transmission via nicotinic and muscarinic pathways in the stellate ganglion of the dog. *J Pharmacol Exp Ther.* 1968;163:266–276.
209. Basta SJ. Modulation of histamine release by neuromuscular blocking drugs. *Curr Opinion Anaesthesiol.* 1992;5:572.
210. Bonner TI, Young AC, Brann MR, Buckley NJ. Cloning and expression of the human and rat m5 muscarinic acetylcholine receptor genes. *Neuron.* 1988;1:403–410.
211. Mak JC, Barnes PJ. Autoradiographic visualization of muscarinic receptor subtypes in human and guinea pig lung. *Am Rev Respir Dis.* 1990;141:1559–1568.
212. Coulson FR, Fryer AD. Muscarinic acetylcholine receptors and airway diseases. *Pharmacol Ther.* 2003;98:59–69.
213. Jooste E, Klafter F, Hirshman CA, Emala CW. A mechanism for rapacuronium-induced bronchospasm: M2 muscarinic receptor antagonism. *Anesthesiology.* 2003;98:906–911.
214. Laxenaire MC, Moneret-Vautrin DA, Widmer S, et al. Anesthetics responsible for anaphylactic shock: a French multicenter study [in French]. *Ann Fr Anesth Reanim.* 1990;9:501–506.
215. Fisher MM, More DG. The epidemiology and clinical features of anaphylactic reactions in anaesthesia. *Anaesth Intensive Care.* 1981;9:226–234.
216. Mertes PM, Laxenaire MC, Alla F. Anaphylactic and anaphylactoid reactions occurring during anesthesia in France in 1999–2000. *Anesthesiology.* 2003;99:536–545.
217. Baldo BA, Fisher MM. Substituted ammonium ions as allergenic determinants in drug allergy. *Nature.* 1983;306:262–264.
218. Mertes PM, Moneret-Vautrin DA, Leynadier F, Laxenaire MC. Skin reactions to intradermal neuromuscular blocking agent injections: a randomized multicenter trial in healthy volunteers. *Anesthesiology.* 2007;107:245–252.
219. Head-Rapson AG, Devlin JC, Parker CJ, Hunter JM. Pharmacokinetics and pharmacodynamics of the three isomers of mivacurium in health, in end-stage renal failure and in patients with impaired renal function. *Br J Anaesth.* 1995;75:31–36.
220. Vandenbrom RH, Wierda JM, Agoston S. Pharmacokinetics and neuromuscular blocking effects of atracurium besylate and two of its metabolites in patients with normal and impaired renal function. *Clin Pharmacokinet.* 1990;19:230–240.
221. Lynam DP, Cronnelly R, Castagnoli KP, et al. The pharmacodynamics and pharmacokinetics of vecuronium in patients anesthetized with isoflurane with normal renal function or with renal failure. *Anesthesiology.* 1988;69:227–231.
222. Sheiner LB, Stanski DR, Vozeh S, Miller RD, Ham J. Simultaneous modeling of pharmacokinetics and pharmacodynamics: application to d-tubocurarine. *Clin Pharmacol Ther.* 1979;25:358–371.
223. Somogyi AA, Shanks CA, Triggs EJ. The effect of renal failure on the disposition and neuromuscular blocking action of pancuronium bromide. *Eur J Clin Pharmacol.* 1977;12:23–29.

17

ANESTHESIA AND DISORDERS OF THE NEUROMUSCULAR SYSTEM

François Donati

Patients with neuromuscular disease present a particular challenge to the anesthesiologist. Decreased muscle power leads to weakness or loss of function of certain muscle groups, particularly those that are responsible for adequate breathing, clearance of secretions, and maintenance of a patent upper airway. Certain conditions are associated with neurological and cardiac symptoms that must be considered in the anesthetic plan. In addition, the presence of neuromuscular disease alters the effects of the anesthetic drugs, particularly neuromuscular blocking agents. The purpose of this chapter is not to list the numerous anesthetic considerations for all these diseases. Rather, the focus will be on the interactions between disease and drugs, as well as the underlying drug mechanism, in particular neuromuscular blocking agents. A summary of interactions between neuromuscular disease and commonly used drugs in anesthesiology can be found in Table 17.1.

Neuromuscular diseases can be classified in many different ways, and changes are made when a new syndrome is described, when similarities are discovered between known entities, or when advances in genetic testing are made. For the purpose of the following discussion, it is convenient to separate the various diseases, syndromes, and conditions according to the primary site of the lesion. Muscle function can be affected because of 1) failure of nerves to supply action potentials to the muscle, 2) a defect in neurotransmission at the neuromuscular junction, or 3) a problem in the muscle itself. Diseases involving the nervous system can be further divided into upper and lower motor neuron disease.

PATHOPHYSIOLOGY

MOTOR UNIT

The control of the motor system in the central nervous system is rather complex, as many parts of the brain are involved in the generation of movement. Usually, however, the connection between the cerebral cortex and the nucleus of the cranial nerve or spinal cord involves just one nerve axon. That single nerve cell synapses with a peripheral motoneuron that exits the central nervous system and forms a long axon without synapsing until it reaches the muscle. Nerve cells are therefore elongated cells that can reach nearly one meter in length and are particularly prone to damage and injury. When it reaches the muscle, the axon branches into several nerve terminals, each of which reaches a muscle cell, or fiber. However, there is only one neuromuscular junction per muscle fiber, so that if a nerve axon is not functional, the muscle fibers it innervates fail to contract. The number of terminal branches depends on the function of the muscle in question. Muscles designed for fine, accurate, and delicate movement may have as few as 3 such branches, while there may be as many as 1000 in strong postural muscles. Muscles of the hand are intermediate. For example, the adductor pollicis is supplied by a mean of 128 nerve fibers, and each of these innervates a mean of 106 muscle fibers,[1] for a total number of 128 x 106 = 13,568 muscle fibers. A motor unit is defined as the nerve cell and all the muscle fibers it innervates. Thus, the adductor pollicis is made up of approximately 128 motor units, with an average size of 106.

DEVELOPMENT

The structural integrity of the neuromuscular junction and muscle depends on muscle activity,[2] which in turn depends on nerve action potential traffic. Therefore, diseases of the nervous system involving the motor system have profound effects on muscle function and structure. It is also useful to distinguish "upper motor neuron" lesions, which affect nerve cells in the central nervous system before they synapse, and "lower motor neuron" lesions, which involve peripheral nerve. With a lower motor neuron lesion, no action potential travels down the nerve to the neuromuscular junction and the muscle exhibits flaccid paralysis.

During development, nicotinic receptors of the fetal or immature type are made up of two α subunits and one each of β, δ, and γ subunits, and are evenly distributed over the whole muscle membrane. With the growth of the nervous system, several nerve terminals reach each muscle fiber, but

Table 17.1 USE OF NEUROMUSCULAR BLOCKING AGENTS AND HALOGENATED AGENTS IN DISORDERS OF NERVE AND MUSCLE

DISORDER	NONDEPOLARIZING NEUROMUSCULAR BLOCKING AGENTS	SUCCINYLCHOLINE	HALOGENATED AGENTS	OTHER DRUGS
MYASTHENIA GRAVIS	Increased sensitivity	Decreased sensitivity	May induce neuromuscular block	Limited effectiveness of anticholinesterase agents if patient taking it already
EATON-LAMBERT MYASTHENIC SYNDROME	Increased sensitivity	Limited data	Limited data	
CONGENITAL MYASTHENIC SYNDROMES	Limited data		Limited data	
LOWER MOTOR NEURON LESION		Contractures		
CHARCOT-MARIE-TOOTH DISEASE	Near normal sensitivity	No abnormal responses reported		
GUILLAIN-BARRÉ SYNDROME	Limited data	Limited data but best avoided		
IMMOBILIZATION	Decreased sensitivity	More subject to hyperkalemia, especially with critical illness		
SPINAL CORD TRAUMA	Decreased sensitivity	High risk of hyperkalemia		
STROKE	Decreased sensitivity, especially on affected side	Risk of hyperkalemia present		
MULTIPLE SCLEROSIS	Near normal sensitivity	No reports of unusual responses		
AMYOTROPHIC LATERAL SCLEROSIS	Limited data	Limited data		
DUCHENNE MUSCULAR DYSTROPHY	Normal or increased sensitivity	Rhabdomyolysis, hyperkalemia	Exacerbates the effect of succinylcholine. May induce rhabdomyolysis of their own.	
BECKER MUSCULAR DYSTROPHY	Normal or increased sensitivity	Rhabdomyolysis, hyperkalemia	Limited data	
OCULO-PHARYNGEAL DYSTROPHY	Increased sensitivity	No adverse effects reported	No adverse effects reported	
CONGENITAL MYOTONIAS	Limited data	Rigidity, contractures	No adverse effects reported in limited series	
MYOTONIC DYSTROPHY DM1 OR STEINERT'S DISEASE	Increased or near normal sensitivity	May produce contractures	May produce hypertonic response	Neostigmine may produce contractures
MYOTONIC DYSTROPHY DM2	Near normal sensitivity, but limited data	Limited data, but contractures are expected	No adverse effects reported, but limited data	Limited data on neostigmine

(Continued)

Table 17.1 (CONTINUED)

DISORDER	NONDEPOLARIZING NEUROMUSCULAR BLOCKING AGENTS	SUCCINYLCHOLINE	HALOGENATED AGENTS	OTHER DRUGS
CRITICAL ILLNESS MYOPATHY	**Increased sensitivity compared with immobilization**	**Risk of hyperkalemia**		
BURNS	**Decreased sensitivity**	**High risk of hyperkalemia**	**No specific risk**	
MALIGNANT HYPERTHERMIA	**Normal sensitivity**	**Potential trigger**	**Potential trigger**	

only one of these eventually develops fully, while the others regress. The area of contact between nerve and muscle, which represents only a tiny fraction of the muscle membrane, develops into a specialized structure called the neuromuscular junction. The number of receptors at the neuromuscular junction increases and the structure of these receptors changes, the γ subunit being substituted for the ε subunit. This new type of receptor, which also responds to acetylcholine, is called the mature, or adult receptor. The endplate, which is the part of the muscle membrane facing the nerve terminal, develops a number of folds. A high density of receptors clusters at the crests of the folds, while the bottom of the folds contains a large number of sodium channels. At the same time, the number of immature, or fetal receptors found elsewhere on the muscle membrane decreases markedly, but their structure remains the same, with a γ subunit.[2,3] Because they are found outside the neuromuscular junction, these immature receptors are also called extrajunctional receptors. In humans, these changes occur in the third trimester and in early postnatal life. Throughout life, the number of receptors at the neuromuscular junction depends on muscle activity. There is a decrease in their numbers (downregulation) when muscle is solicited heavily, as occurs with strenuous exercise, and there is an increase (upregulation) with immobilization or prolonged infusion of neuromuscular blocking agents. Downregulation is associated with an increased sensitivity to nondepolarizing neuromuscular blocking agents and upregulation leads to decreased sensitivity to these agents.[2,4]

DENERVATION

Interruption of nerve action potentials produces the same changes as those observed during development, but in reverse order. Initially, there is upregulation at the neuromuscular junction, with an increase in the number of junctional receptors. Then, extrajunctional receptors start to proliferate, because the nerve no longer provides inhibition of their formation.[4] Another type of receptor, also seen during development, might be seen during denervation. It is made up of five α subunits, and is called α_7.[4] If sufficiently damaged, the nerve axon degenerates, with loss of neuromuscular junction. This leads to muscle fiber degeneration unless there is reinnervation with formation of a new neuromuscular junction. These changes are typical of lower motor neuron lesions. With upper motor neuron lesions, the structural integrity of the lower motoneuron is not affected, and action potentials might be generated either by electrical stimulation or by reflex activation. Upregulation leads to hyperreflexia, and long-term changes such as hypertonicity and rigidity may develop.

MARGIN OF SAFETY

Acetylcholine is synthesized in nerve terminals, packaged into vesicles, and released in the synaptic cleft in response to a nerve action potential. Normally, the quantity of acetylcholine released is in excess of what is required to depolarize the endplate and trigger an action potential in the muscle cell. Furthermore, there are many more receptors available than required to depolarize the endplate.[5] Thus, failure of transmission occurs only when there is a major reduction in the amount of neurotransmitter released or in the number of functional receptors. The actual number of receptors that must be blocked before transmission fails and neuromuscular blockade starts to appear varies between species. There is evidence that in humans the safety margin might be less than in cats and dogs, from which the widely quoted value of 70–75% was derived.[5] Nevertheless, the principle of a safety margin or spare receptors holds true in humans. Also, different muscles have different margins of safety. For example, the diaphragm has a wide margin of safety: it is relatively resistant to the effect of nondepolarizing neuromuscular blocking agents and is affected only in the later stages of myasthenia gravis. In contrast, eye and bulbar muscles have a narrower margin of safety and are particularly affected by nondepolarizing neuromuscular blocking agents and myasthenia gravis. This differential sensitivity cannot be attributed to different cholinergic receptors, because the same adult, ε-type receptor is present at all neuromuscular junctions. Muscle type might explain some of the differences, but geometrical factors probably play a key role. Muscles made up of large fibers having small neuromuscular junctions are likely to have a lower margin of safety than those consisting of smaller fibers and/or larger neuromuscular junctions.[6]

MUSCLE CONTRACTION

If the depolarization at the endplate is sufficient, an action potential that propagates throughout the whole muscle fiber is generated, and this triggers an influx of calcium that initiates muscle contraction involving the interaction between the actin and myosin filaments. Termination of the contraction occurs when calcium is inactivated intracellularly, sequestered in the sarcoplasmic reticulum, or extruded from the cell. Sometimes initiation of contraction is sluggish or inoperative, in which case the electromyographic (EMG) signal, which is the sum of all action potentials in muscle, is normal, but force is abnormal. In other instances relaxation does not proceed normally and a prolonged contraction occurs. A contracture occurs when muscle contracts in the absence of an EMG signal.

DISORDERS OF THE NEUROMUSCULAR JUNCTION

MYASTHENIA GRAVIS

The most common disorder of the neuromuscular junction is myasthenia gravis. It is an autoimmune disorder characterized by the presence of antibodies against cholinergic receptors at the neuromuscular junction. Changes at the neuromuscular junction include a decreased receptor number, with loss of the characteristic folds of the postsynaptic membrane.[7] Onset of the disease may be at any age, but it occurs commonly in the adult years. When onset is before age 40 yr, there is a strong female predominance. Males are more often affected if onset is later. Approximately 80% of patients have measurable antibodies measured by radioimmunoassay.[8] Early symptoms typically involve palpebral, extraocular, and bulbar muscles. Drooped eyelids and diplopia are common and may be the only symptoms (ocular myasthenia). Generalized myasthenia applies to cases in which other muscles are involved. Bulbar involvement may be manifested by difficulty in swallowing, weakness of facial muscles, dysarthria, and aspiration. Respiratory failure is usually a late manifestation of the disease.[9] The sequence of affected muscles is similar to that observed with an increasing dose of nondepolarizing neuromuscular blocking agents: the eye muscles are particularly sensitive, the upper airway musculature is next, and the diaphragm is particularly resistant.

DIAGNOSIS

The diagnosis of myasthenia gravis is based on the same principles as monitoring of intraoperative nondepolarizing blockade: it depends on the detection of fade in response to repetitive stimulation and the action of anticholinesterase agents. When an action potential invades the nerve terminal, a few hundred of the many acetylcholine vesicles located near the synaptic membrane are released simultaneously. If a second action potential arrives shortly thereafter, fewer of these vesicles are present at the release sites, so acetylcholine release is less. If firing from the nerve is sustained, the amount of acetylcholine released with each impulse decreases, until the rate of replenishment of the vesicles balances the rate of release. In normal subjects, the progressive decline in acetylcholine output has no consequence, because there is enough neurotransmitter to depolarize the muscle fiber. In other words, the margin of safety is sufficient for high frequency nerve firing. However, in myasthenia gravis, the number of receptors is reduced, so the amount of acetylcholine release on the first impulse might be just enough to produce depolarization. After subsequent action potentials, there is less and less acetylcholine released, so that depolarization is less and less likely to occur, producing an unsustained response in muscle contraction. This is manifested by fade when the patient is asked to perform a maximum voluntary contraction, or fade with electrical stimulation of the nerve.

TESTS IN MYASTHENIA GRAVIS

There is an obvious analogy between myasthenia gravis and nondepolarizing neuromuscular blockade, which is its pharmacological equivalent. However, whereas nerve stimulation tests have been largely standardized in anesthesia practice, such standardization has not been carried out to the same degree for the diagnosis of myasthenia gravis.[10] For neuromuscular blockade, most experts recommend using the train-of-four, consisting of four impulses delivered at 2 Hz to the ulnar nerve, with observation of the adductor pollicis response. In this case, recovery is regarded as a ratio of the fourth to the first response (train-of-four) greater than 90%. For the diagnosis of myasthenia gravis, many nerve-muscle pairs have been used, with stimulation frequencies ranging from 2 to 5 Hz, a variable number of impulses, and no definite value for the endpoint.[10] Train-of-four ratio in patients with myasthenia gravis presenting for anesthesia is often less than 90%,[11,12] and is related to the severity of disease. Subjects with more severe disease require a smaller dose of nondepolarizing neuromuscular blocking agent. For example, only 20 μg/kg of vecuronium was required to produce 95% block in ocular myasthenia, and 10 μg/kg in generalized myasthenia.[12] In healthy individuals, the dose of vecuronium for 95% block is 45 μg/kg. Another popular test involves assessing the effect of an anticholinesterase agent. Usually, edrophonium is used because of its rapid onset.[10] The patient is asked to perform a task involving sustained muscle contraction, such as hand grip or smiling. Then, 2–10 mg of edrophonium is given intravenously and the task is repeated. Improvement usually indicates the disease is present. A more complicated test involves single nerve fiber stimulation.[10] Investigation of myasthenia gravis is usually completed with measurement of acetylcholine receptor antibodies, which are present in approximately 80% of patients with the disease.[8]

TREATMENT

The mainstay of treatment of myasthenia gravis is administration of anticholinesterase agents. Pyridostigmine is most commonly used for that purpose. The daily dosage of the drug is indicative of the severity of disease and the probability of requirement for mechanical ventilation, with doses > 240–360 mg/day being associated with a greater probability. Neostigmine can also be used, with 15 mg being equivalent to pyridostimine 60 mg by mouth.[9] Corticosteroids are also used frequently, but can produce a myopathy of their own. Immunosuppressant drugs such as azathioprine and cyclosporin may also be used. More invasive forms of treatment include plasmapheresis, with the goal of removing circulating antibodies from the plasma. Thymectomy provides relief in a majority of patients, and anesthesiologists often seen myasthenics presenting for this surgical procedure.[9]

DRUG INTERACTIONS

Anesthesiologists must be aware of the many possible drug interactions in myasthenic patients. Exacerbation of the disease may occur with aminoglycoside antibiotics, local anesthetics, antiarrhythmics, anticonvulsants, and beta blockers.[9] Corticosteroids may aggravate the disease by causing a myopathy of their own, and too much pyridostigmine may be deleterious by producing weakness. Long-term pyridostigmine administration in normal patients causes a downregulation of receptors, with reduction of the number of receptors at the neuromuscular junction, a situation that is analogous to myasthenia gravis. In this case, however, injection of edrophonium usually aggravates the symptoms.

NEUROMUSCULAR BLOCKING AGENTS

The most clinically apparent drug interactions with myasthenia occur during anesthesia. Patients with myasthenia gravis are resistant to the effect of depolarizing neuromuscular blocking agents, so paralysis will occur after a larger than usual dose of succinylcholine.[13] This effect occurs in spite of the inhibiting action of pyridostigmine on plasma cholinesterase, which breaks down succinylcholine. Succinylcholine is not contraindicated in myasthenia gravis and does not cause exaggerated hyperkalemia. In fact, one might suspect that the hyperkalemic response is less than in normal patients, because of the reduction in the number of receptors. On the other hand, this reduced number of receptors at the neuromuscular junction markedly decreases the margin of safety and increases the sensitivity of the patients to nondepolarizing neuromuscular blocking agents.[12] The dose-response curve for all drugs tested is shifted to the left, to an extent that depends on the severity of the disease and the location of the symptoms. For example, patients with ocular myasthenia gravis have been found to have an almost normal response at the adductor pollicis muscle when monitored during anesthesia, but a much reduced twitch height at the orbicularis oculi.[14] Patients with more generalized disease tend to have a decreased train-of-four ratio at the adductor pollicis, even in the absence of neuromuscular blocking agents.[11,12] These individuals are particularly sensitive to nondepolarizing neuromuscular blocking agents.

MAINTENANCE OF ANESTHESIA AND REVERSAL

In patients without myasthenia gravis, inhalational agents potentiate neuromuscular blockade, so it is not surprising that patients with the disease may have more train-of-four fade in the presence of inhalational agents, even in the absence of neuromuscular blocking agents.[11] Recovery may be problematic if reversal is required after giving nondepolarizing neuromuscular blocking agents during anesthesia in patients already taking anticholinesterase drugs. The main mechanism of action of these reversal drugs is inhibition of acetylcholinesterase, the enzyme that breaks down acetylcholine. However, a maximal effect is observed when enzyme inhibition approaches 100%, which might be the case when high preoperative doses are used. Further doses of anticholinesterase agent will not inhibit the enzyme much more, so that the net effect might be negligible. For this reason, some recommend aiming for modest neuromuscular blockade during anesthesia, to anticipate the reduced effectiveness of anticholinesterase agents. Sugammadex might be seen as a suitable option in these patients, but at the time of writing no case reports have been published with this new reversal agent in myasthenic patients. Some authors recommend using total intravenous anesthesia in these patients, with propofol as the main anesthetic. However, most would agree that neuromuscular blocking agents may be used as long as reduced doses are administered, careful monitoring is performed, and the need for postoperative ventilation is anticipated.

EATON-LAMBERT SYNDROME

Several defects of neurotransmission at the neuromuscular junction have been collectively called *myasthenic syndromes*. The defect in these conditions is not an immune reaction to the acetylcholine receptor. The first description of such a syndrome was that of the Eaton-Lambert myasthenic syndrome, which occurs in some patients with some forms of metastatic cancer, typically small cell lung carcinoma.[8] The defect is the production of antibodies directed toward voltage-gated calcium channels, which are essential in the release of acetylcholine.[8] Contrary to myasthenia gravis, train-of-four fade is modest and there is facilitation, not fade, with 50-Hz stimulation.[15] Few case reports have been reported, but it seems prudent to avoid neuromuscular blocking agents.[15]

CONGENITAL MYASTHENIC SYNDROMES

A variety of conditions involving various mutations of the acetylcholine receptor itself, voltage-gated calcium channels, and acetylcholinesterase have been reported. Thus, the defect may be presynaptic, synaptic or postsynaptic.[8,16] The mode of transmission of these genetic defects is autosomal recessive. There are few case reports of myasthenic syndromes and anesthesia.

DISORDERS OF THE NERVE

The functional integrity of the neuromuscular junction is critically dependent on nerve activity. The processes leading to the specialization of the neuromuscular junction, including concentration of receptors, formation of folds, and inclusion of sodium channels, are thought to be orchestrated by agrin, a protein of neural origin that activates muscle-specific kinase (MuSK).[2] Decreased nerve activity leads to upregulation of receptors, proliferation of extrajunctional receptors, and muscle atrophy.

LOWER MOTOR NEURON LESION

Injury to peripheral nerve usually involves only part of the body, so the action of neuromuscular blocking agents is different between affected and nonaffected muscle. This situation normally leads to a decreased sensitivity to nondepolarizing neuromuscular blocking agents in the affected limbs, as long as the nerve and neuromuscular junction do not degenerate. However, in clinical practice neuromuscular blocking agents are not required for relaxation in these limbs, because they are not under central control. The response to succinylcholine is exaggerated, with contractures being prominent. There have been reports of a strong contraction of a limb after injection of succinylcholine with normal response in the other parts of the body.[17]

LOWER MOTOR NEURON DISEASE

Most lower motor neuron conditions develop insidiously, such that gradual changes occur at the neuromuscular junction. For example, sensitivity to neuromuscular blocking agents in muscles affected by *diabetic neuropathy* is increased. This is probably because nerve activity is insufficient to maintain a neuromuscular junction with a high density of receptors. *Spinobulbar muscle atrophy* involves mainly lower motor neurons.[2] There are no reported cases of anesthesia in patients with that disease. *Charcot-Marie-Tooth disease* is a demyelinating disease, but contrary to multiple sclerosis, it targets peripheral nerve. It has a heterogeneous genetic component, tends to target certain muscle groups (peripheral muscle being affected first), and is slowly progressive. Surprisingly, sensitivity to nondepolarizing neuromuscular blocking agents has been found to be normal or near normal in most patients, but this might be due to the choice of monitoring site, the adductor pollicis, which in most cases was not in the areas involved by the disease process.[18] *Guillain-Barré syndrome* involves sensory and motor deficit, probably due to antibodies directed against gangliosides present at the nodes of Ranvier of peripheral nerves and the neuromuscular junction. The disease often occurs after a viral infection. Symptoms are quite variable, with some patients requiring prolonged ventilatory support due to paralysis of upper airway and respiratory muscles. It is prudent to avoid succinylcholine in patients with Guillain-Barré syndrome.[8] To a certain extent, *immobilization* can be considered a lower motor neuron dysfunction. Decreased nerve traffic produces upregulation at the neuromuscular junction, and the sensitivity to neuromuscular blocking agents decreases, so that larger doses of these drugs are needed for the same effect. It is unlikely that the changes are significant enough for an abnormal response to succinylcholine. However, when immobility is combined with other factors, such as *sepsis*, *critical illness myopathy*, and administration of *corticosteroids*, hyperkalemia might follow succinylcholine administration.[2,4]

UPPER MOTOR NEURON DISEASE

The changes that occur with upper motor neuron disease can be best understood by considering the effect of *spinal cord trauma*. Within 24–48 h, lack of incoming nerve activity triggers upregulation, or an increase in the number of receptors at the junction.[4,19] Sensitivity to nondepolarizing neuromuscular blocking agents decreases progressively over the course of several weeks.[19] Normally, nerve activity inhibits formation of extrajunctional receptors; thus, interruption of this activity leads to proliferation of receptors outside the neuromuscular junction, and the number of possible binding sites for succinylcholine is increased. As a consequence, the amount of potassium exiting the intracellular space is increased, because it is proportional to the number of open receptors. These extrajunctional receptors are mainly of the fetal type (with an ε subunit), but others, such as the α_7 type (consisting of five α subunits) may be present as well.[4] Severe hyperkalemia, in some instances leading to cardiac arrest and death, has been reported in patients with spinal cord injury receiving succinylcholine.[20] Other upper motor neuron diseases do not usually lead to such dramatic events. In patients with *stroke*, the response to neuromuscular blocking drugs can be compared in affected and unaffected areas. Response to nondepolarizing neuromuscular blocking agents is usually less in a paretic muscle than in a normal muscle, but the response of the normal muscle is still less than in subjects without stroke.[21] For monitoring purposes, it is recommended to use a normal extremity. Succinylcholine may produce exaggerated hyperkalemia in patients with stroke, especially if many muscles are affected. *Multiple sclerosis* is a demyelinating disease that affects young adults, women more often than men, usually in the 20–40 yr age group. Only myelin in the central nervous system is affected. The course of the disease is highly variable, with alternating cycles of exacerbations and remissions. Later stages are characterized by decreased mobility and contractures. There have been no reports of unusual response to neuromuscular blocking agents in general and to succinylcholine in particular, although the use of succinylcholine is typically not recommended in these patients.[22] In *amyotrophic lateral sclerosis* (Lou Gehrig disease) degeneration of cortical, brainstem, and spinal neurons occurs.[2] Changes in the response to nondepolarizing neuromuscular blocking agents are expected, and it is advisable not to use succinylcholine, but experience with anesthesia in patients with this disease is limited.

DISORDERS OF MUSCLE

Muscle function might be affected in inherited or acquired conditions. The inherited, or genetic, conditions are generally classified as muscle dystrophies or myotonias. Most of the acquired conditions that alter muscle function are drug-induced, or associated with prolonged illness, trauma, sepsis, or a combination of those factors. The neuromuscular junction is not the primary target when these situations arise, and abnormal responses to nondepolarizing neuromuscular blocking agents are usually not seen until late in the development of the disease. However, fragility of the muscle membrane is the rule, making it particularly susceptible to depolarizing neuromuscular blocking drugs and halogenated agents.

MUSCLE DYSTROPHIES

Dystrophin-glycoprotein complex is one of the proteins of the muscle membrane that plays a role in maintaining stability. Muscle dystrophies are a group of diseases in which there is a defect in the formation, regulation, or maintenance of these proteins.[23] *Duchenne muscular dystrophy* is the most common of these diseases. It affects predominantly males and is due to a defect in the dystrophin gene. Symptoms usually appear at age 3–4 yr and the disease is usually fatal by adolescence. Mental retardation is frequent. In *Becker muscular dystrophy*, which is one tenth as common as Duchenne dystrophy, symptoms appear later, usually between the ages of 5 and 15, and progression is slower. As with the Duchenne type, boys are affected, as this is controlled by an X-linked gene. Other less common types are the *fascio-scapulo-humeral*, the *limb-girdle*, and *Emery-Dreyfuss* dystrophies. *Oculo-pharyngeal* dystrophy usually occurs in middle-aged adults; patients have difficulty swallowing and opening their eyes.[24]

In young patients with muscular dystrophy, the major concern is rhabdomyolysis, which is a manifestation of muscle membrane fragility and characterized by leakage of ions, mostly potassium, from the cell. Succinylcholine can trigger rhabdomyolysis, hyperkalemia, and cardiac arrest, especially in the presence of halogenated agents,[25] but such events have been reported to occur also with halogenated agents in the absence of succinylcholine.[26] Cardiac arrest has been reported in apparently healthy children, before the diagnosis of muscular dystrophy was made. Resuscitation was found to be difficult and in some instances unsuccessful when rhabdomyolysis is present.[25] The mechanism for the increase in serum potassium in muscular dystrophies is probably different from that seen in spinal cord injury. Proliferation of extrajunctional receptors probably does not occur, but potassium leaks out of the muscle cell because of abnormal fragility of the muscle membrane, which explains why succinylcholine is not the only agent that can alter membrane integrity. Because of several reports of rhabdomyolysis with halogenated agents, some authors recommend avoiding them in muscular dystrophy patients.[26] Because of the possible occurrence of cardiac arrest following succinylcholine in children with undiagnosed disease, it is recommended to limit the use of succinylcholine in children, especially in boys. It does not appear that patients with muscular dystrophy are at increased risk for malignant hyperthermia.[23] Typically, patients with Duchenne muscular dystrophy have a slightly increased sensitivity to nondepolarizing neuromuscular blocking agents.[27] In oculopharyngeal dystrophy, a modest prolongation of nondepolarizing neuromuscular blocking agents has been found.[28]

General complication rates with both general and regional anesthesia are low.[24]

MYOTONIA AND MYOTONIC DYSTROPHY

Myotonias are a group of disease entities characterized by increased excitability of muscle. In most instances, the disorder is associated with dysfunctions in the chloride, sodium, or calcium channels of the muscle membrane, and there is interference with mechanisms that allow skeletal muscle relaxation.[29] *Neuromyotonias* are separate and less common disease entities in which the defect is hyperexcitability of peripheral nerve, leading to fasciculations, cramps, and contractions.[30] The myotonias affecting muscle directly can be conveniently separated into *congenital myotonias*, in which there is a defect in a gene affecting a channel (usually a chloride channel) in muscle, and *myotonic dystrophies*, where anomalies in gene splicing lead to chloride channel dysfunction, but also to other defects. The two most common forms of congenital myotonia are *Thomsen's* and *Becker's* disease, due to autosomal dominant and recessive transmission, respectively, and in both cases, the chloride channel in muscle is dysfunctional. Succinylcholine has been reported to produce rigidity and contractures.[29] There is debate about the safety of halogenated agents, but it appears that patients with myotonias do not have an increased risk of developing malignant hyperthermia compared to the rest of the population.

In myotonic dystrophy involvement of the chloride channel gives rise to poor relaxation of muscle, but muscle weakness is seen as well. The most common variant is DM1, or *Steinert's disease*, which affects both sexes.[29] Its incidence is approximately 1:8000, with marked variations between countries and populations within a given country. *Proximal myotonic dystrophy*, or DM2 is less common.[31] In DM1, age at onset of symptoms is variable, but the disease occurs often in adolescence or early adulthood. A characteristic feature is the inability to relax after giving a handshake. Cataracts, baldness, cardiac conduction defects, and mental retardation are also seen. Weakness is observed particularly in proximal muscles; facial, bulbar, and respiratory muscles may be particularly affected.[31] Patients with Steinert's disease are reported as having an increased sensitivity to sedatives, opioids, and anesthetic agents, the mechanism of which is not entirely clear. Sensitivity to nondepolarizing neuromuscular blocking agents may be increased.[32] Succinylcholine may produce an increase in muscle tone lasting for a few minutes.[33] Neostigmine has been reported to produce a similar response in some patients.[34] However, these changes might not be observed clinically by the anesthesiologist. In a large series involving 219 patients who had a general anesthetic that often included succinylcholine, nondepolarizing neuromuscular blocking agents, halogenated agents, and reversal drugs, 8.2% had complications, and most of these were postoperative pulmonary complications.[35] Only one subject was described as having a "mild" hypertonic response following succinylcholine. Total intravenous anesthesia has been used successfully in many cases, and propofol appears to produce fewer myotonic responses in vitro in muscle cells with blocked chloride channels.[36] Recently, experience with anesthesia in patients with DM2 has been reported, and no complications related to the disease were observed.[37]

CRITICAL ILLNESS MYOPATHY

In the last two decades of the last century, reports of prolonged weakness associated with the use of nondepolarizing neuromuscular blocking agents in the intensive care unit (ICU) started to emerge. They were first attributed to drugs with a steroid nucleus, such as vecuronium and pancuronium, but case reports involving benzylisoquinoline compounds were also published. This led to a dramatic decrease in the use of neuromuscular blocking agents in the ICU. However, it became apparent that muscle weakness could occur in the absence of neuromuscular blocking agents. Inflammation and the use of corticosteroids most likely play a role.[38] Muscle is probably not the only organ involved; peripheral nerve is also affected. These conditions now are recognized as *critical illness polyneuropathy* and *critical illness myopathy*. The incidence of either or both is 50–70% of patients with systemic inflammatory response syndrome in the ICU. One of the features is a decrease in the compound action potential in muscle, which is indicative of denervation. Contrary to myasthenia gravis, there is no decrement in response to repetitive stimulation, and management is supportive.[39] Patients in the ICU who receive a nondepolarizing neuromuscular blocking agent might initially require larger doses of the drug, because of upregulation of receptors.[19, 39] If polyneuropathy or myopathy develops, an increased sensitivity may be present, which is manifested by prolonged recovery of neuromuscular function.

MISCELLANEOUS

BURNS

Many pathological changes occur in burn injury and muscle function is altered considerably. The response to neuromuscular blocking agents is similar to the situation occurring after spinal cord injury. Within 24–48 hr, decreased sensitivity to nondepolarizing neuromuscular blocking agents develops, and this process continues over several weeks.[19, 40, 41] The reasons for this resistance to nondepolarizing neuromuscular blocking agents is not well understood. It cannot be due to destruction of nerve or nerve endings by the burn injury, as this would produce no twitch response in the muscle. Moreover, some resistance is also observed in muscle groups that are remote from the site of injury.[40] Some kinetic factors may play a role, such as increased protein binding, but do not explain all the changes in sensitivity. The neuromuscular junction might also be altered by mediators involved in inflammation and sepsis. Succinylcholine is best avoided in burn patients, because severe hyperkalemia might occur as early as 48 hr after the onset of injury.[20] The magnitude of this response most likely depends on the extent of the injury. The response to succinylcholine is consistent with proliferation of extrajunctional receptors occurring on at least some of the muscle fibers.

TRAUMA

The changes that occur with trauma may be similar to those seen with burns if trauma is extensive and leads to appreciable tissue damage. If the picture is complicated by sepsis, immobility, or prolonged mechanical ventilation, the same contraindication to the use of succinylcholine might be in order.

CONCLUSION

An understanding the pathophysiology of the diseases of the nervous system, neuromuscular junction, and skeletal muscle helps predict a number of important interactions with drugs given during anesthesia, especially neuromuscular blocking agents. The dose of nondepolarizing neuromuscular blocking agents should be reduced markedly in myasthenia gravis and other diseases of the neuromuscular junction. Succinylcholine may cause hyperkalemia especially in spinal cord injury, burns, muscle dystrophies, but also in upper motor neuron diseases, sepsis, ICU myopathy, and extensive trauma. Halogenated agents are relatively contraindicated in myotonia.

REFERENCES

1. Santo Neto H, Filho JM, Passini R, Marques MJ. Number and size of motor units in thenar muscles. *Clin Anat.* 2004;17:203–211.
2. Naguib M, Flood P, McArdle JJ, Brenner HR. Advances in the neurobiology of the neuromuscular junction: implications for the anesthesiologist. *Anesthesiology.* 2002;96:202–231.
3. Sanes JR, Lichtman JW. Development of the vertebrate neuromuscular junction. *Annu Rev Neurosci.* 1999;22:398–442.
4. Martyn JAJ, Richtsfeld M. Succinylcholine-induced hyperkalemia in acquired pathological states: etiologic factors and molecular mechanisms. *Anesthesiology.* 2006;104:158–169.
5. Wood SJ, Salter CR. Safety factor at the neuromuscular junction. *Prog Neurobiol.* 2001;64:393–429.
6. Slater CR. Structural determinants of the reliability of synaptic transmission at the vertebrate neuromuscular junction. *J Neurocytol.* 2003;32:505–522.
7. Boonyapisit K, Kaminski HJ, Ruff RL. Disorders of neuromuscular junction ion channels. *Am J Med.* 1999;106:97–113.
8. Lang B, Vincent A. Autoimmune disorders of the neuromuscular junction. *Curr Opin Pharmacol.* 2009;9:336–340.
9. Keesey JC. Clinical evaluation and management of myasthenia gravis. *Muscle Nerve.* 2004;29:484–505.
10. Benatar M. A systematic review of diagnostic studies in myasthenia gravis. *Neuromusc Disorders.* 2006;16:459–467.
11. Nitahara K, Sugi Y, Higa K, Shono S, Hamada T. Neuromuscular effects of sevoflurane in myasthenia gravis patients. *Br J Anaesth.* 2007;98:337–341.
12. Itoh H, Shibata K, Nitta S. Difference in sensitivity to vecuronium between patients with ocular and generalized myasthenia gravis. *Br J Anaesth.* 2001;87:885–889.
13. Eisenkraft JB, Book WJ, Mann SM, et al. Resistance to succinylcholine in myasthenia gravis: a dose-response study. *Anesthesiology.* 1988;69:760–763.
14. Itoh H, Shibata K, Yoshida M, Yamamoto K. Neuromuscular monitoring at the orbicularis oculi may overestimate the blockade in myasthenic patients. *Anesthesiology.* 2000;93:1194–1197.
15. Itoh H, Shibata K, Nitta S. Neuromuscular monitoring in myasthenic syndrome. *Anaesthesia.* 2001;56:562–567.
16. Engel AG, Ohno K, Sine SM. Congenital myasthenic syndromes: progress over the past decade. *Muscle Nerve.* 2003;27:4–25.
17. Lee C, Yang E, Katz RL. Focal contracture following injection of succinylcholine in patients with peripheral nerve injury. *Can Anaesth Soc J.* 1977;24:475–478.
18. Schmitt HJ, Münster T. Mivacurium-induced neuromuscular block in adult patients suffering from Charcot-Marie-Tooth disease. *Can J Anaesth.* 2006;53:984–988.
19. Martyn JAJ, White DA, Gronert GA, Jaffe RS, Ward JM. Up-and-down regulation of skeletal muscle acetylcholine receptors. *Anesthesiology.* 1992;76:822–843
20. Gronert GA, Theye RA. Pathophysiology of hyperkalemia induced by succinylcholine. *Anesthesiology.* 1975;43:89–99.
21. Laycock JRD, Smith CE, Donati F, Bevan DR. Sensitivity of the adductor pollicis and diaphragm muscle to atracurium in a hemiplegic patient. *Anesthesiology.* 1987;67:851–853.
22. Dorotta IR, Schubert A. Multiple sclerosis and anesthetic implications. *Curr Opin Anaesthesiol.* 2002;15:365–370.
23. Gurnaney H, Brown A, Litman RS. Malignant hyperthermia and muscular dystrophies. *Anesth Analg.* 2009;109:1043–1048.
24. Pellerin HG, Nicole PC, Trépanier CA, Lessard MR. Postoperative complications in patients with oculopharyngeal muscular dystrophy: a retrospective study. *Can J Anesth.* 2007;54:361–365.
25. Gronert GA. Cardiac arrest after succinylcholine: mortality greater with rhadomyolysis than receptor upregulation. *Anesthesiology.* 2001;94:523–529.
26. Hayes J, Veyckemans F, Bissonnette B. Duchenne muscular dystrophy: an old anesthesia problem revisited. *Ped Anesth.* 2008;18:100–106.
27. Wick S, Muenster T, Schmidt J, Forst J, Schmitt HJ. Onset and duration of rocuronium-induced neuromuscular blockade in patients with Duchenne muscular dystrophy. *Anesthesiology.* 2005;102:915–919.
28. Caron MJ, Girard F, Girard DC, et al. Cisatracurium pharmacodynamics in patients with oculopharyngeal muscular dystrophy. *Anesth Analg.* 2005;100:393–397.
29. Parness J, Brandschapp O, Girard T. The myotonias and susceptibility to malignant hyperthermia. *Anesth Analg.* 2009;109:1054–1064.
30. Ginsburg G, Forde R, Martyn JAJ. Increased sensitivity to a nondepolarizing muscle relaxant in a patient with acquired neuromyotonia. *Muscle Nerve.* 2009;40:139–142.
31. D'Angelo MG, Bresolin N. Cognitive impairment in neuromuscular diseases. *Muscle Nerve.* 2006;34:16–33.
32. Diefenbach C, Lynch J, Abel M, Buzello W. Vecuronium for muscle relaxation in patients with dystrophia myotonica. *Anesth Analg.* 1993;76:872–874.
33. Mitchell MM, Ali HH, Savarese JJ. Myotonia and neuromuscular blocking agents. *Anesthesiology.* 1978;49:44–48.
34. Buzello W, Krieg N, Schlickewei A. Hazards of neostigmine in patients with neuromuscular disorders. *Report of two cases. Br J Anaesth.* 1982;54:529–534.

35. Mathieu J, Allard P, Gobeil G, Girard M, De Braekeleer M, Bégin P. Anesthetic and surgical complications in 219 cases of myotonic dystrophy. *Neurology*. 1997;49:1646–1650.
36. Bandschapp O, Ginz HF, Soule CL, Girard T, Ulwyler A. In vitro effects of propofol and volatile agents on pharmacologically induced chloride channel myotonia. *Anesthesiology*. 2009;111:584–590.
37. Weingarten TN, Hofer RE. Anesthesia and myotonic dystrophy type 2: a case series. *Can J Anesth*. 2010;57:248–255.
38. Bolton CF. Neuromuscular manifestations of critical illness. *Muscle Nerve*. 2005;33:140–163.
39. Murray MJ, Brull SJ, Bolton CF. Nondepolarizing neuromuscular blocking drugs and critical illness myopathy. *Can J Anesth*. 2006; 53:1148–1156.
40. Ibebinjo C, Martyn JAJ. Thermal injury induces greater resistance to d-tubocurarine in local rather than in distal muscles in the rat. *Anesth Analg*. 2000;91:1243–1249.
41. Han TH, Kim HS, Bae JY, Kim KM, Martyn JAJ. Neuromuscular pharmacodynamics of rocuronium in patients with major burns. *Anesth Analg*. 2004;99:386–392.

PART VII

NEURAL TOXICITY

18

ANESTHESIA-MEDIATED NEUROTOXICITY

Vesna Jevtovic-Todorovic

INTRODUCTION

Over the last five decades, the field of clinical anesthesiology has enjoyed enormous growth, evolving into a highly respected specialty with seemingly limitless ability to take care of a variety of patients in all age groups regardless of their health status. As a result, millions of complex surgical procedures are being performed annually. Consequently, human brains are being subjected to a variety of general anesthetics, alone or in combinations.

Despite the widespread use of general anesthetics, their mechanisms of action are not fully understood. Based on studies published over the last few decades, it is becoming increasingly evident that there are specific cellular targets through which general anesthetics act.[1] In general, enhancement of inhibitory synaptic transmission and/or inhibition of excitatory synaptic transmission have been reported. In particular, it is becoming widely accepted that many intravenous anesthetics, among them barbiturates, benzodiazepines, propofol, and etomidate,[1,2] as well as inhalational volatile anesthetics such as isoflurane, sevoflurane, desflurane, and halothane,[3,4] promote inhibitory neurotransmission by enhancing $GABA_A$ (γ-amino-butyric acid)-induced currents in neuronal tissue. For this reason, they are often referred to as GABAergic agents. On the other hand, a small number of intravenous anesthetics (e.g., phencyclidine [PCP] and its derivative, ketamine)[5]and inhalational anesthetics (nitrous oxide and xenon)[6,7] inhibit excitatory neurotransmission by blocking N-methyl-D-aspartate (NMDA) receptors, a subtype of glutamate receptors.

General anesthetics are potent modulators of GABA and glutamate, respectively, the major inhibitory and excitatory neurotransmitters, and thus cause significant imbalance in their functioning. However, only recently has it been recognized that general anesthetics, given in clinically relevant concentrations and combinations, are potentially damaging to neuronal cells in adult and immature brains thus suggesting that these agents are potentially deleterious. In this chapter I will review presently available animal and human findings regarding the neurotoxic potential of commonly used intravenous and inhalational anesthetics.

THE NEUROTOXIC POTENTIAL OF THE NMDA ANTAGONIST CLASS OF GENERAL ANESTHETICS IN THE ADULT MAMMALIAN BRAIN

Two commonly used general anesthetics, ketamine and nitrous oxide, when given systemically to adult rats, have been shown to have acute neurotoxic effects on cerebrocortical neurons.[6,8,9] This neurotoxic reaction, which is mainly confined to specific neurons in the posterior cingulate/retrosplenial cortex (PC/RSC), was initially described as reversible. Consisting of prominent swelling of endoplasmic reticuli and mitochondria, it gives the affected cells a strikingly vacuolated appearance (Figure 18.1). The vacuoles become evident within an hour after the initiation of nitrous oxide or ketamine administration and gradually disappear within several hours after the cessation of administration.[9,10] Our research has subsequently shown that, at higher doses or concentrations as well as after repeated administration, these anesthetics caused irreversible neurodegeneration of neurons in a more disseminated pattern, involving several corticolimbic brain regions in addition to the PC/RSC.[10] These findings signify that the severity of this pathological reaction and its reversibility depends on the duration of NMDA receptor blockade. Of additional interest is the recent finding that nitrous oxide and ketamine, when administered in low, individually nontoxic doses to adult rats, augment one another's reversible neurotoxic effect by an apparently synergistic mechanism.[9] This neurotoxic phenomenon appears to be exaggerated in aging animal brains when ketamine and nitrous oxide, either individually or in combination, are used in clinically relevant concentrations. Specifically, the neurotoxic reaction in the PC/RSC of aged rats is significantly more severe and longer lasting than that in young adult rats, suggesting that the aging brain is more vulnerable to NMDA receptor blockade and consequently more sensitive to the NMDA antagonist class of general anesthetics.[11]

Studies of the ability of other general anesthetics to protect against the neurotoxic effects of NMDA antagonists demonstrated that general anesthetics belonging to

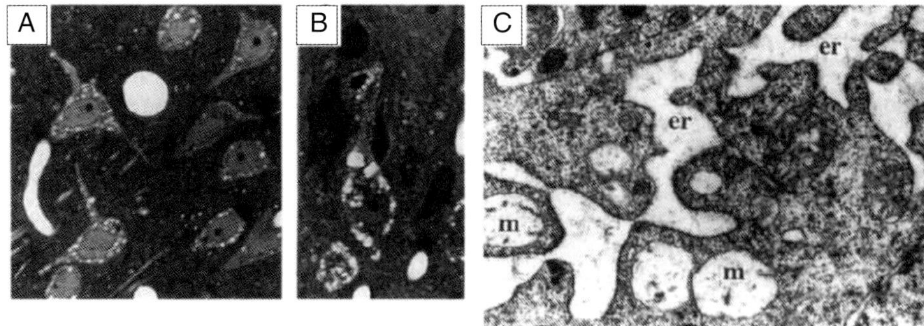

Figure 18.1 *Histological appearance of the PC/RSC neurons in 6-month-old (young adult) rat exposed to nitrous oxide (150-vol%)* (A) and (B): Light micrographs from the PC/RSC after three hours of exposure to nitrous oxide, showing that the vacuole reaction induced by nitrous oxide is severe. Note the many neurons with large multiple and confluent vacuoles and swollen, pale cytoplasm, mainly in pyramidal neurons in layers III and IV (magnification x250 and x400, respectively). (C) Electron micrograph of the vacuolar reaction in a pyramidal neuron from the PC/RSC. Endoplasmic reticulum (er) and mitochondria (m) both contribute to the formation of vacuoles (magnification x18,000). Reprinted by permission from Macmillan Publishers Ltd: *Nature Medicine*. Jevtovic-Todorovic et al . Nitrous oxide is an NMDA antagonist, neuroprotectant and neurotoxin. *Nat Med.* 1998;4:460–463.

GABAergic class of agents are highly effective in protecting against this type of neuronal injury. It has been proposed that glutamate regulates inhibitory tone by tonically stimulating NMDA receptors, located on inhibitory GABAergic neurons. By acting at these NMDA receptors, glutamate maintains tonic inhibition over major excitatory input to PC/RSC neurons. When the NMDA receptors are blocked, tonic inhibition by glutamate is removed, disinhibiting the excitatory pathways that in turn lead to excessive stimulation and injury of PC/RSC neurons. Consistent with this disinhibition hypothesis, GABAergic anesthetics such as barbiturates, benzodiazepines, volatile anesthetics, and propofol, which restore GABA tone, suppress the neurotoxic effects of ketamine and nitrous oxide[10,12,13] (Figure 18.2). Since ketamine and nitrous oxide are commonly used in combination with GABAergic anesthetics, it appears that anesthesia cocktails that were conceived for the purpose of achieving the appropriate plane of general anesthesia are beneficial in protecting with one class of anesthetics the detrimental effects caused by another class of anesthetics.

The cerebrocortical neurotoxic action of NMDA antagonist anesthetics has been shown to be age-dependent: adult animals are highly sensitive, but aging ones are even more so, while very young animals are insensitive.[6,14] Experiments focusing on the reversible vacuole reaction induced in PC/RSC neurons showed that nitrous oxide and ketamine do not induce a significant vacuole reaction in rats under the age of 30 days. The reaction is mild during young adulthood, but reaches peak severity during full adulthood.[8]

Although the changes in animal behavior in response to the administration of ketamine and nitrous oxide appear to be psychotomimetic, it is hard to classify them as schizophrenia-like psychosis. However, schizophrenia-like psychosis has been described in humans being given ketamine or PCP (phencyclidine). PCP is a drug of abuse that was introduced into clinical medicine as a general anesthetic over 50 years ago, but was soon withdrawn because of its potential for abuse and its severe, sometimes long lasting psychotomimetic effects. Ketamine, although a derivative of PCP, is shorter acting and is still in clinical use as an anesthetic because its psychotomimetic effects are less pronounced and shorter lived. It is of interest to note that the troublesome side effects of ketamine could be attenuated and made more manageable by coadministration of GABAergic general anesthetics such as barbiturates, benzodiazepines, and propofol.[15] The clinical observation that adults are more susceptible than children to ketamine-induced "emergence" reactions has resulted in a tendency for ketamine to be used more frequently in pediatric than adult anesthetic practice. Because of its psychoactive potential, ketamine is also a popular drug of abuse and is often called "Special K."

Although the psychoactive effects of nitrous oxide are not considered as profound, it has been known from the early days of its use that this anesthetic gas causes psychotic symptoms that are usually considered pleasurable and exhilarating.[16] Thus, the itinerant showmen introduced the term "laughing gas" well over a century ago to describe the frolicking, drunken-like behavior of a person inhaling nitrous oxide. Like ketamine, nitrous oxide is commonly used as a drug of abuse, especially by health care professionals.

It would be intriguing to propose a causal relationship between the acute swelling of PC/RSC neurons seen in the adult brains of mammals observed in animal studies and the psychotomimetic disturbances observed in human and veterinary medicine after the administration of ketamine or nitrous oxide. We suggest that the clinically observed "emergence" schizophrenia-like reaction that occurs after ketamine administration or the exhilarated behavior observed during nitrous oxide administration could be due, at least in part, to acute swelling of PC/RSC neurons. Interestingly, in 1938, Courville[17] reported a vacuolar reaction in cortical neurons

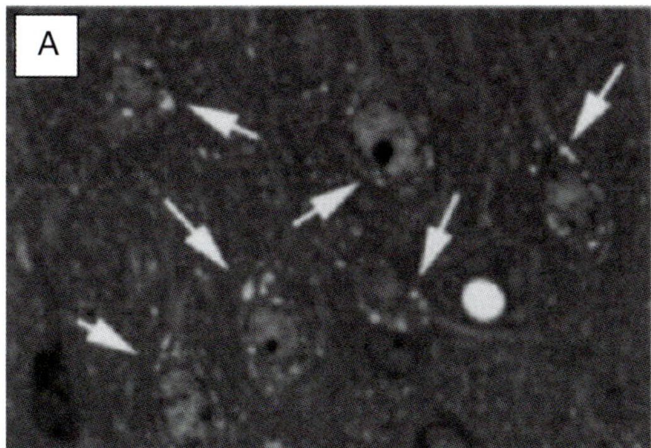

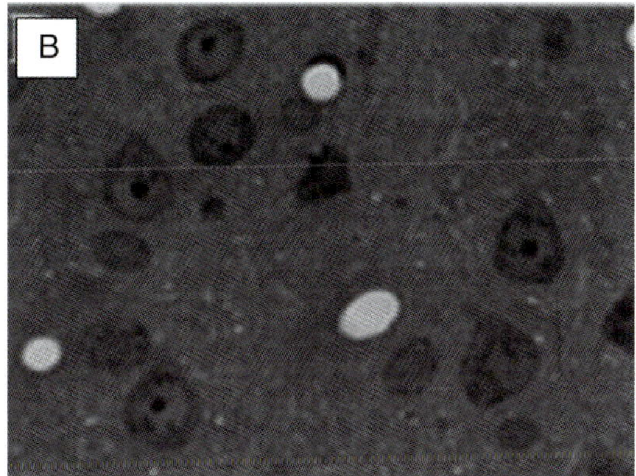

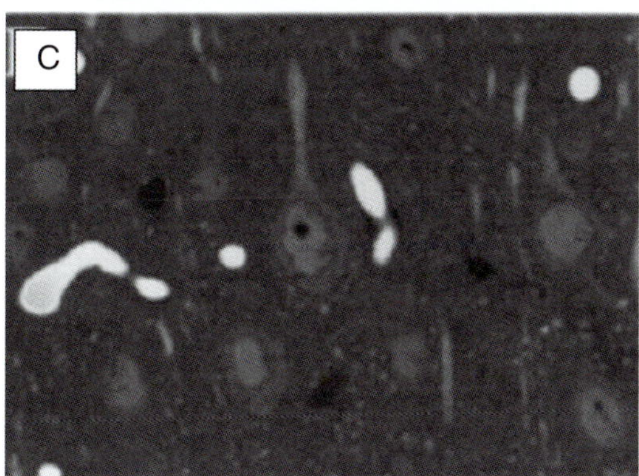

Figure 18.2 *Histological appearance of the PC/RS neurons in 6-month-old (young adult) rat exposed to nitrous oxide (75-vol%) + ketamine (40 mg/kg, i.p.) without (A) and with (B) isoflurane (1.5-vol%)* Isoflurane causes significant amelioration of the vacuolar reaction to nitrous oxide + ketamine. PC/RSC neurons appear normal, showing no difference from controls (exposed to air) (C) (magnification x480). Reprinted with permission from Jevtovic-Todorovic V, Benshoff N, Olney JW. Ketamine potentiates cerebrocortical damage induced by the common anaesthetic agent nitrous oxide in adult rats. *Br J Pharmacol.* 2000;130:1692–1698.

obtained from patients who died after nitrous oxide administration. In the late 1980s, it was hypothesized that NMDA receptor hypofunction might play a role in schizophrenia-like illnesses. To test this hypothesis, several researchers administered very low doses of ketamine (approximately one tenth the dose required for surgical anesthesia) to human subjects and found that it transiently and reversibly triggered mild schizophrenia-like symptoms, including hallucinations, delusions, and related cognitive disturbances.[18,19] It was also demonstrated that that these psychotic symptoms are successfully blocked by the GABAergic class of general anesthetics, a pharmacological strategy that the anesthesiologists had been aware of and had successfully used for several decades to treat the ketamine-induced "emergence" reaction. Evidence that the psychotomimetic effects of ketamine are blocked by benzodiazepines, barbiturates, or propofol, all of which block the neurotoxic effect of ketamine in the adult rat brain, suggests that similar receptor mechanisms underlie the psychotomimetic actions of ketamine in adult humans and the neurotoxic action of ketamine in adult rats. An additional basis for suggesting that similar receptor mechanisms may be the cause of these two phenomena is the similar age-dependency profile for ketamine-induced psychotic reaction in humans and ketamine-induced neurotoxic reaction in rats.

THE NEUROTOXIC POTENTIAL OF GENERAL ANESTHETICS IN THE IMMATURE MAMMALIAN BRAIN

Due to skillful and sophisticated pediatric anesthesia management, the exposure of very young children, including premature babies as young as 20 weeks post conception, to general anesthesia is becoming common, resulting in the annual administration of more than 3 million anesthetics.[20] The frequency of operating suite visits has grown exponentially, as has the length of stays in intensive care units. Heroic attempts to save premature and very ill infants has resulted in prolonged, deep sedation and repeated anesthesia during an extremely delicate period of human development.

In addition to the many unique properties of the physiology and pharmacology of young children, it is becoming clear that the development of all organs is not fully completed at birth. Thus, the first couple of years of postnatal life are an active extension of in utero development. For example, we know that the human central nervous system (CNS) is not fully developed at birth and undergoes rapid growth postnatally.[21,22] In the early stages of in utero life, the CNS goes through extensive neurogenesis, which is almost completed by the end of the second trimester of pregnancy. During the last trimester of pregnancy and the first two years or so of postnatal life, CNS development is marked by synaptogenesis, a process involving massive dendritic branching and the formation of trillions of synapses. This process also coincides with the peak of brain growth.[22] In order for synapses to be formed properly and in timely fashion, several key processes have to occur in synchronized fashion. These include neuronal migration, differentiation, and dendritic arborization, which lead to neuronal maturation and proper formation of circuitries, processes that are tightly controlled by glia, which actively participate in neuron-glia signaling while providing an appropriate milieu for neuron-neuron interaction.[23]

Glutamate promotes all key aspects of neuronal development.[24] It is thought that the fine balance between GABA and glutamate neurotransmission is important for proper and timely formation of neuronal circuitries. Neurons that are not successful in making meaningful connections are considered redundant and are destined to die by programmed cell death, or apoptosis, which occurs naturally during normal development of the CNS. Although this is a physiological process, apoptosis during normal development is tightly controlled, resulting in the removal of only a small percentage of neurons.[25] A disturbance of the fine balance between glutamatergic and GABAergic neurotransmission by excessive depression of neuronal activity and unphysiological changes in the synaptic environment during a crucial stage of brain development may constitute a generic signal for developing neurons to "commit suicide." Since the goal of surgical anesthesia is to render the patient unconscious and insentient to pain, the ultimate question becomes whether general anesthetics at doses that ensure substantial receptor occupancy and profound depression of neuronal activity could be promoting excessive activation of neuroapoptosis and the death of large populations of developing neurons.

Based on recently published findings,[25–29] it is becoming widely accepted that common general anesthetics do indeed cause significant and widespread neuroapoptotic degeneration of developing neurons in various mammalian species, including rats, mice, guinea pigs, and nonhuman primates. The peak of vulnerability to anesthesia-induced neuroapoptosis in each species coincides with its peak of synaptogenesis, with much less vulnerability observed during late stages of synaptogenesis.[28,30] Aside from prominent caspase-3 staining detected at the light microscopic level, detailed examination at the ultrastructural level suggests that the initial insult, visible mainly in the nucleus, is marked by the clamping of chromatin, followed by disruption of the nuclear membrane, intermixing of the cytoplasm and nucleoplasm, and the formation of apoptotic bodies[25] (Figure 18.3). In recent years, we have put considerable effort into elucidating the mechanisms of anesthesia-induced developmental neuroapoptosis and found it to involve several cascades that ultimately lead to neuronal deletion and impairment of proper synapse formation.

GENERAL ANESTHESIA ACTIVATES A MITOCHONDRIA-DEPENDENT APOPTOTIC CASCADE LEADING TO EFFECTOR CASPASE ACTIVATION AND APOPTOTIC NEURODEGENERATION

Apoptosis can occur via different biochemical pathways, resulting in activation of effector caspases as the final step. The mitochondria-dependent pathway, also called the intrinsic pathway, involves the downregulation of anti-apoptotic proteins from the bcl-2 family (e.g., bcl-x_L), an increase in mitochondrial membrane permeability, and increased release of cytochrome c into the cytoplasm. This, in turn, activates caspase-9 and caspase-3, resulting in apoptosis. We have found that general anesthesia administered at the peak of synaptogenesis activates the mitochondria-dependent cascade within the first 2 h after anesthesia exposure and that this activation is characterized by a significant decrease in protein levels of bcl-x_L, a significant rise in cytochrome c, and activation of caspase-9.[30] Melatonin, a sleep hormone known to up regulate bcl-x_L, offers some protection by partially inhibiting anesthesia-induced cytochrome c leakage and caspase-9 activation.[31]

GENERAL ANESTHESIA ACTIVATES A DEATH-RECEPTOR-DEPENDENT APOPTOTIC CASCADE LEADING TO EFFECTOR CASPASE ACTIVATION AND APOPTOTIC NEURODEGENERATION

The extrinsic pathway is initiated by the activation of death receptors. This involves the formation of a death-inducing signaling complex (DISC), which contains Fas, a member of the TNF-α superfamily. DISC formation results in the activation of caspase-8, which activates caspase-3, executing the cell. We found that general anesthesia also activates the extrinsic pathway by causing significant upregulation of Fas protein levels and significant activation of two key effector caspases, caspase-8 and caspase-3.[30] It appears, however, based on timing, that anesthesia-induced activation of the intrinsic pathway occurs before activation of the extrinsic pathway.

GENERAL ANESTHESIA ACTIVATES A NEUROTROPHIC-FACTOR-DEPENDENT APOPTOTIC CASCADE LEADING TO EFFECTOR CASPASE ACTIVATION AND APOPTOTIC NEURODEGENERATION

The neurotrophins, a family of growth factors consisting of nerve growth factor (NGF), brain-derived neurotrophic factor (BDNF), and neurotrophic factor (NT)-3 and NT4/5, support neuronal survival, differentiation, and several forms of synaptic plasticity, and therefore are important in synaptogenesis of the mammalian brain. The signal transduction systems that mediate the diverse biological functions of neurotrophins are initiated by two classes of plasma membrane receptors, the tropomyosin (Trk) receptor kinase receptors and the p75 neurotrophic receptor ($p75^{NTR}$). Current findings suggest that the main physiological functions of $p75^{NTR}$ are not only to regulate Trk receptor activation and signaling, but also to activate the Trk-independent signal transduction cascade.[32] Both Trk-dependent and -independent cascades modulate the activation (phosphorylation) of Akt serine/threonine kinase, the pivotal factor in the major survival pathway for neurons.

Neurotrophins are synthesized and released by neurons; both their biosynthesis and secretion depend on neuronal

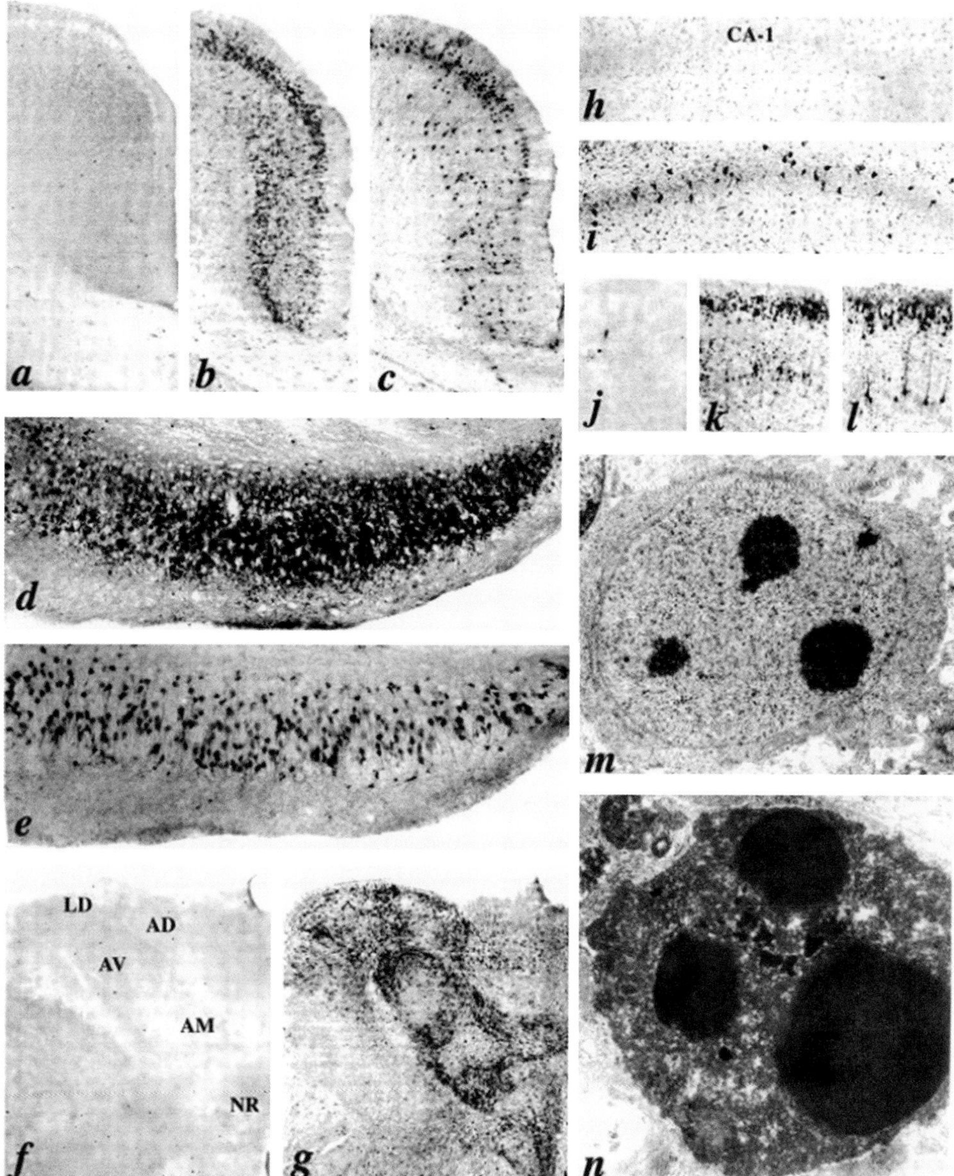

Figure 18.3 *Triple anesthetic cocktail induces apoptotic neurodegeneration* (*a–l*) are light micrographic views of various brain regions of either a control rat (*a, f, h, j*) or a rat exposed to the triple anesthetic cocktail (0.75-vol% isoflurane with midazolam at 9 mg/kg, s.c., and nitrous oxide at 75-vol% for 6 h) (*b–e, g, i, k, l*). Some sections were stained by the DeOlmos silver method (*a, b, d, f, g, k*); the others were immunocytochemically stained to reveal caspase-3 activation (*c, e, h–j, l*). The regions illustrated are the posterior cingulate/retrosplenial cortex (*a–c*), subiculum (*d, e*), anterior thalamus (*f, g*), rostral CA1 hippocampus (*h, i*), and parietal cortex (*j–l*). The individual nuclei shown in the anterior thalamus (*f, g*) are laterodorsal (*LD*), anterodorsal (*AD*), anteroventral (*AV*), anteromedial (*AM*), and nucleus reuniens (*NR*). *m* and *n* are electron micrographic scenes depicting the ultrastructural appearance of neurons undergoing apoptosis. The cell in *m* displays an early stage of apoptosis in which dense spherical chromatin balls are forming in the nucleus while the nuclear membrane remains intact; few changes are evident in the cytoplasm. The cell in *n* exhibits a much later stage of apoptosis in which the entire cell is condensed, the nuclear membrane is absent, and there is intermixing of nuclear and cytoplasmic constituents. These are hallmark characteristics of neuronal apoptosis as it occurs in the in vivo mammalian brain. Reprinted with permission from Jevtovic-Todorovic V, Hartman RE, Izumi Y, et al. Early exposure to common anesthetic agents causes widespread neurodegeneration in the developing rat brain and persistent learning deficits. *J Neurosci*. 2003;23:876–882.

activity. Extensive depression of neuronal activity can impair neurotrophin-regulated survival-promoting signals and consequently promote apoptosis. When clinically used general anesthetics were administered at the peak of synaptogenesis, the observed neuro-apoptotic damage was mediated, at least in part, by a BDNF-modulated apoptotic cascade.[33] Anesthesia-induced disturbances in BDNF-mediated neuronal survival pathways were significant and fairly rapid. Based on the evidence, a dual mechanism was suggested for anesthesia-induced activation of neurotrophin-mediated apoptotic pathways: one via the Trk-dependent and the other via the Trk-independent, $p75^{NTR}$-dependent apoptotic cascade. The importance of both pathways seems to be brain-region-specific. In the thalamus, anesthesia causes a decrease in the protein levels of BDNF and activated Akt levels (without any effects on $p75^{NTR}$ and ceramide levels), resulting in the activation of caspase-9 and -3. In the cerebral cortex, however, anesthesia causes an increase in BDNF levels while decreasing levels of activated Akt and increasing caspase-9 and -3 activity, suggesting that activation of the TrkB signaling pathway is likely overridden by increased production of ceramide via activation of the Trk-independent $p75^{NTR}$-dependent cascade. A sex hormone, β-estradiol, known to upregulate activated Akt levels, offers some protection by partially inhibiting anesthesia-induced caspase-3 activation.[33] The importance of the $p75^{NTR}$ signaling pathway in anesthesia-induced impairment of synaptogenesis was also demonstrated in a study by Head et al, who have shown that isoflurane anesthesia reduces synaptic tPA release and enhanced proBDNF/$p75^{NTR}$-mediated apoptosis both in vivo and in vitro.[34]

GENERAL ANESTHESIA INDUCES SIGNIFICANT NEURONAL DELETION IN VULNERABLE BRAIN REGIONS

An important question regarding the importance of anesthesia-induced neuronal damage during brain development is whether the observed anesthesia-induced apoptosis of developing neurons results in permanent neuronal deletion or is only transient and reversible. The brains of fully developed rats (postnatal day 30)[35] and guinea pigs (first week of postnatal life)[28] that had been exposed to clinically relevant anesthesia at postnatal (P) 7 day (rats) and at 35–40 days in utero (guinea pigs) (a peak of brain vulnerability) were studied and compared to age-matched controls.[28,35] After careful quantification of neuronal densities in the most vulnerable cortical and subcortical regions, it was found that these animals had significant decreases in neuronal densities in these brain regions as compared to their respective controls. Although physiological "pruning" of redundant neurons is commonly observed in the developing mammalian brain, only a small percentage (estimated, with some regional variations, to be approximately less than 1% of the total neuronal population) do not survive normal synaptogenesis. It is of grave concern that clinically relevant general anesthesia severely jeopardizes the survival of many developing neurons, deleting as much as 50% of neurons in vulnerable brain regions.

GENERAL ANESTHESIA INDUCES EFFECTOR CASPASE ACTIVATION AND APOPTOTIC NEURODEGENERATION DESPITE ADEQUATE MAINTENANCE OF CARDIOVASCULAR AND RESPIRATORY HOMEOSTASIS

Of paramount concern in clinical anesthesia practice is the maintenance of adequate oxygenation and ventilation, tissue perfusion, and, ultimately, the stability of vital signs. Due to the technical limitations imposed by the small size of rat and mice pups, these important parameters cannot be continuously monitored and controlled, raising concern that the observed pathomorphological changes in the developing brain could, at least in part, be due to inadequate maintenance of physiological homeostasis. To address this concern, researchers have used larger animals, such as guinea pigs and primates, with which it is technically possible to imitate the clinical anesthesia setup and to tightly control and monitor the adequacy of ventilation, oxygenation, and tissue perfusion. It was found that in spite of strict control of all vital parameters, damage in immature brains was many times greater than that in "true" control brains.[28,29] This strongly suggests that the histomorphological changes observed are caused by general anesthesia per se, rather than by hypoxia, hypercarbia, or metabolic imbalance.[26]

ANESTHESIA-INDUCED IMPAIRMENT OF SYNAPTOGENESIS

Our most recent findings indicate that exposure of immature rats to general anesthesia at the peak of synaptogenesis results in severe, long-lasting functional and ultrastructural abnormalities of developing synapses in young neurons of the hippocampal complex. This was demonstrated as significant decreases in synapse volumetric densities (as much as 40%); the paucity of multiple synaptic boutons on individual neuronal profiles (4 to 5 on average per each control neuronal profile, whereas even normal-looking synapses in experimental rats had one or no boutons) (Figure 18.4); and a long-lasting decrease in the strength of inhibitory synaptic neurotransmission.[36,37] These findings are in agreement with a recently published study showing that exposure of mice to general anesthesia during synaptogenesis results in significant reductions in dendritic filopodial spines and synapse formation both in vivo and in vitro.[34]

LONG-TERM BEHAVIORAL DEFICITS IN ANIMALS

Based on our pathomorphological findings, it is clear that anesthesia exposure results in significant neuronal deletion and long-lasting impairment of synapses in vulnerable brain regions.[28,35] This has led us to propose that the observed pathomorphological findings may have lasting effects on behavior.

Indeed, when rats were exposed to general anesthesia at the peak of synaptogenesis and assessed for cognitive development from early stages into adulthood, we found that their cognitive abilities lagged behind those of controls, with a gap in learning abilities widening in adulthood. For example, although anesthesia-treated rats were able eventually to learn a task in early adulthood, in later adulthood they were not able to master more complicated learning paradigms (Figure 18.5). Our findings indicated that

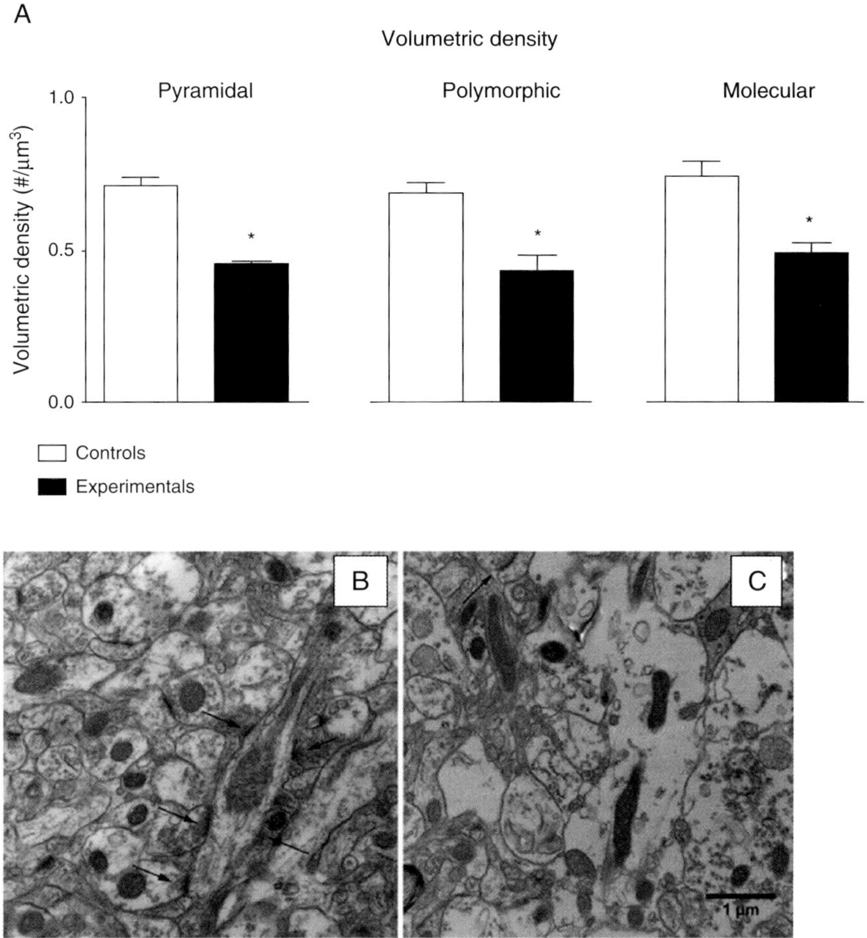

Figure 18.4 *Anesthesia impairs normal synaptogenesis* (A) Anesthesia caused significant decreases in volumetric density in all three subicular layers of 21-day-old rats. When the overall number of synapses per μ^3 was quantified in the pyramidal, polymorphic, and molecular layers, each had, on average, 30–40% less synaptic density than did the corresponding layers in control rats (*pyramidal layer $P < 0.001$; *polymorphic layer and molecular layers, $P < 0.01$) ($n = 4$ control and 4 experimental pups from two litters). When the presence of multiple synaptic boutons (MSBs) on the individual neuronal profiles was assessed it was noted that, unlike the neuronal profile in a control subiculum, which contains an abundance of MSBs (shown with the arrows) (B), there was a substantial lack of synaptic contacts in experimental subiculum (C) (magnification x12,000). With kind permission from Springer Science+Business Media: Lunardi N et al. General anesthesia causes long-lasting disturbances in the ultrastructural properties of developing synapses in young rats. *Neurotox Res*. 2010;17:179–188.

exposure to general anesthesia at the peak of brain development has devastating and long-lasting effects on cognitive development in rats.

During the last several years, behavioral studies of mice have shown that early exposure to intravenously administered general anesthetics in combination, but not singly, significantly alters their behavior during young adulthood (postnatal days 55 to 70). For example, Fredriksson et al[38] have shown that mice exposed at postnatal day 10 to propofol or thiopental in combination with ketamine exhibited altered spontaneous behavior and complete lack of habituation during a 60-min test period; these behavioral changes were demonstrated to be hypoactivity, followed by distinct hyperactivity. These mice also exhibited altered learning and memory when tested in a radial arm maze. Similar behavioral deficits were noted when mice were exposed to a cocktail containing ketamine and diazepam.[39]

Although anesthesia cocktails seem to be most detrimental, ketamine, an intravenous anesthetic, when used alone in rats during early stages of brain development, also caused significant deficits in habituation, marked deficits in acquisition of learning and retention of memory in the radial arm maze-learning task, as well as decreased shift learning in a circular swim maze-learning task.[39] When anesthetic agents with GABAergic and NMDA antagonist properties are combined, which is done frequently in the clinical setting (for example, nitrous oxide and volatile anesthetics or propofol and ketamine) behavioral deficits, including cognitive ones, appear to be profound.[25,38,39] Although it would be difficult to establish a direct causal

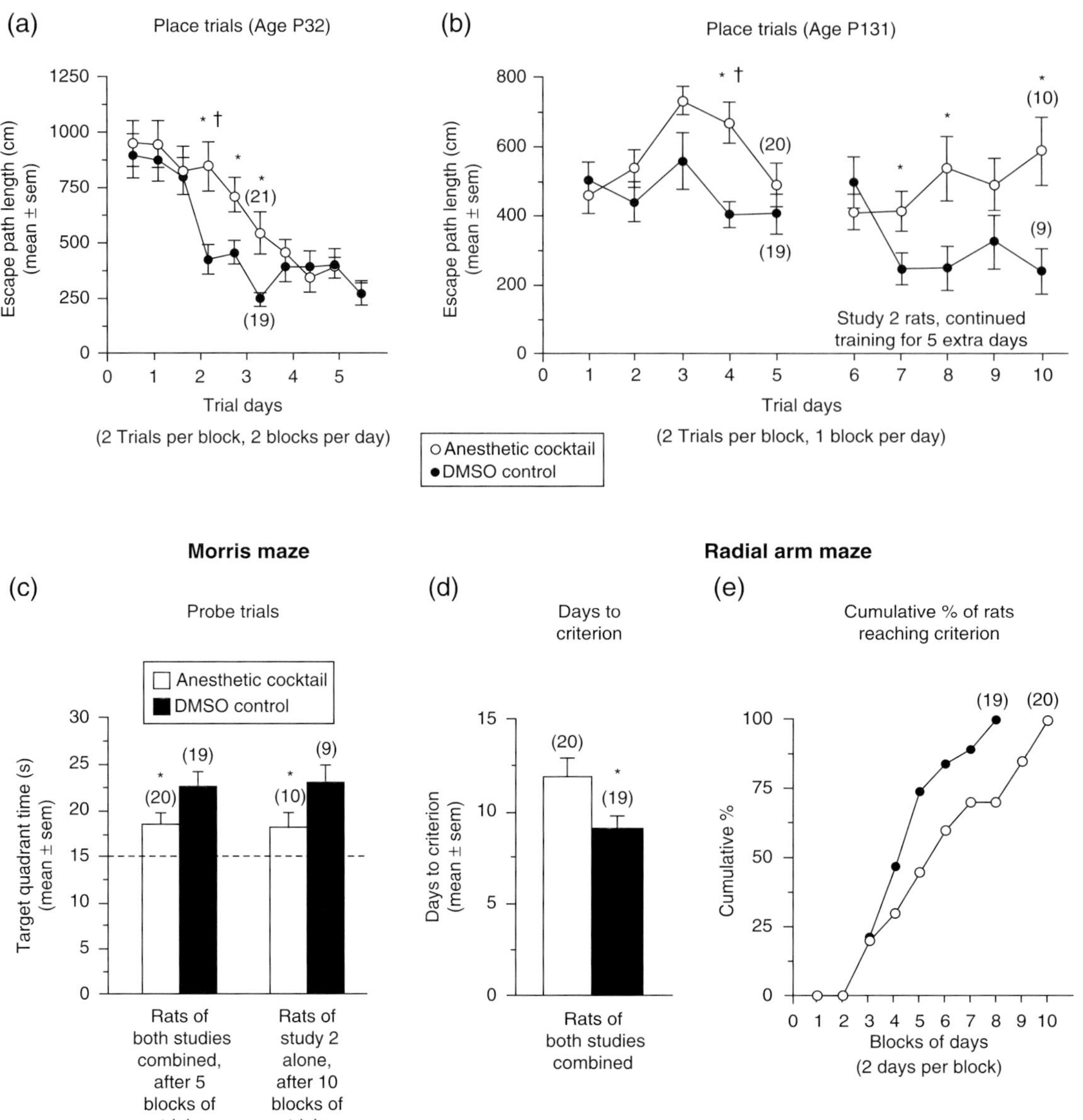

Figure 18.5 *Effects of neonatal triple anesthetic cocktail treatment on spatial learning* (*a*) Rats were tested at P32 for their ability to learn the location of a submerged (not visible) platform. ANOVA analysis of data on the length of escape paths yielded a significant main effect of treatment ($p = 0.032$) and a significant treatment by blocks of trials interaction ($p = 0.024$). These results indicated that the place-training performance of rats given an anesthetic cocktail (0.75-vol% isoflurane with midazolam at 9mg/kg, s.c., and nitrous oxide at 75-vol% for 6 h) was significantly inferior to that of control rats. Subsequent pairwise comparisons indicated that differences were greatest during blocks 4, 5, and 6 ($p = 0.003$, 0.012, and 0.019, respectively). However, rats given the anesthetic cocktail improved their performance to control-like levels during the last four blocks of trials. (*b*) Rats were retested as adults (P131) for their ability to learn a different location of the submerged platform. The graph on the left shows the path-length data from the first five place trials when all rats were tested. ANOVA analysis of these data yielded a significant main effect of treatment ($p = 0.013$), indicating that the control rats, in general, used significantly shorter paths in swimming to the platform than did rats treated with the anesthetic cocktail. Subsequent pairwise comparisons showed that differences were greatest during block 4 ($p = 0.001$).
The graph on the right shows the data from rats given 5 additional training days as adults. During these trials, rats in the control group improved their performance and appeared to reach asymptotic levels, whereas the rats given the anesthetic cocktail showed no improvement. ANOVA analysis of these data yielded a significant main effect of treatment ($p = 0.045$), as well as a significant treatment by blocks of trials interaction ($p = 0.001$). Additional pairwise comparisons showed that group differences were greatest during blocks 7, 8, and 10 ($p = 0.032$, 0.013, and 0.017, respectively). (*c*) Probe trial performance of rats given the anesthetic cocktail and control rats during adult testing. Search behavior of the rats was quantified when the submerged platform was removed from the pool after the last place trials in blocks 5 and 10. The histogram on the left presents data for rats in both studies 1 and 2 combined after five blocks of place trials were completed. The histogram on the right presents data for rats in study 2 alone, after 10 blocks of place trials were completed. The dotted line represents the amount of time that animals would be expected to spend in the target quadrant based on chance alone. Both histograms show that the control rats spent significantly more time in the target quadrant than did the anesthesia-exposed rats, regardless of whether the probe tests were done on both study groups after five blocks or only on the study 2 rats

link, it is reasonable to propose that anesthesia-induced neuroapoptosis, which occurs in immature brains and leads to neuronal deletion, is, at least in part, responsible for the observed cognitive deficits. It remains to be established whether multiple, longer-lasting exposures to anesthesia cocktails during periods of extreme vulnerability have greater effects on neurocognitive development than were initially predicted.

LONG-TERM BEHAVIORAL DEFICITS IN HUMANS

The effects of perioperative events on the psychological and emotional development of children have been known for many decades. For instance, in 1945 Levy's[40] retrospective study was the first to make an association between relatively short surgical procedures, such as tonsillectomy, adenoidectomy, or appendectomy done on otherwise healthy children and these children's development, within the first six postoperative months, of new behavioral problems such as terrors, dependency, destructiveness, and disobedience. These problems were not only quite serious, but uncommon for those children, prompting their parents to seek professional help. Ether, the general anesthetic commonly used at the time, is no longer in use in the United States. Nevertheless, it is noteworthy that the report suggested that the most sensitive children were in the youngest age group. Out of 124 children, 33–58% of them were between 0 and 2 years of age. Several studies over succeeding decades had reported that, on average, the incidence of surgery-associated psychological disturbances in children ranged from 9% to 20%, and also confirmed that children under 2 years of age were at increased risk in spite the variety of anesthetic agents they were given.[40–44] Some of these behavioral disturbances were reported to persist for months and even years. In a prospective multicenter survey of 551 children in 1988, Campbell et al,[45] found a 47% overall incidence of new behavioral problems, including anxiety, nightmares, and attention seeking. In this study age was again an important factor in children's vulnerability to postoperative behavioral changes, with those in the first two years of life having the highest incidence of problems.

Initially, it was assumed that the emotional shocks of hospitalization, separation from family, and the physical trauma of surgical intervention, such as pain, fluid imbalance, nutritional changes, and blood loss, were the main factors in children's regressive behavioral changes. These changes were not linked to a specific anesthesia protocol or technique. Interestingly, however, a careful search of the literature reveals that a possible relationship between anesthesia and personality changes was actually suggested in 1951, when Eckenhoff[42] published a retrospective study of 612 patients under the age of 12 years who had undergone either tonsillectomy or appendectomy. Although different anesthetic agents were used (for example, cyclopropane, nitrous oxide, morphine, and pentobarbital), behavioral changes similar to those reported by Dr. Levy,[40] with the addition of new-onset bed-wetting, occurred, on average, two months after surgery. The highest incidence of behavioral impairments, up to 57%, was again noted in patients younger than 3 years, whereas the lowest incidence, 8%, was reported in those older than 8 years.

The first report to suggest a possible relationship between anesthesia and long-term impairment of cognitive development was that by Backman and Kopf.[44] The surgical procedure, removal of congenital nevocytic nevi, was minor. General anesthesia was induced and maintained with ketamine and halothane, which at that time were relatively new anesthetic agents. Nevertheless, the authors reported an increased incidence of cognitive impairments compared to preoperative baseline. These impairments were described as regressive behavioral changes lasting up to 18 months after anesthesia. Again, children younger than 3 years were the most sensitive. The authors clearly stated that they could not confirm the notion, based on the clinical impressions of many anesthesiologists, that general anesthetics cause no long-term cognitive effect. They did note that they were "....unable to locate any published data concerning the possible long-term effects on memory, problem solving, conceptualization, or learning disabilities in children who have undergone general anesthesia."

The major impetus for methodical investigations into the possibility of anesthesia-induced neurotoxicity in newborns and infants came from several preclinical studies[25,38,39] that clearly implicated anesthetic agents in a variety of

Figure 18.5 *(continued)*
after 10 trials. (*d, e*) Data are shown from the radial arm maze test done on P53 to evaluate spatial working memory capabilities. (*d*) This histogram shows that rats given the anesthetic cocktail required significantly more days to reach a criterion demonstrating learning (8 correct responses out of the first 9 responses for 4 consecutive days) compared with controls. (*e*) This plot shows the days to criterion data as the cumulative percentage of rats reaching criterion in each group as a function of blocks of training days. The acquisition rate of rats given the anesthetic cocktail began to slow around the fourth block of trials and remained slower throughout the rest of the experiment. Numbers in parentheses in each graph indicate sample sizes. $^{*}p < 0.05$; Bonferroni corrected level:$\dagger p < 0.005$ in *a*;$\dagger p < 0.01$ in *b*. Reprinted with permission from Jevtovic-Todorovic V, Hartman RE, Izumi Y, et al. Early exposure to common anesthetic agents causes widespread neurodegeneration in the developing rat brain and persistent learning deficits. *J Neurosci*. 2003;23:876–882.

behavioral disturbances indicative of impaired neurocognitive development. Although such investigations are still at an early stage, the clinical evidence that has emerged over the last few years has begun to point to potentially detrimental effects of anesthetic agents on behavioral development.

Wilder et al,[46] in a population-based retrospective birth-cohort study of 5,357 children, have found that although a single exposure to general anesthesia was not associated with a greater risk of learning disabilities than that in a no-exposure group, children who received two or more general anesthetics before the age of 4 years were at significantly increased risk of learning disabilities. Moreover, that risk increased with longer cumulative duration (more than 2 hours) of anesthesia exposure. Of particular concern is their finding that the cohort exposed to anesthesia before the age of 4 years had actual cognitive scores during their years of schooling that were, on average, two standard deviations below the predicted ones. This suggests that their early exposure to general anesthesia prevented these individuals from reaching their full cognitive potential.

In an even larger population study, Sun et al[47] focused on assessing learning disabilities in 228,961 patients. Again, it was found that children who had received anesthesia before the age of 3 years required higher use of Medicaid services to deal with learning deficits than did children who had not been exposed to anesthesia. Kalkman et al,[48] in the Netherlands, looked at a smaller population of patients who had been exposed to anesthesia very early in life and found a higher incidence of learning deficits during school years.

Several studies of premature infants have suggested that behavioral disabilities later in life are more prevalent among those who were exposed to surgery and general anesthesia during the neonatal period than they are among premature infants who were treated medically. For example, surgically treated premature infants with patent ductus arteriosus[49] or necrotizing enterocolitis[50] had worse neurological outcomes than did premature infants who were treated medically. Although a possible causal link between early exposure to general anesthesia and neurocognitive deficits could be suggested on the basis of these studies, a measure of caution is advisable, since the effects of surgery cannot be clearly separated from the effects of anesthesia.

Although, to date, a few clinical studies suggest that the exposure of infants and neonates to surgery and general anesthetics may cause significant neurocognitive deficits and a variety of behavioral sequelae, those studies were done retrospectively[50–52] and therefore could not control for the many variables that come into play during the perioperative period. However, the complex issues associated with the design of randomized, double-blinded prospective clinical studies of very young patients cannot be underestimated. These issues include, but are not limited to ethical considerations, the lack of biomarkers of apoptosis that can safely be used in a living organism, the complexity and meaningfulness of various clinical outcomes (especially neurocognitive ones), and the lack of appropriate controls.

POTENTIAL CLINICAL IMPORTANCE OF RESEARCH FINDINGS

Although the field of anesthesia-induced neurotoxicity is rapidly emerging, it would be premature to draw definite conclusions regarding the human risk of exposing developing brains to general anesthesia before the clinical relevance of recently published data can be better substantiated. However, it does appear that the timing and duration of anesthesia exposure are important factors that should be carefully considered. Frequent or prolonged exposure at the peak of synaptogenesis seems to be most detrimental. If, indeed, the developing human brain is vulnerable to the apoptogenic cell death observed in developing animal brains, it is of great importance to know, as accurately as possible, when the period of synaptogenesis begins and ends in the developing human brain. In particular, it is crucial to establish when synaptogenesis in the human brain is at the peak, since the vulnerability of mammalian brains to apoptotic neuronal damage coincides with the peak of neuronal development.[28,30] Only a handful of studies have reported regressive behavioral changes in children exposed to general anesthesia, indicating that the most vulnerable age group is younger then 4 years, although the causal relationship between a specific anesthesia protocol and specific cognitive disturbances has never been reported.[40–42,44,46–48]

In view of the rapidly emerging information, it is of paramount importance to pursue a relentless quest for a better grasp of poor neurocognitive outcomes that could be anesthesia-induced. It also is imperative that we improve our understanding of the mechanisms that underlie the neurotoxicity of anesthetic agents. Accordingly, we should be able to develop ways of preventing anesthesia-induced developmental neurotoxicity and, consequently, to use existing anesthetics to their full advantage for therapeutic benefits without the risk of neurotoxic side effects, especially in cases when life-threatening conditions make frequent surgical interventions and prolonged stays in intensive units a necessity that cannot be avoided.

REFERENCES

1. Franks NP. General anaesthesia: from molecular targets to neuronal pathways of sleep and arousal. *Nat Rev Neurosci.* 2008;9: 370–386.
2. Hirota K, Roth SH, Fujimura J, et al.GABAergic mechanisms in the action of general anesthetics. *Toxicol Lett.* 1998;100–101:203–207.
3. Pearce RA: Effects of volatile anesthetics on $GABA_A$ receptors: Electrophysiological studies. In: Moody EJ, Skolnick P, eds. Molecular basis of anesthesia. Boca Raton, FL: CRC Press; 2000.
4. Nishikawa K, Harrison NL. The actions of sevoflurane and desflurane on the gamma-aminobutyric acid receptor type A: effects of TM2

mutations in the alpha and beta subunits. *Anesthesiology.* 2003;99: 678–684.
5. Lodge D, Anis NA. Effects of phencyclidine on excitatory amino acid activation of spinal interneurons in the cat. *Eur J Pharmacol.* 1982;77:203–204.
6. Jevtovic-Todorovic V, Todorovic SM, Mennerick S, et al. Nitrous oxide (laughing gas) is an NMDA antagonist, neuroprotectant and neurotoxin. *Nature Medicine.* 1998;4:460–463.
7. Frank NP, Dickinson R, deSousa SLM, et al. How does xenon produce anesthesia? *Nature.* 1998;396:324.
8. Jevtovic-Todorovic V, Wozniak DF, Benshoff ND, Olney JW. A comparative evaluation of the neurotoxic properties of ketamine and nitrous oxide. *Brain Res.* 2001;895(1–2):264–267.
9. Jevtovic-Todorovic V, Benshoff N, Olney JW. Ketamine potentiates cerebrocortical damage induced by the common anaesthetic agent nitrous oxide in adult rats. *Br J Pharmacol.* 2000;130(7):1692–1698.
10. Jevtovic-Todorovic V, Beals J, Benshoff N, Olney JW. Prolonged exposure to inhalational anesthetic nitrous oxide kills neurons in adult rat brain. *Neuroscience.* 2003;122(3):609–616.
11. Jevtovic-Todorovic V, Carter L.B. The anesthetics nitrous oxide and ketamine are more neurotoxic to old than to young rat brain. *Neurobiology of Aging.* 2005;26(6):947–956.
12. Jevtovic-Todorovic V, Wozniak DW, Powell S, Olney JW. Propofol and sodium thiopental protect against MK-801-induced neuronal necrosis in rat posterior cingulate/retrosplenial cortex. *Brain Res.* 2001;913:185–189.
13. Olney JW, Labruyere J, Wang G, et al. NMDA antagonist neurotoxicity: mechanism and prevention. *Science.* 1991;254(5037): 1515–1518.
14. Farber NB, Wozniak DF, Price MT, et al. Age-specific neurotoxicity in the rat associated with NMDA receptor blockade: potential relevance to schizophrenia? *Biol Psychiatry.* 1995;38(12):788–796.
15. Reich DL, Silvay G. Ketamine: an update on the first twenty-five years of clinical experience. *Can J Anaesth.* 1989;36(2):186–197.
16. Frost EAM. A history of nitrous oxide. In: Eger EI II, ed., *Nitrous Oxide*. New York: Elsevier; 1985:1–22.
17. Courville CD. The pathogenesis of necrosis of the cerebral gray matter following nitrous oxide anesthesia. *Ann Surg.* 1938;107:371.
18. Newcomer JW, Farber NB, Jevtovic-Todorovic V, et al. Ketamine-induced NMDA receptor hypofunction as a model of memory impairment and psychosis. *Neuropsychopharmacology.* 1999;20(2): 106–118.
19. Krystal JH, Karper LP, Seibyl JP, et al. Subanesthetic effects of the noncompetitive NMDA antagonist, ketamine, in humans: psychotomimetic, perceptual, cognitive, and neuroendocrine responses. *Arch Gen Psychiatry.* 1994;51(3):199–214.
20. Calb C. A new study raises questions about the risks to young children. *Newsweek.* Oct 21 2008; Health Section.
21. Brown JK, Omar T, O'Regan M. Brain development and the development of tone and muscle. In: Connolly KJ, Forssberg HF, eds. *Neurophysiology and the Neuropsychology of Motor Development.* London: Mac Keith Press;1997:1–41.
22. Dobbing J, Sands J. The brain growth spurt in various mammalian species. *Early Hum Dev.* 1979;3:79–84.
23. Allen NJ, Barres BA. Signaling between glia and neurons: focus on synaptic plasticity. *Curr Opin Neurobiol.* 2005;15:542–548.
24. Komuro H, Rakic P. Modulation of neuronal migration by NMDA receptors. *Science* 1993;260:95–97.
25. Jevtovic-Todorovic V, Hartman RE, Izumi Y, et al. Early exposure to common anesthetic agents causes widespread neurodegeneration in the developing rat brain and persistent learning deficits. *J Neurosci.* 2003;23:876–882.
26. Loepke AW, Istaphanous GK, McAuliffe JJ 3rd, et al. The effects of neonatal isoflurane exposure in mice on brain cell viability, adult behavior, learning, and memory. *Anesth Analg.* 2009;108:90–104.
27. Young C, Jevtovic-Todorovic V, Qin YQ, et al. Potential of ketamine and midazolam, individually or in combination, to induce apoptotic neurodegeneration in the infant mouse brain. *Br J Pharmacol.* 2005;146:189–197.
28. Rizzi S, Carter LB, Ori C, Jevtovic-Todorovic V. Clinical anesthesia causes permanent damage to the fetal guinea pig brain. *Brain Pathol.* 2008;18:198–210.
29. Slikker W Jr, Zou X, Hotchkiss CE, et al. Ketamine-induced neuronal cell death in the perinatal rhesus monkey. *Toxicol Sci* 2007; 98:145–158.
30. Yon J-H, Daniel-Johnson J, Carter LB, Jevtovic-Todorovic V. Anesthesia induces neuronal cell death in the developing rat brain via the intrinsic and extrinsic apoptotic pathways. *Neuroscience.* 2005;35:815–827.
31. Yon J-H, Carter LB, Reiter RJ, Jevtovic-Todorovic V. Melatonin reduces the severity of anesthesia-induced apoptotic neurodegeneration in the developing rat brain. *Neurobiol Dis.* 2006;21:522–530.
32. Kaplan DR, Miller FD. Neurotrophin signal transduction in the nervous system. *Curr Opin Neurobiol.* 2000;10:381–339.
33. Lu LX, Yon JH, Carter LB, Jevtovic-Todorovic, V. General anesthesia activates BDNF-dependent neuroapoptosis in the developing rat brain. *Apoptosis.* 2006:11;1603–1615.
34. Head BP, Patel HH, Niesman IR, Drummond JC, et al. Inhibition of p75 neurotrophin receptor attenuates isoflurane-mediated neuronal apoptosis in the neonatal central nervous system. *Anesthesiology.* 2009;110:813–825.
35. Nikizad H, Yon J-H, Carter LB, Jevtovic-Todorovic V. Early exposure to general anesthesia causes significant neuronal deletion in the developing rat brain. *Ann N Y Acad Sci.* 2007;1122:69–82.
36. Lunardi N, Joksovic P, Todorovic SM, Erisir A, Jevtovic-Todorovic V. General anesthetics cause structural and functional perturbations of the developing synapses in rat brain. *Soc Neurosci Abst.* 2008, Program-10.13.
37. Lunardi N, Ori C, Erisir A, Jevtovic-Todorovic V. General anesthesia causes long-lasting disturbances in the ultrastructural properties of developing synapses in young rats. *Neurotox Res.* 2009;17:179–188.
38. Fredriksson A, Pontén E, Gordh T, Eriksson P. Neonatal exposure to a combination of N-methyl-D-aspartate and gamma-aminobutyric acid type A receptor anesthetic agents potentiates apoptotic neurodegeneration and persistent behavioral deficits. *Anesthesiology.* 2007;107:427–436.
39. Fredriksson A, Archer T, Alm H, Gordh T, Eriksson P. Neurofunctional deficits and potentiated apoptosis by neonatal NMDA antagonist administration. *Behav Brain Res.* 2004;153: 367–376.
40. Levy DM. Psychic trauma of operations in children and a note on combat neurosis. *Am J Dis Child.* 1945;69:7–25.
41. Jackson K. Psychological preparation as a method of reducing emotional trauma of anesthesia in children. *Anesthesiology.* 1951;12; 293–300.
42. Eckenhoff JE. Relationship of anesthesia to postoperative personality changes in children. *Am J Dis Child.* 1953;86:587–591.
43. Standley K, Soule AB, Copans SA, Klein RP. Multidimensional sources of infant temperament. *Genet Psychol Monogr.* 1978;98: 203–231.
44. Backman ME, Kopf AW. Iatrogenic effects of general anesthesia in children: considerations in treating large congenital nevocytic nevi. *J Dermatol Surg Oncol.* 1986;12:363–367.
45. Campbell IR, Scaife JM, Johnstone JM. Physiological effects of day-case surgery compared with inpatient surgery. *Arch Dis Child.* 1988;63:415–417.
46. Wilder RT, Flick RP, Sprung J, et al. Early exposure to anesthesia and learning disabilities in a population-based birth cohort. *Anesthesiology.* 2009;110:796–804.
47. Sun LS, Li G, Dimaggio C, et al. Anesthesia and neurodevelopment in children: time for an answer? *Anesthesiology.* 2008;109:757–761.
48. Kalkman CJ, Peelen L, Moons KG, et al. Behavior and development in children and age at the time of first anesthetic exposure. *Anesthesiology.* 2009;110:805–812.
49. Chorne N, Leonard C, Piecuch R, Clyman RI. Patent ductus arteriosus and its treatment as risk factors for neonatal and neurodevelopmental morbidity. *Pediatrics.* 2007;119:1165–1174.

50. Hintz SR, Kendrick DE, Stoll BJ, et al. Neurodevelopmental and growth outcomes of extremely low birth weight infants after necrotizing enterocolitis. *Pediatrics.* 2005;115:696–703.
51. Hack M, Taylor HG, Drotar D, et al. Poor predictive validity of the Bayley Scales of Infant Development for cognitive function of extremely low birth weight children at school age. *Pediatrics.* 2005; 116:333–341.
52. Rees CM, Pierro A, Eaton S. Neurodevelopmental outcomes of neonates with medically and surgically treated necrotizing enterocolitis. *Arch Dis Child Fetal Neonatal Ed.* 2007;92: F193–198.

19

POSTOPERATIVE COGNITIVE DISORDERS

Catherine C. Price, Jared J. Tanner, and Terri G. Monk

Almost all clinicians have heard statements that resemble the following:

"Dad has not been the same since his surgery."

or

"I don't feel the same since surgery—I can't focus and have trouble remembering names like I used to."

Postoperative cognitive changes have been reported in elderly patients for over a century, and anesthesia has often been mentioned as a possible cause of this problem. In 1955, Bedford published a retrospective review of 1193 elderly patients who had surgery under general anesthesia during a 5-year period.[1] He identified cognitive problems ranging from mild memory problems to dementia in approximately 10% of older patients after surgery. Bedford concluded that the cognitive decline was related to anesthetic agents and hypotension and that "operations on elderly people should be confined to unequivocally necessary cases." The jury is still out as to whether anesthesia is the culprit for these difficulties. There is supportive evidence that the difficulties encountered after surgery are multifactorial; preoperative, operative, and postoperative factors appear to impact the presence of postoperative cognitive difficulties.

In this chapter we will review two common types of postoperative concerns, particularly for older adults: 1) delirium and 2) postoperative cognitive dysfunction (POCD). We will also review considerations for dementia progression after surgery. First, we provide you with three cases based on our professional experiences exemplifying delirium, POCD, and dementia following surgery.

Case 1 POSTOPERATIVE *DELIRIUM*

An 80-year-old oriented retired economics professor with a history of hypertension, hypercholesterolemia, and longstanding leg edema due to a previous injury underwent right hip replacement surgery with general isoflurane anesthesia and morphine patient-controlled analgesia for postoperative pain relief. Presurgery medications included furosemide that he took daily to assist with his chronic leg edema and hypertension. On the morning of postoperative day 1, he was agitated and reported seeing bugs on the ceiling and rats on the bed. His son found him typing on the bedsheets with his fingers. When questioned, he stated that he was e-mailing the president of the United States to provide him with advice. He remained in this state for five full days. He was continually disoriented to time, slept during the day, and was awake during the night. He was prescribed quetiapine fumate to assist with his symptoms. On postoperative day five, his mental status stabilized such that he could be discharged to an inpatient nursing rehabilitation facility. He additionally developed depression and suicidal ideation during his stay. His quetiapine was monitored and adjusted during this time. Functioning markedly improved after returning home, but remained concerning to family members. He had problems remembering things and required more explanations or time to process information, but was otherwise typically oriented, alert, and free of delusions or hallucinations. Additionally, he was not sleeping regular hours and continued to report depressive symptoms without suicidal ideation. Three months post surgery, formal outpatient neuropsychological, radiological, and neurological evaluations were conducted to rule out dementia. Outpatient neuropsychological testing identified reduced information processing speed but intact memory functions relative to his age-matched peers. Other cognitive abilities were generally consistent with premorbid/presurgery expectations based on family member reports of his presurgery abilities and premorbid cognitive estimates. Brain magnetic resonance imaging (MRI) conducted 2 months post surgery revealed global atrophy but no evidence of acute stroke. There was, however, some evidence of ischemic demyelination suggesting possible long-standing small vessel vascular disease. A behavioral neurological evaluation was largely negative with the exception of some low B12 values during laboratory testing. A consensus meeting among all professionals who had seen him postoperatively (neurology, neuropsychology, radiology) agreed that the diagnosis of *Cognitive Disorder Not Otherwise Specified* was most appropriate, although he clearly had delirium during his inpatient hospitalization. Due to his marked improvement in mental status and superior intellect otherwise, dementia was not a concern. There was, however, concern about his reduced processing speed. The review team attributed this cognitive deficit to surgery and perioperative events interacting with a) his baseline medical factors (mild vascular risk factors including hypercholesterolemia), which can result in altered cerebral arteriole vessel integrity and perfusion to subcortical brain structures (important for processing speed, memory); b) low B12 values that can impact attention and concentration; and c) mild/moderate depression, which can alter sleep-wake cycles and is associated with reduced mental acuity. Follow-up with this patient has indicated continued improvement. Recommendations were to provide him with continuing monitoring at home for instrumental activities of daily living (IADLs) and normal daily rhythms (appetite, hydration, sleep), continuation of B12 supplementation, mood and behavioral sleep management program, and to increase social/mental stimulation. A return neurological and neuropsychological evaluation was encouraged in one year if his functioning did not remain stable.

Case comment: This case demonstrates that even after delirium clears, there can be lingering cognitive difficulties that are concerning to family members, thereby causing concerns for dementia. However, full behavioral and cognitive evaluation could only be conducted when the delirium resolved. Careful consideration with a clinical team ruled out a dementia, but there was concern for his reduced information processing speed (rapid visual-motor coordination, thinking speed). The primary mechanism for his delirium and processing speed reductions remain unknown. There are a number of hypothetical contributors: a) use of general anesthesia (no regional block) may have led to complications with postoperative pain management and induced elements of the delirium, b) abnormal circadian sleep-wake cycles and depression, and c) preexisting small vessel vascular disease on MRI that may have placed him at risk for all of these events. Of note, although quetiapine has been associated with treatment of postoperative delirium in some cases, such effectiveness has not been confirmed by controlled studies.[2] Additionally, it should be noted that the brain MRI was conducted two months after the surgery. An MRI should be conducted within 48 hours (at the latest) to identify a stroke (silent or otherwise) associated with surgery. Thus, it is possible that an arterial ischemic change did occur around the time of surgery and simply was not identifiable via MRI two months post surgery.

Case 2 POSTOPERATIVE COGNITIVE DYSFUNCTION (POCD)

A 60-year-old female underwent general anesthesia with a morphine PCA for a right total knee replacement. She had an uneventful hospital course with no evidence of delirium and was discharged to home on the third postoperative day. She had a successful recovery and was able to play singles tennis by 6 months after surgery. Despite a full recovery, she had difficulty recalling given names. This problem was so severe that she had been unable to remember her mother's given name when introducing her to friends several weeks earlier. She was seen in consultation for this problem and told that mild cognitive decline had been reported following orthopedic surgery and that the etiology for this problem was unknown, but that it might be related to the anesthesia and/or surgery. The patient was scheduled to have a left total knee replacement in several months and when she heard this information, she stated "I am not going to have the other knee done because I can't afford to lose any more of my memory."

Case comment: This case demonstrates mild POCD lasting for 6 months after orthopedic surgery. Despite the fact that the patient had a successful surgical repair and was able to return to an active life style, her mild difficulty remembering names was so distressing that she decided not to have surgery on her other knee. To the observer, she appeared completely normal. Anesthesia providers often see patients who appear normal but complain of memory loss after surgery. It is important that anesthesia providers be empathetic and recognize that mild cognitive disorders may not be obvious to the observer but may still distress the patient. This individual did not have a formal neuropsychological evaluation, so we can only speculate that her difficulty remembering names was likely due to problems suppressing distracting information and multitasking (being in a social situation and unable to quickly recall a name while also smiling, remaining social, and engaging with both her mother and the associated peer at the same time), more so than actual "loss" of her mother's name. Loss of old information (e.g., mother's name) is extremely rare. The inability to learn new information (i.e., remember recent events, places) is more often associated with learning and memory disruption (i.e., pathology in the medial temporal lobe). Interestingly, research has demonstrated that mild memory loss is not associated with functional limitations whereas multitasking and mental flexibility impairment are more serious to patients and the family members.[3]

Case 3 DEMENTIA

A 68-year-old female with 12 years of education, 90 pack years of smoking, previous history of depression and anxiety, and a history of aortic stenosis underwent aortic valve replacement under general anesthesia. Her husband reported that she was "semicomatose" for 5 days after surgery. She had complained of some mild memory problems before her surgery but after the surgery the problem worsened and she started complaining of marked difficulty recalling recent events. Other than memory complaints, her recovery from the surgery was unremarkable. After recovery she was able to perform all activities of daily living (ADLs) but was having some difficulty with IADLs, including grocery shopping and managing finances. Her husband reported that she would occasionally get lost when driving her car to an appointment and, if they were on an extended drive, she would repeatedly ask where they were going. She was referred to neuropsychology three months after her surgery for an assessment of her memory. On testing she was impaired only on memory tests. Her memory score on the Dementia Rating Scale (DRS-2) was impaired; her performance on both verbal and visual memory measures were similarly impaired. However, her performance on all other tests was within normal limits. She was referred for repeat neuropsychological evaluation in order to assess the course of her cognitive impairments. At a 12-month follow-up neuropsychological examination, her memory had declined compared to her initial evaluation. She also was exhibiting difficulty on tests assessing frontal lobe function (mental flexibility, complex mental planning), and she had problems suggesting lateral temporal lobe and parietal lobe involvement (language, recall of word knowledge). She was no longer driving and was having more difficulty with IADLs (cooking, finances). At that time, due to the marked severity of her memory deficits and impairment on other cognitive domains, she was diagnosed with Alzheimer's disease.

Case comment: Her performance at initial neuropsychological evaluation demonstrates impairment in recent memory with relative sparing of other cognitive domains. Her memory complaints started prior to her aortic surgery but markedly worsened after the surgery. However, due to the proximity of the first evaluation to her surgery, sparing of abilities on IADLs, and lack of impairments in multiple cognitive domains, she was not diagnosed with a dementia at that time. She did not have any surgeries between her two neuropsychological evaluations. At follow-up 15 months post surgery, she had impairments in multiple cognitive domains with memory still the most prominent. She also had difficulty performing IADLs, relying more on her husband to manage day-to-day activities. This particular pattern of impairment is indicative of Alzheimer's disease.

It is possible that she suffered an intraoperative complication, but no surgical complications were reported in medical notes or by the family. However, her memory and cognitive deficits did not become pronounced until after the surgery; because they were progressive, it is possible that her surgery presented a risk factor that *contributed* to her to development of an incipient dementia (i.e., Alzheimer's disease).

These three cases provide brief examples of the topics reviewed below. Please refer to Table 19.1 for a summary comparison of delirium, postoperative cognitive dysfunction, and general dementia features.

DELIRIUM

DELIRIUM DEFINED

Delirium is an acute and temporary change in orientation and cognition. It is well defined in the *Diagnostic and Statistical Manual of Mental Disorders* (DSM-IV-TR; American Psychiatric Association; 2000:135; www.dsmivtr.org/), including various subtypes. Delirium can be attributed to an underlying medical condition (*delirium due to a general medical condition*), medications (*substance-induced delirium, substance intoxication delirium*), or withdrawal from medications (*substance withdrawal delirium*). Delirium can also be multifactorial (*delirium due to multiple etiologies*). In addition, *delirium not otherwise specified* is included for presentations in which clinicians are unable to determine a specific etiology.[4] Delirium can be present at hospital admission and presurgically, although it is more often seen in postoperatively managed general medical units, and most frequently in intensive care units (ICUs). In this chapter, we first discuss delirium in the hospitalized patient in general and then focus on postoperative delirium in orthopedic and cardiac surgery.

GENERAL CHARACTERISTICS OF DELIRIUM

Delirium has key characteristics, but can manifest differently depending on patient type. Most common is fluctuating arousal with waxing and waning awareness of orientation. It is often accompanied by altered sleep-wake cycles, and reversed night cycles.[5] Hallucinations and illusions are common. Patients can vary, however, by presenting with hyperactive, hypoactive, or mixed hyper-hypo active cognitive and motor states.[6,7] Hyperactive patients show increased psychomotor activity, such as rapid speech, irritability, and restlessness. These patients can be disruptive, time-consuming, and harmful to staff. They are therefore more readily identified and treated. This type of agitation or delirium postoperatively may involve a substance-induced delirium.[4] Hypoactive patients, by contrast, typically show a calm appearance combined with inattention, decreased mobility, and have difficulty answering simple questions about orientation. Hypoactive delirium may be misdiagnosed as depression or fatigue,[8] when in fact it can be due to acute illness such as intestinal perforation.[9] For these reasons, hypoactive delirium is considered a worse prognosis.

SIGNIFICANCE OF DELIRIUM IN GENERAL MEDICAL PATIENTS VERSUS POSTOPERATIVE PATIENTS:

Although a temporary condition, delirium is a medical and societal stressor from an economic and healthcare standpoint. Delirium occurs in at least 10 to 24% of the general patient population, with reports up to 60% for postoperative patients.[10] One-year medical center costs between 1995 to 1998 have been estimated to be $16,303 to $64,421 per individual with delirium; approximately 2.5 times the costs for those without delirium.[11,12] Patients with delirium after emergent and elective surgery have a median hospital stay of 21 days (range: 1–75 days) compared to a median stay of 8 days (range: 1–79) for those without delirium.[13] Indirect costs of delirium stem from lost work and personal productivity by patients and caregivers. Delirium can have long-lasting implications leading to personal and societal challenges. Moreover, acute postoperative delirium has recently been shown to be an independent predictor of functional decline at one year in a study following patients after cardiac surgery,[14] and with increased morbidity at least among hip surgery patients[15]

Table 19.1 A COMPARISON OF THE CLINICAL FEATURES OF DELIRIUM, POCD, AND GENERAL DEMENTIA*

PARAMETER	DELIRIUM	POCD	DEMENTIA
Onset	**Immediate** **Hours/days**	**Variable** **Days/weeks**	**Insidious and gradual**
Presentation	**Disoriented** **Fluctuating Moods**	**Oriented** **Fully alert** **Vague complaints of attention/memory problems**	**Variable depending on severity and type of dementia**
Course	**Hours/weeks**	**Usually improves; evaluation should be at least 2-weeks after discharge due to confounds from medication and fatigue**	**Slow and continuous with time; insidious when there are no acute strokes (i.e., not multi-infarct dementia)**
Sleep-Wake	**Worse at night, in darkness and on awakening**	**No difficulties**	**> Moderate stage will see evening sundowning, reversed sleep cycles**
Duration	**Hours to < month**	**Improvement by 3-months; if not, then consider cognitive evaluation.**	**Month to years**
Affect	**Labile/variable Fear/panic/euphoria**	**Mild to moderate depression can occur**	**Variable depending on severity and type of dementia** **Can be easily distractible, inappropriate anxiety to apathy**
Assessment	**Confusion Assessment Method**	**Neuropsychological testing**	**Behavioral, Neurological, Neuropsychological**
Disease states to rule out	**Stroke** **Medication toxicity** **Dehydration** **Anemia**	**Transient ischemic attacks** **Fatigue/Pain medications** **Anemia** **B12 deficiency**	**B12 deficiency** **Normal pressure hydrocephalus (NPH)** **Infections and medications**

Some material on delirium and dementia referenced from Capezuti L, et al. *Evidence-Based Geriatric Nursing Protocols for Best Practice*, 3rd ed. New York: Springer Publishing Company; 2008.

ASSESSING DELIRIUM

To assist with diagnosis, a number of investigators have collaborated to develop and validate rapid bedside approaches to diagnose patients at the bedside and ICU. The Confusion Assessment Method (CAM)[16] is the most well known measure for assessing delirium. Based on the *Diagnostic and Statistical Manual of Mental Disorders* (DSM-III-R) criteria for delirium, the CAM assesses four features: acute onset and fluctuating course (feature 1), inattention (feature 2), disorganized thinking (feature 3), and altered level of consciousness (feature 4). The diagnosis of delirium requires the presence of features 1 and 2 and either 3 and 4. (Note that memory impairment is not included, for this is sometimes absent in mild delirium, whereas it is present in other conditions, such as dementia.[16]) Across studies, the CAM has sensitivities of 94% or better, specificities better than 90%, positive and negative predictive accuracy of greater than 90%, and high interrater reliability (kappa = .81 to 1.0).[17]

The Society of Critical Care Medicine has strongly recommended routine evaluation of delirium in ICU patients.[18] For critically ill patients in whom delirium prevalence ranges from 11% to 87%,[19,20] the CAM-ICU (shown in Table 19.2)[21] was designed. It assesses the same four features of the original CAM, but relies more on nonverbal responses. For this examination, patients are assessed for the presence of acute mental status change, inattention, disorganized thinking, and altered levels of consciousness. Ely and colleagues (2001) show this scale to have high sensitivity (93 to 100%), a specificity of 98 to 100%, and high interrater reliability in delirium detection.[21] We encourage you to review some excellent video introductions to the CAM-ICU available via the Internet (www.youtube.com).

The CAM has been translated into 20 other languages including Chinese, Dutch, German, and Spanish.[17] with the CAM-ICU having high validity relative to other delirium scales available in those languages (e.g., Swedish translation[22]). The CAM-ICU, in particular, has been recommended by international guidelines.[18,23] Overall, the CAM and CAM-ICU's simple algorithms allow them to be useful for rapid identification of delirium by both physicians and staff nurses. After training, both scales should take approximately 2 minutes to administer. Because of their ease, these scales have been promoted by organizations such as the Nurses Improving Care for Healthsystem Elders (NICHE) initiative.[24]

The CAM and CAM-ICU are not the only delirium assessment tests available. There are at least six assessment instruments that have gone through validation in critically ill adults.[23,25] Leutz et al have compared the Delirium Detection Score[26] and the Nursing Delirium Screening Scale[27] relative to the CAM-ICU.

PREVALENCE OF DELIRIUM TYPE AND CONSIDERATIONS FOR RISK FACTORS IN GENERAL MEDICAL AND SURGICAL POPULATIONS

An informative study by Lin and colleagues reports on the prevalence of delirium type and associated clinical risk factors.[12] The study is an impressive review of discharge data from the Nationwide Inpatient Sample database, which is funded by the U.S. government's agency for Healthcare Research and Quality and contains discharge data from a stratified, random sample of hospitals across the country. From a total of 1,269,185 adult nonpsychiatric/non–substance abuse general and surgical hospitalizations with at least one delirium code at discharge, the following were identified: first, the infection-related subtype had the largest clinical group (12.5%), with this including respiratory infections, cellulitis, and urinary tract/kidney infections; next, Central Nervous System (CNS) disorder groups were the second most common (10.6%), with this including craniotomy, CNS neoplasms, degenerative nervous system disorders, strokes/transient and other, seizures/headaches, and other nervous system disorders; lastly, delirium in metabolic, cardiovascular, and orthopedic procedures constituted 8.1%, 7.0%, and 6.5%, respectively, of all admissions reviewed.

Lin and colleagues (2010) further divided delirium into three categories: 1) nondementia, nondrug (NDND) delirium (ICD-9 293.0, 293.1); 2) drug-induced delirium (ICD-9 292.81); and 3) any delirium with dementia (ICD-9 codes 290.11, 290.3, 290.41). The most frequent delirium type was *nondementia nondrug delirium,* followed by *drug-induced delirium*, and then *dementia-associated delirium*. NDND delirium had the highest rate of hyponatraemia relative to the other delirium groups. Patients with drug-induced delirium were younger than the other groups (median age of 78 years) and had the lowest proportion of comorbidities. Drug-induced delirium was most common in patients who had lower extremity orthopedic surgery (relative to comparison groups of patients with pneumonia, urinary tract infection, congestive heart failure). This striking finding raises questions about the association between analgesic use in orthopedic and nonorthopedic hospitalizations. Those with dementia-related delirium had a higher rate of admission from long-term facilities, were older (median age of 85 years), had the highest mortality rate, had higher rates of atrial fibrillation, cerebrovascular disease, and had higher rates of pneumonia and urinary tract infections. General delirium risk factors were male sex, increasing age, and cerebrovascular risk factors.

Structural brain disease traits appear to be a viable predictor of delirium, as well. Although studies are of variable quality with regard to imaging methods (e.g., computed tomography versus MRI, subjective rating scales for quantifying white matter abnormalities), studies show

Table 19.2 THE CONFUSION ASSESSMENT METHOD FOR THE INTENSIVE CARE UNIT (CAM-ICU)

FEATURES AND DESCRIPTIONS	ABSENT	PRESENT

I. Acute onset or fluctuating course*

A. Is there evidence of an acute change in mental status from baseline?
B. Or, did the (abnormal) behavior fluctuate during the past 24 hours, that is, tend to come and go and decrease in severity as evidenced by fluctuations on the Richmond Agitation Sedation Scale (RASS) or the Glasgow Coma Scale?

II. Inattention†

Did the patient have difficulty focusing attention as evidenced by a score of less than 8 correct answers on either the visual or auditory components of the Attention Screening Examination (ASE)?

III. Disorganized Thinking

Is there evidence of disorganized or incoherent thinking as evidenced by incorrect answers to 3 or more of the 4 questions and inability to follow the commands?
Questions

1. **Will a stone float on water?**
2. **Are there fish in the sea?**
3. **Does 1 pound weigh more than 2 pounds?**
4. **Can you use a hammer to pound a nail?**

Commands

1. **Are you having unclear thinking?**
2. **Hold up this many fingers. (Examiner holds 2 fingers in front of the patient)**
3. **Now do the same thing with the other hand (without holding the 2 fingers in front of the patient)**

(If the patient is already extubated from the ventilator, determine whether the patient's thinking is disorganized or incoherent, such as rambling or irrelevant conversation, unclear or illogical flow of ideas, or unpredictable switching from subject to subject.)

IV. Altered level of consciousness

Is the patient's level of consciousness anything other than alert, such as being vigilant or lethargic or in a stupor, or coma?

Alert:	**spontaneously fully aware of environment and interacts appropriately**
Vigilant:	**hyperalert**
Lethargic:	**drowsy but easily aroused, unaware of some elements in the environment or not spontaneously interacting with the interviewer; becomes incompletely aware when prodded strongly; can be aroused only by vigorous and repeated stimuli and as soon as the stimulus ceases, stuporous subject lapses back into unresponsive state**
Coma:	**unarousable, unaware of all elements in the environment with no spontaneous interaction or awareness of the interviewer so that the interview is impossible even with maximal prodding**

Overall CAM-ICU Assessment (Features 1 and 2 and either Feature 3 or 4): Yes___ No___

*The scores included in the 10-point RASS range from a high of 4 (combative) to a low of −5 (deeply comatose and unresponsive). Under the RASS system, patients who were spontaneously alert, calm, and not agitated were scored at 0 (neutral zone). Anxious or agitated patients received a range of scores depending on their level of anxiety: 1 for anxious, 2 for agitated (fighting ventilator), 3 for very agitated (pulling on or removing catheters), or 4 for combative (violent and a danger to staff). The scores −1 to −5 were assigned for patients with varying degrees of sedation based on their ability to maintain eye contact: −1 for more than 10 seconds, −2 for less than 10 seconds, and −3 for eye opening but no eye contact. If physical stimulation was required, then the patients were scored as either −4 for eye opening or movement with physical or painful stimulation or −5 for no response to physical or painful stimulation. The RASS has excellent interrater reliability and intraclass correlation coefficients of 0.95 and 0.97, respectively, and has been validated against visual analog scale and geropsychiatric diagnoses in 2 ICU studies.
†In completing the visual ASE, the patients were shown 5 simple pictures (previously published[34]) at 3-second intervals and asked to remember them. They were then immediately shown 10 subsequent pictures and asked to nod "yes" or "no" to indicate whether they had or had not just seen each of the pictures. Since 5 pictures had been shown to them already, for which the correct response was to nod "yes," and 5 others were new, for which the correct response was to shake their heads "no," patients scored perfectly if they achieved 10 correct responses. Scoring accounted for either errors of omission (indicating "no" for a previously shown picture) or for errors of commission (indicating "yes" for a picture not previously shown). In completing the auditory ASE, patients were asked to squeeze the rater's hand whenever they heard the letter *A* during the recitation of a series of 10 letters. The rater then read 10 letters from the following list in a normal tone at a rate of 1 letter per second: *S, A, H, E, V, A, A, R, A, T*. A scoring method similar to that of the visual ASE was used for the auditory ASE testing.

Reproduced with permission: Ely EW, et al. Delirium in mechanically ventilated patients: validity and reliability of the confusion assessment method for the intensive care unit (CAM-ICU). *JAMA.* 2001;286(21):2703–2710.

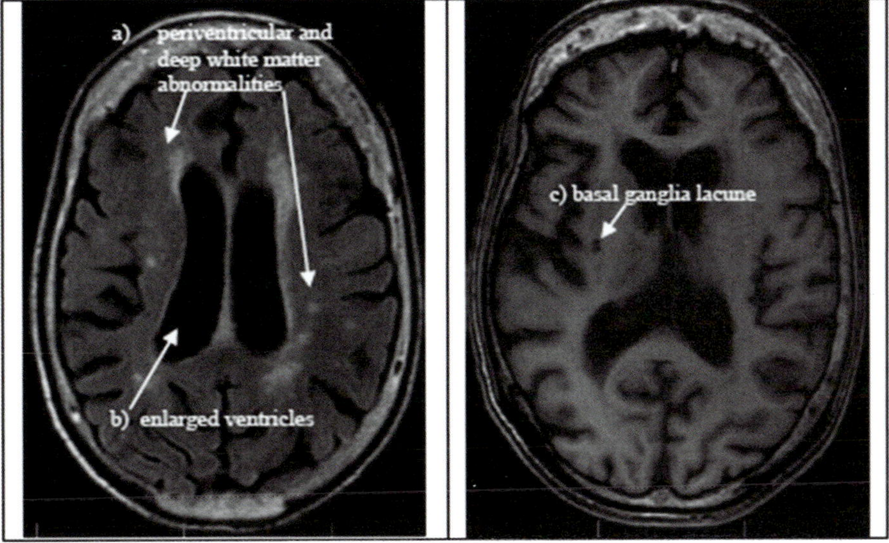

Figure 19.1 Structural brain variables associated with delirium risk: a) white matter abnormalities as seen on T2-weighed Fluid Attentuated Inversion Recovery (FLAIR) scans; b) enlarged ventricles; c) lacunae near/in basal ganglia as seen on standard T1-weighted image.

that delirium patients have preexisting brain disease. Patients with delirium are reported to have preexisting larger ventricle sizes,[28] basal ganglia or caudate lesions/lacunes (see Figure 19.1),[29,30] white matter abnormalities in the periventricular and deep regions of the brain (see Figure 19.1),[29,31] as well as greater cortical[31] and subcortical atrophy.[32] An important caveat, however, is that almost all of these studies are confounded by age; delirium patients are significantly older in age than those without delirium. White matter abnormalities and atrophy increase with age for many individuals, particularly those with hypertension and hypercholesterolemia.[33] Please see Soiza and colleagues' 2008 article for a more thorough review.[34]

Studies of brain risk factors are currently being conducted with more sophisticated structural imaging methods such as diffusion tensor imaging (DTI). Briefly, DTI uses a noninvasive in vivo method to map the microscopic structural information of oriented tissue, such as white matter.[35] The brain's white matter includes afferent and efferent connections between the cortical and subcortical gray matter, thereby supporting numerous hierarchically organized cognitive subsystems.[36] Fractional anisotropy is currently the most commonly used metric for DTI and provides information on how coherent and regular the axons are within each voxel.[37] A recent study by Shioiri and colleagues identified many brain regions with lower fractional anisotropy within the white matter of patients who developed delirium post cardiac surgery.[38] After controlling for age, however, four clusters of brain areas remained significant: left subgyrus of the frontal lobe, right cingulate gyrus, left ventral anterior nucleus of the thalamus, and corpus callosum. These regions are associated with attention, executive function (doing two or more things at the same time, abstract reasoning, planning), and learning. This study lends further support to the hypothesis that there are predisposing brain vulnerability factors, specifically white matter integrity, for the development of delirium.[39]

Brain regions identified in delirium imaging studies to date suggest potential coexisting cerebrovascular disease. White matter abnormalities, lacunes, and subcortical atrophy are developments of subcortical disease states and particularly, small vessel vascular disease. In the general population, small vessel disease and increasing white matter disease are associated with declines in frontal-subcortical functions, i.e., executive functions,[33] as well as depression.[40] These findings correspond with neuropsychological test findings that preoperative executive dysfunction but not global cognitive impairment may identify patients who will develop delirium.[39,41]

In summary, there appears to be convincing evidence from research of general health and brain MRI predictors that vascular disease markers are significant contributors to the development of delirium and specific delirium subtypes. We now turn our attention to discuss risk factors and treatment implications for postoperative delirium in two major surgery types: orthopedic and cardiac surgery.

REDUCING POSTOPERATIVE DELIRIUM: ANESTHETIC CONSIDERATIONS AND PERIOPERATIVE VARIABLES

Postoperative delirium typically presents around 24 hours after surgery and resolves in most by 48 hours,[42] but can last for up to months in some patients.[43] Different risk factors for orthopedic and cardiac surgery have been discussed in the literature and are therefore reviewed separately below.

Specific to Orthopedic Surgery

Although delirium can be noted in elective orthopedic surgery, it is more prominent and concerning among urgent orthopedic surgeries such as hip fracture. Patients who develop delirium after hip fracture surgery are more likely to die, be diagnosed with dementia or mild cognitive impairment, or require institutionalization.[4,15,44] There is an increased need to identify ways to reduce delirium in these patients. Recent randomized controlled studies suggest that analgesia and pain management, as well as depth of general anesthesia, are important modifiable factors for delirium prevalence after hip fracture surgery. A Cochrane review[45] compared outcome differences in hip fracture patients versus regional anesthesia. From five randomized controlled trials meeting inclusion criteria, there were more patients with postoperative confusion in the general anesthesia groups relative to the regional anesthesia groups. The authors concluded that with hip fracture surgery, regional anesthesia relative to general anesthesia results in a 2-fold reduction of acute delirium. Moreover, a recent study by Marino and colleagues reports regional anesthesia techniques significantly reduced total hydromorphone consumption and delirium (disorientation to time and/or place) compared with patient-controlled analgesia alone after unilateral hip replacement.[46]

Sieber[43] however, in a very thorough review of some of the most the most prominent studies to date examining delirium incidence in regional versus general anesthesia,[47–53] pointed out that all studies failed to attend to sedation during regional anesthesia with postoperative pain management also uncontrolled. He lends credibility to this argument in a recently published study. Using a double blind, randomized control trial for elderly patients without preoperative delirium or severe dementia, Sieber and colleagues demonstrate that anesthetic propofol sedation depth with spinal anesthesia is a contributor to delirium frequency after hip fracture repair.[54] Elderly patients without preoperative delirium or severe dementia who were randomized to "deep sedation" (Bispectral Index, approximately 50, which is consistent with general anesthesia) had higher rates of delirium (40%) than the light sedation group (Bispectral Index, ≥ 80; 19%). They authors report that 1 incident of delirium will be prevented for every 4.7 patients treated with light sedation. Clearly, further work is needed to clarify the role of sedation depth in combination with or without spinal anesthesia. We encourage readers to review a clear discussion on the benefits of regional anesthesia and analgesia by Halaszynski[55] and to consider the role of regional anesthesia and sedation depth on delirium outcome in patients.

Identifying and treating delirium risk factors in patients *prior* to surgery may also be a method for reducing postoperative delirium. For hip surgery patients, Bjorkelund and colleagues[56] have shown that decreased postoperative oxygen saturation (SpO2 < 90%), fasting time 12 h or more, dementia, postoperative anemia (hemoglobin < 6.2mmol/l), postoperative transfusion, preoperative use of four or more prescribed drugs, and difficulties walking without assistance strongly associate with delirium development. These researchers subsequently conducted a quasi-experimental intervention study[57] where preoperative patients with hip fractures admitted to the hospital were either treated with a multifactorial intervention program (n = 131) or served as a control group (n = 132). The multifactorial intervention program included 1) the use of supplemental oxygen perioperatively, 2) intravenous fluid supplementation and extra nutrition, 3) increased monitoring of vital physiological parameters starting at the place of injury until the postoperative period 4) adequate pain relief immediately after admission, 5) efficient transfer logistics, 6) daily delirium screening, 7) avoidance of polypharmacy including sedatives/hypnotics and anticholinergic medications, and 8) anesthesia recommendations (premedication with acetaminophen, propofol and/or alfentanil IV on arrival to operating suite, spinal anesthesia with bupivacaine). Findings showed less delirium in the intervention group relative to the control group, suggesting the value of *multifactorial perioperative intervention approaches* rather than the use of one or two therapies alone.

Specific to Cardiac Surgery

Delirium after cardiac surgery has been reported for years, but has recently been shown to be a strong independent predictor of mortality for up to 10 years postoperatively, even in younger individuals and in those without prior stroke.[58] Coronary artery bypass graft or valve surgery is also associated with risk of functional decline at one month after discharge, with this outcome independent of comorbidity, baseline function, and cognition.[14] These two recent studies highlight the need to identify risk factors and conduct intervention trials to preserve short- and long-term function.

To date, identified preoperative risk factors are very similar across studies. They primarily include increased age, cerebrovascular disease, and dementia. As also mentioned above in our discussion of general risk factors, preoperative white matter fractional anisotropy[59] may serve as an important risk factor and indicate reduced frontal-subcortical functions and early markers of brain cerebrovascular disease. Operative risk factors include impaired left ventricular ejection fraction, time on cardiopulmonary bypass, high perioperative transfusion requirement, and postoperative hypertension. Microemboli, common to all cardiac surgical procedures[60–64] has not, to date, been specifically associated with delirium[65] although it continues to be considered a potential contributor when other variables and stressors such as hypoperfusion and psychoactive medications are involved.[58]

There may be specific modifiable risk factors for delirium after cardiopulmonary bypass. In a group of individuals receiving standardized surgery, anesthesia, postoperative pain management protocols, and daily delirium evaluations, Burkhart and colleagues identified that delirium risk factors were 1) the dose of fentanyl per kilogram of body weight administered during the operation, 2) the duration of mechanical ventilation, and 3) maximum value of C-reactive protein measured postoperatively.[66] The authors pose that fentanyl, with questionable anticholinergic effects,[67,68] may be a modifiable risk factor; alternatives such as remifentanil or other opioids may be worth considering for intervention trials. Duration of mechanical ventilation requires sedation and therefore may be a consequence of the specific drugs used to maintain sedation. Sedation depth may also be worth considering, such as proposed by Sieber.[43,54] Postoperative rates of C-reactive protein suggest a systemic inflammatory response to surgery. This may indicate a relationship to endotoxin, a common consequence of coronary artery bypass grafting and trauma-induced intra-abdominal infections.[69] Burkhart and colleague's C-reactive protein findings,[66] coupled with other findings that cortisol levels also correlate with postoperative delirium,[70,71] suggest that these areas need further investigation. Clearly, there is a specific need for intervention trials with potentially modifiable risk factors in cardiac patients. Furthermore, anesthetic and surgical interventions targeting biological stress responses for both cardiac and noncardiac surgeries may be appropriate.

CONSIDERATIONS FOR ANTICHOLINERGIC MEDICATIONS AND ANESTHESIA

Anticholinergic drugs and/or interaction of these drugs with anesthetic agents is considered a probable factor for postoperative delirium (see excellent review and neurobiological discussion of theories by Pratico et al,[72] as well as by Cancelli et al[73] and Fong et al.[74] Anticholinergic drugs compete for acetylcholine receptor subtypes (nicotinic and muscarinic), antagonize the effects of acetylcholine, and impair memory performance. High serum levels of anticholinergic drugs are associated with delirium and cognitive impairment.[75,76] Unfortunately, these medications are commonly taken by older adults, prescribed often by general practitioners, and are often missed as a general cause of memory difficulties. Common anticholinergic medications include tricyclic antidepressants used to treat mood but also pain and sleep (e.g. amitriptyline), antihistamines, and antibiotics (e.g. cephalosporin, third generation). Anesthesiologists should identify patients on anticholinergic medications prior to surgery. At least one potential mechanism for anesthetic action is via the suppression of cholinergic cells (e.g. isoflurane and sevoflurane suppress acetylcholine release[72]). Thus, there is potential for more pronounced reduction of cholinergic activity. Randomized prospective studies are needed to identify the extent to which presurgery anticholinergic medications interact with anesthesia to induce delirium and even postoperative cognitive dysfunction. There have been attempts to prevent postoperative delirium with cholinesterase inhibitors (e.g., rivastigmine) in randomized treatment trials. Unfortunately, to date, these have been largely unsuccessful for both elective total joint replacement[77,78] and cardiopulmonary bypass.[79] Additional large interventional trials are needed.

POSTOPERATIVE COGNITIVE DYSFUNCTION (POCD)

POCD DEFINED

POCD is a subtle impairment of memory, concentration, and information processing that is distinct from delirium and dementia. Despite the fact that POCD is not a formal psychiatric diagnosis, the term is commonly used in current literature and POCD is considered to be a mild neurocognitive disorder. The DSM-IV-TR states that a mild neurocognitive disorder can only be diagnosed if the cognitive disturbance does not meet the criteria for three other conditions (delirium, dementia, or amnestic disorder).[80] The diagnosis of a mild neurocognitive disorder must be corroborated by the results of neuropsychological testing showing that an individual has a new onset of deficits in at least two areas of cognitive functioning lasting for a period of at least two weeks. These diagnostic criteria make it virtually impossible to make a clinical diagnosis of POCD during the hospital stay.

SIGNIFICANCE OF POCD

Due to the subtle nature of POCD, the patient, partner, or close friends are often the first to notice the problem. The symptoms vary from mild memory loss to the inability to efficiently process information, concentrate, and self-monitor. Price et al[3] analyzed the type and severity of pre- to postoperative cognitive decline in 77 patients exhibiting POCD at 3 months after major noncardiac surgery. In the impaired patients, 42 (55%) had memory decline, 26 (34%) had executive function problems (problems with processing speed and ignoring distracting information), and 9 (11%) had a combined memory and executive function impairment. Executive and combined impairments were associated with significant functional limitations.[3]

POCD can also influence long-term outcomes in elderly adults. Monk et al[81] found that cognitive decline in the first 3 months after major noncardiac surgery was associated with increased mortality for 1 year after surgery. A second study confirmed that POCD at 3 months after noncardiac surgery was associated with increased mortality for as long as 8 years after surgery and that POCD at 1 week was associated with the risk of early retirement and dependency on social transfer payments.[82]

ASSESSING POCD

POCD is not a formal diagnosis and has no formal criteria. Most of the published studies report preoperative and postoperative neurocognitive results for patients and define POCD based on severity of test decline. Unfortunately there is significant variation among studies describing POCD with one publication describing nine different definitions of neuropsychological deficits that have been used to diagnose POCD.[83] Other methodological problems complicating research in this area include learning effects with repeated testing, baseline testing performance, loss of patients during follow-up, reliability of testing if patients are experiencing pain or are on analgesic medications, and the timing of postoperative testing.[84]

CURRENT RESEARCH ON POCD

Several prospective studies have presented evidence that postoperative cognitive decline is indeed a reality. A prospective longitudinal study of 261 patients who underwent coronary artery bypass surgery found that 53% of the patients had cognitive decline at hospital discharge, 36% at 6 weeks, 24% at 6 months, and 42% at 5 years after surgery.[85] These investigators evaluated predictors of cognitive decline at 5 years after surgery and found that cognitive impairment at hospital discharge was a significant predictor of long-term cognitive impairment.

A second multinational, prospective study reported on postoperative cognitive decline following noncardiac surgery. In this study, Moller et al[86] evaluated cognitive function in patients aged 60 years or older after major abdominal and orthopedic surgery. These patients completed a battery of psychometric tests prior to surgery and at one week and three months after surgery. In this study, 25% of the patients had measurable cognitive dysfunction a week after the operation, and 10% had cognitive changes three months after surgery. Perioperative hypoxemia and hypotension were studied as potential causative factors for postoperative cognitive decline, but the investigators found no evidence that either of these factors correlated with the occurrence of POCD. The only risk factor for prolonged POCD was advancing age, with an incidence of 7% for patients between the ages of 60 to 69 years compared to 14% of the patients aged 70 or older.

A third study evaluated the incidence of POCD following noncardiac surgery in patients aged 18 years and older.[81] These investigators demonstrated that POCD is common in all age groups at hospital discharge, ranging from 37% of young patients (aged 18 to 39 years), 30% in middle-aged patients (aged 40 to 59 years), to 41% in elderly patients (aged 60 years and older). However, at 3 months after surgery, cognitive decline occurred in 13% of elderly patients compared to 6% in young and middle-aged patients. This difference was significant, demonstrating that the risk of long-term POCD (3 months after surgery) is low for patients younger than 60 years. This study also found that advancing age, lower educational level, a history of previous stroke with no residual impairment, and POCD at hospital discharge were the most important factors predicting long-term cognitive decline for patients after major noncardiac surgery.

Several studies have failed to demonstrate any long-term differences in postoperative cognitive function between general and regional anesthesia. Williams-Russo and colleagues[47] examined 262 patients over the age of 40 who were undergoing total knee arthroplasty. The patients were randomly assigned to either epidural or general anesthesia. This investigation found no differences between the patients in the two anesthesia groups for either cognitive or cardiovascular outcome. Rather, at 2 weeks postoperatively, both anesthetic groups had significant declines from their preoperative neurocognitive tests scores. At 6 months postoperatively, both groups improved on their cognitive scores, but the incidence of long-term postoperative cognitive deficit at this testing period remained at 5% regardless of anesthesia group.

In a slightly larger study, Rasmussen and colleagues[87] randomly allocated patients aged 60 years or older to general or regional anesthesia for major noncardiac surgery. They demonstrated that a substantial proportion of patients experienced postoperative cognitive dysfunction at 1 week and 3 months post surgery (incidence rate ranged from 10% to 20%). There was no significant difference in the incidence of POCD between the groups at 3 months after surgery.

POTENTIAL MECHANISMS FOR POCD

The mechanisms responsible for postoperative cognitive decline after noncardiac surgery are unknown, but potential risk factors can be classified into patient, surgical, and anesthetic categories. It is likely that the etiology of POCD in the elderly patient is multifactorial and may include the preoperative health status of the patient, the patient's preoperative level of cognition, intraoperative events related to the surgery itself, and neurotoxic effects of anesthetic agents.

At this time there are no definitive conclusions regarding the effects of anesthesia on learning and memory—additional research is needed to clarify the relationship between anesthetic agents and postoperative cognitive changes. In vitro studies have shown that the inhalational anesthetic isoflurane enhances oligomerization and cytotoxicity of amyloid β peptides, a protein change associated with Alzheimer's disease.[88] However, several studies (see above) report that the risk of postoperative cognitive problems is the same for regional and general anesthesia, which suggests that inhalational anesthesia is not responsible for these problems.[47,87] Additional randomized clinical trials are needed to determine the best (if any) anesthetic techniques for older patients.

While it may seem obvious that intraoperative hypotension would be associated with increased postoperative cognitive problems, the literature does not support this theory. Williams-Russo et al[89] randomized older adults undergoing total hip replacement to either normotension (mean arterial pressure of 55–70) or deliberate hypotension (mean arterial pressure of 45–55) during surgery. At 4 months after surgery, there were no significant differences in the rates of POCD between the groups, as well as no significant differences in other complications including cardiac, renal, and thromboembolic events. These findings are in agreement with an earlier longitudinal study that found no relationship between intraoperative hypotension or hypoxemia and POCD in elderly patients.[86]

It has also been hypothesized that hyperventilation and the resultant decrease in cerebral blood flow might result in insufficient cerebral oxygenation and cause POCD. In a study of patients undergoing cataract surgery, patients were randomized to 3 groups: general anesthesia and ventilation to 4.9 kPa (37 torr) versus general anesthesia and hyperventilation to 2.9 kPa (22 torr) versus local anesthesia with spontaneous ventilation.[90] There were no significant differences in cognitive outcome among the groups at 4 days and 4 weeks after surgery.

CONSIDERATIONS FOR POSTOPERATIVE DEMENTIA DEVELOPMENT OR PROGRESSION

THRESHOLD AND BRAIN/ COGNITIVE RESERVE

The concept of a threshold and brain/cognitive reserve is often mentioned when attempting to explain why 1) certain individuals develop delirium or postoperative cognitive dysfunction, and 2) certain patients may proceed to an irreversible dementia. We provide a brief review of the threshold and reserve concepts below.

Roth and colleagues[91–93] first introduced the concept of a "threshold" in their postmortem Newcastle-Upon-Tyne studies. These researchers attended to observations between senile plaque counts and measures of disease/dementia severity. They noted that, in Parkinson's disease, clinical parkinsonism does not appear until 85% of the cells of the nigrostriatal system are depleted and dopamine has declined in a similar proportion.[94] A similar pattern was reported in Alzheimer's disease with regard to neurofibrillary plaques and tangles.[95]

Satz contributed significantly to the concept of a threshold by formally providing some general properties for a threshold theory and reserve.[96] Satz outlines two postulates: A) how greater brain reserve (as measured by premorbid intellectual abilities, academic abilities, or current intelligence) serves as a protective factor to a lesion or pathology, and B) how lesser brain reserve serves as a vulnerability factor to lesion or pathology. He also provides subpostulates discussing the effects of aggregate lesions, disease progression, and challenge. See Figure 19.2 for a modified figure depicting Satz's Postulate A and B.

We can apply Satz's postulates[96] to the topics of delirium and POCD. Using Figure 19.2, you can see that Patient A has greater reserve (which can be measured in a number of ways: education level, intelligence, etc) relative to Patient B. Both experience an insult to the brain that results in a similarly sized "lesion." Patient A, however, because of cognitive reserve, does not demonstrate delirium or postoperative cognitive change; Patient A remains above the critical threshold for identifying a measurable change in behavior. By contrast, Patient B with less preoperative "reserve" falls below this critical threshold and demonstrates significant changes in function.

We could further hypothesize that Patient A may eventually develop cognitive impairment if he experiences an additional lesion (e.g., another surgical event, a motor vehicle accident, etc). The aggregate effect of the two lesions eliminates the remaining reserve for Patient A; he now presents with clinical symptoms of cognitive impairment. This pattern resembles what would be hypothesized for an individual with a prodromal disease state (i.e., Mild Cognitive Impairment–Amnestic being a precursor to Alzheimer's disease[97]; consider case three from the beginning of the chapter). Clinical manifestation of memory impairment may remain at subthreshold until there is a summation of perioperative factors (preoperative medications,

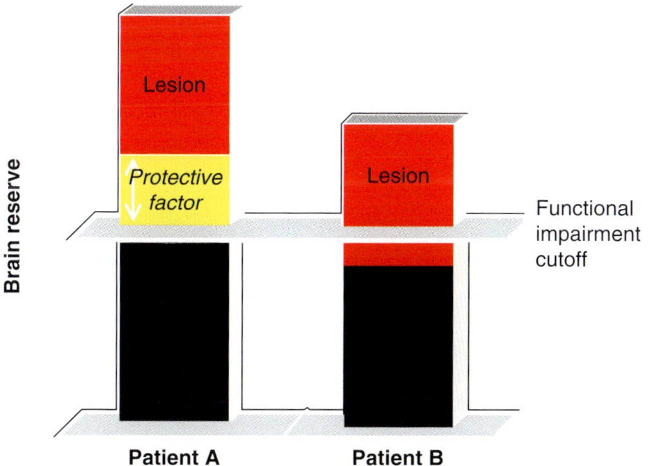

Figure 19.2 Brain reserve capacity and threshold concept discussed by Paul Satz (1993). Adapted from Satz P. Brain reserve capacity on symptom onset after brain injury: a formulation and review of evidence for threshold theory. *Neuropsychology.* 1993;7(3): 273–295, based on permission authorization through APA Journal.

anesthesia, anemia) that places him below the functional impairment cutoff. For high functioning individuals, Satz also postulates that a lesion may remain at subthreshold until the person is presented with a specific challenge (i.e., a certain neuropsychological test or environmental demand is encountered thereby requiring demonstration of certain cognitive abilities).

Unfortunately, it is difficult to define and measure reserve and use the concept to predict risk for delirium or POCD. Some researchers propose that education is a surrogate marker for reserve. The concept of education is multifold, however. Education may signify more neuronal connections, but also it may simply mark better test taking abilities, better social networks, and healthcare. For these reasons, reserve has been extensively studied beyond that of education alone. According to Stern, there are at least two forms of reserve. Reserve can be characterized 1) as simply "brain reserve" (essentially brain structure), or 2) as "cognitive reserve" represented by neural function and compensation. Unfortunately, operationally defining both brain and cognitive reserve remains challenging and are topics worthy of longitudinal investigation. We encourage you to become familiar with the topic of reserve subtypes[98,99] as well as discussions on reserve and postoperative disorders.[100]

Interestingly, much work needs to be done with regard to the topic of reserve and delirium; we were surprised to learn that most delirium research fails to even mention the topic of education as a risk factor. This may be due to the nature of large delirium "risk factor" studies; most are retrospective and education is not a common variable acquired in preoperative and postoperative hospital settings. Prospective research integrating the topics of threshold and reserve with traditional (i.e., education based) or other variables (i.e., questionnaires addressing lifestyle issues that may impact reserve) with regard to delirium and POCD is clearly warranted.

At least one group of researchers is attempting to address the concepts of reserve and delirium. Max Gunther and colleagues have outlined an interesting hypothesis for delirium that they are currently investigating with functional magnetic resonance imaging (see Figure 19.3).

Gunther and coinvestigators propose a circuit of change between the ascending reticular activity system (ARAS), medial temporal/hippocampal region (MTL), posterior parietal cortex (PPC), and dorsal prefrontal cortex (PFC). Older age and particularly certain dementias such as Alzheimer's disease are associated with changes to the integrity of the MTL, PPC, and PFC. The MTL is particularly important for new learning, the PPC is important for components of language as well as spatial awareness, and the PFC is essential for multitasking, working memory, planning, and organizing general information for learning to occur. As we age, these regions of the brain may change normally or abnormally, depending on disease status. Gunther and colleagues hypothesize that anesthetics and sedative agents impacting the brainstem may lead to disruption of the ARAS leading to fluctuating arousal, sensorium, and attention. This may cause additional stress on already compromised MTL, PPC, and PFC systems thereby leading to reduced awareness and interpretation of surroundings, impaired learning, and poor higher level functions (planning, organization). As Gunther and colleagues insightfully point out, this hypothesized circuit may be particularly true for individuals with reduced "reserve" in the MTL, PPC, and PFC regions–such as those with Alzheimer's disease or APO-e4 genotype. For more information on this group's research, please see http://www.icudelirium.org/.

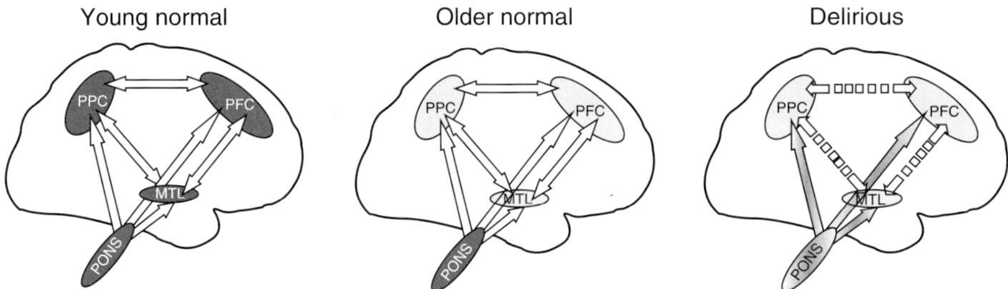

Figure 19.3 (1) YOUNG NORMAL: In healthy individuals there is normal and consistent connectivity between the PPC, MTL, and PFC. This circuit is innervated, activated, and maintained by the ARAS arising from the brainstem; (2) OLDER NORMAL: elderly individuals begin to show signs of grey matter atrophy in the PPC, MTL, and PFC. Although functional connectivity between these regions remains intact, the strength of the connections is no longer as robust as it once was in the healthy CNS. This circuit continues to be activated and maintained by the ARAS directly and via the thalamus; (3) DELIRIOUS: individuals treated in the ICU are subject to a number of medical and pharmacological challenges that may disrupt normal CNS connectivity. Serious illnesses such as sepsis, ARDA, and ALI as well as sedative and analgesic medications commonly prescribed in the ICU have the potential to weaken functional links between the cortical regions depicted above. This is particularly likely for processes impacting the ARAS. Fluctuations in activation arising from the brainstem may be sufficient in elderly individuals to cause a disruption which surpasses a critical threshold of threats to neurocognitive function, prolonged decoupling of this circuit may lead to deleterious neurodegenerative consequences such as excitotoxicity. Over time this has the potential to result in apoptosis and long-term cognitive impairment. Note: PPC, posterior parietal cortex; PFC, prefrontal cortex; MTL, medial temporal lobe; ARAS, ascending reticular activating system. Reprinted from Gunther ML, Jackson JC, Ely EW. Loss of IQ in the ICU brain injury without the insult. *Medical Hypotheses.* 2007;69:1180, with permission from Elsevier.

Through this type of research we may be able to eventually predict the *type* of dysfunction that will develop and type of cognitive-behavioral intervention needed. There is some evidence that POCD can manifest differently for older adults after noncardiac surgery: some individuals present with memory problems, some present with problems in multitasking, while other present with both memory and multitasking problems.[3] Patients with both memory and multitasking difficulties are more likely to develop difficulties with IADLs. Individuals with memory problems may be more likely to develop Alzheimer's disease. Those with multitasking difficulties are more likely to develop vascular dementia, while those with both may have mixed pathologies. Based on the threshold theory and reserve hypothesis, these findings may suggest those individuals with postoperative memory difficulties had preoperative vulnerability in regions of the brain required for memory (i.e., early forms of Alzheimer's disease; also known as Mild Cognitive Impairment, amnestic subtype[97]). Alternatively, those who developed more difficulties with multitasking may have risk factors for dementias that impact frontal-subcortical circuits or frontal cortical regions. These statements, however, are hypothetical and need to be formally investigated. Thus, we encourage longitudinal research studies examining postoperative cognitive domains (e.g., memory, multitasking, language, visuospatial functions) and changes in these cognitive domains for patients with either or both delirium/POCD. Examining cognitive domain vulnerability to perioperative variables will facilitate research on biological-neuronal-perioperative interactions.

CONCLUSION

There is growing evidence that postoperative delirium and POCD can result in reduction in acute and long-term function for some individuals, especially older adults. Delirium and POCD can therefore be interpreted as representing an insult to the brain. The development of interventions to prevent and treat these conditions is essential with our increasingly older adult population.

REFERENCES

1. Bedford P. Adverse cerebral effects of anaesthesia on old people. *Lancet*. 1955;2:758–861.
2. Khouzam HR. Quetiapine in the treatment of postoperative delirium: a report of three cases. *Compr Ther*. 2008;34(3–4):207–217.
3. Price CC, Garvan CW, Monk TG. Type and severity of cognitive decline in older adults after noncardiac surgery. *Anesthesiology*. 2008;108(1):8–17.
4. Deiner S, Silverstein JH, Postoperative delirium and cognitive dysfunction. *Br J Anaesth*. 2009;103(Suppl 1):i41–46.
5. Trzepacz P. Delirium—advances in diagnosis, pathophysiology, and treatment. *Psychiatry Clinical North America*. 1996;19:429–449.
6. Lipowski Z. Delirium in the elderly patient. *N Engl J Med*. 1989; 320:578–582.
7. Meagher DJ, Trezepacz T. Motoric subtypes of delirium. *Semin Clinic Neuropsychiatry*. 2000;5:75–85.
8. Spiller JA, Keen, J C. Hypoactive delirium: assessing the extent of the problem for impatient specialist palliative care. *Palliative Medicine*. 2006;20(1):17–23.
9. Morita T, et al. Hypoactive delirium as a clinical symptom of intestinal perforation. *Psychosomatics*. 1999;40(2):130–131.
10. Maldonado JR. Delirium in the acute care setting: characteristics, diagnosis and treatment. *Crit Care Clin*. 2008;24(4):657–722, vii.
11. Inouye SK, et al. Does delirium contribute to poor hospital outcomes? a three-site epidemiologic study. *J Gen Intern Med*. 1998; 13(4):234–242.
12. Lin RY, Heacock LC, Fogel JF. Drug-induced, dementia-associated and non-dementia, non-drug delirium hospitalizations in the United States, 1998–2005: an analysis of the national inpatient sample. *Drugs Aging*. 2010;27(1):51–61.
13. Ansaloni L, et al. Risk factors and incidence of postoperative delirium in elderly patients after elective and emergency surgery. *Br J Surg*. 2010;97(2):273–280.
14. Rudolph JL, et al. Delirium: an independent predictor of functional decline after cardiac surgery. *J Am Geriatr Soc*. 2010;58(4):643–649.
15. Kat MG, Vreeswijk R, de Jonghe JFM. Long-term cognitive outcome of delirium in elderly hip surgery patients. *Dement Geriatr Cogn Dis*. 2008;26:1–8.
16. Inouye SK, et al. Clarifying confusion: the confusion assessment method; a new method for detection of delirium. *Ann Intern Med*. 1990;113(12):941–948.
17. Wei LA, et al. The confusion assessment method: a systematic review of current usage. *J Am Geriatr Soc*. 2008;56(5):823–830.
18. Jacobi J, et al. Clinical practice guidelines for the sustained use of sedatives and analgesics in the critically ill adult. *Crit Care Med*. 2002;30(1):119–141.
19. Aldemir M, et al. Predisposing factors for delirium in the surgical intensive care unit. *Crit Care*. 2001;5(5):265–270.
20. Ely EW, et al. The impact of delirium in the intensive care unit on hospital length of stay. *Intensive Care Med*. 2001;27(12):1892–1900.
21. Ely EW, et al. Delirium in mechanically ventilated patients: validity and reliability of the confusion assessment method for the intensive care unit (CAM-ICU). *JAMA*. 2001;286(21):2703–2710.
22. Larsson C, Axell AG, Ersson A. Confusion assessment method for the intensive care unit (CAM-ICU): translation, retranslation and validation into Swedish intensive care settings. *Acta Anaesthesiol Scand*. 2007;51(7):888–892.
23. Luetz A, et al. Different assessment tools for intensive care unit delirium: which score to use? *Crit Care Med*. 2010;38(2):409–418.
24. Fletcher K, et al. Using nurse practitioners to implement best practice care for the elderly during hospitalization: the NICHE journey at the University of Virginia Medical Center. *Crit Care Nurs Clin North Am*. 2007;19(3):321–37, vii.
25. Devlin J, et al. Delirium assessment in the critically ill. *Intensive Care Med*. 2007;33:929–940.
26. Sander M, et al. Alcohol use disorder: risks in anesthesia and intensive care medicine. *Internist (Berl)*. 2006;47(4):332, 334–336, 338, passim.
27. Lutz A, et al. The nursing delirium screening scale (Nu-DESC)—Guideline conformal translation for the German language space. *Anasthesiologie Intensivmedizin Notfallmedizin Schmerztherapie*. 2008;43(2):98–102.
28. Koponen H, Hurri L, Stenback U, Mattila E, Soinien H, Riekkinen PJ. Computed-tomography findings in delirium. *J Nerv Ment Dis*. 1989;177:226–231.
29. Figiel GS, et al. Radiologic correlates of antidepressant-induced delirium: the possible significance of basal-ganglia lesions. *J Neuropsychiatry Clin Neurosci*. 1989;1(2):188–190.
30. Figiel GS, Krishnan KRR, Doraiswamy M. Subcortical structural changes in ECT-induced delirium *J Geriatr Psychiatry Neurol*. 1990;3:172–176.

31. Henon H, Lebert F, Durieu I, et al. Confusional state in stroke-relation to pre-existing dementia, patient characteristics, and outcome. *Stroke*. 1999;30:773–779.
32. Samton JB, Fernando, S J, Sanelli P, Karimi S, Raiteri V, Barnhill, J W. The clock drawing test: diagnostic, functional and neuroimaging correlates in older medically ill adults. *J Neuropsychiatry Clin Neurosci*. 2005;17:533–540.
33. Libon DJ, et al. From Binswanger's disease to leuokoaraiosis: what we have learned about subcortical vascular dementia. *Clin Neuropsychol*. 2004;18(1):83–100.
34. Soiza RL, Sharma V, Ferguson K, Shenkin SD, Seymour DG, MacLullich AMJ. Neuroimaging studies of delirium: a systematic review. *J Psychosom Res*. 2008;65:239–248.
35. Sullivan EV, Pfefferbaum A. Diffusion tensor imaging and aging. *Neurosci Biobehav Rev*. 2006;30(6):749–761.
36. Felleman DJ, Van Essen DC. Distributed hierarchical processing in the primate cerebral cortex. *Cereb Cortex*. 1991;1(1):1–47.
37. Klingberg T, et al. Myelination and organization of the frontal white matter in children: a diffusion tensor MRI study. *Neuroreport*. 1999;10(13):2817–2821.
38. Shioiri A, et al. White matter abnormalities as a risk factor for postoperative delirium revealed by diffusion tensor imaging. *Am J Geriatr Psychiatry*. 2010;18(8):743–751.
39. Greene NH, et al. Measures of executive function and depression identify patients at risk for postoperative delirium. *Anesthesiology*. 2009;110(4):788–795.
40. de Groot JC, et al. Cerebral white matter lesions and depressive symptoms in elderly adults. *Arch Gen Psychiatry*. 2000;57(11): 1071–1076.
41. Smith PJ, et al. Executive function and depression as independent risk factors for postoperative delirium. *Anesthesiology*. 2009;110(4): 781–787.
42. Duppils GS, Wikblad K. Acute confusional states in patients undergoing hip surgery: a prospective observation study. *Gerontology*. 2000;46(1):36–43.
43. Sieber FE. Postoperative delirium in the elderly surgical patient. *Anesthesiol Clin*. 2009;27(3):451–464, table of contents.
44. Bickel H, Gradinger R, Kochs E, Forstl H. High risk of cognitive and functional decline after postoperative delirium. *Dement Geriatr Cogn Dis*. 2008;26:420–426.
45. Parker MJ, Handoll HH, Griffiths R. Anaesthesia for hip fracture surgery in adults. *Cochrane Database Syst Rev*. 2004; (4):CD000521.
46. Marino J, et al. Continuous lumbar plexus block for postoperative pain control after total hip arthroplasty: a randomized controlled trial. *J Bone Joint Surg*. 2009;91:29–37.
47. Williams-Russo P, et al. Cognitive effects after epidural vs general anesthesia in older adults: a randomized trial. *JAMA*. 1995;274(1): 44–50.
48. Chung FF, et al. Comparison of perioperative mental function after general anaesthesia and spinal anaesthesia with intravenous sedation. *Can J Anaesth*. 1989;36(4):382–387.
49. Berggren D, et al. Postoperative confusion after anesthesia in elderly patients with femoral neck fractures. *Anesth Analg*. 1987;66(6): 497–504.
50. Crul BJ, Hulstijn W, Burger IC. Influence of the type of anaesthesia on post-operative subjective physical well-being and mental function in elderly patients. *Acta Anaesthesiol Scand*. 1992;36(7): 615–620.
51. Campbell DN, et al. A prospective randomised study of local versus general anaesthesia for cataract surgery. *Anaesthesia*. 1993;48(5): 422–428.
52. Bigler D, et al. Mental function and morbidity after acute hip surgery during spinal and general anaesthesia. *Anaesthesia*. 1985; 40(7):672–676.
53. Cook PT, et al. A prospective randomised trial comparing spinal anaesthesia using hyperbaric cinchocaine with general anaesthesia for lower limb vascular surgery. *Anaesth Intensive Care*. 1986; 14(4):373–380.
54. Sieber FE, et al. Sedation depth during spinal anesthesia and the development of postoperative delirium in elderly patients undergoing hip fracture repair. *Mayo Clin Proc*. 2010;85(1):18–26.
55. Halaszynski TM. Pain management in the elderly and cognitively impaired patient: the role of regional anesthesia and analgesia. *Curr Opin Anaesthesiol*. 2009;22:594–599.
56. Bjorkelund KB, et al. Factors at admission associated with 4 months outcome in elderly patients with hip fracture. *AANA J*. 2009; 77(1):49–58.
57. Bjorkelund KB, et al. Reducing delirium in elderly patients with hip fracture: a multi-factorial intervention study. *Acta Anaesthesiol Scand*. 2010;54(6):678–688.
58. Gottesman RF, et al. Delirium after coronary artery bypass graft surgery and late mortality. *Ann Neurol*. 2010;67(3):338–344.
59. Shioiri A, Kurumaji A, Takeuchi T, Matsuda H, Arai H, Nishikawa T. White matter abnormalities as a risk factor for postoperative delirium revealed by diffusion tensor imaging. *Am J Geriatr Psychiatry*. 2010;18(8):743–751.
60. Restrepo M, et al. Diffusion- and perfusion- weighted magnetic resonance imaging of the brain before and after coronary artery bypass grafting surgery. *Stroke*. 2002;33:2909–2915.
61. Jacobs A, et al. Alterations of neuropsychological function and cerebral glucose metabolism after cardiac surgery are not related only to intraoperative microembolic events. *Stroke*. 1998;29(3): 660–667.
62. Pugsley W, et al. The impact of microemboli during cardiopulmonary bypass on neuropsychological functioning. *Stroke*. 1994; 25(7):1393–1399.
63. Lund C, et al. Comparison of cerebral embolization during off-pump and on-pump coronary artery bypass surgery. *Ann Thorac Surg*. 2003;76(3):765–770; discussion 770.
64. Diegeler A, et al. Neuromonitoring and neurocognitive outcome in off-pump versus conventional coronary bypass operation. *Ann Thorac Surg*. 2000;69(4):1162–1166.
65. Rudolph JL, et al. Microemboli are not associated with delirium after coronary artery bypass graft surgery. *Perfusion*. 2009;24(6): 409–415.
66. Burkhart CS, et al. Modifiable and nonmodifiable risk factors for postoperative delirium after cardiac surgery with cardiopulmonary bypass. *J Cardiothorac Vasc Anesth*. 2010;24(4):555–559.
67. Han L, et al. Use of medications with anticholinergic effect predicts clinical severity of delirium symptoms in older medical inpatients. *Arch Intern Med*. 2001;161(8):1099–1105.
68. Chew ML, et al. Anticholinergic activity of 107 medications commonly used by older adults. *J Am Geriatr Soc*. 2008;56(7):1333–1341.
69. Dellinger EP. Can one use biologic modifiers to prevent multiple organ dysfunction syndrome after abdominal infections? *Surg Infect (Larchmt)*. 2000;1(3):239–248.
70. Kudoh A, et al. Postoperative interleukin-6 and cortisol concentrations in elderly patients with postoperative confusion. *Neuroimmunomodulation*. 2005;12(1):60–66.
71. McIntosh TK, et al. Beta-endorphin, cortisol and postoperative delirium: a preliminary report. *Psychoneuroendocrinology*. 1985; 10(3):303–313.
72. Pratico C, et al. Drugs of anesthesia acting on central cholinergic system may cause post-operative cognitive dysfunction and delirium. *Med Hypotheses*. 2005;65(5):972–982.
73. Cancelli I, et al. Drugs with anticholinergic properties: a potential risk factor for psychosis onset in Alzheimer's disease? *Expert Opin Drug Saf*. 2009;8(5):549–557.
74. Fong TG, et al. Delirium accelerates cognitive decline in Alzheimer disease. *Neurology*. 2009;72(18):1570–1575.
75. Flacker JM, et al. The association of serum anticholinergic activity with delirium in elderly medical patients. *Am J Geriatr Psychiatry*. 1998;6(1):31–41.

76. Mussi C, et al. Importance of serum anticholinergic activity in the assessment of elderly patients with delirium. *J Geriatr Psychiatry Neurol.* 1999;12(2):82–86.
77. Liptzin B, et al. Donepezil in the prevention and treatment of post-surgical delirium. *Am J Geriatr Psychiatry.* 2005;13(12):1100–1106.
78. Sampson EL, et al. A randomized, double-blind, placebo-controlled trial of donepezil hydrochloride (Aricept) for reducing the incidence of postoperative delirium after elective total hip replacement. *Int J Geriatr Psychiatry.* 2007;22(4):343–349.
79. Gamberini M, et al. Rivastigmine for the prevention of postoperative delirium in elderly patients undergoing elective cardiac surgery—a randomized controlled trial. *Crit Care Med.* 2009; 37(5):1762–1768.
80. APA. *Diagnostic and Statistical Manual of Mental Disorders (DSM-IV-TR), Fourth Edition Text Revision.* Washington, DC: American Psychiatric Association; 2000.
81. Monk TG, et al. Predictors of cognitive dysfunction after major noncardiac surgery. *Anesthesiology.* 2008;108(1):18–30.
82. Steinmetz J, et al. Long-term consequences of postoperative cognitive dysfunction. *Anesthesiology.* 2009;110(3):548–555.
83. Rasmussen LS, et al. The assessment of postoperative cognitive function. *Acta Anaesthesiol Scand.* 2001;45(3):275–289.
84. Funder KS, Steinmetz J, Rasmussen LS. Methodological issues of postoperative cognitive dysfunction research. *Semin Cardiothorac Vasc Anesth.* 2010;14(2):119–122.
85. Newman MF, et al. Longitudinal assessment of neurocognitive function after coronary-artery bypass surgery. *N Engl J Med.* 2001; 344(6):395–402.
86. Moller JT, et al. Long-term postoperative cognitive dysfunction in the elderly ISPOCD1 study. ISPOCD investigators. International Study of Post-Operative Cognitive Dysfunction. *Lancet.* 1998; 351(9106):857–861.
87. Rasmussen LS, et al. Does anaesthesia cause postoperative cognitive dysfunction? a randomised study of regional versus general anaesthesia in 438 elderly patients. *Acta Anaesthesiol Scand.* 2003;47(3):260–266.
88. Eckenhoff RG, et al. Inhaled anesthetic enhancement of amyloid-beta oligomerization and cytotoxicity. *Anesthesiology.* 2004;101(3): 703–709.
89. Williams-Russo P, et al. Randomized trial of hypotensive epidural anesthesia in older adults. *Anesthesiology.* 1999;91(4):926–935.
90. Jhaveri RM. The effects of hypocapnic ventilation on mental function in elderly patients undergoing cataract surgery. *Anaesthesia.* 1989;44(8):635–640.
91. Blessed G, Tomlinson BE, Roth M. The association between quantitative measures of dementia and of senile change in the cerebral grey matter of elderly subjects. *Br J Psychiatry.* 1968;114(512): 797–811.
92. Roth AM. Classification and etiology in mental disorders of old age: some recent developments. *Br J Psychiatry,* Special Publication. 1971;6:1–18.
93. Roth M, Tomlinson BE, Blessed G, The relationship between quantitative measures of dementia and of degenerative changes in the cerebral grey matter of elderly subjects. *Proc R Soc Med.* 1967; 60(3):254–260.
94. Quinn NP, Rossor MN, Marsden CD, Dementia and Parkinson's disease—pathological and neurochemical considerations. *Br Med Bull.* 1986;42(1):86–90.
95. Roth M. The association of clinical and neurological findings and its bearing on the classification and aetiology of Alzheimer's disease. *Br Med Bull.* 1986;42(1):42–50.
96. Satz P. Brain reserve capacity on symptom onset after brain injury: a formulation and review of evidence for Threshold Theory. *Neuropsychology* 1993;7(3):273–275.
97. Petersen RC, et al. Mild cognitive impairment: clinical characterization and outcome. *Arch Neurol.* 1999;56(3):303–308.
98. Stern Y. Cognitive reserve. *Neuropsychologia.* 2009;47(10): 2015–2028.
99. Stern Y. The concept of cognitive reserve: a catalyst for research. *J Clin Exp Neuropsychol.* 2003;25(5):589–593.
100. Jones RN, et al. Aging, brain disease, and reserve: implications for delirium. *Am J Geriatr Psychiatry.* 2010;18(2):117–127.

20

ANESTHESIA AND NEURODEGENERATIVE DISORDERS

Zhongcong Xie and Yiying (Laura) Zhang

Alzheimer's disease, Parkinson's disease, and Huntington's disease are some of the most common neurodegenerative disorders. The mechanisms and risk factors for these diseases remain largely to be determined. Recent studies have indicated that anesthesia and surgery may have an impact on the development of these diseases. With the increase in the number of older adults, anesthesiologists will encounter more and more surgical patients who have these common neurodegenerative disorders. Therefore, it is important to understand the effects of anesthesia on the neuropathogenesis of these disorders, and to start the discussion of how best to provide anesthesia care for surgical patients who suffer from neurodegenerative disease.

ALZHEIMER'S DISEASE

GENERAL INFORMATION

Alzheimer's disease (AD), also called Alzheimer disease, Senile Dementia of the Alzheimer Type, or simply Alzheimer's, is the most common form of dementia. AD has become one of the greatest public health problems in the United States, and its impact will only increase with the demographic changes anticipated in the coming decades.[1] Currently, AD affects 5.3 million Americans. It is estimated that the number of AD patients will reach 13.2 million in the United States by 2050 if no treatments are found. According to the data presented by the Alzheimer's Association in 2009, there is a new AD case every 70 seconds in the United States, and AD is the 6th leading cause of death in the United States. In addition, there are 9.9 million unpaid caregivers and the annual cost for AD is 148 billion dollars in the United States.[2]

Clinically, AD patients usually present with a subtle onset of memory loss followed by a slow progression of dementia over several years. The initial symptoms include impairment of attention, planning, and thinking, as well as difficulties in language, executive function, perception, and movement. Symptoms of moderate dementia include wandering, irritability, labile affect, crying, aggression, resistance to caregiving, sundowning, illusions, and delusions. Finally, AD patients develop complete loss of speech, extreme apathy and exhaustion, becoming totally dependent on caregivers. AD patients usually do not die from the disease itself, but rather from associated complications, such as ulcers and pneumonia.[3]

Genetically, identification of four AD genes has provided a foundation for rapid progress in understanding neuropathogenesis. PSEN 1 (located in chromosome 14), PSEN2 (located in chromosome 1), and amyloid precursor protein (APP) (located in chromosome 21) are genes that—when mutated—may very likely lead to early-onset familial AD. On the other hand, the APOE-ε4 gene, located in chromosome 19, is only a risk factor for the development of late-onset AD. The other risk factors for AD are age, family history, head injury, vascular disease, and diabetes.[4] Many investigators have been actively searching for new AD genes and risk factors.

The diagnosis of AD includes obtaining a history from the patient and from relatives, excluding other neurological disorders, and assessing the patient using neuropsychological tests. The diagnostic criteria are the presence of cognitive impairment and a suspected dementia syndrome, which can be confirmed by neuropsychological testing. Recent developments have suggested that imaging studies could also help the diagnosis of AD.[3]

There is no cure for AD, but current pharmacologic interventions may be able to attenuate the symptoms. These medicines include cholinesterase inhibitors donepezil, galantamine, and rivastigmine, and the non-competitive *N*-methyl-*D*-aspartate (NMDA) glutamate receptor antagonist memantine. In addition, it is important to employ psychosocial interventions, including behavior, emotion cognition, or stimulation interventions. Finally, caregivers play an essential role in the treatment of AD patients.[3]

NEUROPATHOGENESIS

AD neuropathogenesis still remains largely to be determined. Recent studies have suggested that processing of amyloid precursor protein and accumulation of β-amyloid protein (Aβ), tau protein phosphorylation, synaptic dysfunction, oxidative stress and mitochondrial failure, neuroinflammation, and many other factors contribute to AD neuropathogenesis.[5]

Aβ is the key component of senile plaques in AD dementia patients and was first isolated from meningovascular amyloid deposits in AD and Down's syndrome patients.[6,7] These findings led to the cloning of the AD gene APP,[8,9] which further led to many studies of APP and Aβ at the genetic, protein, and cellular levels, as well as at the level of animal-based model systems. The results from these studies have led to the formation of the amyloid hypothesis first initiated by Glenner and Wong[10] and further supported by many other AD researchers since (see reviews[11,12]). According to the amyloid hypothesis, the imbalance between the Aβ generation and Aβ clearance is the molecular basis of AD neuropathogenesis.

Aβ is produced via serial proteolysis of amyloid precursor protein (APP) by aspartyl protease β-site APP-cleaving enzyme (BACE), or β-secretase, and γ-secretase. BACE cleaves APP to generate a 99-residue membrane-associated C-terminus fragment (APP-C99). APP-C99 is further cleaved by γ-secretase to release 4 kDa Aβ and β-amyloid precursor protein intracellular domain.[13–15] γ-Secretase is a detergent-sensitive, high molecular weight complex[16] that includes at least four proteins, presenilin 1/presenilin 2 (PS1/PS2), nicastrin (NCSTN)/APH2, APH-1, and PEN-2 (see Figure 20.1).[17–20]

Increasing evidence suggests a role for caspase activation and apoptosis in AD neuropathogenesis.[21,22] Even though studies have suggested that apoptosis is involved in AD neuropathogenesis, the contribution of apoptosis to AD neuropathology remains controversial.[21–24] This could be due to the long duration of AD and very rapid clearance of apoptotic cells from organs. Specifically, caspase-3 activation, caspase-3-cleaved-β-actin and caspase-cleaved-APP have been found in brains of AD patients.[25–28] There have also been autopsy data to indicate some other apoptotic characteristics in the brains of AD patients.[29,30] Recent studies have suggested initiator phases, but not the terminal commitment phase, of apoptosis are involved in AD neuropathogenesis.[22]

Another histopathological hallmark of AD is intraneuronal neurofibrillary tangles. The tangles are mainly composed of abnormally hyperphosphorylated tau protein,[12] which has been shown to induce synaptic and cell loss.[31] However it is still controversial whether tau protein is neurotoxic, protective, or simply a marker of AD.[32] Nevertheless, recent studies have shown that activation of a mutant tau gene in mice results in neuronal loss, brain atrophy, and memory impairment; whereas inhibition of the mutant tau gene leads to cessation of neuronal loss, decreased brain atrophy, and improvement in memory.[33]

Synapse loss and dysfunction contribute to AD neuropathogenesis. It has been hypothesized that Aβ can compromise

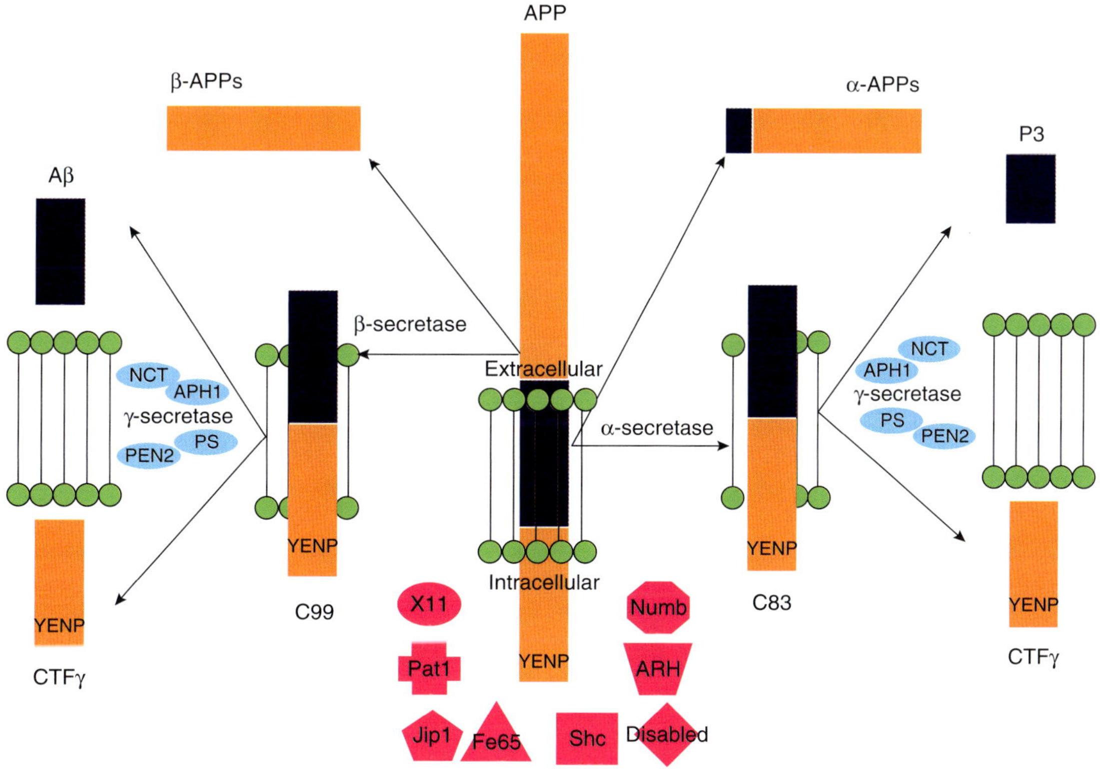

Figure 20.1 Amyloid precursor protein (APP) processing and Aβ generation. Aβ is produced from APP through proteolytic processing by two proteases, β-secretase and γ-secretase. The cleavage by β-secretase generates APP-C99, which is further cleaved by γ-secretase to release 4 kDa Aβ. γ-secretase consists of presenilins, nicastrin/APH2, APH-1, and PEN-2. Reprinted from Xie Z, Tanzi RE. Alzheimer's disease and post-operative cognitive dysfunction. *Exp Gerontol.* 2006;41:346–359, with permission from Elsevier.

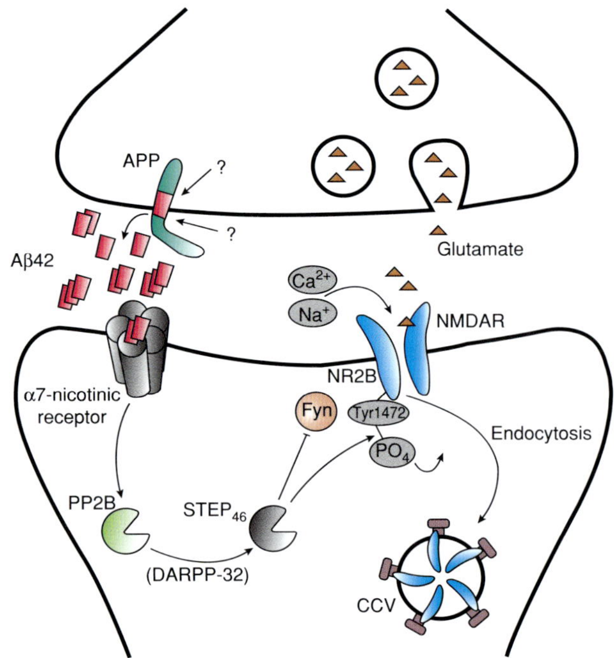

Figure 20.2 Synaptic dysfunction. Aβ, which is secreted into the synaptic cleft via cleavage of APP, can promote the endocytosis of N-methyl-D-aspartate (NMDA) receptors, reduce the density of NMDA receptors at synapses, and decrease glutamatergic transmission, leading to impairment of synaptic plasticity. Reprinted with permission from Macmillan Publishers Ltd: *Nat Neurosci*. Tanzi RE. The synaptic amyloid beta hypothesis of Alzheimer disease. *Nat Neurosci*. 2005;8:977–979.

synaptic function and decrease long-term potentiation, leading to the clinical dementia associated with AD (this is referred to as the synaptic Aβ hypothesis of AD).[34] Recently, it has been shown that Aβ can facilitate NMDA receptor endocytosis and inhibit NMDA-evoked currents, which may likely cause learning and memory impairment (Figure 20.2).[35]

Aβ can induce mitochondrial damage and inhibit mitochondrial enzymes, leading to further cytotoxicity.[5] Specifically, Aβ has been reported to inhibit cytochrome c oxidase,[36] which leads to impairment of electron transport, ATP production, oxygen consumption, and mitochondrial membrane potential. Aβ can also induce the generation of reactive oxygen species[37] and reactive nitrogen species.[38] Ultimately, these changes will lead to apoptosis and cell death. Recent studies further suggest that the involvement of mitochondrial dysfunction precedes other aspects of AD neuropathogenesis.[39]

Finally, neuroinflammation has been suggested to play a role in AD.[40–43] Specifically, a recent Framingham study by Tan et al.[44] suggests that elevated blood levels of tumor necrosis factor-α and interleukin 1, the proinflammatory cytokines, are associated with increased risk of developing AD. Microglia cells may have contradictory roles in AD neuropathogenesis. On the one hand, microglia cells can engulf and degrade Aβ (eliminating Aβ); on the other hand, chronically activated microglia cells can release cytokines (releasing pro-inflammatory molecules), which may lead to cell damage.[40] The exact role of inflammation in AD neuropathogenesis and the application of anti-inflammatory agents in the treatment of AD remain to be further investigated.[5]

EFFECTS OF ANESTHESIA AND SURGERY ON THE NEUROPATHOGENESIS

In 1998 and 2001, Moller et al. and Newman et al. reported a delayed and long-lasting postoperative cognitive dysfunction (POCD) following noncardiac[45] and cardiac[46] surgery, respectively.[1] Since then, there have been many studies evaluating the etiology of POCD, including the investigation of whether anesthetics and other perioperative factors can lead to POCD. Given that Aβ accumulation, tau hyperphosphorylation, synaptic dysfunction, apoptosis, and neuroinflammation are part of the AD neuropathogenesis, many studies focused on the assessment of the effects of anesthetics on these biochemical changes.

Among these studies, Eckenhoff et al. have reported that the commonly used inhalation anesthetic isoflurane can enhance the Aβ oligomerization and potentiate the Aβ-induced cytotoxicity in cultured cells.[47] Culley et al. showed that isoflurane induced learning and memory impairment in aged rats.[48] Xie et al. reported that hypocapnia may induce apoptosis and increase levels of Aβ in vitro[49] in 2004. In 2005, Wei et al. reported that isoflurane can cause cell death in vitro.[50] In 2006, 2007, and 2008, Xie and colleagues performed a series of experiments to assess the effects of isoflurane on AD neuropathogenesis and found that isoflurane can induce apoptosis, promote APP processing, and increase Aβ generation both in vitro[51–53] and in the brain tissue of mice.[54] Moreover, they found that isoflurane may induce neuroinflammation and tau protein phosphorylation (unpublished results). In the up-stream mechanism studies, they reported that isoflurane may increase the generation of reactive oxygen species, cause mitochondrial damage, and initiate the mitochondria pathway of apoptosis, leading to cell death.[55] This group has also reported that while sevoflurane can induce apoptosis and Aβ generation in vitro and in vivo,[56] desflurane can only induce apoptosis and Aβ generation under hypoxic conditions in vitro.[57] The combination of nitrous oxide plus low concentration isoflurane induces apoptosis and increases Aβ levels in vitro.[58] Meanwhile, Bianchi et al. showed that isoflurane can increase the amount of amyloid plaque in brain tissues of mice as well as induce learning and memory impairment in mice.[59] Planel et al. illustrated that anesthesia and anesthesia-induced hypothermia can induce AD-associated tau metabolism.[60–62] At this time, there are many ongoing studies in this field and we may learn more regarding whether anesthetics can promote AD neuropathogenesis in the coming years (Figure 20.3).

The findings that commonly used inhalation anesthetics may promote AD neuropathogenesis may make

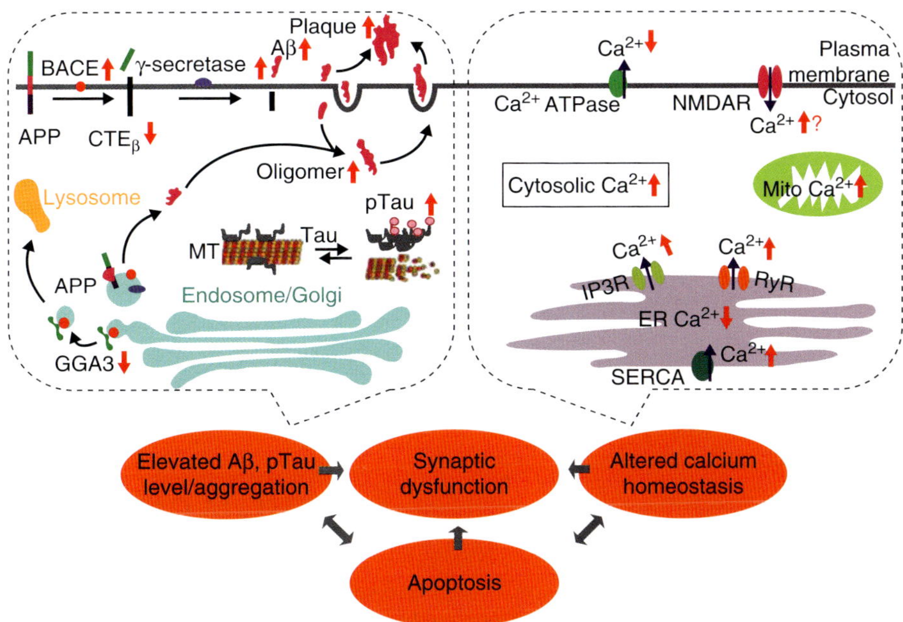

Figure 20.3 Anesthesia and Alzheimer disease (AD) neuropathogenesis. In the amyloid and tau pathway, on the left, anesthetics can induce caspase activation and apoptosis, which decrease the levels of adaptor protein GGA3, leading to decreased β-site APP-cleaving enzyme (BACE) lysosomal degradation and consequent increase in BACE levels. The increased BACE levels will lead to Aβ accumulation. Inhalation anesthetics also interact with the Aβ monomers to promote the formation of small soluble oligomers. These oligomers further associate to form fibrils and extracellular plaque, which have been found to be increased in mice with transgenic AD after exposure to anesthetic. Microtubule-bound tau becomes hyperphosphorylated and detached by anesthetics and hypothermia, resulting in tau aggregates and decreased microtubule stability. On the right side of the figure, anesthetics increase cytosolic calcium via several mechanisms. Increased cytosolic calcium levels can lead to apoptosis directly. Both the Aβ/tau and calcium pathways contribute to synaptic dysfunction and learning/memory impairment. Reprinted with permission from Tang J, Eckenhoff MF, Eckenhoff RG. Anesthesia and the old brain. *Anesth Analg*. 2010;110:421–426.

both patients and physicians worry that anesthesia and surgery may be another risk factor of AD. In fact, it has been reported that age of onset of AD in patients is inversely related to cumulative exposure to anesthesia and surgery before age 50,[63] even though anesthesia and surgery may not increase the incidence of AD.[64] Patients having coronary artery bypass graft surgery under general anesthesia have been reported to have increased risk for AD as compared to those having percutaneous transluminal coronary angioplasty under local anesthesia.[65] However, some other human studies have suggested that there is little or no relationship between anesthesia and AD,[66–68] and other studies have shown that anesthetics do not prompt the biochemical changes associated with AD neuropathogenesis. More studies, especially adequately powered prospective human studies, are needed before we can make any conclusion regarding the potential association of anesthesia and AD.[69] At this moment, it is premature to recommend changes in clinical practice, but additional studies are warranted and needed.[70]

Intraoperatively, anesthetic drugs may affect the postoperative course of AD patients. Therefore, short acting drugs, which have quick onset and offset, are generally good choices. It has been reported that desflurane and remifentail are good choices for elderly patients and AD patients.[71,72] However, there is no single "best" anesthetic for AD patients. Each patient must be managed individually. However, it has been well acknowledged that glycopyrrolate, an anticholinergic drug that does not cross blood-brain barrier, is preferable to scopolamine or atropine.

AD drugs can also modulate the effects of anesthetics. Specifically, the AD drug donepezil can block acetylcholine hydrolysis and antagonize the effects of atracurium, and the AD drug galantamine can reverse neuromuscular paralysis.[73,74]

Postoperatively, adequate analgesia, early ambulation, and proper pulmonary care are important for elderly and AD patients. The AD patient may have a delayed recovery from anesthesia; therefore, such patients may require prolonged observation in the recovery room.

PARKINSON'S DISEASE

GENERAL INFORMATION

Parkinson's disease (also known as Parkinson disease or PD) is a degenerative disorder of the central nervous system, which can affect all cultures and races.[75] It is estimated that 6.3 million people in the world have PD and 1 to 1.5 million Americans have it. Men are slightly more likely than women to have PD.

PD primarily affects movement. The common motor symptoms are tremor, rigidity (joint stiffness and increased muscle tone), bradykinesia (slowness of movement), and postural instability (failure of postural reflexes). Most PD patients do not have any specific etiology (idiopathic PD). However, genetic factors, head trauma, cerebral anoxia, and toxins may also lead to PD.

The diagnosis of PD is based on medical history and physical examination. The current treatments for PD include levodopa, bromocriptine, pergolide, pramipexole, ropinirole, piribedil, cabergoline, apomorphine, lisuride, and monoamine oxidase-B (MAO-B) inhibitors selegiline and rasagiline. Deep brain stimulation, surgical resection of the subthalamic nucleus and the internal segment of the globus pallidus, can also be used to treat PD.[3]

NEUROPATHOGENESIS

The loss of dopaminergic neurons in the pars compacta region of the substantia nigra disrupts the activity of the neural circuits within the basal ganglia that regulate movement, which eventually leads to a hypokinetic movement disorder.

The mechanism underlying the loss of the dopaminergic neurons is not clear. It has been suggested that the abnormal accumulation of the protein alpha-synuclein may lead to the damage of dopaminergic neurons. Alpha-synuclein binds to ubiquitin to form a complex, which cannot be directed to the proteosome. This protein accumulation forms proteinaceous cytoplasmic inclusions called Lewy bodies. Alpha-synuclein may induce a defect in the machinery that transports proteins between two major cellular organelles—the endoplasmic reticulum and the Golgi apparatus, which leads to the death of dopaminergic neurons. In addition, the disturbance of calcium homeostasis may also lead to the death of dopaminergic neurons. Recent studies have also suggested that the genes α-synuclein, parkin, PTEN induced Putative Kinase 1, DJ-1, Leucine Rich Repeat Kinase 2, and ATP13A2 may be also involved in PD.[76]

EFFECTS OF ANESTHESIA AND SURGERY ON THE NEUROPATHOGENESIS

Anesthesia has been suggested to be potentially associated with PD. Specifically, anesthesiologists who are exposed to anesthetic gases may develop PD symptoms, and parkinsonian symptoms can be triggered by general anesthesia.[77] Another retrospective study investigated PD mortality among large cohorts of male U.S. anesthesiologists (n = 33,040) and internal medicine physicians (n = 33,044). The findings from the study suggested that the anesthesiologists may have a significantly elevated risk for PD as an underlying cause of death as compared to internal medicine physicians. Interestingly, PD mortality for any mention on a death certificate was lower than rates in U.S. men during the same period of time for both groups. The study, however, has some significant limitations, as the authors acknowledged.[78]

In contrast to AD neuropathogenesis, there have been no studies to suggest that anesthetics can promote the PD neuropathogenesis in vitro or in vivo. However, anesthetics have been shown to induce apoptosis (see review[70]) and to disturb calcium homeostasis (see review[79]); both apoptosis and calcium dyshomeostasis have been suggested to be involved in PD neuropathogenesis.[76] Thus, it is possible that anesthetics can also affect PD neuropathogenesis. More studies to determine the potential effects of anesthesia and other perioperative factors on PD neuropathogenesis are warranted.

ANESTHESIA CARE FOR PARKINSON'S DISEASE PATIENTS

Perioperatively, it is important for PD patients to continue taking the medications, e.g., levodopa, to avoid the progression of PD symptoms.[71] Anesthesiologists should be aware that respiratory impairment can occur in PD patients[71,80] because they may have dysfunction of laryngeal and respiratory muscles, leading to reduced lung compliance, retained secretions, and upper airway obstruction. Levodopa and bromocriptine can cause orthostatic hypotension; it is therefore important to prevent and treat the hypotensive episodes that may occur in the perioperative period for PD patients.[71,81]

It has been reported in PD patients that the combination of levodopa and halothane can sensitize the heart to catecholamine, fentanyl can cause muscle rigidity, alfentanil can induce dystonia,[82] and morphine can reduce dyskinesia and dystonia.[83] These findings may help anesthesiologists to choose suitable opiates for PD patients. MAOI type A drugs and opiates can have adverse interactions. Combination of MAOI type B, e.g., selegiline, with meperidine can lead to agitation, muscular rigidity, sweating, hyperpyrexia, and yet more severe events.[84] Therefore, it is prudent to avoid the combination of meperidine with MAO inhibitors.[71]

HUNTINGTON'S DISEASE

GENERAL INFORMATION

Huntington's disease (HD) is a rare (5 to 7 per 100,000 individuals) and incurable neurodegenerative genetic disorder, affecting muscle coordination and some cognitive functions. HD typically becomes manifest in middle age. The disease has an autosomal dominant mode of transmission and is caused by a mutation of the gene Huntingtin (*HTT*) on chromosome 4. The disease is characterized by degeneration of striatal neurons.

The symptoms of HD include jerky, random, and uncontrollable movements called chorea.[85] Initially, chorea presents as general restlessness, small unintentionally initiated or uncompleted motions, lack of coordination, or slowed saccadic eye movements. Later on, the symptoms include rigidity, writhing motions or abnormal posture, physical instability, abnormal facial expressions, and difficulties chewing, swallowing, and speaking. Eating difficulties can lead to malnutrition and weight loss.[86] Sleep disturbances can also occur.[87]

Although there is no cure for HD, some treatments may reduce the severity of the symptoms. Tetrabenazine, a newly approved medicine (2008), can specifically reduce the severity of chorea in HD.[85] Neuroleptics and benzodiazepines may also reduce the degree of chorea, antiparkinsonism drugs can treat hypokinesia and rigidity, and valproic acid can treat myoclonic hyperkinesia. Anxiety, depression, and other mood disorders also need to be treated.

NEUROPATHOGENESIS

All humans have the Huntingtin gene (*HTT*), which codes for the protein huntingtin (HTT). HD patients have mutant HTT (mHTT), which is characterized by an enlarged polyglutamine repeat section. The mHTT is believed to cause the pathological changes underlying HD. The exact function of mHTT still remains to be investigated, but mHTT has been reported to induce cell damage (gain of toxic function of mHTT) in the brain areas of striatum, substantia nigra, cerebral cortex, hippocampus, Purkinje cells in the cerebellum, lateral tuberal nuclei of the hypothalamus, and parts of the thalamus.[85] The mHTT may interact with chaperone proteins and caspases to cause cell damage. The mHTT may also affect glutamate, energy production within cells, and expression of other genes, leading to cell damage. Protein Rhes has been reported to be able to enhance the cytotoxic effects of mHTT.[88] Mitochondrial dysfunction has also been suggested to contribute to HD neuropathogenesis.[89]

EFFECTS OF ANESTHESIA AND SURGERY ON THE NEUROPATHOGENESIS

There are very few studies to assess the effects of anesthetics on HD neuropathogenesis. Overactivation of IP3 receptors and increases in calcium release from the endoplasmic reticulum via the IP3 receptors may contribute to HD neuropathogenesis.[90] In an in vitro study,[91] it has been shown that the common inhalation anesthetic isoflurane can induce more cell damage in HTT knockin striatal cells than in the corresponding wild-type striatal cells. Meanwhile, isoflurane can induce a greater degree of elevation of cytosolic calcium in HTT knockin striatal cells than in the wild-type cells. These findings suggest that anesthetics may affect HD neuropathogenesis.

In an in vivo experiment, a recent study[92] employed a unilateral quinolinic acid-induced excitotoxic lesion rat model of HD and found that isoflurane, as compared to ketamine, can induce greater ipsilateral rotation behavior, larger striatal lesions, and significant differences in other measurements reflecting the extent of the lesion.

More studies that determine the potential effects of anesthetics on the HD neuropathogenesis may emerge in the near future, which could include investigating the effects of anesthetics on the expression of HD gene *HTT* and function of HD protein mHTT.

ANESTHESIA CARE FOR HUNTINGTON'S DISEASE PATIENTS

Early studies suggested prolonged paralysis and sedation following succinylcholine, sodium thiopental, and midazolam in HD patients. These findings have led to recommendations that these drugs should not be used in HD patients. However, the prolonged action could be due to the larger dose used in HD patients. Many other studies and a recent report have shown that HD patients have a normal response to general anesthesia.[93] It therefore remains debatable as to whether we should be able to use succinylcholine, sodium thiopental, and midazolam in HD patients.

HD patients are at increased risk for aspiration due to bulbar muscle dysfunction. It has been recommended to avoid the use of the promotility drugs that act on central dopamine receptors, e.g., metoclopramide, because these drugs may aggravate chorea symptoms of HD.[94]

SUMMARY

In summary, more and more patients may have neurodegenerative diseases (e.g., one in ten Americans aged 71 and older have AD[95]). Anesthesiologists frequently provide perioperative care for patients with neurodegenerative disorders. Special considerations should be given to these patients and their caregivers. There have been ongoing studies to determine whether anesthetics and perioperative factors can affect the neuropathogenesis of AD, PD, and HD.[96] However, the answer is uncertain, and at this stage it is premature to conclude that any anesthetic is dangerous to use in these patients. Further studies are needed before any conclusion regarding the contribution of anesthesia and/or surgery to the neuropathogenesis of neurodegenerative disorders.

REFERENCES

1. Xie Z, Tanzi RE. Alzheimer's disease and post-operative cognitive dysfunction. *Exp Gerontol.* 2006;41:346–359.
2. Alzheimer's Association. 2009 Alzheimer's disease facts and figures. *Alzheimer's and Dementia: The Journal of the Alzheimer's Association.* 2009;5(3):234–270.
3. Weiner CM, Bloomfield G, Harrison TR, et al. *Harrison's Principles of Internal Medicine, 17th Edition.* New York: McGraw Hill Medical;2008.

4. Tanzi RE, Bertram L. Alzheimer's disease: the latest suspect. *Nature.* 2008;454:706–708.
5. Querfurth HW, LaFerla FM, et al. Alzheimer's disease. *N Engl J Med.* 2010;362:329–344.
6. Glenner GG, Wong CW. Alzheimer's disease and Down's syndrome: sharing of a unique cerebrovascular amyloid fibril protein. *Biochem Biophys Res Commun.* 1984;122:1131–1135.
7. Goate A, Chartier-Harlin MC, Mullan M, et al. Segregation of a missense mutation in the amyloid precursor protein gene with familial Alzheimer's disease. *Nature.* 1991;349:704–706.
8. Kang J, Lemaire HG, Unterbeck A, et al. The precursor of Alzheimer's disease amyloid A4 protein resembles a cell-surface receptor. *Nature.* 1987;325:733–736.
9. Tanzi RE, Gusella JF, Watkins PC, et al. Amyloid beta protein gene: cDNA, mRNA distribution, and genetic linkage near the Alzheimer locus. *Science.* 1987;235:880–884.
10. Glenner GG, Wong CW. Alzheimer's disease: initial report of the purification and characterization of a novel cerebrovascular amyloid protein. *Biochem Biophys Res Commun.* 1984;120:885–890.
11. Bertram L, Tanzi RE. Thirty years of Alzheimer's disease genetics: the implications of systematic meta-analyses. *Nat Rev Neurosci.* 2008;9:768–778.
12. Selkoe DJ. Alzheimer's disease: genes, proteins, and therapy. *Physiol Rev.* 2001;81:741–766.
13. Gu Y, Misonou H, Sato T, Dohmae N, Takio K, Ihara Y. Distinct intramembrane cleavage of the beta-amyloid precursor protein family resembling gamma-secretase-like cleavage of Notch. *J Biol Chem.* 2001;276:35235–35238.
14. Sastre M, Steiner H, Fuchs K, et al. Presenilin-dependent gamma-secretase processing of beta-amyloid precursor protein at a site corresponding to the S3 cleavage of Notch. *EMBO Rep.* 2001;2:835–841.
15. Yu C, Kim SH, Ikeuchi T, et al. Characterization of a presenilin-mediated amyloid precursor protein carboxyl-terminal fragment gamma: evidence for distinct mechanisms involved in gamma -secretase processing of the APP and Notch1 transmembrane domains. *J Biol Chem.* 2001;276:43756–43760.
16. Li YM, Lai MT, Xu M, et al. Presenilin 1 is linked with gamma-secretase activity in the detergent solubilized state. *Proc Natl Acad Sci U S A.* 2000;97:6138–6143.
17. Edbauer D, Winkler E, Regula JT, Pesold B, Steiner H, Haass C. Reconstitution of gamma-secretase activity. *Nat Cell Biol.* 2003;5:486–488.
18. Steiner H, Winkler E, Edbauer D, et al. PEN-2 is an integral component of the gamma-secretase complex required for coordinated expression of presenilin and nicastrin. *J Biol Chem.* 2002;277:39062–39065.
19. Francis R, McGrath G, Zhang J, et al. aph-1 and pen-2 are required for Notch pathway signaling, gamma-secretase cleavage of betaAPP, and presenilin protein accumulation. *Dev Cell.* 2002;3:85–97.
20. De Strooper B. Aph-1, Pen-2, and nicastrin with presenilin generate an active gamma-secretase complex. *Neuron.* 2003;38:9–12.
21. Mattson MP. Contributions of mitochondrial alterations, resulting from bad genes and a hostile environment, to the pathogenesis of Alzheimer's disease. *Int Rev Neurobiol.* 2002;53:387–409.
22. Raina AK, Hochman A, Ickes H, et al. Apoptotic promoters and inhibitors in Alzheimer's disease: who wins out? *Prog Neuropsychopharmacol Biol Psychiatry.* 2003;27:251–254.
23. LeBlanc AC. The role of apoptotic pathways in Alzheimer's disease neurodegeneration and cell death. *Curr Alzheimer Res.* 2005;2:389–402.
24. Cribbs DH, Poon WW, Rissman RA, Blurton-Jones M. Caspase-mediated degeneration in Alzheimer's disease. *Am J Pathol.* 2004;165:353–355.
25. Gervais FG, Xu D, Robertson GS, et al. Involvement of caspases in proteolytic cleavage of Alzheimer's amyloid-beta precursor protein and amyloidogenic A beta peptide formation. *Cell.* 1999;97:395–406.
26. Masliah E, Mallory M, Alford M, Tanaka S, Hansen LA. Caspase dependent DNA fragmentation might be associated with excitotoxicity in Alzheimer disease. *J Neuropathol Exp Neurol.* 1998;57:1041–1052.
27. Shimohama S, Tanino H, Fujimoto S. Changes in caspase expression in Alzheimer's disease: comparison with development and aging. *Biochem Biophys Res Commun.* 1999;256:381–384.
28. Yang F, Sun X, Beech W, et al. Antibody to caspase-cleaved actin detects apoptosis in differentiated neuroblastoma and plaque-associated neurons and microglia in Alzheimer's disease. *Am J Pathol.* 1998;152:379–389.
29. Su JH, Anderson AJ, Cummings BJ, Cotman CW. Immunohistochemical evidence for apoptosis in Alzheimer's disease. *Neuroreport.* 1994;5:2529–2533.
30. Su JH, Deng G, Cotman CW. Bax protein expression is increased in Alzheimer's brain: correlations with DNA damage, Bcl-2 expression, and brain pathology. *J Neuropathol Exp Neurol.* 1997;56:86–93.
31. Small SA, Duff K. Linking Abeta and tau in late-onset Alzheimer's disease: a dual pathway hypothesis. *Neuron.* 2008;60:534–542.
32. Tanzi RE. Tangles and neurodegenerative disease—a surprising twist. *N Engl J Med.* 2005;353:1853–1855.
33. Santacruz K, Lewis J, Spires T, et al. Tau suppression in a neurodegenerative mouse model improves memory function. *Science.* 2005;309:476–481.
34. Tanzi RE. The synaptic Abeta hypothesis of Alzheimer disease. *Nat Neurosci.* 2005;8:977–979.
35. Snyder EM, Nong Y, Almeida CG, et al. Regulation of NMDA receptor trafficking by amyloid-beta. *Nat Neurosci.* 2005;8:1051–1058.
36. Caspersen C, Wang N, Yao J, et al. Mitochondrial Abeta: a potential focal point for neuronal metabolic dysfunction in Alzheimer's disease. *FASEB J.* 2005;19:2040–2041.
37. Hensley K, Carney JM, Mattson MP, et al. A model for beta-amyloid aggregation and neurotoxicity based on free radical generation by the peptide: relevance to Alzheimer disease. *Proc Natl Acad Sci U S A.* 1994;91:3270–3274.
38. Combs CK, Karlo JC, Kao SC, Landreth GE. beta-Amyloid stimulation of microglia and monocytes results in TNFalpha-dependent expression of inducible nitric oxide synthase and neuronal apoptosis. *J Neurosci.* 2001;21:1179–1188.
39. Yao J, Irwin RW, Zhao L, Nilsen J, Hamilton RT, Brinton RD. Mitochondrial bioenergetic deficit precedes Alzheimer's pathology in female mouse model of Alzheimer's disease. *Proc Natl Acad Sci U S A.* 2009;106:14670–14675.
40. Akiyama H, Barger S, Barnum S, et al. Inflammation and Alzheimer's disease. *Neurobiol Aging.* 2000;21:383–421.
41. Heneka MT, O'Banion MK. Inflammatory processes in Alzheimer's disease. *J Neuroimmunol.* 2007;184:69–91.
42. Sastre M, Klockgether T, Heneka MT. Contribution of inflammatory processes to Alzheimer's disease: molecular mechanisms. *Int J Dev Neurosci.* 2006;24:167–176.
43. Cameron B, Landreth GE. Inflammation, microglia, and Alzheimer's disease. *Neurobiol Dis.* 2009;37(3):503.
44. Tan ZS, Beiser AS, Vasan RS, et al. Inflammatory markers and the risk of Alzheimer disease: the Framingham study. *Neurology.* 2007;68:1902–1908.
45. Moller JT, Cluitmans P, Rasmussen LS, et al. Long-term postoperative cognitive dysfunction in the elderly ISPOCD1 study. ISPOCD investigators. International Study of Post-Operative Cognitive Dysfunction. *Lancet.* 1998;351:857–861.
46. Newman MF, Kirchner JL, Phillips-Bute B, et al. Longitudinal assessment of neurocognitive function after coronary-artery bypass surgery. *N Engl J Med.* 2001;344:395–402.
47. Eckenhoff RG, Johansson JS, Wei H, et al. Inhaled anesthetic enhancement of amyloid-beta oligomerization and cytotoxicity. *Anesthesiology.* 2004;101:703–709.
48. Culley DJ, Baxter MG, Yukhananov R, Crosby G. Long-term impairment of acquisition of a spatial memory task following isoflurane-nitrous oxide anesthesia in rats. *Anesthesiology.* 2004;100:309–314.

49. Xie Z, Moir RD, Romano DM, Tesco G, Kovacs DM, Tanzi RE. Hypocapnia induces caspase-3 activation and increases abeta production. *Neurodegener Dis.* 2004;1:29–37.
50. Wei H, Kang B, Wei W, et al. Isoflurane and sevoflurane affect cell survival and BCL-2/BAX ratio differently. *Brain Res.* 2005;1037: 139–147.
51. Xie Z, Dong Y, Maeda U, et al. The common inhalation anesthetic isoflurane induces apoptosis and increases amyloid beta protein levels. *Anesthesiology.* 2006;104:988–994.
52. Xie Z, Dong Y, Maeda U, et al. Isoflurane-induced apoptosis: a potential pathogenic link between delirium and dementia. *J Gerontol A Biol Sci Med Sci.* 2006;61:1300–1306.
53. Xie Z, Dong Y, Maeda U, et al. The inhalation anesthetic isoflurane induces a vicious cycle of apoptosis and amyloid beta-protein accumulation. *J Neurosci.* 2007;27:1247–1254.
54. Xie Z, Culley DJ, Dong Y, et al. The common inhalation anesthetic isoflurane induces caspase activation and increases amyloid beta-protein level in vivo. *Ann Neurol.* 2008;64:618–627.
55. Zhang Y, Dong Y, Wu X, et al. The mitochondrial pathway of anesthetic isoflurane-induced apoptosis. *J Biol Chem.* 2010;285: 4025–4037.
56. Dong Y, Zhang G, Zhang B, et al. The common inhalational anesthetic sevoflurane induces apoptosis and increases beta-amyloid protein levels. *Arch Neurol.* 2009;66:620–631.
57. Zhang B, Dong Y, Zhang G, et al. The inhalation anesthetic desflurane induces caspase activation and increases amyloid beta-protein levels under hypoxic conditions. *J Biol Chem.* 2008;283: 11866–11875.
58. Zhen Y, Dong Y, Wu X, et al. Nitrous oxide plus isoflurane induces apoptosis and increases beta-amyloid protein levels. *Anesthesiology.* 2009;111:741–752.
59. Bianchi SL, Tran T, Liu C, et al. Brain and behavior changes in 12-month-old Tg2576 and nontransgenic mice exposed to anesthetics. *Neurobiol Aging.* 2008;29:1002–1010.
60. Planel E, Bretteville A, Liu L, et al. Acceleration and persistence of neurofibrillary pathology in a mouse model of tauopathy following anesthesia. *FASEB J.* 2009;23:2595–2604.
61. Planel E, Krishnamurthy P, Miyasaka T, et al. Anesthesia-induced hyperphosphorylation detaches 3-repeat tau from microtubules without affecting their stability in vivo. *J Neurosci.* 2008;28: 12798–12807.
62. Planel E, Richter KE, Nolan CE, et al. Anesthesia leads to tau hyperphosphorylation through inhibition of phosphatase activity by hypothermia. *J Neurosci.* 2007;27:3090–3097.
63. Bohnen N, Warner MA, Kokmen E, Kurland LT. Early and midlife exposure to anesthesia and age of onset of Alzheimer's disease. *Int J Neurosci.* 1994;77:181–185.
64. Bohnen NI, Warner MA, Kokmen E, Beard CM, Kurland LT. Alzheimer's disease and cumulative exposure to anesthesia: a case-control study. *J Am Geriatr Soc.* 1994;42:198–201.
65. Lee TA, Wolozin B, Weiss KB, Bednar MM. Assessment of the emergence of Alzheimer's disease following coronary artery bypass graft surgery or percutaneous transluminal coronary angioplasty. *J Alzheimers Dis.* 2005;7:319–324.
66. Knopman DS, Petersen RC, Cha RH, Edland SD, Rocca WA. Coronary artery bypass grafting is not a risk factor for dementia or Alzheimer disease. *Neurology.* 2005;65:986–990.
67. Gasparini M, Vanacore N, Schiaffini C, et al. A case-control study on Alzheimer's disease and exposure to anesthesia. *Neurol Sci.* 2002; 23:11–14.
68. Avidan MS, Searleman AC, Storandt M, et al. Long-term cognitive decline in older subjects was not attributable to noncardiac surgery or major illness. *Anesthesiology.* 2009;111:964–970.
69. Harris RA, Eger EI 2nd. Alzheimer's disease and anesthesia: out of body, out of mind or not? *Ann Neurol.* 2008;64:595–597.
70. Culley DJ, Xie Z, Crosby G. General anesthetic-induced neurotoxicity: an emerging problem for the young and old? *Curr Opin Anaesthesiol.* 2007;20:408–413.
71. Burton DA, Nicholson G, Hall GM. Anaesthesia in elderly patients with neurodegenerative disorders: special considerations. *Drugs Aging.* 2004;21:229–242.
72. Conzen P, Peter K. Inhalation anaesthesia at the extremes of age: geriatric anaesthesia. *Anaesthesia.* 1995;50 Suppl:29–33.
73. Fernandez CR, Fields A, Richards T, Kaye AD. Anesthetic considerations in patients with Alzheimer's disease. *J Clin Anesth.* 2003;15:52–58.
74. Fodale V, Quattrone D, Trecroci C, Caminiti V, Santamaria LB. Alzheimer's disease and anaesthesia: implications for the central cholinergic system. *Br J Anaesth.* 2006;97:445–452.
75. Jankovic J. Parkinson's disease: clinical features and diagnosis. *J Neurol Neurosurg Psychiatry.* 2008;79:368–376.
76. Yang YX, Wood NW, Latchman DS. Molecular basis of Parkinson's disease. *Neuroreport.* 2009;20:150–156.
77. Muravchick S, Smith DS. Parkinsonian symptoms during emergence from general anesthesia. *Anesthesiology.* 1995;82:305–307.
78. Peretz C, Alexander BH, Nagahama SI, Domino KB, Checkoway H. Parkinson's disease mortality among male anesthesiologists and internists. *Mov Disord.* 2005;20:1614–1617.
79. Wei H, Xie Z. Anesthesia, calcium homeostasis and Alzheimer's disease. *Curr Alzheimer Res.* 2009;6:30–35.
80. Vincken WG, Gauthier SG, Dollfuss RE, Hanson RE, Darauay CM, Cosio MG. Involvement of upper-airway muscles in extrapyramidal disorders: a cause of airflow limitation. *N Engl J Med.* 1984;311:438–442.
81. Hutchinson RC, Sugden JC. Anaesthesia for Shy-Drager syndrome. *Anaesthesia.* 1984;39:1229–1231.
82. Mets B. Acute dystonia after alfentanil in untreated Parkinson's disease. *Anesth Analg.* 1991;72:557–558.
83. Berg D, Becker G, Reiners K. Reduction of dyskinesia and induction of akinesia induced by morphine in two Parkinsonian patients with severe sciatica. *J Neural Transm.* 1999;106:725–728.
84. Zornberg GL, Bodkin JA, Cohen BM. Severe adverse interaction between pethidine and selegiline. *Lancet.* 1991;337:246.
85. Walker FO. Huntington's disease. *Lancet.* 2007;369:218–228.
86. Aziz NA, van der Marck MA, Pijl H, Olde Rikkert MG, Bloem BR, Roos RA. Weight loss in neurodegenerative disorders. *J Neurol.* 2008;255:1872–1880.
87. Gagnon JF, Petit D, Latreille V, Montplaisir J. Neurobiology of sleep disturbances in neurodegenerative disorders. *Curr Pharm Des.* 2008; 14:3430–3445.
88. Subramaniam S, Sixt KM, Barrow R, Snyder SH. Rhes, a striatal specific protein, mediates mutant-huntingtin cytotoxicity. *Science.* 2009;324:1327–1330.
89. Quintanilla RA, Johnson GV. Role of mitochondrial dysfunction in the pathogenesis of Huntington's disease. *Brain Res Bull.* 2009;80: 242–247.
90. Tang TS, Tu H, Chan EY, et al. Huntingtin and huntingtin-associated protein 1 influence neuronal calcium signaling mediated by inositol-(1,4,5) triphosphate receptor type 1. *Neuron.* 2003;39: 227–239.
91. Wei H, Liang G, Yang H, et al. The common inhalational anesthetic isoflurane induces apoptosis via activation of inositol 1,4,5-trisphosphate receptors. *Anesthesiology.* 2008;108:251–260.
92. Jiang W, Buchele F, Papazoglou A, Dobrossy M, Nikkhah G. Ketamine anaesthesia interferes with the quinolinic acid-induced lesion in a rat model of Huntington's disease. *J Neurosci Methods.* 2009;179:219–223.
93. Kivela JE, Sprung J, Southorn PA, Watson JC, Weingarten TN. Anesthetic management of patients with Huntington disease. *Anesth Analg.* 2010;110:515–523.
94. Giroud M, Fabre JL, Putelat R, et al. Can metoclopramide reveal Huntington's disease? *Lancet.* 1982;2:1153.
95. CNN, Sep. 23 2009.
96. Tang J, Eckenhoff MF, Eckenhoff RG. Anesthesia and the old brain. *Anesth Analg.* 2010;110:421–426.

INDEX